NATIONAL LIBRARY of MEDICINE CLASSIFICATION

A Scheme for the Shelf Arrangement of Library Materials in the Field of Medicine and Its Related Sciences

Fifth Edition 1994

Revised 1999

U.S. DEPARTMENT OF HEALTH AND HUMAN SERVICES
Public Health Service
National Institutes of Health

NATIONAL LIBRARY OF MEDICINE
8600 Rockville Pike
Bethesda, Maryland 20894

NIH Publication No. 00-1535

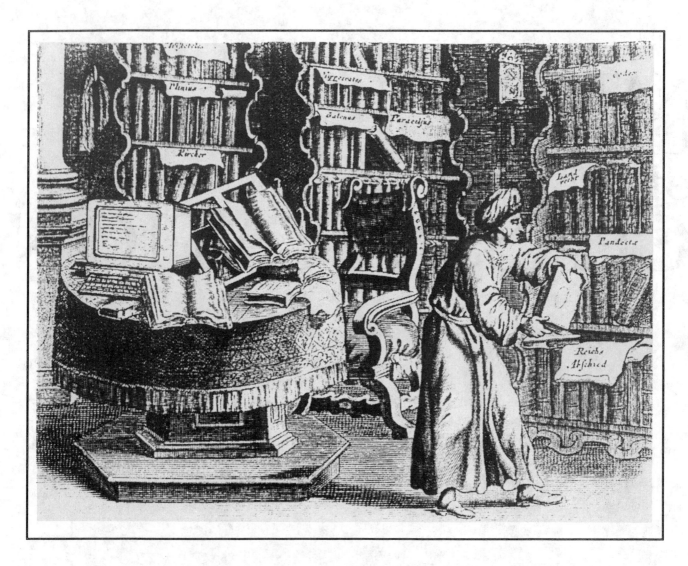

Early Library in: Franciscus Phillippus Florinus [pseud.] Oeconumus prudens et legais Nurnberg, 1722.
p. 125 18th c. (modified, 1994)

NATIONAL LIBRARY of MEDICINE
CLASSIFICATION

**A Scheme for the Shelf Arrangement
of Library Materials in the Field of
Medicine and Its Related Sciences**

Fifth Edition, 1994
Revised 1999

U.S. DEPARTMENT OF HEALTH
AND HUMAN SERVICES
Public Health Service
National Institutes of Health

NATIONAL LIBRARY OF MEDICINE
8600 Rockville Pike
Bethesda, Maryland 20894

NIH Publication No. 00-1535

First edition 1951
Second edition 1958
Third edition 1964
Third edition (with supplement 1969)
Fourth edition 1978
Fourth edition, revised 1981
Fourth edition, revised, second printing 1992
Fifth edition, 1994
Fifth edition, revised, 1999

National Library of Medicine Cataloging in Publication

National Library of Medicine (U.S.)
    National Library of Medicine classification : a scheme for the shelf arrangement of library materials in the field of medicine and its related sciences. – 5th ed., rev. – Bethesda. Md. : U.S. Dept. of Health and Human Services, Public Health Service, National Institutes of Health, National Library of Medicine ; Washington, D.C. : For sale by the Supt. of Docs., U.S., G.P.O., 1999.

  -- (NIH publication ; no. 00-1535)

Includes bibliographic references and index.

1. Classification. 2.Medicine. I. Title II. Series

Z 697.M4 U63c 1999

Cit. No. 100901931

This book is printed on acid-free paper for permanence.

∞ ™

The Secretary of Health and Human Services has determined that the publication of this monograph is necessary in the transaction of the public business required by law of this Department. Use of funds for printing this monograph has been approved by the Director of the Office of Management and Budget through September 30, 2000.

For sale by the U.S. Government Printing Office
Superintendent of Documents, Mail Stop: SSOP, Washington, DC 20402-9328
ISBN 0-16-050261-6

TABLE OF CONTENTS

PREFACE
Fifth Edition, Revised

This 1999 revision of the *NLM Classification* incorporates all additions and changes to the classification schedules since the fifth edition was published in 1995. These changes have previously appeared in the *NLM Technical Bulletin*. In addition, several hundred new entry terms, published from 1994 through 1999 in the *NLM Medical Subject Headings Annotated Alphabetic List* (MeSH®), have been added to the Index of this revised edition.

Ms. Wen-min Kao, retired Principal Cataloger, coordinated the update of the index terminology. The Cataloging Section is grateful for her contribution. Ms. Christa Hoffmann, Head, Cataloging Section, managed and edited this revision.

PREFACE

The 1994 fifth edition of the *NLM Classification* updates the fourth revised edition published in 1981 and reprinted in 1992. The fifth edition contains a number of new classification numbers for new concepts and knowledge; however few changes were made to existing numbers. The Index to the Classification schedules was significantly expanded with descriptors from the Medical Subject Headings (MeSH ®) vocabulary.

Many people, but above all NLM Cataloging Section's staff, contributed to the revision of the *Classification*. Wen-min Kao, Principal Cataloger, was its editor. Christa Hoffmann, Head Cataloging Section, managed the project and worked with John Cox, Office of Computer and Communications Systems, to make essential programming and database changes which assisted in a more systematic updating and verification of data against MeSH. Senior Cataloging staff - Evelyn Bain, Chong Chung, Grace Rawsthorne and Sharon Willis - reviewed MeSH vocabulary for inclusion in the Index and assigned appropriate class numbers to the terms. Other staff members of the Cataloging Section provided valuable intellectual and editorial assistance. Peri Schuyler, Head Medical Subject Headings Section, and her staff of subject specialists; Dr. Elizabeth Van Lenten, Index Section; and Dr. Sue Goo Rhee from the NIH/National Heart Lung and Blood Institute, contributed their subject expertise. Ronald Gordner, NLM Reference Section, provided the public services point of view. Pauline Cochrane, University of Illinois at Urbana-Champaign GSLIS, performed important preliminary work that assisted in developing the update and revision process.

The following reviewed and commented on the *Classification* schedules, and many of their constructive suggestions were incorporated into the final publication:

Wilma Bass
   Georgetown University, Dahlgren Memorial Library
Elizabeth Crabtree
   American Hospital Association, AHA Resource Center
Susan L. Gullion
   University of California Los Angeles, L. Darling Biomedical Library
Lynn El-Hoshy
   Library of Congress, Cataloging Policy & Support Office
Mary Kreinbring
   Northwestern University, The Dental School Library
Robert Pisciotta
   University of Kansas Medical Center, Dykes Library
Wendy Skinner
   Crouse Irving Memorial Hospital, School of Nursing Library
Margaret Stangohr
   East Carolina University, Health Sciences Library
Steven Squires
   University of North Carolina at Chapel Hill, Health Sciences Library
Margaret Wineburgh-Freed
   University of Southern California, Norris Medical Library

The revision of the *National Library of Medicine Classification* benefits both NLM and the many health science libraries in the United States and abroad which use it to arrange their materials or to browse their online catalogs. All who contributed to its successful completion deserve our gratitude and commendation.

Donald A.B. Lindberg,, M.D.
Director
National Library of Medicine

INTRODUCTION

The *National Library of Medicine Classification* covers the field of medicine and related sciences, utilizing schedules QS-QZ and W-WZ permanently excluded from the *Library of Congress (LC) Classification* schedules. The various schedules of the *LC Classification* supplement the *NLM Classification* for subjects bordering on medicine and for general reference materials. The LC schedules for Human Anatomy (QM), Microbiology (QR) and Medicine (R) are not used at all by the National Library of Medicine since they overlap the *NLM Classification*.

The genesis of the *NLM Classification* is a Survey Report on the Army Medical Library, published in 1944, which recommended that the "Library be reclassified according to a modern scheme," and that the new scheme be a mixed notation (letters and numbers) resembling that of the Library of Congress. Subsequently a classification committee was formed, chaired by Keyes D. Metcalf and including Mary Louise Marshall who compiled the schedules. Medical specialists acted as consultants to the committee. Based on the consultants' advice, that of the committee and of the NLM cataloging staff, Ms. Marshall produced a preliminary edition of the Library's Classification which was issued in 1948.

The preliminary edition was revised by Frank B. Rogers and the first edition of the new classification was published in 1951 as the *U.S. Army Medical Library Classification*. It firmly established the current structure of the classification and NLM's classification practices. The headings for the individual schedules were given in brief form (e.g., WE - Musculoskeletal System; WG - Cardiovascular System) and together they provided an outline of the subjects that constitute the *National Library of Medicine Classification*. These headings were interpreted broadly as including the physiological system, the specialty or specialties connected with them, the regions of the body chiefly concerned and subordinate related fields. Within each schedule, division by organ usually has priority. All schedules, including some of their sections, are preceded by a group of form numbers ranging generally from 1-39 which are employed as mnemonic devices throughout the *Classification*.

Scope of Revision

The objectives of the fifth revised edition were to incorporate additions and changes made to schedules since 1995 and to update the Index with appropriate MeSH terminology through 1999. The fifth edition incorporated all additions and changes made since publishing the fourth revised edition. Selected schedules that needed updating were revised and new MeSH descriptors used in cataloging were integrated and the terminology used in the index, captions and scope note were revised to conform to current usage. New classification numbers for new concepts were introduced following guidelines designed to maintain the structure of the *Classification*. In general, new numbers were added when:

a) there was no suitable number available for a subject; for example, WL 103.7 was added to cover the new discipline of Psychoneuroimmunology. In addition, new numbers were added by expanding the use of subdivision by special topics where needed and by adding new "A-Z" entries under established lists of Special Topics. For example, QT 37.5 for specific Biomedical and biocompatible materials was added with the special topics Ceramics (.C4) and Polymers (.P7)

b) there was scattered placement of a subject in many different numbers; for example, WB 101 was added for Ambulatory care (General) to provide a classification for ambulatory care beyond the hospital setting.

c) a classification number was heavily used and needed to be further broken down; for example, the new form number "18.2 Educational materials" was established to separate materials about education from materials used in education. This separation of Education and Educational materials is employed in all schedules throughout the Classification.

d) there was sufficient material on diseases already classified with materials on the specialty and/or organ system under "General works" to warrant a new classification number for the diseases; for example WG 210 was added for Heart diseases, WH 120 for Hematologic diseases, WL 140 for Nervous system diseases, etc.

e) form numbers not previously assigned to a schedule or section were incorporated; for example, "17" for Atlases.

In keeping with the structure of the *NLM Classification*, preference was given to the use of whole numbers over decimals when establishing a new classification number. However, logical placement of a subject or publication form was the predominant factor when introducing a new classification number into an established range of numbers. Whenever possible the mnemonic characteristic for a form number was maintained. For example, the number "17" is used to identify classification numbers for atlases. Atlases on Operative dentistry are classed in WU 317 and atlases on Orthodontics in WU 417. Some exceptions to this principle are WU 507 for atlases on Prosthodontics and WU 600.7 for atlases on Oral surgery. In the former case, the number "507" is used to insert the form number for atlases on prosthodontics between WU 500 General Works and WU 515 Partial dentures... , and in the latter case, the number "600.7" is used to insert the form number for atlases on oral surgery between WU 600 General Works and WU 605 Tooth extraction.

Relationship to MeSH

The schedules with their special requirements for use with all types and forms of materials preclude strict adherence to the hierarchical arrangement of the Medical Subject Headings (MeSH), the Library's thesaurus for indexing and cataloging. The schedules maintain their own character in order to provide for material, old as well as new, acquired for the collection, including dictionaries, atlases, directories and other items which are not suitable for the arrangements found in MeSH. However, an effort was made to make schedule headings, subheadings and class number captions compatible with MeSH terminology. The MeSH Tree Structures were used extensively to determine the proper placement of a concept in a schedule and to relate index headings to one another. Since the representation of subjects in the schedules of the *NLM Classification* is intentionally broad, the captions do not enumerate all of the subordinate concepts that are to be classified in a given number. MeSH descriptors for these subordinate concepts do appear in the index with the appropriate references to the classification numbers.

Index

The Index to the *NLM Classification* provides access to classification numbers through the terminology of Medical Subject Headings (MeSH). Index entries were updated to reflect additions and changes to the MeSH vocabulary through 1999. Because resource limitations did not permit the verification of all classification numbers that previously appeared in see references in the Index, the classification numbers were removed from these entries. For additional information on the Index see the Introduction to the Index to the Classification, p. I-i.

NLM CLASSIFICATION PRACTICES

GENERAL

The Library applies subject classification primarily to materials treated as monographs. Serial publications are separated by form and are assigned classification numbers within several broad categories.

The classification practices outlined below are current conventions. They are provided as explanation, stating NLM's general classification approach using the National Library of Medicine's and the Library of Congress's schedules, rather than 'how to classify' instructions.

Basic Rules

The classification number assigned to a work is determined by the main focus or subject content of the work.

A work dealing with several subjects that fall into different areas of the classification is classed by emphasis, or if emphasis is lacking, by the first subject treated in the work.

A work on a particular disease is classified with the disease which in turn is classified with the organ or region chiefly affected, regardless of special emphasis on diet, drug, or other specific form of therapy.

Form Numbers

Each schedule, as well as some sections within a schedule (e.g., WO 201-233.1), contains a group of form numbers, generally 1 through 39, that are used to classify material by publication type within the general subject area of the schedule. In general, classification by publication type takes precedence over classification by subject.

Special cases for classification by form number:

1. Collections by several authors or by individual authors, and works comprised of addresses, essays, and lectures are classed in their respective form numbers when the works cover the overall subject of the schedule. Collections of works or essays that cover a particular subject within the schedule are classed by subject. For example, Psychiatry - Collected Works is classified in WM 5 or 7 while Psychotherapy - Collected Works is classified in WM 420.

2. Some numbers in the range of 1 through 39 are not true form numbers, that is, they are used to classify material with a special emphasis, such as 26.5 for Medical informatics, computers, and automatic data processing (General) when the emphasis applies to the overall subject of the schedule. If the material covers a particular aspect of the overall subject, it is classified by subject. For example, Computers in cardiology is classified in WG 26.5 while Computers in heart surgery is classified in WG 169.

3. In general, the form number 11 is used for works dealing with the history of any aspect of a subject within a classification schedule. For example, WM 11 is used for both Psychiatry - history and Psychotherapy - history. There are exceptions to the use of the form number for history which are generally noted under the particular form number or in the Index. Furthermore, the form number 11 is not assigned to the schedules W and WB. The history of health professions and the practice of medicine are instead classified in the WZ schedule.

Because many form numbers correlate with a publication type that is added to subject headings in cataloging, the definitions for publication types given in the section on "Publication Types – Genres' of the current *Medical Subject Headings -- Annotated Alphabetic List*, may assist in determining when to classify by form number.

Table G

Geographic subdivision is provided for certain subjects in the NLM schedules by the application of Table G *(see p. xix)*. The use of geographical breakdown is restricted to those classes which are annotated with "Table G" in the schedules and includes both monographs and serials.

If a work on a subject that is geographically subdivided covers an area larger than what is represented in a Table G notation it is classified in the General coverage (Not Table G) number, directly following the class number that provides for geographic subdivision. For example WG 11 History (Table G) is the number for the history of cardiology in particular geographic areas and WG 11.1 General coverage (Not Table G) is the number for books with general coverage of the history of cardiology.

SPECIAL PLANS

Several types of monographic publications are classified according to special plans: Nineteenth century titles, Early printed books, and Bibliographies. Classification numbers for these publications do not appear in the Index.

Nineteenth Century Titles

A simplified subject classification derived from the letters that represent the preclinical and clinical subjects covered by the *NLM Classification* is used for nineteenth century (1801-1913) monographs. This abbreviated classification is limited to combinations of letters and the classification notations W1-6, W 600, WX 2 and the form number 22 that appears throughout the schedule. In addition, the entire WZ schedule, History of Medicine, is used for nineteenth century titles. When the subject falls outside of the schedules of the *NLM Classification*, only the letters of the LC schedule representing the subject are used, e.g., BF Psychology, SF Veterinary Medicine, etc. Facsimiles and reprints of entire nineteenth century works are classified in the 19th Century Schedule. Bibliographies imprinted in the nineteenth century use the special plan for Bibliographies rather than the 19th Century Schedule.

Early Printed Books

Works published before 1801 and Americana, i.e., early imprints from North, South and Central America and the Caribbean islands, are considered early printed books and are classified in a special part of the WZ schedule, WZ 220-270. These books are arranged alphabetically by author within each century or in the Americana number. (See WZ 270 for specific guidance by state for the coverage of Americana.) Reprints and translations of pre-1801 works are classified in WZ 290.

Bibliographies

A bibliography within the scope of the *NLM Classification* is classified in the number for the subject, prefixed by a capital Z. Bibliographies outside the scope of the NLM Classification are classed in LC's Z schedule for Bibliography. Numbers for bibliographies are seldom given in the Index but are derived by using the instructions below for formulating the call number of a bibliography. Unless otherwise noted, the classification numbers for bibliographies may be used for both monographs and serials.

BIBLIOGRAPHIES – Classification	**CLASS NUMBERS**
General medical serials	ZW 1
General medical serials in one library	ZW 1
General medical monographs and/or serials issued periodically	ZW 1
Monographic works on general medicine	ZWB 100 (monographs only)

General holdings of libraries in special fields (including private libraries)	[Not LC practice]
Chiropractic	Z 675.C48
Dentistry	Z 675.D3
Hospital	Z 675.H7
Medicine	Z 675.M4
Mental health	Z 675.M43
Nursing	Z 675.N8
Occupational health	Z 675.O22
Pharmacy	Z 675.P48
Veterinary medicine	Z 675.V47
Others, A-Z as listed in LC's Z schedule under Z 675	
General monographic holdings of non-specialized libraries, university, public, etc., by country	Z 881-977
General serials holdings of non-specialized libraries and union lists of serials	Z 6945
Specific topics in medicine and allied fields	Z + NLM schedule letters
Specific topics in fields outside scope of NLM classification	Z 5051-7999

Exception: ZQ 1 is used for bibliography of general scientific periodicals and ZSF [and number] for subjects in the SF schedules. Other exceptions made in the past will no longer be used.

General materials published in a particular country (national bibliographies)	Z 1201-4980
General serials published in a particular country	Z 6947-6964
Private library catalogs, other than those in Z 675	Z 997
Booksellers catalogs	
Monographs	Z 998-1000.5
Serials	Z 6946-6964
Dissertations	
General	Z 5053-5055
Of schools of dentistry, medicine, nursing, pharmacy, public health, veterinary medicine, etc.	
Foreign	
Individual (with the university)	W4
Collective	ZW 4
United States (by subject)	ZSF, ZQS-ZWZ
General bibliographies of periodicals	Z 6941

SERIAL PUBLICATIONS

NLM follows the *Anglo-American Cataloguing Rules*, second edition, revised 1998, in defining serials. A serial is a "... publication in any medium issued in successive parts bearing numeric or chronological designations and intended to be continued indefinitely. Serials include periodicals; newspapers; annuals (reports, yearbooks, etc.); the journals, memoirs, proceedings, transactions, etc. of societies; and numbered monographic series."

Serials are classified in the form number W1 with the exceptions noted below.

Exceptions

Government Administrative Reports or Statistics (W2)
Serial government publications that are administrative or statistical in nature are classed in W2. Integrated reports of administrative and/or statistical information on several hospitals under government administration are classed in W2. Serials classified in W2 are sub-arranged by jurisdiction according to "Table G."

Hospital Administrative Reports or Statistics (WX 2)
Serial hospital publications that are administrative or statistical in nature, including reports of single government hospitals, are classed in WX 2. Serials classified in WX 2 are sub-arranged geographically according to "Table G."

Directory, Handbooks, etc.
Certain publication types, such as directories, handbooks, etc., issued serially are classed in form numbers used also for monographs. For example, Directory, whether monographic or serial in nature, are classed in form number 22. Numbers used for both types of publications are identified in the schedules with an asterisk (*). The appropriate LC schedule is used for the above defined publication types when their subject falls outside the scope of the *NLM Classification*.

Bibliographies and Indexes
Serial publications of bibliographies or indexes are classed according to the instructions in the section on Bibliographies above.

LIBRARY OF CONGRESS CLASSIFICATION SCHEDULES

The LC schedules for Human anatomy (QM), Microbiology (QR) and Medicine (R) are not used at all by the National Library of Medicine since they overlap the *NLM Classification*. Otherwise, the Library of Congress schedules augment the *NLM Classification* for subjects related to medicine. NLM rarely uses LC's schedule for Law (K) except for general works. Legal works related to medicine are classified with the subject rather than the law.

LC class numbers are provided in the Index to the *NLM Classification*. Although these numbers were verified against the LC schedules for this revision, the pertinent LC schedules should also be consulted since the numbers may change over time.

Special Instructions

Below are listed those LC schedules with special instructions for subjects that fall within both the NLM and LC schedules.

QD - Chemistry -- Use QU or QV if any portion of a work is devoted to biochemistry or pharmacology.

QH - Natural Sciences (General) -- Classify here general works on genetics and evolution.

QL - Zoology -- Classify here non-pathogenic invertebrates. Pathogenic invertebrates are classed in NLM's QX schedule.
     Vertebrates -- Anatomy and physiology of domestic animals are classed in SF (see below). Care and clinical use of laboratory animals in QY 50-60. Works on experimental studies in the interest of learning more about human disease are classed in the appropriate NLM schedule numbers.

QP - Physiology -- Classify here physiology of wild animals in general. Physiology of domestic animals is classed in SF. Special topics in this area, when applicable to humans, are for the most part classed in the appropriate NLM numbers; for example, Altitude, WD 710-715, Body temperature regulation, QT 165.

SF - Animal culture -- Classify here anatomy and physiology of domestic animals.

T - Technology -- Classify here Human engineering TA, Biotechnology TP; however, works on Biomedical engineering are classed in NLM's QT schedule.

U - Military Science -- Classify here Military medicine.

CHANGES IN CLASSIFICATION PRACTICES

Numbered Congresses -- W3, W 3.5 and ZW 3

NLM no longer classifies serial publications of congresses or sequentially issued, numbered and dated monographic congresses in W3. All newly acquired monographic congresses, including those of named meetings previously classified in W3, are classed in the appropriate subject classification number. Serial publications that are proceedings or reports of meetings are classified in W1.

Nurses' instruction

Since 1984 background materials on specific subjects, in any format, prepared for a nursing audience have been classified with the subject with the form subdivision "nurses' instruction" added to the subject headings. Prior to 1984 these materials were classified in the WY schedule together with materials dealing with nursing techniques in special fields of medicine.

TABLE G

General

Table G is a system of notations that provides geographical or jurisdictional arrangement of materials under specific class numbers in the *NLM Classification*. The use of Table G permits a shelving order that is controlled geographically and alphabetically. Table G is applied only when a class number heading is annotated by "(Table G)." When *LC Classification* numbers are used, the geographical breakdown or tables provided in the LC schedules are applied.

The geographic tables of the *NLM Classification* consist of nine geographic regions. Additionally, special provision is made for international agencies that frequently publish materials related to medicine. Each region or group is identified by a letter.

A – United States	J – Middle East and Asia
D – Americas	K – Australasia
F – Great Britain	L – Islands of the Pacifica and Indian Oceans
G – Europe	M – International Agencies
H – Africa	P – Polar Regions

The notation is composed of two letters and one or two numbers from the Cutter-Sanborn tables. The first letter of a notation represents the geographical region or jurisdiction, and the second one is the first letter of the name of a country or, in case of the states of the United States, a state.

New geographic notations are interpolated into Table G when needed following the established pattern. When a country changes its name a Table G notation is assigned to the new name. The notation for the latest form of a name is used regardless of which form of name is found in the item or when the item was produced.

United States -- Special Instructions

Special provisions are made for United States government documents published at the federal, state or local level. Works pertaining to the internal affairs of the various departments or agencies of the U.S. Federal Government, with the exception of the Armed Forces, take the designation "A."

Publications pertaining to the internal affairs of the Armed Forces take the following designations:

A1 Department of Defense
A2 Department of the Army
A3 Army Air Forces (to 1947)
A4 Department of the Air Force
A5 Department of the Navy

AA1 is used for materials pertaining to the United States as a whole but not to the internal affairs of the government. AA1 is also used for materials that span four or more states or territories, unless there is a number for the region.

As noted above, each state is provided with a separate number. The only city appearing in Table G is New York City. For other subordinate political units in the United States, it is the individual state number which is so modified, as indicated above.

Subordinate Political Units

The Table provides a state or political unit break down only for the United States and Great Britain. A work that is limited to a city, or a state, province or its equivalent, takes the geographic notation for the state or country, or for the smallest area below the national level that has its own notation.

Examples:

AM3 – Maryland	DC2 — Canada	FE5 — England
AM3.1 M7 — Montgomery County	DC2.1 B8 — British Columbia	FE5.1 M6 -- Middlesex
AM3.2 B2 — Baltimore	DC2.2 V2 — Vancouver	FE5.2 L6 – London

Other heavily used state or country notations may be modified to form county (province, state, etc.) or city notations by the addition of .1 (county) or .2 (city) to the appropriate notation.

The expanded country notation below for Australia is an example of how a cataloging agency may expand the notation of a state, country, etc. when the need arises. NLM has used this method; however, since these expansions are infrequent and on an ad hoc basis they are not printed in the *Classification*.

Example:

KA8   Australia
.C6 Commission of Inquiry into Poverty
.D3 Department of Health
.D32 Department of Labor and Immigration
.D34 Department of Science
.D4 Department of Social Security
.H6 Hospitals and Health Services
etc.

KA8.1
A8 Australian Capital Territory
.N3 New South Wales
.N6 Northern Territory
.Q3 Queensland
etc.

KA8.2
.A3 Adelaide
.B8 Brisbane
.C2 Canberra
etc.

This kind of pattern can be used for any single country number.

Table G notations no longer in use are found below under the heading "Obsolete Table G Notations."

Examples for Applying Table G

1.   Application of Table G to monographic materials.

United States
WZ 70   Hume, Ruth Fox, 1922-
AM3   Medicine in Maryland

WA 546   Ziegler, Mark V., 1891-
AM3.1   A survey of the Health Department of Montgomery
M7   County, Maryland / ...

WA 546   United States. Bureau of the Census
AC2.2   Social and health indicators system, Los Angeles
L86

Foreign
WZ 70   Anning, Stephen T.
FE5   The history of medicine of Leeds

WM 11   Psychoanalyse in Berlin
GG4

WA 900   Health on the march, 1948-1960, West Bengal
JI4.1   ("W5" represents West Bengal, the state)
W5

2.   The application of Table G to serial documents (W2)

United States
W2   United States. Army. Air Corps. Materiel Division
A3   Air Corps technical report

W2   Connecticut Commission on Alcoholism
AC   Annual report

Foreign
W2   Great Britain. General Register Office
FA1   Quarterly return of marriages, births, and death ...

W2   Saskatchewan. Bureau of Public Health
DC2.1   Annual report
S2

3.   The application of Table G to hospital reports
        As instructed in the WX schedule under "WX 2   Serial hospital reports" these serials are arranged geographically and cuttered for the hospital. Decimal subdivisions .1 and .2 for subordinate political divisions are not used, but a notation is added to represent the city.

Civilian hospitals
WX   Cedars of Lebanon Hospital (Los Angeles, Calif.)
2   Staff journal
AC2
L8

WX   Hahnemann Hospital tidings
2
AP4
P5

WX   Lasarettet i Landskrona
2   Aarsberättelse
GS8
L2

WX   St. Luke's Hospital (Jacksonville, Fla.)
2   Annual report
AF4
J2

U.S. Military Hospitals.
        Named hospitals have fixed locations and are cuttered the same way as civilian hospitals except that the military symbol precedes the geographical notation. Numbered hospitals do not have fixed locations and geographical notation is not applied to them.

WX   United States. Army. Walter Reed Army Hospital, Washington, D.C.
2   Annual report
A2
D6

WX   United States. Army. General Hospital No. 141
2   Year book
A2
141

TABLE G Continued

I. SUMMARY

A--United States (Federal Government)
AA1--United States (as geographical area)
D--Americas
F--Great Britain
G--Europe
H--Africa

J--Middle East and Asia
K--Australasia
L--Islands of the Pacific and Indian Oceans
M--International Agencies
P--Polar Regions

II. UNITED STATES (Federal Government)

A--United States (as author)
A1--Department of Defense
A2--Department of the Army

A3--Army Air Forces (to 1947)
A4--Department of the Air Force
A5--Department of the Navy

III. UNITED STATES

AA1--United States
AA4--Alabama
AA5--Alaska
AA6--Appalachian Region
AA7--Arizona
AA8--Arkansas
AC2--California
AC6--Colorado
AC8--Connecticut
AD4--Delaware
AD6--District of Columbia
AF4--Florida
AG4--Georgia
AG7--Great Lakes Region
AH3--Hawaii
AI2--Idaho
AI3--Illinois
A16--Indiana
A18--Iowa
AK3--Kansas
AK4--Kentucky
AL6--Louisiana
AM2--Maine
AM3--Maryland
AM4--Massachusetts
AM5--Michigan
AM53--Mid-Atlantic Region
AM56--Midwestern United States
AM6--Minnesota
AM7--Mississippi

AM8--Missouri
AM9--Montana
AN1--Nebraska
AN2--Nevada
AN25--New England
AN3--New Hampshire
AN4--New Jersey
AN5--New Mexico
AN6--New York (State)
AN7--New York City
AN8--North Carolina
AN9--North Dakota
AO3--Ohio
AO5--Oklahoma
AO7--Oregon
AP4--Pennsylvania
AR4--Rhode Island
AS6--South Carolina
AS8--South Dakota
AS9--Southeastern United States
AS95--Southwestern United States
AT2--Tennessee
AT4--Texas
AU8--Utah
AV5--Vermont
AV8--Virginia
AW2--Washington
AW4--West Virginia
AW6--Wisconsin
AW8--Wyoming

IV. AMERICAS

DA1--Americas
DA15--Latin America
DA2--North America
DA3--Central America
DA4--South America
DA7--Argentina
DB3--Bahamas
DB34--Barbados
DB38--Belize
DB4--Bermuda
DB6--Bolivia
DB8--Brazil
    British Guiana see Guyana
    British Honduras see Belize
DC2--Canada
DC3--Caribbean Region
DC5--Chile
DC7--Colombia
DC8--Costa Rica
DC9--Cuba
DD6--Dominican Republic
    Dutch Guiana see Suriname
DE2--Ecuador
DF3--Falkland Islands

DG4--Grenada
DG5--Guatemala
DG6--Guyana
DG8--French Guiana
DH2--Haiti
DH7--Honduras
DJ2--Jamaica
DM3--Martinique
DM4--Mexico
DN4--Netherlands Antilles
DN5--Nicaragua
DP2--Panama
DP3--Panama Canal Zone
DP4--Paraguay
DP6--Peru
DP8--Puerto Rico
DS2--Salvador
DS9--Suriname
DT7--Trinidad and Tobago
DU7--Uruguay
DV4--Venezuela
DV5--Virgin Islands
DW5--West Indies

V. GREAT BRITAIN

FA1--Great Britain
FE5--England
FG9--Guernsey
FI7--Northern Ireland

FM2--Isle of Man
FS2--Scotland
FW3--Wales

VI. EUROPE

GA1-- Europe
GA4--Albania
GA5--Andorra
GA7--Armenia
GA8--Austria
GA85--Azerbaijan
GA9--Azores
GB4--Belgium
GB5--Bosnia-Herzegovina
GB8--Bulgaria
GB9--Byelarus
GC5--Croatia
GC7--Cyprus
GC75--Czech Republic
GD4--Denmark

GE7--Estonia
GF5--Finland
GF7--France
GG3--Georgia (Republic)
GG4--Germany
GG5--Gibraltar
GG6--Greece
GG7--Greenland
GH8--Hungary
GI3--Iceland
GI6--Ireland
GI8--Italy
GL3--Latvia
GL4—Liechtenstein
GL5--Lithuania

TABLE G Continued

EUROPE Continued

GL8--Luxembourg
GM2--Macedonia (Republic)
GM3--Malta
GM35--Mediterranean Region
GM4--Moldova
GM5--Monaco
GM6--Montenegro
GN4--Netherlands
GN6—Norway
GP6--Poland

GP7--Portugal
GR8--Romania
GR9--Russia
GS3--Scandinavia
GS4--Serbia
GS45--Slovakia
GS5--Slovenia
GS6--Spain
GS8--Sweden
GS9--Switzerland
GU5--Ukraine
GY8--Yugoslavia

VII. AFRICA

HA1--Africa
HA12--Africa South of the Sahara
HA14--Central Africa
HA15--Eastern Africa
HA2--North Africa
HA21--Western Africa
HA4--Algeria
HA6--Angola
HA7--African Atlantic Islands
HA71--Ascension
HA72--St. Helena
HA73--Tristan de Cunha
    Basutoland see Lesotho
    Bechuanaland see Botswana
    Belgian Congo see Congo (Democratic Republic)
HB35--Benin
HB4--Botswana
HB8--Burundi
HC3--Cameroon
HC4--Cape Verde Islands
HC43--Central African Republic
HC45--Chad
HC5--Congo (Brazzaville)
    Congo (Kinshasa) see Congo (Democratic Republic)
HC6--Congo (Democratic Republic)
HC7--Côte d'Ivoire
    Dahomey see Benin
    Democratic Republic of the Congo see Congo (Democratic Republic)
HD6--Djibouti
HE3--Egypt
HE6--Equatorial Guinea
HE7--Eritrea
HE8--Ethiopia
    French Somaliland see Djibouti

HG2—Gabon
HG3--Gambia
HG6--Ghana
HG66--Guinea
HG7--Guinea-Bissau
HG9--Equatorial Guinea
    Ivory Coast see Côte d'Ivoire
HK4--Kenya
HL3--Lesotho
HL5--Liberia
HL6--Libya
HM3--Madagascar
    Malagasy Republic see Madagascar
HM4—Malawi
HM45--Mali
HM48--Mauritania
HM5--Morocco
HM7--Mozambique
HN2--Namibia
HN4--Niger
HN5--Nigeria
    Nyasaland see Malawi
    Portuguese Guinea see Guinea-Bissau
    Rhodesia, Northern see Zambia
    Rhodesia, Southern see Zimbabwe
HR8--Rwanda
HS1--Senegal
HS3--Sierra Leone
HS5--Somalia
HS8--South West Africa
    Spanish Guinea see Equatorial Guinea
HS86--Sudan
HS9--Swaziland
    Tanganyika see Tanzania
HT3--Tanzania
HT6—Togo

TABLE G Continued

AFRICAN Continued

HT8--Tunisia

HU4--Uganda

HU5--South Africa

    Zaire see Congo (Democratic Republic)

HZ2--Zambia

    Zanzibar see Tanzania

HZ7--Zimbabwe

VIII. MIDDLE EAST AND ASIA

JA1--Asia

JA2--Middle East

JA4--Afghanistan

JA7--Arabia

JB1--Bahrain

JB2--Bangladesh

    Burma see Myanmar

JC2--Cambodia

    Ceylon see Sri Lanka

JC6--China

    Formosa see Taiwan

JH6--Hong Kong

JI4--India

JI5--Indochina

JI7--Iran

JI8--Iraq

JI9--Israel

JJ3--Japan

JJ6--Jordan

JK2--Kazakhstan

JK6--Korea

JK8--Kuwait

JK9--Kyrgyzstan

JL2--Laos

JL4--Lebanon

JM1--Macao

JM2--Malaysia

    Malaya see Malaysia

    Manchuria see China

JM6--Mongolia

JM9--Myanmar

JN4--Nepal

JP2--Palestine

JP3--Pakistan

JQ2--Qatar

JS2--Saudi Arabia

JS6--Singapore

JS8--Sri Lanka

JS9--Syria

JT2--Taiwan

JT23--Tajikistan

JT3--Thailand

JT5--Tibet

JT8--Turkey

JT9--Turkmenistan

JU9--Uzbekistan

JV6--Vietman

JY4--Yemen

IX. AUSTRALASIA

KA8—Australia

KN4—New Zealand

X. ISLANDS OF THE PACIFIC AND INDIAN OCEANS

LA1--Pacific Islands

LA2--Indian Ocean Islands

LB6--Borneo

LB7--Brunei

LC7--Comoros

LF4--Fiji

LI4--Indonesia

LM4--Mauritius

LM6—Micronesia

LN6--New Caledonia

LP2--Papua New Guinea

LP5--Philippines

LP7--Polynesia

LR4--Reunion

LS5--Seychelles

LV2--Vanuatu

TABLE G Continued

XI. INTERNATIONAL AGENCIES

M--International agencies
    (General or not listed below)
MA4--Allied Forces
MF6--Food and Agricultural Organization
    of the United Nations
MI3--International Labour Office
ML4--League of Nations
MP2--Pan American Sanitary Bureau
MP3--Pan American Union

MP4--Pan American Zoonoses Center
MS7--SEATO (South East Asia Treaty
    Organization)
MS9--Supreme Commander of the Allied
    Powers
MU5--United Nations
MU7--Unesco
MU8--Unicef
MW6--World Health Organization

XII. POLAR REGIONS

PA6—Antarctic

PA7--Arctic

OBSOLETE *TABLE G* NOTATIONS

Obsolete Notation	Geographical Names	New Notation
AMERICAS		
DA5	Lesser Antilles	None
DG7	Dutch Guiana	DS9
DH8	British Honduras	DB38
EUROPE		
GC8	Czechoslovakia	GC75, GS45
GT8	Turkey	JT8
AFRICA		
HB3	Basutoland	HL3
HF4	French Equatorial Africa	None
HF8	French West Africa	None
HM6	Spanish Morocco	None
HN8	Nyasaland	HM4
HR4	Rhodesia	None
HR5	Rio de Oro	HM48
HS6	French Somaliland	HD6
HT4	Tangier	None
HZ15	Zaire	HC6
HZ3	Zanzibar	HT3

TABLE G Continued

Obsolete Notation	Geographical Names	New Notation
	MIDDLE EAST AND ASIA	
JB8	Burma	JM9
JC4	Ceylon	JS8
JF6	Formosa	JT2
JM3	Manchuria	JC6
JT7	Trans-Jordan	None
	ISLANDS OF THE PACIFIC AND INDIAN OCEANS	
LN4	Netherlands East Indies	LI4
	INTERNATIONAL AGENCIES	
MI8	Islamic Countries	None

OUTLINE OF SCHEDULES

PRECLINICAL SCIENCES

MEDICINE AND RELATED SUBJECTS

QS

HUMAN ANATOMY

Classify here general material on normal human anatomy including that of men, women, or children treated separately. Classify material on anatomy of a part of the body with the part, on surgical anatomy in WO 101, on artistic anatomy of human or animal in NC 760–783.8, on anatomy of animals in QL or SF.

QS 1–132	**Anatomy**
QS 504–539	**Histology**
QS 604–681	**Embryology**

ANATOMY

Note that other form numbers are used under Histology (QS 504–539) and under Embryology (QS 604–681).

* 1   **Societies (Cutter from the name of society)**
Includes ephemeral membership lists issued serially or separately. Classify substantial lists with directories. Classify annual reports, journals, etc., in W1.

4   **General works**
Classify here works on regional anatomy. If written for the surgeon, classify in WO 101 Surgical anatomy. Classify material on comparative anatomy in QS 124.

Collections (General)
5   **By several authors**
7   **By individual authors**

9   **Addresses. Essays. Lectures (General)**

11   **History (Table G)**
11.1   **General coverage (Not Table G)**

* 13   **Dictionaries. Encyclopedias**

* 15   **Classification. Nomenclature. Terminology**

* 16   **Tables. Statistics**

17   **Atlases. Pictorial works**

*NUMBER CAN BE USED FOR BOTH MONOGRAPHS AND SERIALS.

18 **Education**
Classify here works about education.

* 18.2 **Educational materials**
Classify here educational materials, e.g., outlines, questions and answers, programmed instruction, catalogs, computer–assisted instruction, etc., regardless of format. Classify textbooks, regardless of format, by subject.

20.5 **Research (General)**
Classify here works about research in general. Classsify works about research on a particular subject by subject.

21 **Anatomy as a profession**

* 22 **Directories (Table G)**
* 22.1 **General coverage (Not Table G)**

Laboratories, institutes, etc.
23 **Collective**
24 **Individual (Cutter from name of agency)**

25 **Laboratory manuals. Technique**

* 26 **Equipment and supplies**
Classify catalogs here.

26.5 **Medical informatics. Automatic data processing. Computers (General)**
Classify works on use for special subjects by subject.

Museums, exhibits, etc.
27 **Collective (Table G)**
27.1 **General coverage (Not Table G)**
28 **Individual (Table G)**

[32] **[This number not used]**
Classify laws on dissection in QS 132.

* 39 **Handbooks. Resource guides**

124 **Comparative anatomy of humans and animals**
Classify works on artistic anatomy of humans and animals in NC 760–783.8; on comparative anatomy limited to animals in QL 801–950.9.

130 **Dissection manuals**

*NUMBER CAN BE USED FOR BOTH MONOGRAPHS AND SERIALS.

* 132　　Laws concerning dissection.　Discussion of law

HISTOLOGY

504　　General works

　　　　Collections (General)
505　　　　By several authors
507　　　　By individual authors

509　　Addresses.　Essays.　Lectures (General)

511　　History (Table G)
511.1　　General coverage (Not Table G)

* 513　　Dictionaries.　Encyclopedias

* 515　　Classification.　Nomenclature.　Terminology

* 516　　Tables.　Statistics

517　　Atlases.　Pictorial works

518　　Education
　　　　Classify here works about education.

* 518.2　　Educational materials
　　　　Classify here educational materials, e.g., outlines, questions and answers, programmed instruction, catalogs, computer–assisted instruction, etc., regardless of format. Classify textbooks, regardless of format, by subject.

520　　Research (General)
　　　　Classify here works about research in general.　Classify works about research on a particular subject by subject.　Cf. 530 Experimental histology.

521　　Histology as a profession

* 522　　Directories (Table G)
* 522.1　　General coverage (Not Table G)

Tissue banks

523   Collective

524   Individual (Cutter from name of bank)

525   Laboratory manuals.   Technique

* 526   Equipment and supplies
            Classify catalogs here.

526.5   Medical informatics.   Automatic data processing.   Computers (General)
            Classify works on use for special subjects by subject.

* 529   Handbooks.   Resource guides

530   Experimental histology
            Classify works on cytology of normal tissue in QH.   Classify works about research
              in QS 520.

531   Histocytochemistry

532   Types of normal tissue (General)
            Classify works on aging tissue of the elderly in WT 104; on lymphoid tissue in WH
              700; on fetal membranes in WQ 210 or in QS 645 if written for the embryologist.

532.5   Specific types of tissue, A–Z

          .A3   Adipose tissue
          .C7   Connective tissue
          .E5   Elastic tissue
          .E7   Epithelium
          .M3   Membranes (General)
          .M8   Mucous membrane
          .N3   Nerve tissue

EMBRYOLOGY

604   General works

Collections (General)

605   By several authors

607   By individual authors

609   Addresses.   Essays.   Lectures (General)

611 History (Table G)
611.1   General coverage (Not Table G)

* 613 Dictionaries. Encyclopedias

* 615 Classification. Nomenclature. Terminology

* 616 Tables. Statistics

617 Atlases. Pictorial works

618 Education
Classify here works about education.

* 618.2 Educational materials
Classify here educational materials, for example, outlines, questions and answers, programmed instruction, catalogs, computer–assisted instruction, etc., regardless of format. Classify textbooks, regardless of format, by subject.

620 Research (General)
Classify here works about research in general. Classify works about research on a particular subject by subject.

621 Embryology as a profession

* 622 Directories (Table G)
* 622.1   General coverage (Not Table G)

625 Laboratory manuals. Technique

* 626 Equipment and supplies
Classify catalogs here.

626.5 Medical informatics. Automatic data processing. Computers (General)
Classify works on use for special subjects by subject.

* 629 Handbooks. Resource guides

638 Sex determination (Embryogenic)

640 Sex differentiation

642 Twinning

*NUMBER CAN BE USED FOR BOTH MONOGRAPHS AND SERIALS.

645   **Placentation.   Fetal membranes**

675   **Congenital abnormalities (General or not elsewhere classified)**
> *Classify works on specific abnormalities with anatomical part involved, e.g., Cleft lip WV 440. Classify works on inborn errors of metabolism, general and systemic, in WD 205, etc.*

677   **Chromosome abnormalities, including experimental works**
> *Classify works on chromosome aberrations in QH 462.*

679   **Drug–induced abnormalities, including experimental works**

681   **Radiation–induced abnormalities, including experimental works**
> *Classify works on specific abnormalities with anatomical part involved, e.g., of the central nervous system in WL 101.*

QT

PHYSIOLOGY

Classify here material on general physiology; classify physiology of a part of the body with the part; classify animal physiology in QP, QL, or SF. The last part of QT covers the broad areas of hygiene.

QT 1–33.1	General
QT 34–37.5	Physics, Mathematics, and Engineering
QT 104–172	Human Physiology
QT 180–275	Physiology and Hygiene

GENERAL

* 1   **Societies (Cutter from name of society)**
Includes ephemeral membership lists issued serially or separately. Classify substantial lists with directories. Classify annual reports, journals, etc., in W1.

4   **General works, including comparative physiology**
Classify material on comparative physiology limited to animals in QP.

Collections (General)
5   **By several authors**
7   **By individual authors**

9   **Addresses. Essays. Lectures (General)**

11   **History (Table G)**
11.1   **General coverage (Not Table G)**

* 13   **Dictionaries. Encyclopedias**

* 15   **Classification. Nomenclature. Terminology**

* 16   **Tables. Statistics**

17   **Atlases. Pictorial works**

18   **Education**
         Classify here works about education.

* 18.2   **Educational materials**
         Classify here educational materials, e.g., outlines, questions and answers, programmed instruction, catalogs, computer–assisted instruction, etc., regardless of format. Classify textbooks, regardless of format, by subject.

* 19   **Schools, departments, and faculties of physiology or physical education**

20.5   **Research (General)**
         Classify here works about research in general. Classify works about research on a particular subject by subject. Cf. QT 25 Experimental physiology.

21   **Physiology as a profession. Ethics. Peer review**

* 22   **Directories (Table G)**
* 22.1   **General coverage (Not Table G)**

         Laboratories, institutes, etc.
23   **Collective**
24   **Individual (Cutter from name of agency)**

25   **Laboratory manuals. Experimental physiology. Technique**

* 26   **Equipment and supplies**
         Classify catalogs here.

26.5   **Medical informatics. Automatic data processing. Computers (General)**
         Classify works on use for special subjects by subject.

         Museums, exhibits, etc.
27   **Collective**
28   **Individual (Cutter from name of museum, etc.)**

* 29   **Handbooks. Resource guides**

* 32   **Laws (Table G)**
* 32.1   **General coverage (Not Table G)**

* 33   **Discussion of law (Table G)**
* 33.1   **General coverage (Not Table G)**

*NUMBER CAN BE USED FOR BOTH MONOGRAPHS AND SERIALS.

PHYSICS, MATHEMATICS, AND ENGINEERING

Include here only general works on physics, mathematics, and engineering as applied to physiological and medical phenomena. Classify works on their applications to specific problems by subject.

34   **Biophysics**
         Cf. WN   Radiology.   Diagnostic imaging

35   **Biomedical mathematics**
         Cf. WA 950   Theory or methods of medical statistics.   Classify works for the biologist in QH 323.5.

36   **Biomedical engineering**

37   **Biomedical and biocompatible materials**
         Classify works on dental materials in WU 180–190.

37.5   **Specific materials, A–Z**

         .C4   **Ceramics**
         .P7   **Polymers**

HUMAN PHYSIOLOGY

104   **General works**

120   **Homeostasis (General)**

140   **Environmental exposure.   Physiological adaptation**

145   **Acclimatization**

150   **Hot climates**

160   **Cold climates**

Environmental exposure. Physiological adaptation – Continued

162   **Other environmental factors acting on human physiology, A–Z**

Classify works on animals in general and on wild animals in QP 82–82.2; on domestic animals in SF 768–768.2. Classify works on environmental factors relating to personal health and hygiene in QT 230; to disease, in QZ 57; to public health, in WA. For other environmental factors not listed here, consult the Index to the classification.

       .A5   **Air ionization**
       .E4   **Electrolytes**
       .G7   **Gravitation**
       .H8   **Humidity**
       .L5   **Light**
       .M3   **Magnetics**
       .S8   **Stress**
       .U4   **Ultraviolet rays and other non–ionizing radiation not classified elsewhere.**

Cf. WB 117 for general medical use; WB 288 for diagnostic use; WB 480 for therapeutic use; WD 605 for adverse effects.

165   **Body temperature regulation**

167   **Physiological periodicity**

172   **Exocrine glands (General)**

Classify works on specific glands with the system where located, e.g., Sebaceous glands WR 410.

PHYSIOLOGY AND HYGIENE

180   **Physiology. General hygiene**

Include college level texts.

200   **Teachers' manuals, books for nurses, etc., on physiology and hygiene**

Classify works about study and teaching of public health in WA 18. Classify works on informal health education (community, radio, etc.) in WA 590.

     School texts of physiology and hygiene

Classify material on hygiene of adolescence in WS 460.

210   **Secondary**

215   **Juvenile**

225   **Sex education**

Classify in HQ material on sex education other than school texts.

230   **Lighting. Air. Sunlight. Living space**

235   **Diet**
Classify works on particular foods and beverages in the numbers for diet in health and disease, WB 400–449; on diets for particular diseases with the disease.

240   **Cleanliness**

245   **Clothing**

250   **Recreation. Outdoor activities**

255   **Physical fitness. Gymnastics. Physical education**
Cf. WB 541 Medical gymnastics.

260   **Athletics. Sports**
Classify works on first aid in WA 292.

260.5   **Special activities, A–Z**

.B2	Baseball
.B3	Basketball
.B5	Bicycling
.B7	Boxing
.D6	Diving
.F6	Football
.G6	Golf
.H6	Hockey
.J6	Jogging
.M3	Martial arts
.M9	Mountaineering
.R9	Running
.S6	Skiing
.S7	Soccer
.S9	Swimming
.T3	Tennis
.T7	Track and field
.W2	Walking
.W4	Weight lifting
.W9	Wrestling

261   **Sports medicine**
Classify works on first aid in WA 292; on specific pathological conditions with the condition.

265   **Relaxation. Rest. Sleep (Hygiene)**
Classify works on therapeutic use of rest, etc., in WB 545; on disorders of sleep in WM 188; on physiology of sleep in WL 108.

275   **Hygienic aspects of beauty culture**
Classify works on hair care in WR 465; on public health aspects of barber shops, beauty salons, and cosmetics in WA 744.

QU

BIOCHEMISTRY

* 1   **Societies (Cutter from name of society)**
Includes ephemeral membership lists issued serially or separately. Classify substantial lists with directories; annual reports, journals, etc. in W1.

4   **General works**

          Collections (General)
5   **By several authors**
7   **By individual authors**

9   **Addresses. Essays. Lectures (General)**

11   **History (Table G)**
11.1   **General coverage (Not Table G)**

* 13   **Dictionaries.   Encyclopedias**

* 15   **Classification.   Nomenclature.   Terminology**

* 16   **Tables.   Statistics**
Classify nutrition tables or food value tables in QU 145–145.5.

17   **Atlases.   Pictorial works**

18   **Education**
Classify here works about education.

* 18.2   **Educational materials**
Classify here educational materials, e.g., outlines, questions and answers, programmed instruction, catalogs, computer-assisted instruction, etc., regardless of format. Classify textbooks, regardless of format, by subject.

20   **Research (General)**
Classify here works about research in general. Classify works about research on a particular subject by subject.

21   **Biochemistry as a profession**

* 22	**Directories (Table G)**
* 22.1	**General coverage (Not Table G)**

Laboratories, institutes, etc.

23	**Collective**
24	**Individual (Cutter from name of agency)**

25   **Laboratory manuals. Technique**

* 26   **Equipment and supplies**
Classify catalogs here.

26.5   **Medical informatics. Automatic data processing. Computers (General)**
Classify works on use for special subjects by subject.

* 32   **Laws (Table G)**
* 32.1   **General coverage (Not Table G)**

* 33   **Discussion of law (Table G)**
* 33.1   **General coverage (Not Table G)**

34   **Biochemical phenomena (General or not elsewhere classified)**
Classify here works on binding sites, diffusion, energy transfer, osmosis, etc., when related to biochemistry in general.

* 39   **Handbooks. Resource guides**

50   **Chemistry of food substances (General)**

54   **Nitrogen and related compounds (General or not elsewhere classified)**
Classify works on nitrogen compounds that work primarily on a particular body system in QV.

55   **Proteins (General or not elsewhere classified)**
Classify here works on proteins in general or those in foods. Classify works on proteins that work primarily on a particular body system in QV; on those that are localized, by site, e.g., eye proteins in WW 101; on those that are enzymes or coenzymes in QU 135–141 or with the system acted upon; on blood proteins in WH or in clinical pathology QY 455; on immunoglobulins in QW 601; on other immunoproteins in appropriate QW number.

56   **Nucleoproteins**

57   **Nucleosides. Nucleotides**

58   Nucleic acids and derivatives (General or not elsewhere classified)
               Classify works on derivatives acting on blood and blood formation in QV 185.

58.5   DNA

58.7   RNA

60   Amino acids (General or not elsewhere classified)

61   Amines. Amidines (General or not elsewhere classified)
               Classify works on catecholamines in WK 725; on amino alcohols in QV 82–84.

62   Amides (General or not elsewhere classified)

65   Heterocyclic compounds associated with amino acid synthesis and metabolism
               e.g., Allantoin. Indoleacetic acids

68   Peptides (General or not elsewhere classified)

70   Nitrogen fixation

75   Carbohydrates
               Cf. QY 470 under Blood chemistry.

83   Polysaccharides and derivatives
                  e.g., Dextrins. Glycogen

84   Sugar acids and their salts and esters (General or not elsewhere classified)

85   Lipids (General or not elsewhere classified)
               Cf. QY 465 under Blood chemistry.

86   Fats. Oils

87   Lipotropic factors
                  Classify works on methionine in QU 60.

90   Fatty acids

93   Phospholipids
                  e.g., Phosphatidylethanolamines

Lipids – Continued

95   **Sterols**
          e.g., Cholesterol

98   **Carboxylic acids and their salts and esters (General or not elsewhere classified)**

99   **Aldehydes (General or not elsewhere classified)**

100   **Body composition**

105   **Body fluids**
          Classify here works on acid–base equilibrium, hydrogen–ion concentration, and water–electrolyte balance in body fluids. Cf. WD 220 Water–electrolyte imbalance, etc.

107   **Growth substances. Growth inhibitors (General or not elsewhere classified)**

110   **Pigments (General or not elsewhere classified)**

120   **Metabolism**
          Classify works on metabolism of a particular substance with the substance, e.g., Metabolism of proteins in QU 55.

125   **Energy metabolism. Calorimetry**

130   **Inorganic substances (General or not elsewhere classified)**
          Cf. QY 480 under Blood chemistry.

130.5   **Trace elements**

131   **Organometallic compounds. Organophosphorus compounds. Organothiophosphorus compounds (General or not elsewhere classified)**

133   **Colloids (General or not elsewhere classified)**

135   **Enzymes. Coenzymes (General or not elsewhere classified). Enzymology**
          Classify works on enzyme deficiency in WD 105 or with the diseases resulting.

136   **Hydrolases (General or not elsewhere classified)**

137   **Isomerases (General or not elsewhere classified)**

Enzymes. Coenzymes. Enzymology – Continued

138   **Ligases (General or not elsewhere classified)**

139   **Lyases (General or not elsewhere classified)**

140   **Oxidoreductases (General or not elsewhere classified)**

141   **Transferases (General or not elsewhere classified)**

142   **Enzyme precursors (General or not elsewhere classified)**

143   **Enzyme inhibitors (General or not elsewhere classified)**

144   **Enzyme reactivators (General or not elsewhere classified)**

145   **Nutrition. Nutritional requirements**
Classify works on infant nutrition in WS 115–125; on child nutrition in WS 115–130; on geriatric nutrition in WT 115.

145.5   **Nutritive values of food**

146   **Nutritional surveys (Table G)**
146.1   **General coverage (Not Table G)**

160   **Vitamins. Vitamin requirements**
Cf. QY 350 Assay of vitamins; QZ 109 Vitamin deficiencies; SF 98.V5 Vitamins in animal nutrition; WD 105 Deficiency diseases.

165   **Fat soluble vitamins**

167   **Vitamin A, A1, etc.**

173   **Vitamin D, D2, etc.**

179   **Vitamin E**

181   **Vitamin K**

185   **Water soluble vitamins**

187   **Vitamin B complex (General)**

Vitamins.   Vitamin requirements
Water soluble vitamins
Vitamin B complex – Continued

QV

PHARMACOLOGY

Classify here works on pharmacology in general or on the pharmacology of individual drugs or types of drugs grouped according to their specific action. Classify works on an individual drug according to its principal action. Classify works on the use of an individual drug in the treatment of a particular disease with the disease. Classify works on the purely chemical or technological use of chemicals in the QD or the T schedules. Classify a drug derived from a plant with the drug.

Classify works on vitamins in QU; on endocrine preparations (including synthetic substitutes) in WJ, WK, or WP; and non–endocrine biologicals in QW. Note that occasionally agents are classed together because they are frequently treated together regardless of their different actions, e.g., sulfur and sulfur compounds in QV 265. Classify works dealing with the general aspects of pharmacy and pharmaceutics in the section beginning with QV 701. Note that Pharmacy and Pharmaceutics section also has many of the early range or form numbers found under Pharmacology.

QV 1–370	General
QV 600–667	Toxicology
QV 701–835	Pharmacy and Pharmaceutics

GENERAL

* 1   **Societies (Cutter from name of society)**
Includes ephemeral membership lists issued serially or separately. Classify substantial lists with directories; annual reports, journals, etc., in W1.

4   **General works**

Collections (General)
5   **By several authors**
7   **By individual authors**

9   **Addresses. Essays. Lectures (General)**

11   **History (Table G)**
11.1   **General coverage (Not Table G)**
Classify works on the history of a specific drug with the drug.

* 13   **Dictionaries. Encyclopedias**

* 15   **Classification. Nomenclature. Terminology**

*NUMBER CAN BE USED FOR BOTH MONOGRAPHS AND SERIALS.

* 16   **Tables. Weights and measures. Statistics**

17   **Atlases. Pictorial works**
Classify pictorial works on medicinal plants or materia medica in QV 717.

18   **Education**
Classify here works about education.

* 18.2   **Educational materials**
Classify here educational materials, e.g., outlines, questions and answers, programmed instruction, catalogs, computer–assisted instruction, etc., regardless of format. Classify textbooks, regardless of format, by subject.

* 19   **Schools and colleges**
Classify courses of study, catalogs, etc., in W 19.5.

20   **Graduate and continuing education in pharmacy (including fellowships, internships, residencies, etc.)**

20.5   **Research (General)**
Classify here works about research in general. Classify works about research on a particular subject by subject. Cf. QV 34 Experimental pharmacology.

21   **Pharmacology as a profession. Pharmacy as a profession. Ethics. Peer review**

21.5   **Pharmacists' aides**

* 22   **Directories (Table G)**
* 22.1   **General coverage (Not Table G)**

     Laboratories, institutes, etc.
23   **Collective**
24   **Individual (Cutter from name of agency)**

25   **Laboratory manuals, including those on microscopic and chemical analysis. Technique**
Cf. QV 744 Pharmaceutical chemistry.

* 26   **Equipment and supplies**
Classify drug catalogs in QV 772. Cf. QV 785–835 for pharmaceutical supplies.

26.5   **Medical informatics. Automatic data processing. Computers (General)**
Classify works on use for special subjects by subject.

Museums, exhibits, etc.

27   Collective
28   Individual (Cutter from name of museum, etc.)

29   Registration of pharmacists (Table G)
29.1   General coverage (Not Table G)

* 32   Laws (Table G)
* 32.1 General coverage (Not Table G)

* 33   Discussion of law. Jurisprudence (Table G)
* 33.1 General coverage (Not Table G)

34   Experimental pharmacology (General)
      Classify here works that discuss the experimental work itself. Classify works about research in QV 20.5. Classify works on specific subjects by subject.

38   Drug action (including absorption, distribution, excretion of drugs; mechanism of drug action; synergism, antagonism, tolerance; factors modifying drug action, including genetic factors)

* 39   Handbooks. Resource guides

50   Dental pharmacology
      Cf. WU 180–190 Dental materials.

55   Drugs (General)
      Cf. QV 38 Drug action; QV 704 Pharmacy; QY 450–490 Blood chemistry.

60   Dermatologic agents
      Classify works on topical anti–inflammatory agents here. Cf. QV 247 for other anti–inflammatory agents. Classify works on local anti–infective agents in QV 220.

63   Protectives
      e.g., Adsorbents. Demulcents. Emollients

65   Irritants. Astringents

66   Gastrointestinal agents (General or not elsewhere classified)
      Cf. WI 703 Bile acids, salts, etc.

69   Antacids. Anti–ulcer agents

71   Antidiarrheals

*NUMBER CAN BE USED FOR BOTH MONOGRAPHS AND SERIALS.

Gastrointestinal agents – Continued

73	**Emetics. Antiemetics**
75	**Cathartics**
76	**Antitussive agents**
76.5	**Neuropharmacology. Drugs acting on the nervous system (General or not elsewhere classified)**
77	**Psychopharmacology**
77.2	**Psychotropic drugs (General or not elsewhere classified)**
77.5	**Antidepressive agents**
77.7	**Hallucinogens**
77.9	**Tranquilizers**

80   **Depressants of the central nervous system**
Note that some of the agents classed in this group of numbers, QV 80–98, are here because of their relation to the depressant listed.

81   **Agents of general anesthesia**
Classify here works on anesthetics in general also. Cf. QV 110–115 Local anesthetics. Classify works on the barbiturates (except hexobarbital) in QV 88.

82	**Alcohols**
83	**Methyl**
84	**Ethyl**
85	**Hypnotics. Sedatives. Anticonvulsants**
87	**Bromides**

88   **Barbiturates**
Classify works on hexobarbital in QV 81.

Depressants of the central nervous system – Continued

89   **Opioid analgesics. Narcotics and narcotic antagonists**
Cf. QV 95 Anti–inflammatory analgesics.

90   **Opium alkaloids**

92   **Morphine and derivatives**

95   **Anti–inflammatory analgesics. Non–narcotic analgesics**
Classify general works on analgesics here. Cf. QV 89 Opioid analgesics; WO 234 Preanesthetic medication.

98   **Gout suppressants**

100   **Stimulants of the central nervous system**

101   **Analeptics**

102   **Amphetamines**

103   **Convulsants**

107   **Xanthines**
e.g., Caffeine. Theobromine. Theophylline

110   **Local anesthetics (General or not elsewhere classified)**

113   **Cocaine and derivatives**

115   **Synthetic local anesthetics**

120   **Autonomic agents (General or not elsewhere classified)**
Classify general works on bronchodilator agents here. Classify works on theophylline in QV 107. Classify works on autonomic agents that are also anti–inflammatory agents in QV 247; that are also histamine antagonists in QV 157; that are also sympathomimetics in QV 129; that are also vasodilator agents in QV 150.

122   **Parasympathomimetics**
e.g., Pilocarpine

124   **Cholinesterase inhibitors and reactivators**

Parasympathomimetics – Continued

126   **Neurotransmitters (General or not elsewhere classified)**
Classify works on epinephrine, norepinephrine, and other catecholamines in WK 725.

129   **Sympathomimetics**
e.g., Ephedrine
See note under QV 126 above. Classify works on amphetamines in QV 102.

132   **Sympatholytics. Parasympatholytics**
Classify works on cholinesterase reactivators in QV 124.

134   **Atropine and allied compounds**

137   **Nicotine**

138   **Non–metallic elements and their compounds, A–Z**
The substances classed here are used largely in experimental pharmacology, toxicology, and/or biochemistry for various purposes. Classify by specific use where possible.

     .C1   **Carbon**
     .P4   **Phosphorus**
     .S5   **Selenium**

140   **Neuromuscular agents**
e.g., Curare
Classify works on tranquilizers in QV 77.9.

150   **Drugs acting on the cardiovascular system**

153   **Digitalis. Cardiac glycosides**

155   **Quinidine and related compounds**

156   **Nitrates, nitrites, etc.**

157   **Histamine. Histamine antagonists. Histamine receptor blockaders**

160   **Diuretics. Antidiuretics**

170   **Drugs acting on the reproductive organs**

173   **Oxytocics**

Drugs acting on the reproductive organs
Oxytocics – Continued

174   **Ergot and its derivatives**

175   **Abortifacient agents**

177   **Contraceptives (including those with indirect action)**
           Classify works on contraceptive devices in WP 640.

180   **Drugs acting on blood cells and blood formation (General or not elsewhere classified)**
           Classify works on folic acid and vitamin B12 in QU 188 and QU 194, respectively.

181   **Hematinics**

183   **Iron. Iron salts**

184   **Liver extracts**

185   **Nucleic acid derivatives**
           Cf. QU 58 for works on biochemistry of nucleic acid derivatives.

190   **Drugs affecting blood coagulation**

193   **Anticoagulants**
           e.g., Coumarins. Heparin

195   **Hemostatics. Coagulants**

220   **Local anti–infective agents. Disinfectants (General or not elsewhere classified)**

223   **Phenols. Cresols (General or not elsewhere classified)**

225   **Formaldehyde. Nitrofurazone**

229   **Oxidizing antiseptics**
           e.g., Hydrogen peroxide. Potassium permanganate

231   **Halogen antiseptics**
           e.g., Iodine

233   **Detergents and other surface–active agents**

Local anti-infective agents. Disinfectants – Continued

235   **Dyes**
          Cf. QV 240 for general works on the pharmacology of dyes, etc.

239   **Boron compounds**

240   **Dyes and related compounds used in diagnosis or as reagents, indicators, etc.**

241   **Tars. Balsams**

243   **Urinary anti–infective agents**
          e.g., Methenamine. Mandelic acids

247   **Anti–inflammatory agents (General or not elsewhere classified)**
          Classify works on anti–inflammatory analgesics in QV 95; on topical anti–inflammatory agents in QV 60.

250   **Anti–infective agents (General or not elsewhere classified)**
          Classify works on local anti–infective agents in QV 220–239.

252   **Antifungal agents. Antifungal antibiotics**

253   **Anthelmintics**

254   **Antiprotozoal agents (General or not elsewhere classified)**

255   **Amebicides**

256   **Antimalarials**

257   **Cinchona and its derivatives**

258   **Synthetic drugs**

259   **Leprostatic agents**
          e.g., Chaulmoogra oil

261   **Antisyphilitics**
          e.g., Mercury compounds. Bismuth compounds. Iodides

262   **Arsenicals (General or not elsewhere classified)**

Anti-infective agents – Continued

265   **Sulfonamides. Sulfur and other sulfur compounds (General or not elsewhere classified)**

268   **Antitubercular agents. Antitubercular antibiotics**
Cf. WF 360 Drug therapy of pulmonary tuberculosis. Classify works on streptomycin in QV 356.

268.5   **Antiviral agents (General or not elsewhere classified)**

269   **Antineoplastic agents. Antineoplastic antibiotics**
Cf. QZ 267 Drug therapy of neoplasms. Classify works on azaserine in QV 252 Antifungal antibiotics or in QW 920 Immunosuppressive agents.

270   **Water. Inorganic ions. Electrolytes (General or not elsewhere classified)**
Cf. QU 105 Water-electrolyte balance; WD 220 Water-electrolyte imbalance.

273   **Water. Sodium salts**

275   **Cations and related compounds. Alkali and alkaline earth metals (General or not elsewhere classified)**
Cf. QV 290–298 Heavy metals and their compounds.

276   **Calcium**

277   **Potassium**

278   **Magnesium**

280   **Anions. Halogens**
Classify works on antiseptic halogens in QV 231.

282   **Fluorine. Fluorides**
Cf. QV 50 Dental pharmacology.

283   **Iodine. Iodides and related compounds**
Cf. QV 231 for iodines, etc. as antiseptics.

285   **Phosphates**
Classify works on sugar phosphates in QU 75.

290   **Heavy metals and their compounds (General or not elsewhere classified)**
Include works on rare earth metals not indexed elsewhere. Classify works on toxicological effects here also. Classify here works on chelating agents in general, but classify works on particular chelating agents with specific metal.

Heavy metals and their compounds – Continued

292	Lead
293	Mercury (General or compounds not elsewhere classified)
294	Arsenic (General or compounds not elsewhere classified)
295	Antimony
296	Gold
297	Silver
298	Zinc
310	Gases and their compounds (General or not elsewhere classified)
312	Oxygen and its compounds (General or not elsewhere classified)
314	Carbon dioxide
318	Helium

350   Antibiotics (General or not elsewhere classified)
Classify works on antifungal, antineoplastic, and antitubercular antibiotics in QV 252, QV 269, and QV 268, respectively.

350.5   Specific drugs, A–Z

         .C3   Cephalosporins
         .C5   Chloramphenicol
         .E7   Erythromycin
         .G3   Gentamicins

354	Penicillins
356	Streptomycin
360	Tetracyclines

370   **Tissue extracts**
Classify works on tissue therapy in WB 391; on therapy of specific diseases with the disease. Classify works on liver extracts in QV 184.

TOXICOLOGY

Classify general works on industrial poisons and poisoning in WA 465; general works on food poisoning in WC 268; on public health aspects of food poisoning in WA 695–722; on animal poisons in WD 400–430; on plant poisons in WD 500–530; on poisons acting on plants or animals in the appropriate LC schedules (See Index to this Classification). Classify works on agents that are primarily air, water, or soil pollutants in WA or WN. Classify works on chemicals used extensively in drug therapy or in experimental pharmacology in the pharmacology numbers.

600   **General works**

601   **Antidotes and other therapeutic measures**

602   **Detection of poisons. Tests. Laboratory manuals. Technique**
Classify works on medicolegal aspects in W 750.

* 605   **Directories of poison control centers. Lists of poisons, antidotes, etc. (Table G)**
* 605.1   **General coverage (Not Table G)**

* 607   **Handbooks. Resource guides**

610   **Inorganic poisons**

612   **Acids. Alkalies**

618   **Irritant poisons**
Cf. QV 664 Lung irritants; QV 666 Irritant gases.

627   **Organic poisons**

628   **Alkaloids**

632   **Non–alkaloids**

633   **Hydrocarbons. Volatile poisons. Solvents**

662 **Gas poisons and poisoning**
 Cf. QV 81 Anesthetic gases; QV 310 Gases used in therapy.

663 **Chemical warfare agents**
 Classify here works on the agent even if its war use is not part of the discussion.

664 **Lung irritants**
 e.g., Chloropicrin. Phosgene
 Cf. QV 666 for works on irritant gases.

665 **Tear gases. Toxic smokes**

666 **Irritant gases**
 Cf. QV 644 for general works on lung irritants.

667 **Systemic poisons. Paralysants**

PHARMACY AND PHARMACEUTICS

Classify works on pharmacy as a profession in QV 21; on pharmacy education in QV 18–20.

* 701 **Societies (Cutter from name of society)**
 Includes ephemeral membership lists issued serially or separately. Classify substantial lists with directories. Classify annual reports, journals, etc., in W1.

704 **General works**

Collections (General)
705 **By several authors**
707 **By individual authors**

709 **Addresses. Essays. Lectures (General)**

711 **History (Table G)**
711.1 **General coverage (Not Table G)**

* 715 **Classification. Nomenclature. Terminology**

717 **Atlases. Pictorial works**

* 722   **Directories (Table G)**
* 722.1   **General Coverage (Not Table G)**

* 732   **Laws (Table G)**
* 732.1   **General coverage (Not Table G)**

* 733   **Discussion of law. Jurisprudence (Table G)**
* 733.1   **General coverage (Not Table G)**

* 735   **Handbooks. Resource guides**

736   **Drug industry. Economics of pharmacy. Advertising**

737   **Pharmaceutical services. Community pharmacy services. Pharmacies**
             Classify works on hospital pharmacy service in WX 179; on public health aspects in WA 730.

* 738   **Pharmacopoeias (Official, i.e., one adopted by a government or other authoritative pharmaceutical body) (Table G)**
* 738.1   **General coverage (Not Table G)**

* 740   **Dispensatories, formularies, etc. (Unofficial) (Table G)**
* 740.1   **General coverage (Not Table G)**

744   **Pharmaceutical chemistry**
             Classify works on techniques of drug analysis and laboratory manuals in QV 25.

746   **Drug incompatibility (Pharmaceutical aspects)**

748   **Prescription writing. Dosage**

752   **Pharmacognosy. Natural history of drugs**

754   **Collection and preservation of drugs**
             Cf. QV 820 Preservatives.

760   **Materia medica**

* 766   **Medicinal plants (General and without geographic application)**

767   **Herbs**

Medicinal plants – Continued

770	**Geographic distribution (Table G)**
770.1	**General coverage (Not Table G)**
	General geographic coverage with more than three areas.

771   **Standardization and evaluation of drugs**
Classify works on monitoring drugs in WB 330; on monitoring those used for a particular disease, with the disease.

* 772   **Commercial preparations. Patent medicines**
Include here drug catalogs issued singly or serially.

773   **Fraud in manufacturing of drugs**

778   **Pharmaceutical processes. Drug compounding**

785   **Types of pharmaceutical preparations. Dosage forms (General or not elsewhere classified)**

786   **Solutions**

787   **Tablets**

800   **Vehicles. Pharmaceutic aids**

810   **Flavoring agents**

820   **Preservatives**
Cf. QV 754 Collection and preservation of drugs.

825   **Packaging**

835   **Labels and labeling**

QW

MICROBIOLOGY AND IMMUNOLOGY

Classify works on a particular species of bacteria with the order to which that species belongs, according to the classification in Bergey's Manual of Determinative Bacteriology.

QW 1–300	**Microbiology**
QW 501–949	**Immunology**

MICROBIOLOGY

* 1   **Societies (Cutter from name of society)**
Includes ephemeral membership lists issued serially or separately. Classify substantial lists with directories. Classify annual reports, journals, etc., in W1.

4   **General works**
Classify here works on microbiology as a whole. Classify works on bacteriology alone in QW 50; on virology alone in QW 160–170; on mycology alone in QW 180–180.5, or appropriate LC numbers.

Collections (General)
5   **By several authors**
7   **By individual authors**

9   **Addresses. Essays. Lectures (General)**

11   **History (Table G)**
11.1   **General coverage (Not Table G)**

* 13   **Dictionaries. Encyclopedias**

* 15   **Classification. Nomenclature. Terminology**

* 16   **Tables. Statistics**

17   **Atlases. Pictorial works**

18   **Education**
Classify here works about education.

*NUMBER CAN BE USED FOR BOTH MONOGRAPHS AND SERIALS.

* 18.2   **Educational materials**
Classify here educational materials, e.g., outlines, questions and answers, programmed instruction, catalogs, computer–assisted instruction, etc., regardless of format. Classify textbooks, regardless of format, by subject.

20.5   **Research (General)**
Classify here works about research in general. Classify works about research on a particular subject by subject.

21   **Microbiology and immunology as professions**

* 22   **Directories (Table G)**
* 22.1   **General coverage (Not Table G)**

Laboratories, institutes, etc.
23   **Collective**
24   **Individual (Cutter from name of agency)**

25   **Laboratory manuals. Technique**

25.5   **Specific techniques, A–Z**

     .M6   **Microbial sensitivity tests**
     .V7   **Virus cultivation**

* 26   **Apparatus, equipment, etc.**
Classify catalogs here.

26.5   **Medical informatics. Automatic data processing. Computers (General)**
Classify works on use for special subjects by subject.

Museums, exhibits, etc.
27   **Collective**
28   **Individual (Cutter from name of museum, etc.)**

* 32   **Laws (Table G)**
* 32.1   **General coverage (Not Table G)**

* 33   **Discussion of law (Table G)**
* 33.1   **General coverage (Not Table G)**

* 39   **Handbooks. Resource guides**

50   **Bacteria (General). Bacteriology**

*NUMBER CAN BE USED FOR BOTH MONOGRAPHS AND SERIALS.

51   **Morphology and variability of bacteria. Bacterial genetics**
         Classify works on fungi in QW 180; on viruses in QW 160 or with the specific fungi or virus group.

52   **Physiology and chemistry of bacteria. Metabolism**
         Classify works on fungi in QW 180; on viruses in QW 160 or with the specific fungi or virus group.

55   **Environmental microbiology**

60   **Plant and soil microbiology**
         Classify works on specific microorganisms by subject, e.g., Plant viruses QW 163.

65   **Dental microbiology**

70   **Veterinary microbiology**

75   **Industrial microbiology**

80   **Water and sewage microbiology**

82   **Air microbiology**

85   **Microbiology of food, milk, and other beverages**

115   **Actinomycetes and related organisms**

118   **Coryneform group**

120   **Propionibacteriaceae**

125   **Actinomycetales**

125.5   **Specific organisms, A–Z**

           .A2   **Actinomycetaceae**
           .M9   **Mycobacteriaceae**
           .S8   **Streptomycetaceae**

127   **Bacillaceae**

Bacillaceae – Continued

127.5   Specific groups, A–Z

         .B2   Bacillus
         .C5   Clostridium

128   Gliding bacteria

131   Gram–negative bacteria (General). Gram–negative aerobic bacteria (include cocci and rods)

133   Gram–negative anaerobic bacteria (include cocci and rods)

135   Gram–negative chemolithotrophic bacteria

137   Gram–negative facultatively anaerobic rods (General or not elsewhere classified)

138   Enterobacteriaceae

138.5   Specific organisms, A–Z

         .E5   Enterobacter
         .E8   Escherichia
         .K5   Klebsiella
         .P7   Proteus
         .S2   Salmonella
         .S3   Serratia
         .S4   Shigella
         .Y3   Yersinia

139   Haemophilus

140   Pasteurella

141   Vibrionaceae

142   Gram–positive bacteria (General or not elsewhere classified)

142.5   Specific organisms, A–Z

         .A8   Asporogenous rods
         .C6   Cocci

143   **Mollicutes**

145   **Phototrophic bacteria**

149   **Rickettsias and chlamydias**

150   **Rickettsiales**

152   **Chlamydiales**

153   **Sheathed bacteria. Budding or appendaged bacteria**

154   **Spiral and curved bacteria**

155   **Spirochaetales**

160   **Viruses (General). Virology**
        Classify works about a virus disease with the disease.

161   **Bacteriophages**

161.5   **Specific phages, A–Z**

        .C6   **Coliphages**
        .M9   **Mycobacteriophages**
        .S8   **Staphylococcus phages**

162   **Insect viruses**
        Classify works on diseases of insects in SB 942.

163   **Plant viruses**
        Classify works on virus diseases of plants in SB 736.

164   **Vertebrate viruses**

165   **DNA viruses**

165.5   **Specific DNA groups, A–Z**

        .A3   **Adenoviridae**
        .H3   **Herpesviridae**

Vertebrate viruses
  DNA viruses
    Specific DNA groups, A-Z – Continued

.I6	Iridoviridae
.P2	Papovaviridae
.P3	Parvoviridae
.P6	Poxviridae

166   **Oncogenic viruses**

168   **RNA viruses**

168.5   **Specific RNA groups, A–Z**

.A7	Arboviruses
.A8	Arenaviridae
.B9	Bunyaviridae
.C8	Coronaviridae
.H6	HIV
.O7	Orthomyxoviridae
.P2	Paramyxoviridae
.P4	Picornaviridae
.R15	Reoviridae
.R18	Retroviridae
.R2	Rhabdoviridae
.R8	Rubivirus. Rubella virus

169   **Vertebrate viruses, unclassified**

170   **Hepatitis viruses**

180   **Pathogenic fungi. Mycology**
Classify general non–medical works on mycology and non–pathogenic fungi in QK 600–635.

180.5   **Specific fungi, A–Z**

.A8	Ascomycetes
.B2	Basidiomycota
.D3	Dermatophytes
.D38	Deuteromycetes
.M9	Myxomycetes
.P4	Phycomycetes
.Y3	Yeasts

Classify specific yeasts under the appropriate number for the class.

190   **Bacterial and fungal spores**
Classify works on bacterial spores alone in QW 51; on fungal spores alone in QW 180.

300   Biological warfare

IMMUNOLOGY

Classify works on immunologic diseases in WD 300–330.

* 501   **Societies (Cutter from name of society)**
Includes ephemeral membership lists issued serially or separately. Classify substantial lists with directories. Classify annual reports, journals, etc., in W1.

504   **General works**

504.5   **Immunochemistry. Immunohistochemistry**

Collections (General)
505   By several authors
507   By individual authors

509   **Addresses. Essays. Lectures (General)**

511   **History (Table G)**
511.1   General coverage (Not Table G)

* 513   **Dictionaries. Encyclopedias**

* 515   **Classification. Nomenclature. Terminology**

* 516   **Tables. Statistics**

517   **Atlases. Pictorial works**

518   **Education**
Classify here works about education.

* 518.2   **Educational materials**
Classify here educational materials, e.g., outlines, questions and answers, programmed instruction, catalogs, computer–assisted instruction, etc., regardless of format. Classify textbooks, regardless of format, by subject.

520   **Research (General)**
Classify here works about research in general. Classify works about research on a particular subject by subject.

*NUMBER CAN BE USED FOR BOTH MONOGRAPHS AND SERIALS.

[521]	[This number not used] *Classify works on immunology as a profession in QW 21.*

* 522	Directories (Table G)
* 522.1	General coverage (Not Table G)

           Laboratories, institutes, etc.

523	Collective
524	Individual (Cutter from name of agency)

525	Laboratory manuals. Technique *Classify works on immunodiagnostic tests in QY 250–275.*

525.5	Specific techniques, A–Z

.E6	Enzyme–linked immunosorbent assay
.F6	Fluorescent antibody technique
.I3	Immunoassay
.I32	Immunoblotting
.I34	Immunoenzyme techniques
.I36	Immunophenotyping
.L6	Leukocyte adherence inhibition test
.R15	Radioallergosorbent test
.R2	Radioimmunoassay

* 526	Equipment and supplies *Classify catalogs here.*

* 539	Handbooks. Resource guides

540	Immunity (General or not elsewhere classified)

541	Natural immunity. Immunogenetics

545	Autoimmunity

551	Acquired immunity. Artificial immunity *Classify preparations producing artificial immunity in QW 800–815.*

552	Active immunity

553	Passive immunity

563	Local immunity

*NUMBER CAN BE USED FOR BOTH MONOGRAPHS AND SERIALS.

568   **Cellular immunity. Immunologic cytotoxicity. Immunocompetence. Immunologic factors (General or not elsewhere classified)**

570   **Antigens. Antibodies. Serology**

573   **Antigens**

573.5   **Specific antigens, A–Z**

          .H6   **Ilistocompatibility antigens**
          .H7   **HLA antigens**

575   **Antibodies**

575.5   **Specific antibodies, A–Z**

          .A6   **Antibodies, Monoclonal**

601   **Immunoglobulins**

630   **Toxins. Antitoxins**
          Classify works on toxoids, antitoxins, etc., as preparations producing immunity in QW 800–815.

630.5   **Specific toxins and antitoxins, A–Z**

          .B2   **Bacterial toxins**
          .C9   **Cytotoxins**
          .E5   **Endotoxins**
          .E6   **Enterotoxins**
          .I3   **Immunotoxins**
          .M3   **Marine toxins**
          .M9   **Mycotoxins**
          .N4   **Neurotoxins**
          .R5   **Ricin**

640   **Agglutination. Precipitation**
          Classify works on immunodiagnostic tests in QY 265.

660   **Lysis and bacterial action**

680   **Complement. Complement fixation**
          Classify works on immunodiagnostic tests in QY 265.

690   **Phagocytosis**

700   **Infection.   Mechanisms of infection and resistance**

730   **Virulence.   Invasiveness**

800   **Biological products producing immunity**
          Classify works on vaccines and vaccination for a specific disease, with the disease, e.g., Smallpox vaccination, WC 588.

805   **Vaccines.   Antitoxins.   Toxoids**
          Classify works on toxins or antitoxins formed in the body in QW 630–630.5.

806   **Vaccination**

815   **Immune serums**

900   **Anaphylaxis and hypersensitivity.   Allergens**
          Classify works on diseases of hypersensitivity in general in WD 300–375.   Classify specific allergic reactions with the system affected.

920   **Immunosuppression.   Immunosuppressive agents**
          Classify transplantation immunology in WO 680.

940   **Immunotherapy**
          Classify works on therapy of a particular disease with the disease.

945   **Serotherapy**

949   **Active immunotherapy**

QX

PARASITOLOGY

* 1   **Societies (Cutter from name of society)**
Includes ephemeral membership lists issued serially or separately. Classify substantial lists with directories. Classify annual reports, journals, etc., in W1.

4   **General works**

        Collections (General)
5   **By several authors**
7   **By individual authors**

9   **Addresses. Essays. Lectures (General)**

11   **History (Table G)**
11.1   **General coverage (Not Table G)**

* 13   **Dictionaries. Encyclopedias**

* 15   **Classification. Nomenclature. Terminology**

* 16   **Tables. Statistics**

17   **Atlases. Pictorial works**

18   **Education**
Classify here works about education.

* 18.2   **Educational materials**
Classify here educational materials, e.g., outlines, questions and answers, programmed instruction, catalogs, computer–assisted instruction, etc., regardless of format. Classify textbooks, regardless of format, by subject.

* 19   **Schools, departments, and faculties of parasitology**

20   **Research (General)**
Classify here works about research in general. Classify works about research on a particular subject by subject.

21	Parasitology as a profession

* 22	Directories (Table G)
* 22.1	General coverage (Not Table G)

Laboratories, institutes, etc.

23	Collective
24	Individual (Cutter from name of agency)

25	Laboratory manuals. Technique

* 26	Equipment and supplies

Classify catalogs here.

26.5	Medical informatics. Automatic data processing. Computers (General)

Classify works on use for special subjects by subject.

Museums, exhibits, etc.

27	Collective
28	Individual (Cutter from name of museum, etc.)

* 32	Laws (Table G)
* 32.1	General coverage (Not Table G)

* 33	Discussion of law (Table G)
* 33.1	General coverage (Not Table G)

* 39	Handbooks. Resource guides

45	Host–parasite relations

50	Protozoa

55	Sarcodina (Amoebae)

70	Mastigophora

e.g., Giardia. Trichomonas. Trypanosoma. Leishmania

123	Sporozoa

135	Plasmodia

Protozoa
    Sporozoa – Continued

140	Toxoplasma
151	Ciliata
195	Cnidaria
200	Helminths
203	Nematoda
207	Trichuroidea
243	Strongyloidea
248	Trichostrongyloidea
271	Oxyuroidea
277	Ascaroidea
301	Filarioidea
350	Platyhelminths
352	Turbellaria
353	Trematoda
355	Schistosoma
365	Fasciola
400	Cestoda
442	Echinococcus
451	Annelida
460	Arthropods

Arthropods – Continued

463   **Crustacea**

467   **Arachnida**

469   **Scorpions**

471   **Spiders**

473   **Acari**

475   **Sarcoptidae (Mites)**
            e.g., Sarcoptes scabiei

479   **Ticks**

483   **Trombiculid mites**

500   **Insects**
      Classify works on diseases of insects in SB 942.

501   **Phthiroptera**

502   **Lice**

503   **Hemiptera**
        e.g., Bedbugs

505   **Diptera**

510   **Mosquitoes**

515   **Anopheles**

525   **Aedes**

530   **Culex**

550   **Siphonaptera (Fleas)**

555   **Coleoptera (Beetles)**

Insects – Continued

560   **Lepidoptera (Moths.   Butterflies)**

565   **Hymenoptera (Bees.   Wasps.   Ants)**

570   **Orthoptera**
          e.g., Grasshoppers

600   **Insect control.   Tick control**
          Classify works on pest control in general and other public health aspects in WA 240.

650   **Insect vectors**

675   **Mollusca**

QY

CLINICAL PATHOLOGY

Classify here works on general clinical pathology and diagnostics. Classify works on tests for a particular disease or for diseases of a particular system with the disease or system, except for works on syphilis tests, which are classed here.

QY 1–350   **General**
QY 400–490   **Blood**

GENERAL

* 1   **Societies (Cutter from name of society)**
      Includes ephemeral membership lists issued serially or separately. Classify annual reports, journals, etc., in W1.

4   **General works**

      Collections (General)
5   **By several authors**
7   **By individual authors**

9   **Addresses. Essays. Lectures (General)**

11   **History (Table G)**
11.1   **General coverage (Not Table G)**

* 13   **Dictionaries. Encyclopedias**

* 15   **Classification. Nomenclature. Terminology**

* 16   **Tables. Statistics**

17   **Atlases. Pictorial works**

18   **Education**
      Classify here works about education.

*NUMBER CAN BE USED FOR BOTH MONOGRAPHS AND SERIALS.

48

*	18.2	**Educational materials** *Classify here educational materials, e.g., outlines, questions and answers, programmed instruction, catalogs, computer-assisted instruction, etc., regardless of format. Classify textbooks, regardless of format, by subject.*
*	19	**Schools and colleges** *Classify courses of study, catalogs, etc., in W 19.5.*
	20	**Research (General)** *Classify here works about research in general. Classify works about research on a particular subject by subject.*
	21	**Medical laboratory technology as a profession. Ethics. Peer review**
*	22	**Directories of medical laboratory technology (Table G)** *Classify directories of all pathologists in QZ 22.*
*	22.1	**Directories of medical laboratory technology (Not Table G)**

Laboratories, institutes, etc.
Classify hospital laboratories in WX 207.

	23	**Collective**
	24	**Individual (Cutter from name of agency)**
	25	**Laboratory manuals. Technique** *Classify works on specific tests by type.*
*	26	**Equipment and supplies** *Classify catalogs here.*
	26.5	**Medical informatics. Automatic data processing. Computers (General)** *Classify works on use for special subjects by subject.*

Museums, exhibits, etc.

	27	**Collective**
	28	**Individual (Cutter from name of museum, etc.)**
*	32	**Laws (Table G)**
*	32.1	**General coverage (Not Table G)**
*	33	**Discussion of law (Table G)**
*	33.1	**General coverage (Not Table G)**
	35	**Molding and casting of anatomic models. Moulages**
*	39	**Handbooks. Resource guides**

50   **Laboratory animals (General or not elsewhere classified)**
Classify works on diseases of laboratory animals in SF 996.5; on vivisection as experimental surgery in WO 50; and on antivivisection in HV 4905–4959.

52   **Acquisition and transportation**
Classify catalogs in QY 26; directories of users and sources for obtaining, in QY 22.

54   **Care and breeding**

56   **Environment**
e.g., Germ-free life

58   **Experimental techniques**
Cf. QY 25 Laboratory manuals.

60   **Special classes of animals, A–Z**

         .A6   **Amphibia**
         .B4   **Birds**
         .C2   **Cats**
         .D6   **Dogs**
         .F4   **Fishes**
         .L3   **Lagomorpha (Rabbits, etc.)**
         .M2   **Mammals (General or not elsewhere classified)**
         .P7   **Primates**
         .R6   **Rodents**
         .S8   **Swine**

90   **Chemical techniques**

95   **Cytological techniques**
Cf. QH 585 Methods in cytology.

100   **Bacteriological techniques**

110   **Methods in medical mycology**

120   **Sputum**

125   **Saliva**

130   **Gastric and duodenal contents**

140	Liver tests
143	Bile pigments
147	Function tests
160	Feces
175	Kidney function tests
185	Urinalysis
190	Semen
210	Puncture fluids (Peritoneal. Pleural. Pericardial)
220	Cerebrospinal fluid
250	Immunodiagnostic tests

250   *Cf. QW 525 for techniques of administering other immunologic tests.*

260	Diagnostic skin tests
265	Agglutination, precipitation, flocculation, and complement fixation tests
275	Serodiagnostic tests for syphilis
330	Assay of hormones
335	Pregnancy tests
350	Assay of vitamins

BLOOD

400   **General works**
     Classify works on morphology, physiology, and clinical aspects of diseases of blood in WH. Cf. WG for works on the cardiovascular system.

402   **Cellular elements**

408   **Physical examination**
         e.g., Sedimentation. Volume index, etc.

410   **Coagulation**
         e.g., Bleeding time, clotting time, etc.

415   **Typing**

450   **Blood chemistry**

455   **Nitrogenous constituents**

465   **Lipids**

470   **Carbohydrates**

480   **Inorganic substances**

490   **Enzymes**

QZ

PATHOLOGY

* 1   **Societies (Cutter from name of society)**
        Includes ephemeral membership lists issued serially or separately. Classify substantial lists with directories. Classify annual reports, journals, etc., in W1.

  4   **General works**
        Classify material on comparative pathology in QZ 33.

        Collections (General)
  5   **By several authors**
  7   **By individual authors**

  9   **Addresses. Essays. Lectures (General)**

  11   **History (Table G)**
  11.1   **General coverage (Not Table G)**

  11.5   **Paleopathology**

* 13   **Dictionaries. Encyclopedias**

* 15   **Classification. Nomenclature. Terminology**

* 16   **Tables. Statistics**

  17   **Atlases. Pictorial works**
        Classify here atlases on tissue pathology in disease.

  18   **Education**
        Classify here works about education.

* 18.2 **Educational materials**
        Classify here educational materials, e.g., outlines, questions and answers, programmed instruction, catalogs, computer-assisted instruction, etc., regardless of format. Classify textbooks, regardless of format, by subject.

* 19   **Schools, departments, and faculties of pathology**

20.5   **Research (General)**
            Classify material on cancer research in QZ 206.

21   **Pathology as a profession. Ethics. Peer review**

* 22   **Directories (Table G)**
* 22.1   **General coverage (Not Table G)**

            Laboratories, institutes, etc. Cancer hospitals
23   **Collective**
24   **Individual (Cutter from name of agency)**

25   **Laboratory manuals. Technique**

* 26   **Equipment and supplies**
            Classify catalogs here.

26.5   **Medical informatics. Automatic data processing. Computers (General)**
            Classify works on use for special subjects by subject.

            Museums, exhibits, etc.
27   **Collective**
28   **Individual (Cutter from name of agency)**

* 32   **Laws (Table G)**
* 32.1   **General coverage (Not Table G)**

* 32.3   **Discussion of law (Table G)**
* 32.4   **General coverage (Not Table G)**

33   **Comparative pathology**

35   **Postmortem examination**
            Classify works on examination of dead bodies for medicolegal purposes in W 800–867.

* 39   **Handbooks. Resource guides**

40   **Pathogenesis of disease**
            Classify here works on causative factors and development. Classify works on diagnosis, therapy, etc., of the resultant disease with the disease or system.

42   **Iatrogenic disease (General). Adverse effects of drugs. Medication errors**
            Classify works with emphasis on drug action in QV 38.

Pathogenesis of disease – Continued

45	**Developmental defects**
50	**Heredity. Body constitution. Medical genetics** *Classify works on pharmacogenetics in QV 38.*
53	**Age factors. Sex factors** *Classify works on age factors or sex factors relating to a particular disease, with the disease.*
55	**Trauma (Physical)**
57	**Physical agents** e.g., Light. Vibration *Cf. QT 162 for physiological effects.*
59	**Chemical agents**
65	**Bacteria. Fungi. Viruses. Rickettsia (General)** *Classify works on specific organisms in QW regardless of the subject.*
85	**Animal parasites**
105	**Nutrition disorders** *Cf. WD 100–175 for clinical aspects.*
109	**Vitamin deficiencies**
140	**General manifestations of disease**
150	**Local reactions to injury and disease**
160	**General reactions to injury and disease. Stress**
170	**Circulatory disorders**
180	**Degenerative processes. Disorders of metabolism** *Cf. WD 200–226 for clinical aspects.*
190	**Local disorders of growth** e.g., Hyperplasia
200	**Neoplasms. Cysts (General)** *Classify works on neoplasms by site or tissue if applicable.*

Neoplasms. Cysts – Continued

201   **Popular works**
Classify here popular works on all aspects of neoplasms.

202   **Etiology. Metastasis. Regression. Invasiveness**

204   **Precancerous conditions**

206   **Research (General)**
Classify works on specific topics by subject, e.g., on experimental work on the etiology of neoplasms in QZ 202.

241   **Diagnosis**

266   **Therapy**

267   **Drug therapy**

268   **Surgical techniques**

269   **Radiotherapy**

275   **Pediatric oncology. Adolescent oncology (General)**
Classify here all aspects of pediatric and adolescent neoplasms in general; classify works on particular neoplasms with the neoplasm. Classify works on neoplasms by site or tissue if applicable.

Specific types of neoplasms
Classify books on neoplasms by site when possible, especially when the emphasis is on dysfunction, symptomatology, and treatment. Emphasis in this section is on the pathology of tissues rather than on organ. Classify works on dental or oral tissue in WU 280.

310   **Embryonal and mixed tumors**

340   **Connective, muscle, and vascular tissues**

345   **Sarcoma**

350   **Leukemia. Lymphoma. Hematologic neoplasms**
Cf. WH 250 and WH 525 for clinical aspects.

365   **Glandular epithelial tissues. Carcinoma (General or not elsewhere classified)**

Neoplasms. Cysts
    Specific types of neoplasms – Continued

380   **Nerve tissue**

W

HEALTH PROFESSIONS

Classify here general and miscellaneous material relating to the health professions.

W 1–96   General
W 100–275   Medical, Dental, and Pharmaceutical Service Plans
W 322–323   Other Medical Services
W 601–925   Forensic Medicine and Dentistry

GENERAL

* 1   Serials. Periodicals

* 2   Serial documents (Table G)
Classify here government administrative reports and statistics, including administrative reports and statistics on several hospitals under governmental administration. Cf. WX 2 Hospital administrative reports and statistics.

* 3   Congresses
Classify here monographic and serial publications of recurring congresses on medicine and related subjects. Note that as of July 1, 1988, NLM no longer assigns W3 to newly acquired publications, with the exception of analytics to ongoing serial publications already classified in W3.

* 3.5   Directories of congresses
Classify bibliographies of congress publications in ZW3. Note that as of July 1, 1988, NLM no longer assigns W 3.5 or ZW 3 to newly acquired publications.

* 4   Dissertations, by university

* 4A   American dissertations, by author
Classify dissertations which qualify as Americana in WZ 270.

Collections (General)
5   By several authors
6   Pamphlet volumes. Miscellaneous reprint volumes
7   By individual authors

9   Addresses. Essays. Lectures (General)
Classify works on specific topics by subject.

*NUMBER CAN BE USED FOR BOTH MONOGRAPHS AND SERIALS.

10 Voyages. Expeditions. Travels

* 13 Dictionaries. Encyclopedias
Classify material on medical shorthand here if it is the primary subject of book.

* 15 Nomenclature. Terminology
Classify works on classification of disease and on disease eponyms in WB 15.

* 16 Tables. Statistics

18 Education
Classify here works about education.

* 18.2 Educational materials
Classify here educational materials, e.g., outlines, questions and answers, programmed instruction, catalogs, computer-assisted instruction, etc., regardless of format. Classify textbooks, regardless of format, by subject.

* 19 Schools and colleges

* 19.5 Courses of study, catalogs, announcements, etc., of all schools (including schools of dentistry, nursing, etc.) (Table G)

20 Graduate and continuing medical education (including fellowships, internships, residencies, etc.)

20.5 Medical research (General)
Classify here material on the various aspects and accomplishments of medical research. Classify works on research limited to a particular subject with the subject.

20.55 Special topics, A–Z

.A5 Animal testing alternatives
.H9 Human experimentation

20.9 Fraternities in medicine and allied fields (Cutter from name of fraternity)

21 Medicine as a profession. Peer review
Classify here works about medical careers. Classify those about other specific careers with the specialty, e.g., those about nursing in WY 16. Classify works on the specialities in general in W 87.

21.5   **Allied health personnel. Allied health professions**
            *Classify here works about supply and distribution as well as those about careers.
            Classify works on specific personnel in more specific number when available, e.g.,
            those on nurses aides in WY 193. Classify works on health manpower
            including physicians in W 76.*

* 22   **Directories (Table G)**
* 22.1   **General coverage (Not Table G)**

            Laboratories, institutes, etc.
23   **Collective**
24   **Individual (Cutter from name of agency)**

* 26   **Equipment and supplies**
            *Classify here medical and surgical supply and instrument catalogs as well as catalogs
            of special equipment, e.g., tables and chairs in doctors' waiting rooms. Include
            works on history of instruments in general.*

26.5   **Medical informatics. Health informatics**
            Classify works on use for special subjects by subject.

26.55   **Special topics, A–Z**

            .A7   **Artificial intelligence. Expert systems**
            .A9   **Automatic data processing**
            .C7   **Computers**
            .D2   **Decision making, Computer–assisted**
                     *Classify works on computer–assisted diagnosis (general) in WB 141; on
                     computer–assisted therapy (general) in WB 300.*
            .I4   **Information systems. Information storage and retrieval**
            .S6   **Software**

            Museums, exhibits, etc.
27   **Collective**
28   **Individual (Cutter from name of agency or exhibit)**

* 32   **Laws (General) (Table G)**
* 32.1   **General coverage (Not Table G)**

* 32.5   **Discussion of law. Medical jurisprudence (General) (Table G)**
            *Include here works on legal advice, court decisions and opinions, legal rights and
            obligations. Cf. W 700, etc., Forensic medicine.*
* 32.6   **General coverage (Not Table G)**

* 33   **Laws governing medical practice (Table G)**
* 33.1   **General coverage (Not Table G)**

40   **Licensure (Table G)**

*NUMBER CAN BE USED FOR BOTH MONOGRAPHS AND SERIALS.

         Laws
             Licensure – Continued

40.1   General coverage (Not Table G)

44   Malpractice (Table G)
44.1   General coverage (Not Table G)

* 49   Handbooks.   Resource guides

50   Medical ethics

58   Advertising.   Fee–splitting

61   Medical philosophy and logic

62   Social relations of the physician (including relations with patients; relations with public, clubs, societies, etc.)   Attitude

64   Referral and consultation (General)
           Classify here works on referral, etc., initiated by the physician. Classify works on particular medical problems by subject; works on problems referred by specialists with the specialty.

74   Medical economics.   Health care costs (General)
           Cf. W 58 for economic aspects of medical ethics.

76   Health manpower and services, distribution and characteristics
           Classify works limited to allied health manpower in W 21.5.

79   Income of physicians

80   Practice management (including business administration)
           Classify here medical secretaries' handbooks.

82   Medical technology (General)

83   Telemedicine (General) (Table G)
           Classify works on telemedicine relating only to private practice in WB 50.
83.1   General coverage (Not Table G)

84   Health services.   Quality of health care (General) (Table G)
           Classify works on public health administration in appropriate WA number. Classify works on quality of health care relating only to private practice in WB 50.
84.1   General coverage (Not Table G)
84.3   Research (General)

Health services. Quality of health care – Continued

84.5 **Comprehensive health care. Community medicine**
Cf. WA 546 Community health service.

84.6 **Primary health care**

84.7 **Patient care planning. Progressive health care (General)**
Classify works on care of hospital patients in WX 162.

84.8 **Patient care team**
Classify works on hospital teams in WX 162.5.

85 **Patients. Attitude and compliance. Satisfaction**
Classify works on attitude toward particular subject with the subject.

85.5 **Right to die. Advance directives. Living wills**
Cf. WB 310 Hospice care. Terminal care.

87 **Professional practice**
Cf. W 21 Medicine as a profession. Include here general works about types of practice in medicine and allied fields. Classify works on specific medical specialties or allied fields by subject, e.g., on surgery in WO 21; on nursing in WY 101-145, etc.

88 **Administrative work. Teaching. Research**
Classify here works about planning for administrative, teaching, or research careers. Classify works on practice management in W 80, etc.; on education and how to teach in W 18, etc.; on research itself in W 20.5, etc.

89 **Family practice (As a specialty) Private practice**
Classify texts and treatises for general practitioner or family doctor in WB 110.

90 **Specialism (General)**
Classify works on a particular specialty with the specialty.

92 **Group practice. Partnership practice**

94 **Government services**

96 **Institutional practice**

MEDICAL, DENTAL, AND PHARMACEUTICAL SERVICE PLANS

Classify works on Medicare and medical care plans for the aged in WT 31.

100   **General works**
            Cf. W 275   General service plans by country.

125   **Voluntary pre–payment plans (General or not elsewhere classified)
                (Table G)**
125.1   **General coverage (Not Table G)**

130   **Managed care plans (General or not elsewhere classified) (Table G)**
130.1   **General coverage (Not Table G)**

132   **Health maintenance organizations (Table G)**
132.1   **General coverage (Not Table G)**

160   **Hospitalization insurance. Major medical insurance. Long–term care
                insurance. Medigap insurance (Table G)**
160.1   **General coverage (Not Table G)**

185   **Compulsory pre–payment plans (not a function of the state) (General or not
                elsewhere classified) (Table G)**
185.1   **General coverage (Not Table G)**

225   **Medicine as function of the state (Table G)**
            *Classify here material on health protection for everyone as a function of the state,
                supported by taxation, with medical services subject to regulation by the state.*
225.1   **General coverage (Not Table G)**

250   **Medical care for low–income and indigent groups. Medicaid (Table G)**
250.1   **General coverage (Not Table G)**

255   **Nursing insurance**

260   **Dental insurance. State dentistry (Table G)**
260.1   **General coverage (Not Table G)**

265   **Pharmaceutical insurance (Table G)**
265.1   **General coverage (Not Table G)**

270   **Psychiatric insurance (Table G)**
270.1   **General coverage (Not Table G)**

275   **Medical, dental, pharmaceutical and/or psychiatric service plans, by country (Table G)**
Classify here works covering both compulsory and voluntary plans.   Cf. W 100 General works.

OTHER MEDICAL SERVICES

322   **Medical social work**
Include works on social service in hospitals here.   Cf. WM 30.5 Psychiatric social work.

323   **Medical missions**
Classify biographical or autobiographical works of medical missionary doctors and nurses in WZ 100.

FORENSIC MEDICINE AND DENTISTRY

* 601   **Societies (Cutter from name of society)**
Includes ephemeral membership lists issued serially or separately.   Classify substantial lists with directories.   Classify annual reports, journals, etc., in W1.

          Collections (General)
605   **By several authors**
607   **By individual authors**

609   **Addresses. Essays. Lectures (General)**

611   **History (Table G)**
611.1   **General coverage (Not Table G)**

* 613   **Dictionaries. Encyclopedias**

* 615   **Classification. Nomenclature. Terminology**

* 616   **Tables. Statistics**

617   **Atlases. Pictorial works**
Classify here atlases and pictorial works on any phase of forensic medicine, etc.

618   **Education**
Classify here works about education.

*NUMBER CAN BE USED FOR BOTH MONOGRAPHS AND SERIALS.

* **618.2** **Educational materials**
Classify here educational materials, e.g., outlines, questions and answers, programmed instruction, catalogs, computer–assisted instruction, etc., regardless of format. Classify textbooks, regardless of format, by subject.

* **622** **Directories (Table G)**
* **622.1** **General coverage (Not Table G)**

Laboratories, institutes, etc.
623 **Collective**
624 **Individual (Cutter from name of agency)**

625 **Laboratory manuals. Technique**

626 **Equipment and supplies**
Classify catalogs in W 26.

626.5 **Medical informatics. Automatic data processing. Computers (General)**
Classify works on use for special subjects by subject.

Museums, exhibits, etc., on medicolegal subjects
627 **Collective**
628 **Individual (Cutter from name of agency, exhibit, etc.)**

[632] **[This number not used]**
Classify works on medical jurisprudence only, in W 32.5–32.6. Cf. W 700.

* **639** **Handbooks. Resource guides**

700 **General works**
Classify here works on medical and pathological examination of criminal evidence, as well as works including material on medical jurisprudence. Classify works on medical jurisprudence only, in W 32.5–32.6.

705 **Medicolegal dentistry**

725 **Medical evidence in the establishment of responsibility**

740 **Forensic psychiatry**
Classify works on commitment in WM 32–33.

750 **Examination of evidential material. Forensic chemistry**

775 **Medicolegal examination**

*NUMBER CAN BE USED FOR BOTH MONOGRAPHS AND SERIALS.

Medicolegal examination – Continued

780   Examination of the living

783   Malingering

786   Identification

789   Legal establishment of the beginning of life

791   Consanguinity. Paternity. Pregnancy

795   Rape. Sexual offenses

800   Examination of dead bodies. Duties of coroners

820   Signs of death. Time of death. Sudden death

822   Destruction and attempted destruction of the human body

825   Determination of cause of death. Medicolegal autopsy

843   Trauma

860   Criminal violence. Homicide

864   Suicide

867   Criminal abortion. Infanticide
                   Cf. WQ 225 for spontaneous abortion; WQ 440 for medical aspects of
                   therapeutic or induced abortion; HQ 767 for social aspects of induced
                   abortion.

900   Medicolegal aspects of insurance
                Classify works on liability insurance in form number 44 with malpractice when
                available in NLM schedules or in HG 9990 if general material.

910   Medicolegal aspects of compensation to victims of criminal violence

925   Medicolegal aspects of occupational disease and injury
                Cf. WV 32 for estimation of disability in otolaryngology; WW 32 for estimation of
                disability in ophthalmology.

WA

PUBLIC HEALTH

GENERAL

* 1   Societies (Cutter from name of society)
        Include ephemeral membership lists issued serially or separately. Classify substantial lists with directories. Classify annual reports, journals, etc., in W1.

4   Works on general hygiene (including in one volume personal hygiene, public health, etc.)
        Classify general works on public health in WA 100.

        Collections (General)
5   By several authors
7   By individual authors

9   Addresses. Essays. Lectures (General)

11   History (Table G)
11.1   General coverage (Not Table G)

* 13   Dictionaries. Encyclopedias

* 15   Classification. Nomenclature. Terminology

* 16   Tables. Statistics

17   Atlases. Pictorial works

18   **Education**
Classify here works about education.

* 18.2   **Educational materials**
Classify here educational materials, e.g., outlines, questions and answers, programmed instruction, catalogs, computer–assisted instruction, etc., regardless of format. Classify textbooks, regardless of format, by subject.

* 19   **Schools, colleges, and specialized departments and facilities**
Classify courses of study, college catalogs, etc., in W 19.5.

20.5   **Research (General)**
Classify here works about research in general. Classify research limited to a particular subject with the subject.

21   **Public health as a profession. Ethics. Peer review**

* 22   **Directories (Table G)**
* 22.1   **General coverage (Not Table G)**

     Laboratories, institutes, etc.
23   **Collective**
24   **Individual (Cutter from name of agency)**

25   **Laboratory manuals. Technique**

26   **Equipment and supplies**
Classify catalogs in W 26. Classify works on safety equipment in general in WA 260; on industrial safety equipment in WA 485.

26.5   **Medical informatics. Automatic data processing. Computers (General)**
Classify works on use for special subjects by subject.

     Museums, exhibits, etc.
27   **Collective**
28   **Individual (Cutter from name of museum or exhibit)**

30   **Social, economic, and environmental factors in public health (General)**
Classify works on rural health and hygiene in WA 390; on urban health and hygiene in WA 380.

30.5   **Environmental medicine. Environmental illness**

31   **Social medicine. Medical sociology**

* 32   **Laws (Table G)**
            Classify pure food laws in WA 697.
* 32.1   **General coverage (Not Table G)**

* 33   **Discussion of law (Table G)**
* 33.1   **General coverage (Not Table G)**

* 39   **Handbooks. Resource guides**

54   **Registration and certification of the dead**

55   **Registration of notifiable diseases**

100   **General works**

105   **Epidemiology**
            Classify statistics in WA 900.

106   **Disease reservoirs**

PREVENTIVE MEDICINE

108   **Preventive health services. Preventive medicine (General)**

110   **Prevention and control of communicable diseases. Transmission of infectious diseases**
            Classify works on immunological aspects in QW 700; on parasitological aspects of insect control in QX 600; on control of sexually transmitted diseases in WC 142.

230   **Quarantine**
            Classify material on laws in WA 32–33.

234   **Port and maritime quarantine**

240   **Disinfection. Disinfestation. Pesticides (Including diseases caused by)**
            Classify works on immunological aspects in QX 650. Classify works on ectoparasitic infestations and disinfestations in WC 900.

243   **Diagnostic services**
            Classify works on mass chest X-ray in WF 225; on mobile health units in WX 190.

*NUMBER CAN BE USED FOR BOTH MONOGRAPHS AND SERIALS.

Diagnostic services – Continued

245   Mass screening.   Multiphasic screening

PREVENTION OF ACCIDENT AND OF INJURY

250   General works
Classify works on occupational accidents and their prevention in WA 485.

260   Protective devices (General)

275   Traffic accidents.   Public health aspects of automobile driving

288   Accidents in the home, office, etc.   Consumer protection and product safety (General)
Include works on household articles and products as causes of accidents

292   First aid in illness and injury, e.g., Bandaging.   Minor injuries
Classify works on resuscitation in anesthesiology in WO 250; on resuscitation of the newborn in WQ 450.   Classify military first aid manuals in UH 396.

HEALTH PROBLEMS OF SPECIAL POPULATION GROUPS

300   General works
Classify general works on diseases generally associated with particular ethnic groups in WB 720.   Include works on particular groups not elsewhere classified.

305   Mental health of special population groups
Classify works on particular diseases in WM.   Cf. WM 105 for general works on mental health.

308   Family health
Cf. W 89 Family practice as a specialty; WB 110 for works for the family doctor.

309   Women's health
Cf. WA 491   Protection of women in the workplace.

310   Maternal welfare.   Maternal and child welfare.   Maternal health services

320   Child welfare.   Child abuse.   Child health services

330	**Adolescent health services**
350	**School health and hygiene services. School dental health services** *Classify works on diseases of school children in WS. Cf. WU 113 for dental hygiene.*
351	**Universities and colleges**
352	**School mental health services** *Classify works on diseases in WM.*
353	**Universities and colleges**
380	**Urban health and hygiene** *Cf. WA 546 Local health administration.*
390	**Rural health and hygiene** *Classify agricultural workers' diseases in WA 400.*
395	**Health in developing countries**

OCCUPATIONAL MEDICINE, HEALTH AND HYGIENE

400	**General works (including occupational diseases)** *Classify works on particular diseases by system, etc. Cf. WF 405 Tuberculosis in the workplace; WR 600 Occupational dermatitis; WW 505 Occupational ophthalmology.*
412	**Medical and dental services**
440	**Prevention and control of occupational diseases**
450	**Control of atmospheric conditions**
465	**Industrial poisons and poisoning (General)** *Classify works on toxicology of chemicals with no industrial health emphasis and on specific chemicals in QV 600–662; or if insecticides in WA 240.*
470	**Illumination. Noise. Radiation. Vibration**
475	**Occupational fatigue and its prevention**

485   Occupational accidents. Safety equipment

487   Accidents in professional work
             Use only for works on professions not ordinarily considered industrial

487.5   By profession, A–Z

             .A78   Art
             .D4   Dancing
             .F4   Firefighting

491   Protection of women in the workplace
             Cf. WA 309 Women's health.

495   Occupational mental health services

HEALTH ADMINISTRATION AND ORGANIZATION

525   General works

530   International health administration (Table G)
530.1   General coverage (Not Table G)

540   National and state health administration (Table G)
540.1   General coverage (Not Table G)

541   Regional health planning (Table G)
541.1   General coverage (Not Table G)

546   Local health administration. Community health services (Table G)
546.1   General coverage (Not Table G)

590   Health education
             *Classify here works on informal health education (community, radio, etc.). Classify
             works on study and teaching of public health in WA 18; classify teachers' manuals
             on physiology and hygiene in QT 200.*

SANITATION AND ENVIRONMENTAL CONTROL

670   General works

671   **Sanitary engineering. Environmental control (General)**
Classify works on entraterrestrial environment in WD 758; on sealed cabin ecology in WD 756.

672   **Inspection. Surveys (Table G)**
Classify works on inspection in particular areas by subject.

672.1   **General coverage (Not Table G)**

675   **Water. Water supply. Sources**
Include works on sanitary aspects of ice and ice making here.

686   **Analysis**
Cf. QW 80 Water microbiology.

687   **Saline water conversion**

689   **Pollution**
Classify works on radioactive pollution in WN 615; general works on industrial seawater pollution in WA 788; on pollution of bathing beaches in WA 820.

690   **Purification**

695   **Food. Food supply. Food inspection**

697   **Pure food laws**
Classify here food and drug laws discussed together. Classify works on drug laws alone in QV 32–33.

701   **Adulteration and contamination**
Classify works on radioactive contamination in WN 612.

703   **Fresh foods (Vegetables. Fruits. Eggs. Fish)**

707   **Meat and poultry inspection**

710   **Preserved foods (canned, dried, frozen, salted, smoked, etc.)**

712   **Food additives**

715   **Milk. Milk supply. Dairy products**

716   **Analysis**

Food. Food supply. Food inspection
Milk. Milk supply. Dairy products – Continued

719   Pasteurization

722   Fats. Oils. Margarine

730   Drugs. Drug adulteration and contamination. Pharmacies
           Classify here works on refrigeration of biological products. Classify works on fraud in QV 773; on drug legislation in QV 32–33.

744   Cosmetics. Barber shops. Beauty salons

750   Air sanitation and hygiene

754   Pollution and pollutants
           Cf. QW 82 Air microbiology; WA 450 Industrial pollution. Classify works on radioactive pollutions and pollutants in WN 615. Classify works on agents used extensively in biochemistry or pharmacology in QU or QV.

770   Ventilating. Heating

774   Air conditioning

776   Noise and noise abatement

778   Waste products. Waste disposal

780   Refuse and garbage disposal

785   Sewage disposal. Soil pollution
           Classify works on radioactive pollution and pollutants in WN 615.

788   Hazardous waste. Industrial waste (including radioactive waste)
           Cf. WN 650 for general works on radiation safety.

790   Medical waste. Dental waste

795   Housing

799   Public buildings. Restaurants

810   Public transportation

820   Bathing beaches. Public baths. Swimming pools

830   **Toilet facilities**

840   **Mortuary practice**

844   **Embalming**

846   **Burial. Cemeteries**

847   **Cremation**

STATISTICS AND SURVEYS

900   **Public health statistics (including narrative reports on health conditions and health surveys) (Table G)**
        Classify mortality statistics with causes of death here. Classify works on mortality statistics alone in HB. Classify works on nutrition surveys in QU 146–146.1.

900.1   **General coverage (Not Table G)**

950   **Theory or methods of medical statistics**
        Classify works on biometry in its broader sense in QH 323.5.

WB

PRACTICE OF MEDICINE

WB 1–130   **General**
WB 141–293   **General Diagnosis**
WB 300–962   **Therapeutics**

GENERAL

* 1   **Societies (Table G)**
Includes ephemeral membership lists issued serially or separately. Classify substantial lists with directories. Classify annual reports, journals, etc., in W1.

Collections (on clinical medicine, diagnosis, special therapeutic systems)
Classify collections on a specific subject with the subject. Cf. W5–7 on the medical profession.
5   **By several authors**
7   **By individual authors**

9   **Addresses. Essays. Lectures (General)**

[11]   **[This number not used]**
Use WZ for history of medical practice. Classify works on the history of special systems of therapeutics in the numbers for those specialities (WB 900–962). The latter are the only numbers used for history in the WB schedule.

13   **Encyclopedias**
Classify dictionaries in W 13.

* 15   **Classification. Nomenclature. Terminology**
Classify works that consist of general medical nomenclature or terminology in W 15.

* 16   **Tables. Statistics**

17   **Atlases. Pictorial works**
e.g., those on special devices or forms of therapy, such as Acupuncture.
Cf. QZ 17 for tissue pathology of disease.

18   **Education**
Classify here materials on education in the special systems of therapeutics or other topics specific to this schedule. Classify materials on general medical education in W 18.

* 18.2   **Educational materials**
Classify here educational materials, e.g., outlines, questions and answers, programmed instruction, catalogs, computer–assisted instruction, etc., regardless of format. Classify textbooks, regardless of format, by subject.

* 22   **Directories (of health resorts and/or special systems of therapeutics) (Table G)**
ᵗ 22.1   **General coverage (Not Table G)**

        Institutes. Laboratories of experimental research
23   **Collective**
24   **Individual (Cutter from name of agency)**

25   **Technique of research in internal medicine**
Classify works on technique of research limited to a particular subject with the subject.

26   **Equipment and supplies**
Classify medical and surgical supply and instrument catalogs in W 26. Classify works on self help devices in WB 320.

[26.5]   **[This number not used]**
Classify works on medical informatics, data processing or computers used in medicine in W 26.5 or by subject.

        Hospitals, dispensaries and clinics for specialized types of therapy e.g., Homeopathy. Diathermy. Hydrotherapy
Classify works on general hospitals in WX; others in specialty numbers.
27   **Collective (Table G)**
27.1   **General coverage (Not Table G)**
28   **Individual (Table G)**

29   **Rehabilitation centers. Residential facilities. Sheltered workshops**
Cf. WM 29–29.1 Mental health facilities.

* 32   **Laws relating to special systems of therapeutics (Table G)**
* 32.1   **General coverage (Not Table G)**

* 33   **Discussion of law (Table G)**
* 33.1   **General coverage (Not Table G)**

* 39   **Handbooks. Resource guides**

*NUMBER CAN BE USED FOR BOTH MONOGRAPHS AND SERIALS.

50   **Medical practice (Table G)**
Classify here works dealing only with private practice. Classify works on health services in general in W 84–84.3.

50.1   **General coverage (Not Table G)**

100   **General works**

101   **Ambulatory care (General)**
Cf. WX 205 Hospital outpatient clinics, ambulatory care facilities.

102   **Clinical medicine**

103   **Behavioral medicine**

104   **Medical psychology**

105   **Emergency medicine. Medical emergencies**
Classify works on emergency hospital service in WX 215; on first aid in WA 292.

110   **Family practice (including general practice)**
Classify works on general or family practice as a specialty in W 89.

115   **Internal medicine**

117   **Medical uses of non–ionizing radiation (General)**
Cf. WB 288 for diagnostic use; WB 480 for therapeutic use.

120   **Popular medicine (General)**
e.g., Household medical books. Self medication
Example: Mayo Clinic family health book computer file.

130   **General works for laymen**
Classify here books on general medicine written in style suitable for laymen. Example: The frontiers of medicine.

GENERAL DIAGNOSIS

141   **General works**
Cf. QY 4 General works on clinical pathology.

141.4   **Health status**

141.5   **Differential diagnosis**

THERAPEUTICS

300   General works

305   Instructions or non–drug prescriptions for devices or therapy (General)
       Classify specific devices or therapies by subject.

310   Hospice care. Palliative care. Terminal care
       Cf. W 85.5 Right to die; WY 152 Nursing care of terminal patients.

320   Rehabilitation of the disabled (General)
       *Classify here works on physical and medical rehabilitation in general as well as those
       that include in addition educational, social, and vocational rehabilitation. Classify
       works on specific types, by type, e.g., Physical therapy WB 460. Classify works
       with no medical slant in HD 7255–7256.*

325   Aftercare
       *Cf. WM 29–29.1 for mental patients; WO 183 Postoperative care; WY 100 Nursing
       care.*

327   Self care

330   Drug therapy
       Cf. QV Pharmacology.

340   Administration of medicine

342   Inhalation. Intranasal

344   Rectal

350   Oral

354   Injections. Infusions

356   Blood transfusion

365   Various other therapeutic and diagnostic procedures (General or not elsewhere
       classified)

369   Acupuncture. Moxibustion

Various other therapeutic and diagnostic procedures – Continued

371   Cupping.   Counterirritation
  e.g., Mustard plasters

373   Punctures (General or not elsewhere classified)

377   Spinal, cisternal and ventricular puncture

379   Biopsy

381   Bloodletting.   Phlebotomy

391   Tissue therapy.   Organotherapy

400   Dietetics.   Diet therapy
  Classify works on diets to be used with particular diseases with the disease, e.g., atherogenic diet in WG 550.   Classify works on nutrition and food values in QU 145–145.5.

405   Dietary cookbooks (General)

410   Special methods of feeding, e.g., parenteral; tube

420   Fasting

422   Macrobiotic diet

424   Low sodium diets.   Salt–free diets

425   Fat control
  Classify works on reducing diets in WD 210–212.

426   Meat diets.   Protein control

427   Carbohydrate control

428   Milk diets.   Calcium control

430   Vegetable diets.   Fruit diets

431   Cereals.   Grains.   Seeds.   Breads

Dietetics. Diet therapy – Continued

432	Raw food diets
433	Beverages
438	Coffee. Tea. Chocolate
442	Water. Mineral waters *Classify general works on hydrotherapy in WB 520.*
444	Wines. Liquors. Cordials. Beer
447	Miscellaneous food preparations e.g., Yeast
449	Diet fads (Critical and historical material)
460	Physical medicine. Physical therapy
469	Heat therapy. Induced hyperthermia
473	Cryotherapy. Therapeutic use of cold
480	Ultraviolet therapy. Sunlight. Light therapy
495	Electric stimulation therapy
510	Diathermy
515	Ultrasonic therapy
520	Hydrotherapy (General)
525	Balneology
535	Mechanotherapy. Massage, exercise, rest, etc., treated together
537	Massage
541	Exercise therapy. Medical gymnastics *Cf. QT 255 Physical education*

Physical medicine. Physical therapy
Mechanotherapy. Massage, exercise, rest, etc. treated together – Continued

545   **Rest. Relaxation**
          Classify works on hygienic aspects of rest and relaxation in QT 265.

550   **Therapeutic use of music**
          Classify works on therapeutic use of music in psychiatry in WM 450.5.M8.

555   **Occupational therapy**
          Classify works on occupational therapy in psychiatry in WM 450.5.O2.

700   **Medical climatology. Geography of disease**

710   **Diseases of geographic areas**

720   **Diseases of ethnic groups (General or not elsewhere classified)**
          Classify here works on diseases that are associated primarily with a particular ethnic group, when treated as such. Classify works on general health problems of ethnic groups in WA 300–305. Classify works on specific diseases with the disease.

750   **Climatotherapy**
          Cf. WF 330 Climatotherapy of pulmonary tuberculosis.

760   **Health resorts (Table G)**
          Includes history.
760.1   **General coverage (Not Table G)**

880   **Mental healing**

885   **Faith healing. Christian Science healing**

890   **Special systems of therapeutics. Alternative medicine (General or not elsewhere classified)**
          Classify works on cupping in WB 371; on diet fads in WB 449; on vegetarianism in WB 430; on mental healing in WB 880–885. Classify works on a specific disease with the disease.

900   **History of special systems or alternative medicine (General or not elsewhere classified)**

903   **Anthroposophy (used in medicine)**
          Cf. BP 595–597 General works.

905   **Chiropractic**

905.6   **History and philosophy**

Special systems of therapeutics. Alternative medicine
Chiropractic – Continued

905.7   Chiropractic as a profession. Ethics. Peer review
Classify works on education in WB 18.

905.8   Diagnosis

905.9   Therapeutics

920   Eclecticism

925   Herbal medicine

930   Homeopathy

935   Naturopathy

940   Osteopathy

960   Radiesthesia

962   Reflexotherapy

WC

COMMUNICABLE DISEASES

Classify here all major systemic infectious diseases with the exception of tuberculosis, which classes in WF 200–415. A few infectious diseases, usually local in character, are classed with the part affected (e.g., those classed in Dermatology, WR 220–245). Classify diseases for which no specific class number exists here on the basis of likeness, e.g. pseudoglanders with glanders in WC 330. Note that some related diseases are classed together regardless of the affecting organism, e.g., the pneumonias (WC 202–209) and the dysenteries (WC 280–285). Classify works on an infection which affects a single organ with the organ.

* 1   **Societies (Cutter from name of society)**
       Includes ephemeral membership lists issued serially or separately. Classify substantial lists with directories. Classify annual reports, journals, etc., in W1.

       Collections (General)
5   **By several authors**
7   **By individual authors**

9   **Addresses. Essays. Lectures (General)**

11   **History (General) (Table G)**
       Classify history of a single infectious disease with the disease.
11.1   **General coverage (Not Table G)**

* 13   **Dictionaries. Encyclopedias**

* 15   **Classification. Nomenclature. Terminology**

* 16   **Tables. Statistics**

17   **Atlases. Pictorial works**
       Classify here also atlases on single infectious diseases.

18   **Education**
       Classify here works about education.

* 18.2 **Educational materials**
       Classify here educational materials, e.g., outlines, questions and answers, programmed instruction, catalogs, computer–assisted instruction, etc., regardless of format. Classify textbooks, regardless of format, by subject.

*NUMBER CAN BE USED FOR BOTH MONOGRAPHS AND SERIALS.

* 19   **Schools, colleges, and specialized departments and facilities**

20   **Research (General)**
Classify here works about research in general. Classify works about research on a particular subject by subject.

* 22   **Directories (Table G)**
* 22.1   **General coverage (Not Table G)**

          Laboratories, institutes, etc.
23   **Collective**
24   **Individual (Cutter from name of agency)**

25   **Laboratory manuals. Technique**

26   **Equipment and supplies**
Classify catalogs in W 26.

26.5   **Medical informatics. Automatic data processing. Computers (General)**
Classify works on use for special subjects by subject.

          Isolation and quarantine hospitals, leprosaria, prophylaxis stations, clinics, dispensaries, etc.
27   **Collective (Table G)**
27.1   **General coverage (Not Table G)**
28   **Individual (Table G)**

[32]   **[This number not used]**
Classify laws relating to infectious diseases under appropriate topics in WA Public Health.

[33]   **[This number not used]**
Classify discussion of laws relating to infectious diseases under appropriate topics in WA Public Health.

* 39   **Handbooks. Resource guides**

100   **General works**

140   **Sexually transmitted diseases**
Classify works on AIDS and HIV infections in WC 503–503.7.

142   **Control measures**

144   **Prevention**

*NUMBER CAN BE USED FOR BOTH MONOGRAPHS AND SERIALS.

150   **Gonorrhea**
Classify works on gonorrhea in the female in WP 157.

155   **Chancroid**

160   **Syphilis**

161   **Congenital**

162   **Primary. Secondary**

164   **Tertiary**

165   **Neurosyphilis. Paresis**
Cf. WM 220 for general works on organic psychoses.

168   **Cardiovascular**

170   **Treatment**

180   **Granuloma inguinale**

185   **Lymphogranuloma venereum**

195   **Infection. Cross infection. Laboratory infection**
Cf. WX 167 for prevention and control of cross infection in hospitals; WU 29 for prevention and control of cross infection in dental health facilities or in the provision of dental care.

200   **Bacterial infections (General or not elsewhere classified)**
Classify works on localized bacterial infections by site.

202   **Pneumonia (General)**

204   **Pneumococcal pneumonia. Staphylococcal pneumonia**

207   **Viral pneumonia**

209   **Other**

210   **Streptococcal infections (General or not elsewhere classified)**
Classify works on endocarditis in WG 285; on impetigo in WR 225.

Bacterial infections
    Streptococcal infections – Continued

214   Scarlet fever

217   Pneumococcal infections
          Classify works on lobar pneumonia in WC 204.

220   Rheumatic fever.   Chorea in rheumatic fever
          Classify works on rheumatic heart disease in WG 240.

230   Focal infection
          Cf. WU 290 in dentistry.

234   Erysipelas

240   Bacteremia.   Septicemia.   Toxemias
          Classify works on pregnancy toxemias in WQ 215.

242   Listeria infections

245   Meningococcal infections

246   Mycoplasmatales infections

250   Staphylococcal infections
          Classify works on infectious skin diseases in WR; on hordeolum in WW 205; on staphylococcal pneumonia in WC 204; on food poisoning in WC 268.

255   Wound infection
          Cf. WO 185   Surgical wound infection.

260   Enterobacteriaceae and other enteric infections
          Classify works on Yersinia infections in WC 350.

262   Cholera

264   Epidemics

266   Paratyphoid fevers

268   Bacterial food poisoning
          Classify works on contamination of food by specific chemicals with the chemical involved.   Classify works on food poisoning caused by pesticides in WA 240. Classify works on plant poisoning in WD 500–530.

Bacterial infections
Enterobacteriaceae and other enteric infections – Continued

269   **Salmonella infections**
Classify works on salmonella food poisoning in WC 268; on paratyphoid fevers in WC 266.

270   **Typhoid**

280   **Dysentery**

282   **Bacillary dysentery**

285   **Amebic dysentery. Amebiasis**
Classify works on amebic liver abscess in WI 730.

290   **Escherichia coli infections**

302   **Actinomycetales infections. Mycobacterium infections**
Classify works on leprosy in WC 335; on maduromycosis in WR 340; on tuberculosis in WF, etc.

305   **Anthrax**

310   **Brucellosis**

318   **Corynebacterium infections**

320   **Diphtheria**

330   **Pseudomonas infections. Glanders**

335   **Leprosy**

340   **Bordetella infections. Whooping cough**

350   **Yersinia infections. Plague**

355   **Epidemics**

368   **Clostridium infections**
Classify works on botulism in WC 268; on bacillary hemoglobinuria in WJ 344.

370   **Tetanus. Trismus**

Bacterial infections
  Clostridium infections – Continued

375   Gas gangrene

380   Tularemia

390   Rat–bite fever

400   Spirochete infections

406   Borrelia infections. Lyme disease

410   Relapsing fever

420   Leptospirosis. Weil's disease

422   Treponemal infections
               Classify works on syphilis in WC 160–170.

425   Yaws

450   Mycoses (General or not elsewhere classified)
             Classify works on dermatomycoses in WR 300–340; on fungal lung diseases in WF 652.

460   Coccidioidomycosis. Paracoccidioidomycosis

465   Histoplasmosis

470   Candidiasis
             Classify works on cutaneous candidiasis in WR 300.

475   Cryptococcosis. Sporotrichosis

500   Virus diseases (General or not elsewhere classified)

501   RNA virus infections (General or not elsewhere classified)

502   Retroviridae infections (General or not elsewhere classified)

503   Acquired immunodeficiency syndrome. HIV infections

Virus diseases
    RNA virus infections
        Retroviridae infections
            Acquired Immunodeficiency syndrome. HIV infections – Continued

503.1	Diagnosis
503.2	Therapy
503.3	Etiology. Transmission
503.4	Epidemiology (Table G)
503.41	General Coverage (Not Table G)
503.5	Complications
503.6	Prevention and control
503.7	Psychosocial aspects
505	Viral respiratory tract infections (General or not elsewhere classified)
510	Common cold
512	Orthomyxoviridae infections (General or not elsewhere classified)
515	Influenza
518	Paramyxovirus infections (General or not elsewhere classified)
	Classify works on measles in WC 580.
520	Mumps
522	Infectious mononucleosis
524	Arbovirus infections (General or not elsewhere classified)
	Classify works on epidemic encephalitis in WC 542; on lymphocytic choriomeningitis in WC 540.
526	Phlebotomus fever
528	Dengue
530	Yellow fever

Virus diseases
  Arbovirus infections
    Yellow fever – Continued

532   Epidemics

534   Viral hemorrhagic fevers

536   Human viral hepatitis

540   Neurotropic virus diseases (General or not elsewhere classified)

542   Epidemic encephalitis.   Equine encephalomyelitis (in humans)
          Classify works on encephalomyelitis of the horse in SF 959.E5.

550   Rabies

555   Poliomyelitis

556   Prevention and control

570   Infectious viral skin diseases (General or not elsewhere classified)

571   Herpesviridae infections (General or not elsewhere classified)
          Classify works on infectious mononucleosis in WC 522; on Burkitt's lymphoma
          in WH 525; on other infections with no skin manifestations in WC 500.

572   Chickenpox

575   Herpes zoster

578   Herpes simplex

580   Measles

582   Rubella

584   Poxviridae infections (General or not elsewhere classified)

585   Smallpox

588   Prevention and control

590   Epidemics

Virus diseases
Infectious viral skin diseases - Continued

593   **Cat–scratch disease**

600   **Rickettsial and chlamydial infections. Tick–borne diseases (General or not elsewhere classified)**

602   **Trench fever**

605   **Epidemic louse–borne typhus**

610   **Epidemics**

615   **Endemic flea–borne typhus**

620   **Rocky Mountain spotted fever**

625   **Other tick–borne rickettsial infections**
          e.g., Q fever

630   **Scrub typhus**

635   **Other mite–borne rickettsial infections**
          e.g., Rickettsialpox

640   **Bartonellaceae infections**

660   **Ornithosis**

680   **Tropical diseases (General)**
          Cf. WR 350   Tropical diseases of the skin.

695   **Parasitic diseases (General or not elsewhere classified)**
          Classify general works on localized infections by site, e.g., Parasitic skin diseases in WR 345.

698   **Parasitic intestinal diseases (General or not elsewhere classified)**
          Classify works on amebic dysentery in WC 285.

700   **Protozoan infections (General or not elsewhere classified)**
          Classify works on amebiasis in WC 285; on trichomonas vaginitis in WP 258. See also other localized infections indexed.

705   **Trypanosomiasis**

Parasitic diseases
    Protozoan infections – Continued

715   **Visceral leishmaniasis**
                 Classify general works on leishmaniasis and on mucocutaneous leishmaniasis in WR 350.

725   **Toxoplasmosis (General or not elsewhere classified)**

730   **Coccidiosis**

735   **Balantidiasis**

750   **Malaria**

755   **Epidemiology**

765   **Prevention and control**

770   **Therapy**

800   **Helminthiasis (General or not elsewhere classified)**

805   **Trematode infections (General or not elsewhere classified)**

810   **Schistosomiasis**

830   **Cestode infections (General or not elsewhere classified)**

838   **Cysticercosis. Taeniasis**

840   **Echinococcosis**
                 Classify works on hepatic echinococcosis in WI 700; on pulmonary echinococcosis in WF 600.

850   **Nematode infections (General or not elsewhere classified)**

855   **Trichinosis**

860   **Trichuriasis. Oxyuriasis**

865   **Strongyloidiasis**

Parasitic diseases
Helminthias
Nematode infections – Continued

870 Ascariasis

880 Filariasis and related conditions (General or not elsewhere classified)

885 Onchocerciasis

890 Hookworm infections (General or not elsewhere classified)

900 Ectoparasitic infestations (General or not elsewhere classified)
Disinfestation
Classify works on pediculosis in WR 375; on scabies in WR 365 or if veterinary in SF 810. Cf. WC 625 and WC 635 for tick and mite–borne rickettsial infections.

950 Zoonoses (General)
Classify work on specific diseases of animals in SF.

WD

The WD schedule consists of a series of small tables which deal with subjects that cannot be readily integrated into other schedules because of the underlying framework of the Classification. Classify works on history or societies in the general number for each table.

WD 100–175   Nutrition Disorders
WD 200–226   Metabolic Diseases
WD 300–375   Immunologic and Collagen Diseases. Hypersensitivity
WD 400–430   Animal Poisons
WD 500–530   Plant Poisons
WD 600–670   Diseases and Injuries Caused by Physical Agents
WD 700–758   Aviation and Space Medicine

NUTRITION DISORDERS

Classify works on nutrition disorders in infancy and childhood in WS 115–130; in the aged in WT 115.

100   **General works**
Classify here works on particular nutrition disorders not included below or elsewhere classified.

* 101   **Handbooks. Resource guides**

105   **Deficiency diseases (General or not elsewhere classified)**
Classify works on deficiency of hormones in WK; on deficiencies as etiological factors in particular diseases with the disease.

110   **Vitamin A deficiency**
e.g., Night blindness

120   **Vitamin B deficiency**

122   **Thiamine deficiency**
e.g., Beriberi

124   **Riboflavin deficiency**

*NUMBER CAN BE USED FOR BOTH MONOGRAPHS AND SERIALS.

Deficiency diseases
  Vitamin B deficiency– Continued

126   Pellagra

140   Ascorbic acid deficiency
             e.g., Scurvy

145   Vitamin D deficiency
             e.g., Rickets

150   Vitamin E deficiency

155   Vitamin K deficiency

175   Celiac disease. Sprue

METABOLIC DISEASES

200   General works
          *Classify works on diabetes and related conditions in WK; on achlorhydria in WI
          308.*

* 200.1 Handbooks. Resource guides

200.5   Specific diseases or groups of diseases not classified elsewhere, A–Z

          .C2   Calcium metabolism disorders
                    Classify works on deficiency diseases in WD 100–175.
          .H8   Hyperlipemia
          .H9   Hyperprolactinemia
          .I7   Iron metabolism disorders
          .M2   Malabsorption syndromes
                    *Classify works on celiac disease and sprue in WD 175. Classify works
                    for the gastroenterologist in WI 500.*
          .P4   Phosphorus metabolism disorders
          .P7   Protein–losing enteropathies

205   Inborn errors of metabolism (General)
          *Classify works on the hemolytic anemias in WH 170; on chronic idiopathic jaundice
          in WI 703; on errors of renal tubular transport in WJ 301.*

205.5   Specific errors or groups of errors not elsewhere classified, A–Z

          .A5   Amino acid metabolism
                    Classify works on albinism in WR 265.
          .A6   Amyloidosis

*NUMBER CAN BE USED FOR BOTH MONOGRAPHS AND SERIALS.

Inborn errors of metabolism
Specific errors or groups of errors not elsewhere classified, A-Z – Continued

.C2 Carbohydrate metabolism
.H9 Hyperbilirubinemia, Hereditary
.L5 Lipid metabolism
.M3 Metal metabolism (General)
   Classify works on specific disorders separately.
.M4 Minerals
.P2 Paralysis, Familial periodic
.P6 Porphyria
.P8 Purine–pyrimidine metabolism
   Classify works on gout in WE 350.
.X2 Xanthomatosis

210 Obesity
Classify works on reducing diets here or in WD 212 below.

212 Popular works

214 Adiposis dolorosa. Lipomatosis. Lipodystrophy
Classify works on panniculitis in WR 220; on lipochondrodystrophy in WD 205.5.C2.

220 Water–electrolyte imbalance. Acid–base imbalance
Classify works on water–electrolyte balance and acid base equilibrium in QU 105.

222 Acidosis
Classify works on diabetic acidosis in WK 830; on renal tubular acidosis in WJ 301; on respiratory acidosis in WF 140.

226 Alkalosis

IMMUNOLOGIC AND COLLAGEN DISEASES. HYPERSENSITIVITY

This schedule is for works on diseases that are largely systemic. Classify works on the hematologic diseases in WH; on disorders associated with transplantation in WO 680; on phagocytic bactericidal dysfunction and associated conditions in QW 690.

300 General works
Classify works on asthma in WF 553; on hay fever in WV 335; on dermatitis in WR 160; on respiratory hypersensitivity in WF 150.

* 301 Handbooks. Resource guides

305 Autoimmune diseases (General)

*NUMBER CAN BE USED FOR BOTH MONOGRAPHS AND SERIALS.

308   **Immune complex disease. Immunologic deficiency syndromes (General or not elsewhere classified)**
        Classify works on acquired immunodeficiency syndrome (AIDS) and other HIV infections in WC 503–503.7.

310   **Food hypersensitivity**

320   **Drug hypersensitivity**

330   **Serum sickness**

375   **Collagen diseases and other connective tissue diseases (General)**
        Cf. WE 346 Rheumatoid arthritis; WG 240 Rheumatic heart disease; WC 220 Rheumatic fever; WG 518 Periarteritis nodosa; WG 520 Thromboangiitis obliterans; WR 152 Lupus erythematosus, Systemic; WR 260 Scleroderma, Systemic.

ANIMAL POISONS

400   **General works**

* 401   **Handbooks. Resource guides**

405   **Marine forms**

410   **Reptiles**

420   **Spiders. Scorpions. Centipedes. Leeches**

430   **Insects**

PLANT POISONS

500   **General works**
        Cf. QV 627 Organic poisons.

* 501   **Handbooks. Resource guides**

505   **Ergotism**

515	Favism

| 520 | Mushroom poisoning |

| 530 | Milk sickness |

DISEASES AND INJURIES CAUSED BY PHYSICAL AGENTS

600   **General works**
Classify material on burns in WO 704; on blast injuries in WO 820; on radiation injuries in WN 610.

* 601   **Handbooks.   Resource guides**

602   **Electric injuries**

605   **Non–ionizing radiation injuries (General)**

610   **Heat exhaustion.   Sunstroke**

630   **Motion sickness**
e.g., Seasickness.   Airsickness

640   **Vibration disorders (General)**
Classify works on vibration as a cause of disease in QZ 57; on aviation effects in WD 735; on control in industry in WA 470; on therapeutic use in WB 535.

650   **High air pressure.   Submarine medicine**

655   **Anoxia.   Anoxemia**
Cf. WF 143   Respiratory symptoms; WD 715   Aviation medicine.

670   **Hypothermia**
Classify here works written for the practicing physician, such as those on diagnosis, treatment, etc.   Classify works on pathogenesis of hypothermia in QZ 57; studies of normal physiological effects of cold in QT 160; on induced hypothermia in WO350.

AVIATION AND SPACE MEDICINE

Classify work combining both atmospheric and space flight in WD 700-745; on space flight alone in WD 750-759. Classify here works on diseases associated with high altitude on earth as well as in the air.

AVIATION MEDICINE

700   **General works**
Classify material on aerotitis media in WV 232; on vision in WW.

* 701   **Handbooks. Resource guides**

* 703   **Dictionaries. Encyclopedias**

704   **Research (General)**
Classify here works about research in general, in aviation medicine alone or in aviation medicine and space medicine combined. Classify works about research in space medicine alone in WD 751. Classify works about research on a particular subject, by subject.

705   **Personnel selection and fitness. Physical standards**

710   **Altitude effects**

712   **Decompression sickness**

715   **Anoxia. Inert gas narcosis**

720   **Speed. Acceleration. Deceleration. Gravitation. Rotation**
e.g., G force
Classify works on airsickness in WD 630.

730   **Psychological aspects**
e.g., Fear. Stress

735   **Fatigue. Effect of noise. Effect of vibration**

740   **Aviation accidents. Protective devices**

745   **Aviation dentistry**

SPACE MEDICINE

750   **General works (including works on broad aspects of space flight)**

*NUMBER CAN BE USED FOR BOTH MONOGRAPHS AND SERIALS.

751   **Research (General)**
Classify works about research on a particular subject by subject.

751.6   **Medical informatics.   Automatic data processing.   Computers (General)**
Classify works on use for special subjects by subject.

752   **Physiological aspects**

754   **Psychological aspects**

756   **Closed ecological systems**

758   **Extraterrestrial environment**

WE

MUSCULOSKELETAL SYSTEM

Classify general works on the musculoskeletal system and its diseases in WS 270 when related to children; in WY 157.6 when related to nursing. Classify works on nursing of patients with specific diseases in WY also. Classify works on skindiseases in WR.

WE 1–190   **General**
WE 200–600   **By Tissue**
WE 700–890   **By Region**

GENERAL

* 1   **Societies (Cutter from name of society)**
          Includes ephemeral membership lists issued serially or separately. Classify substantial lists with directories. Classify annual reports, journals, etc., in W1.

          Collections (General)
5   **By several authors**
7   **By individual authors**

9   **Addresses. Essays. Lectures (General)**

11   **History (Table G)**
11.1   **General coverage (Not Table G)**

* 13   **Dictionaries. Encyclopedias**

* 15   **Classification. Nomenclature. Terminology**

* 16   **Tables. Statistics**

17   **Atlases. Pictorial works**
          Classify atlases limited to a particular part of the system here also.

18   **Education**
          Classify here works about education.

*NUMBER CAN BE USED FOR BOTH MONOGRAPHS AND SERIALS.

* 18.2 **Educational materials**
Classify here educational materials, e.g., outlines, questions and answers, programmed instruction, catalogs, computer–assisted instruction, etc., regardless of format. Classify textbooks, regardless of format, by subject.

* 19 **Schools, departments and faculties of orthopedics**

20 **Research (General)**
Classify here works about research in general. Classify works about research on a particular subject by subject.

21 **Orthopedics as a profession. Ethics. Peer review**

* 22 **Directories (Table G)**
* 22.1 **General coverage (Not Table G)**

Laboratories, institutes, etc.
23 **Collective**
24 **Individual (Cutter from name of agency)**

25 **Laboratory manuals. Technique**

26 **Equipment and supplies**
Classify catalogs in W 26. Classify works on bone plates and screws in WE 185.

26.5 **Medical informatics. Automatic data processing. Computers (General)**
Classify works on use for special subjects by subject.

Hospitals, clinics, dispensaries, etc.
27 **Collective (Table G)**
27.1 **General coverage (Not Table G)**
28 **Individual (Table G)**

* 32 **Laws (Table G)**
* 32.1 **General coverage (Not Table G)**

* 33 **Discussion of law (Table G)**
* 33.1 **General coverage (Not Table G)**

* 39 **Handbooks. Resource guides**

100 **General works**
Classify works on specialty and on the specialty and diseases here. Classify works on diseases alone in WE 140.

101   **Anatomy. Histology. Embryology (General)**

102   **Physiology. Biochemistry**

103   **Movement. Locomotion. Posture. Exertion**

104   **Kinesthesis. Weight perception**

140   **Diseases (General)**

141   **Examination. Diagnosis. Diagnostic methods. Radiography**
           Classify material on a single organ with the organ.

168   **Orthopedics (General)**

170   **Amputation**

172   **Prosthesis**
           Classify catalogs in W 26.

175   **Fractures. Dislocations. Sprains**

180   **Fractures**

182   **Open fractures**

185   **Fracture fixation**

190   **Reconstructive orthopedics. Transplantation of bone and bones**

BY TISSUE

200   **Bone and bones (General)**
           Include works on structure and function of bones in general. Classify works on specific bones with part or system involved.

225   **Bone diseases**
           Classify works on eosinophilic granuloma in WH 650.

Bone diseases – Continued

250   **Congenital abnormalities.   Disorders of metabolism, growth, or development**
Classify works on abnormalities of specific bones or regions with the bone or region. Classify works on systemic metabolic disorders involving the bones in WD 200–205.5.

251   **Osteomyelitis and other infectious diseases**

253   **Tuberculosis of bones and joints**

258   **Neoplasms.   Cysts**
Classify works on neoplasms of specific bones by site.

259   **Osteochondritis**

300   **Joints.   Ligaments.   Synovial membranes and fluid.   Cartilage**

304   **Joint diseases**

312   **Surgery (including arthrodesis and arthroplasty) (General)**

344   **Arthritis**

346   **Rheumatoid arthritis.   Ankylosis**
Cf. WU 140   Temporomandibular joint ankylosis; WE 725   Ankylosing spondylitis.

348   **Degenerative joint disease.   Osteoarthritis**

350   **Gout**

400   **Bursae**

500   **Muscles.   Fascia**
Include works on structure and function.   Classify works on diseases in general in WE 550.   Classify works on specific muscles with part or system involved.

544   **Myositis.   Fibrositis.   Rheumatism**

545   **Contracture**
Classify works on muscle contraction in WE 500; on muscle cramp and myoclonus in WE 550.

Muscles. Fascia – Continued

550   **Muscular diseases. Neuromuscular diseases**
           Classify works on neuromuscular diseases of the eye in WW 400–475.

555   **Myasthenia gravis**

559   **Muscular dystrophy**

600   **Tendons. Tendon sheaths**

BY REGION

700   **Head and trunk**

705   **Head. Face**
           Cf. WU 101 works for the dentist. Classify works on the jaw in WU; on the temporal bone written for the otolaryngologist in WV 201.

706   **Injuries**

707   **Neoplasms (Head and neck)**

708   **Neck**

715   **Thorax. Ribs**
           Classify material on anatomy and physiology here as well as that on bone disorders and malformations. Classify material on diseases of organs or systems within the thoracic cavity, as well as thoracic surgery, in WF.

720   **Back**

725   **Spine. Vertebrae**
           Classify works on lumbar and sacral vertebrae in WE 750; on spinal tuberculosis in WE 253.

730   **Congenital anomalies**
           e.g., Spinal dysraphism

735   **Curvatures**
           e.g., Scoliosis. Kyphosis. Lordosis

740   **Intervertebral disks**

750   Lumbosacral region. Sacrococcygeal region. Pelvis

755   Low back pain. Sciatica

800   Extremities

805   Upper extremity

810   Shoulder. Upper arm

812   Axilla

820   Elbow. Forearm

830   Wrist. Hand

832   Infections of the hand

835   Fingers. Toes

850   Lower extremity
            Classify works on varicose veins in WG 620.

855   Hip. Upper leg

860   Hip joint

865   Femur. Thigh

870   Knee. Lower leg

880   Ankle. Foot
            Classify works on toes in WE 835.

883   Deformities
            e.g., Clubfoot

886   Flat feet

890   Podiatry

WF

RESPIRATORY SYSTEM

Classify general works on the respiratory system and its diseases in WS 280 when related to children; in WY 163 when related to nursing. Classify works on nursing of patients with specific diseases in WY also.

WF 1–900	**General**
WF 970–985	**Thorax and Thoracic Surgery**

GENERAL

* 1   **Societies (Cutter from name of society)**
Includes ephemeral membership lists issued serially or separately. Classify substantial lists with directories. Classify annual reports, journals, etc., in Wl.

Collections (General)
5   **By several authors**
7   **By individual authors**

9   **Addresses. Essays. Lectures (General)**

11   **History (Table G)**
11.1   **General coverage (Not Table G)**

* 13   **Dictionaries. Encyclopedias**

* 15   **Classification. Nomenclature. Terminology**

* 16   **Tables. Statistics**

17   **Atlases. Pictorial works**
Classify atlases limited to a particular part of the system here also.

18   **Education**
Classify here works about education.

* 18.2   **Educational materials**
Classify here educational materials, e.g., outlines, questions and answers, programmed instruction, catalogs, computer–assisted instruction, etc., regardless of format. Classify textbooks, regardless of format, by subject.

* 19   **Schools, colleges, and specialized departments and facilities**

20   **Research (General)**
Classify here works about research in general. Classify works about research on a particular subject by subject.

21   **Pneumology as a profession. Ethics. Peer review**

* 22   **Directories (Table G)**
* 22.1   **General coverage (Not Table G)**

Institutes. Laboratories of experimental research
23   **Collective**
24   **Individual (Cutter from name of agency)**

25   **Laboratory manuals. Technique**

26   **Equipment and supplies**
Classify catalogs in W 26.

26.5   **Medical informatics. Automatic data processing. Computers (General)**
Classify works for use on special subjects by subject.

Hospitals, sanatoriums, clinics, etc.
27   **Collective (Table G)**
27.1   **General coverage (Not Table G)**
28   **Individual (Table G)**

* 32   **Laws (Table G)**
Classify legislation on tuberculosis in WF 200.
* 32.1   **General coverage (Not Table G)**

* 33   **Discussion of law (Table G)**
* 33.1   **General coverage (Not Table G)**

* 39   **Handbooks. Resource guides**

100   **General works**
Classify works on specialty and on the specialty and diseases here. Classify works on diseases alone in WF 140.

101   **Anatomy. Histology. Embryology. Abnormalities**

102   **Physiology of respiration**

110   **Biochemistry of respiration and the respiratory system**

140   **Diseases of the respiratory system (General)**

141   **Examination. Diagnosis. Radiography. Monitoring**

141.5   **Specific techniques, A–Z**

         .B8   **Bronchial provocation tests**
         .C2   **Capnography**
         .P7   **Plethysmography, Whole body**

143   **Signs and symptoms**

145   **Therapeutics**

150   **Respiratory hypersensitivity (General)**
         Classify localized reactions with organs affected, e.g., Hay fever in WV 335.

200   **Tuberculosis (General)**
         Classify works on tuberculosis of organs of other systems, with the organ or system.
         Classify here also legislation on tuberculosis.

205   **Epidemiology**

215   **Pathology**

220   **Diagnosis. Prognosis**

225   **Mass chest X-ray**

250   **Immunological aspects**
         e.g., BCG vaccine

290   **Lymph node tuberculosis. Scrofula**

300   **Pulmonary tuberculosis**
       Classify works on silicotuberculosis in WF 654.

310   **Therapy**

315   **Diet. Rest. Exercise. Home care**

330   **Hospitalization. Climatotherapy. Heliotherapy**

350   **Surgery**

360   **Drug therapy**

380   **Miliary tuberculosis**

390   **Pleural tuberculosis**

405   **Tuberculosis in the workplace**

415   **Tuberculosis in childhood**

450   **Neoplasms (General)**

490   **Pharynx. Trachea**
       *Classify works for the otolaryngologist in WV 410. Classify works on
       tracheoesophageal fistula in WI 250.*

500   **Bronchi**

544   **Bronchiectasis**

546   **Bronchitis. Tracheitis**

553   **Asthma**

600   **Lungs**
       *Classify works on the pneumonias in WC 202–209; on pulmonary tuberculosis in
       WF 300–360.*

645   **Atelectasis**

Lungs – Continued

648   **Emphysema**

651   **Lung abscess**

652   **Fungal lung diseases**

654   **Pneumoconiosis**

658   **Neoplasms**
        Include works on lung neoplasms of bronchial origin.

668   **Surgery**
        e.g., Pneumonectomy

700   **Pleura.   Pleural cavity**

744   **Pleurisy.   Pleuritis**

745   **Empyema**

746   **Pneumothorax.   Hemothorax**

768   **Artificial pneumothorax**

800   **Diaphragm**

805   **Functional disorders**
        e.g., Hiccup

810   **Diaphragmatic hernia**

900   **Mediastinum**

THORAX AND THORACIC SURGERY

970   **General works**
        Classify here works on two or more systems within the thoracic cavity, e.g., on respiratory and cardiovascular systems. Classify works on anatomy, physiology, bone structure and abnormalities of the skeletal portion of the thorax in WE 715.

975   Diagnosis.   Radiography

980   Surgery

985   Injuries

WG

CARDIOVASCULAR SYSTEM

Classify general works on the cardiovascular system and its diseases in WS 290 when related to children; in WY 152.5 when related to nursing. Classify works on nursing of patients with specific diseases in WY also. Classify works on blood supply of specific parts of other body systems with the system or part.

WG 1–170	**General**
WG 200–460	**Heart**
WG 500–700	**Blood Vessels**

GENERAL

* 1   **Societies (Cutter from name of society)**
Includes ephemeral membership lists issued serially or separately. Classify substantial lists with directories. Classify annual reports, journals, etc. in W1.

    Collections (General)
5   **By several authors**
7   **By individual authors**

9   **Addresses. Essays. Lectures (General)**

11   **History (Table G)**
11.1   **General coverage (Not Table G)**

* 13   **Dictionaries. Encyclopedias**

* 15   **Classification. Nomenclature. Terminology**

* 16   **Tables. Statistics**

17   **Atlases. Pictorial works**
Classify atlases limited to a particular part of the system here also.

18   **Education**
Classify here works about education.

* 18.2   **Educational materials**

Classify here educational materials, e.g., outlines, questions and answers, programmed instruction, catalogs, computer–assisted instruction, etc., regardless of format. Classify textbooks, regardless of format, by subject.

* 19   **Schools, colleges, and specialized departments and facilities**

20   **Research (General)**

Classify here works about research in general. Classify works about research on a particular subject by subject. Cf. WG 110 Experimental studies.

21   **Cardiology as a profession. Ethics. Peer review**

* 22   **Directories (Table G)**
* 22.1   **General coverage (Not Table G)**

     Institutes. Laboratories of experimental research
23   **Collective**
24   **Individual (Cutter from name of agency)**

25   **Laboratory manuals. Technique**

Cf. WG 140 for clinical examination and diagnosis.

26   **Equipment and supplies**

Classify catalogs in W 26. Classify works on artificial and mechanical hearts in WG 169.5. Classify works on artificial pacemakers here. Cf. WG 168 for artificial cardiac pacing.

26.5   **Medical informatics. Automatic data processing. Computers (General)**

Classify works on use for special subjects by subject.

     Hospitals, clinics, dispensaries, etc.
27   **Collective (Table G)**
27.1   **General coverage (Not Table G)**
28   **Individual (Table G)**

* 32   **Laws (Table G)**
* 32.1   **General coverage (Not Table G)**

* 33   **Discussion of law (Table G)**
* 33.1   **General coverage (Not Table G)**

* 39   **Handbooks. Resource guides**

100   **General works**
Classify works on specialty and on the specialty and diseases here. Classify works on diseases alone in WG 120.

101   **Anatomy. Histology. Embryology**

102   **Physiology. Biochemistry**

103   **Circulation (General)**
Classify works on blood circulation of a system or part with system or part.

104   **Microcirculation (General)**

106   **Hemodynamics. Blood velocity, volume, pressure, etc.**
Classify works on hypertension and hypotension in WG 340; on measurement of blood pressure in clinical diagnosis in WB 280.

110   **Experimental studies**
Classify here works that discuss the experimental work itself. Classify works about research in WG 20. Classify works on specific subjects by subject.

113   **Popular works**
Classify here works on heart and vascular diseases in general or on coronary disease and congestive heart failure in particular. Classify works on other specific disorders with the disorder.

120   **Cardiovascular diseases (General or not elsewhere classified)**

140   **Electrocardiography. Vectorcardiography. Monitoring (General)**

141   **Examination. Diagnosis. Diagnostic methods (General and heart specifically)**

141.5   **Specific diagnostic methods, A–Z**

         .A3   **Angiocardiography**
         .A9   **Auscultation, Heart**
         .B2   **Ballistocardiography**
         .C15   **Cardiography, Impedance**
         .C2   **Catheterization, Heart**
         .E2   **Echocardiography**
         .F9   **Function tests, Heart (General)**
         .K5   **Kinetocardiography**
         .K9   **Kymography**
         .P4   **Phonocardiography**
         .P7   **Plethysmography**

Examination. Diagnosis. Diagnostic methods
Special diagnostic methods, A-Z - Continued

.R2	Radiography (General)
.R3	Radionuclide imaging
.T6	Tomography

142   **Pathology**

166   **Therapeutics**
Classify works on drugs acting on the cardiovascular system in QV 150.

166.5   **Specific therapeutic methods, A–Z**

.A3	Angioplasty
.A5	Angioplasty, Laser
.B2	Balloon dilatation. Balloon angioplasty

168   **Cardiovascular surgery. Artificial cardiac pacing**
Classify works on surgery for a particular disorder with the disorder.

169   **Heart surgery. Heart transplantation**
Classify works on surgery of coronary vessels in general, heart valves, myocardium, etc., here. Classify works on surgery of the aorta in WG 410. Classify works on surgery of a particular disorder with the disorder.

169.5   **Artificial heart. Heart–lung machine**

170   **Vascular surgery**
Classify works on surgery of arteries and veins in general here. Cf. WG 410 Aorta and numbers for other specific vessels.

HEART

200   **General works**
Note that popular works are classed in WG 113; works on examination, in WG 140–141.5; on surgery, in WG 169–169.5.

201   **Anatomy. Histology. Embryology**

202   **Physiology. Mechanism of the heart beat**

205   **Cardiac emergencies**

210   **Heart diseases (General or not elsewhere classified)**

220   **Congenital heart disease. Abnormalities of the heart and the cardiovascular system (General)**

240   **Rheumatic heart disease**

260   **Valves**

262   **Mitral**

265   **Aortic**

268   **Tricuspid**

269   **Pulmonary**

275   **Pericardium**

280   **Myocardium**
        Classify material on myocardial infarct in WG 300.

285   **Endocardium**

298   **Angina pectoris**

300   **Coronary vessels. Coronary disease**

320   **Functional heart disease**
        e.g., Neurocirculatory asthenia

330   **Disorders of the heart beat**

340   **Hypertension. Hypertensive heart disease. Hypotension**

370   **Congestive heart failure**

410   **Aorta**
        Cf. WC 168 for aortic involvement in syphilis.

420   **Pulmonary embolism and related disorders. Pulmonary heart disease**

460   **Special cardiac problems in anesthesia, dentistry, surgery**
         e.g., Choice of anesthetic
         Cf. WO 235 for general works on choice of anesthetic. Classify works on problems
         in pregnancy in WQ 244; in labor specifically in WQ 330.

BLOOD VESSELS

Classify works on blood supply of the extremities here, but classify works on blood supply
of specific parts of other body systems with that system or part. Classify works on
coronary vessels in WG 300; on the aorta specifically in WG 410; on circulation
in WG 103–104; on vascular resistance in WG 106; on vascular surgery in WG 170.

500   **General works. Radiography**

510   **Arteries (General or not elsewhere classified)**

515   **Inflammation**

518   **Polyarteritis nodosa**

520   **Thromboangiitis obliterans**

530   **Immersion foot. Frostbite**

540   **Arterial embolism. Arterial thrombosis**

550   **Arteriosclerosis and related disorders**

560   **Vasomotor regulation and disorders**
         Classify material on carotid sinus syndrome here.

570   **Raynaud's disease**

578   **Vasodilator disorders**

580   **Aneurysms**
         Classify works on aortic aneurysm in WG 410; on heart aneurysm in WG 300;
         on cerebral aneurysm in WL 354–355.

590   **Arteriovenous anastomosis. Arteriovenous fistula**

Arteries – Continued

595   **Specific arteries, A–Z**
Classify works on the aorta in WG 410; on coronary arteries in WG 300.

.A9	Axillary artery
.B2	Basilar artery
.B7	Brachial artery
.B72	Brachiocephalic trunk
.B76	Bronchial arteries
.C2	Carotid arteries
.C3	Celiac artery
.C37	Cerebral arteries
.F3	Femoral artery
.H3	Hepatic artery
.I5	Iliac artery
.M2	Maxillary artery
.M3	Meningeal arteries
.M38	Mesenteric arteries
.O7	Ophthalmic artery
.P6	Popliteal artery
.P8	Pulmonary artery
.R3	Renal artery
.R38	Retinal artery
.S7	Splenic artery
.S8	Subclavian artery
.T3	Temporal arteries
.T4	Thoracic arteries
.U6	Umbilical arteries
.V3	Vertebral artery

600   **Veins**

610   **Thrombosis. Phlebothrombosis. Thrombophlebitis and related disorders**

620   **Varicose veins**

625   **Specific veins, A–Z**
Classify works on coronary veins in WG 300; on the portal system in WI 720.

.A9	Axillary vein
.A99	Azygos vein
.B7	Brachiocephalic veins
.C3	Cerebral veins
.C7	Cranial sinuses
.F3	Femoral vein
.H3	Hepatic veins
.I5	Iliac vein
.J8	Jugular vein
.P6	Popliteal vein
.P8	Pulmonary veins
.R3	Renal veins

Veins
Specific veins, A-Z – Continued

.R38	Retinal vein
.S2	Saphenous vein
.S8	Subclavian vein
.V3	Venae cavae

700 **Capillaries**
Classify works on capillary resistance in WG 106; on microcirculation in WG 104.

WH

HEMIC AND LYMPHATIC SYSTEMS

Classify general works on the hemic and lymphatic systems and their diseases in WS 300 when related to children; in WY 152.5 when related to nursing. Classify works on nursing of patients with specific diseases in WY also.

* 1   **Societies (Cutter from name of society)**
             Includes ephemeral membership lists issued serially or separately. Classify substantial lists with directories. Classify annual reports, journals, etc., in W1.

             Collections (General)
5   **By several authors**
7   **By individual authors**

9   **Addresses. Essays. Lectures (General)**

11   **History (Table G)**
11.1   **General coverage (Not Table G)**

* 13   **Dictionaries. Encyclopedias**

* 15   **Classification. Nomenclature. Terminology**

* 16   **Tables. Statistics**

17   **Atlases. Pictorial works**
             Classify atlases limited to a particular part of the system here also.

18   **Education**
             Classify here works about education.

* 18.2   **Educational materials**
             Classify here educational materials, e.g., outlines, questions and answers, programmed instruction, catalogs, computer-assisted instruction, etc., regardless of format. Classify textbooks, regardless of format, by subject.

* 19   **Schools, departments and faculties of hematology**

20   **Research (General)**
             Classify here works about research in general. Classify works about research on a particular subject by subject.

*NUMBER CAN BE USED FOR BOTH MONOGRAPHS AND SERIALS.

21   Hematology as a profession.   Ethics.   Peer review

* 22   Directories (Table G)
* 22.1   General coverage (Not Table G)

Institutes.   Laboratories of experimental research.   Blood banks
23   Collective
24   Individual (Cutter from name of agency)

25   Laboratory manuals.   Technique
            Classify works on laboratory examination of blood in QY 400–490.

26   Equipment and supplies
            Classify catalogs in W 26.

26.5   Medical informatics.   Automatic data processing.   Computers (General)
            Classify works on use for special subjects by subject.

Hospitals, clinics, etc.
28   Individual (Table G)

* 32   Laws (Table G)
* 32.1   General coverage (Not Table G)

* 33   Discussion of law (Table G)
* 33.1   General coverage (Not Table G)

* 39   Handbooks.   Resource guides

100   General works
            Classify works on specialty and on the specialty and diseases here.   Classify works
            on diseases alone in WH 120.

120   Hematologic diseases (General or not elsewhere classified)

140   Hematopoietic system and hematopoiesis.   Developmental theories.   Blood cells (General)
            Classify material on blood chemistry in QY 450.

150   Erythrocytes

155   Anemia
            Classify works on neonatal anemia in WS 420; on splenic anemia in WH 600;
            on blood group incompatibility in WH 420.

*NUMBER CAN BE USED FOR BOTH MONOGRAPHS AND SERIALS.

Erythrocytes
Anemia – Continued

160   **Hypochromic anemia**

165   **Macrocytic anemia. Pernicious anemia**

170   **Hemolytic anemia**
         e.g., Sickle cell anemia
         Classify works on favism in WD 515; on hemoglobinuria in WJ 344; on
         kernicterus in WL 362.

175   **Anemias of bone marrow dysfunction**
         e.g., Aplastic anemia

180   **Polycythemia. Polycythemia vera**

190   **Hemoglobin and other hemeproteins. Porphyrins (Associated with**
         hemoglobin)
         Classify general works on porphyrins in QU 110; on porphyria in WD 205.5.P6.

200   **Leukocytes. Leukocyte disorders (General)**

250   **Leukemia**
         Classify works on histology and pathology of leukemia in QZ 350.

300   **Blood platelets**

310   **Mechanism of blood coagulation. Hemostasis**
         Classify works on blood coagulation disorders in WH 322–325.

312   **Hemorrhagic disorders (General)**
         Classify works on blood platelet disorders in WH 300.

314   **Purpura (General)**

315   **Thrombopenic purpura**

320   **Non–thrombopenic purpuras**

322   **Blood coagulation disorders (General)**

325   **Hemophilia. Hemarthrosis**

380   **Bone marrow. Bone marrow diseases (General or not elsewhere classified) Sternal puncture**
Cf. WH 175 Anemias; WH 180 Polycythemia vera.

400   **Fluid elements. Plasma. Serum. Blood proteins. Blood protein disorders**
Classify works on blood chemistry in QY 450–490; on inborn errors of protein metabolism in WD 205–205.5. Cf. WH 540 Multiple myeloma.

420   **Blood groups. Blood group incompatibility (General)**
Classify works on blood typing in QY 415; on medicolegal examination in W 791.

425   **Rh–Hr blood group system. Fetal erythroblastosis**
Classify works on kernicterus in WL 362.

450   **Whole blood. Blood derivatives. Plasma substitutes. Blood expanders**

460   **Blood bank procedures**
e.g., Procurement, processing, preservation, storage, shipment, etc. Blood donors. Plasmapheresis
Classify material on blood banks in WH 23 or WH 24; on blood transfusion in WB 356.

500   **Hodgkin's disease**

525   **Hematologic neoplasms (General). Lymphoma**
Classify works on hematologic neoplasms in general here. Classify here also works which deal collectively with subjects classed in WH 250 Leukemia, WH 500 Hodgkin's disease, and WH 525 Lymphoma. Classify works on histology and pathology of hematologic neoplasms or lymphomas in QZ 350.

540   **Multiple myeloma**

600   **Spleen**

650   **Reticuloendothelial system**
Classify works on the lipoidoses alone in WD 205.5.L5.

700   **Lymphatic system. Lymphatic diseases (General)**
Classify works on cells in general in WH 140; on blood cells by type in the numbers provided above.

WI

DIGESTIVE SYSTEM

Classify general works on the digestive system and its diseases in WS 310–312 when related to children; in WY 156.5 when related to nursing. Classify works on nursing of patients with specific diseases in WY number also. Classify works on liver and biliary tract treated together in WI 700–740 and in WI 770 if applicable. Classify works on gallbladder and other specific parts in WI 750–765 as indicated.

WI 1–250	General
WI 300–387	Stomach
WI 400–575	Intestines
WI 600–650	Anus and Rectum
WI 700–770	Liver and Biliary Tract
WI 800–830	Pancreas
WI 900–970	Abdomen and Abdominal Surgery

GENERAL

* 1   **Societies (Cutter from name of society)**
Includes ephemeral membership lists issued serially or separately. Classify substantial lists with directories. Classify annual reports, journals, etc., in W1.

          Collections (General)
5   **By several authors**
7   **By individual authors**

9   **Addresses. Essays. Lectures (General)**

11   **History (Table G)**
11.1   **General coverage (Not Table G)**

* 13   **Dictionaries. Encyclopedias**

* 15   **Classification. Nomenclature. Terminology**

* 16   **Tables. Statistics**

17   **Atlases. Pictorial works**
Classify atlases limited to a particular part of the system here also.

18   **Education**
Classify here works about education.

* 18.2   **Educational materials**
Classify here educational materials, e.g., outlines, questions and answers, programmed instruction, catalogs, computer–assisted instruction, etc., regardless of format. Classify textbooks, regardless of format, by subject.

* 19   **Schools, departments, and faculties of gastroenterology**

20   **Research (General)**
Classify here works about research in general. Classify works about research on a particular subject by subject.

21   **Gastroenterology as a profession. Ethics. Peer review**

* 22   **Directories (Table G)**
* 22.1   **General coverage (Not Table G)**

Laboratories, institutes, etc.
23   **Collective**
24   **Individual (Cutter from name of agency)**

25   **Laboratory manuals. Technique**

26   **Equipment and supplies**
Classify catalogs in W 26.

26.5   **Medical informatics. Automatic data processing. Computers (General)**
Classify works on use for special subjects by subject.

Hospitals, clinics, etc.
27   **Collective (Table G)**
27.1   **General coverage (Not Table G)**
28   **Individual (Table G)**

* 32   **Laws (Table G)**
* 32.1   **General coverage (Not Table G)**

* 33   **Discussion of law (Table G)**
* 33.1   **General coverage (Not Table G)**

* 39   **Handbooks. Resource guides**

100   **General works**
Classify works on surgery of the digestive or gastrointestinal system in general in WI 900.

101   **Anatomy. Histology. Embryology. Abnormalities**

102   **Physiology. Biochemistry. Digestion**

113   **Popular works (General). Hygiene**

140   **Diseases (General)**

141   **Examination. Diagnosis. Diagnostic methods. Monitoring (General)**
Classify works on examination of organ with the organ.

143   **Signs and symptoms**

145   **Dyspepsia and related conditions**

146   **Nausea. Vomiting**

147   **Abdominal pain**

149   **Neoplasms**
Classify works on neoplasms of specific organ with the organ.

150   **Functional disorders**

200   **Lips. Mouth**
Classify works for the dentist in WU 140; on neoplasms written for the dentist in WU 280.

210   **Tongue. Taste buds**

230   **Salivary glands**

250   **Esophagus**

STOMACH

300	**General works**
	Classify works on analysis of stomach contents in QY 130.
301	**Anatomy. Histology. Embryology. Congenital abnormalities**
302	**Physiology**
308	**Achlorhydria**
310	**Gastritis**
320	**Neoplasms**
350	**Peptic ulcer**
360	**Stomach ulcer**
370	**Duodenal ulcer**
380	**Surgery. Postgastrectomy syndromes**
387	**Pylorus. Pyloric antrum. Pyloric stenosis**

INTESTINES

400	**General works**
402	**Physiology**
405	**Signs and symptoms**
407	**Diarrhea**
409	**Constipation**
412	**Congenital malformations**

420   **Inflammation**
         e.g., Enteritis; inflammatory bowel diseases
         Classify works on regional enteritis in WI 512.

425   **Diverticulitis. Diverticulosis**

430   **Polyps. Polyposis**

435   **Neoplasms**

450   **Intussusception**

460   **Intestinal obstruction. Ileus**

480   **Surgery (General)**

500   **Small intestine. Mesentery**

505   **Duodenum**
         Classify works on duodenal ulcer in WI 370; on analysis of duodenal contents
            in QY 130.

510   **Jejunum**

512   **Ileum**

520   **Colon**
         Classify works on diverticulitis and diverticulosis in WI 425. Cf. WC 280 Dysentery.

522   **Inflammation**
         e.g., Colitis

528   **Megacolon**
         e.g., Hirschsprung's disease

529   **Neoplasms. Polyps**
         Classify works on colorectal neoplasms here.

530   **Cecum**

535   **Appendix**

560   Sigmoid

575   Peritoneum.   Omentum.   Peritoneal cavity.   Retroperitoneal space

ANUS AND RECTUM

600   **General works**

605   Hemorrhoids.   Fissure in ano.   Rectal fistula

610   Neoplasms
        Classify works on colorectal neoplasms in WI 529.

620   Proctoscopy.   Sigmoidoscopy

650   Proctological surgery

LIVER AND BILIARY TRACT

700   **General works**

702   Physiology.   Liver circulation

703   Bile.   Bile acids, alcohols, and salts.   Jaundice (General or not elsewhere classified)

704   Liver function in food metabolism

715   Hepatitis (General or not elsewhere classified)

720   Circulatory disorders.   Portal system.   Portal hypertension

725   Cirrhosis

730   Abscess

735   Neoplasms

740   Degenerative diseases.   Hepatolenticular degeneration

750   Gallbladder.   Bile ducts.   Vater's ampulla.   Cholecystography

755   Cholecystitis.   Cholelithiasis

765   Neoplasms

770   Surgery (General)

PANCREAS

800   General works
       Classify works on the islands of Langerhans in WK 800–885.

802   Physiology.   Secretions

805   Pancreatitis

810   Neoplasms.   Cysts

820   Cystic fibrosis

830   Surgery (General)

ABDOMEN AND ABDOMINAL SURGERY

Classify works on surgery of the digestive or gastrointestinal system in general here.

900   General works

940   Umbilical region

950   Hernia

955   Ventral

Hernia – Continued

960   Inguinal

965   Femoral

970   Neoplasms

WJ

UROGENITAL SYSTEM

Classify general works on the urogenital system and its diseases in WS 320–322 when related to children; in WY 164 when related to nursing. Classify works on nursing of patients with specific diseases in WY numbers also.

WJ 1–190	General
WJ 300–378	Kidney
WJ 400	Ureter
WJ 500–504	Bladder
WJ 600	Urethra
WJ 700–875	Male Genitalia

GENERAL

* 1 **Societies (Cutter from name of society)**
    Includes ephemeral membership lists issued serially or separately. Classify substantial lists with directories. Classify annual reports, journals, etc., in W1.

    Collections (General)
5   **By several authors**
7   **By individual authors**

9 **Addresses. Essays. Lectures (General)**

11 **History (Table G)**
11.1   **General coverage (Not Table G)**

* 13 **Dictionaries. Encyclopedias**

* 15 **Classification. Nomenclature. Terminology**

* 16 **Tables. Statistics**

17 **Atlases. Pictorial works**
    Classify atlases limited to a particular part of the system here also.

18 **Education**
    Classify here works about education.

* **18.2**   **Educational materials**
Classify here educational materials, e.g., outlines, questions and answers, programmed instruction, catalogs, computer–assisted instruction, etc., regardless of format. Classify textbooks, regardless of format, by subject.

* **19**   **Schools, departments, and faculties of urology**

20   **Research (General)**
Classify here works about research in general. Classify works about research on a particular subject by subject.

21   **Urology as a profession. Ethics. Peer review**

* **22**   **Directories (Table G)**
* **22.1**   **General coverage (Not Table G)**

Laboratories, institutes, etc.
23   **Collective**
24   **Individual (Cutter from name of agency)**

25   **Laboratory manuals. Technique**

26   **Equipment and supplies**
Classify catalogs in W 26.

26.5   **Medical informatics. Automatic data processing. Computers (General)**
Classify works on use for special subjects by subject.

Hospitals, clinics, dispensaries, etc.
27   **Collective (Table G)**
27.1   **General coverage (Not Table G)**
28   **Individual (Table G)**

* **32**   **Laws (Table G)**
* **32.1**   **General coverage (Not Table G)**

* **33**   **Discussion of law (Table G)**
* **33.1**   **General coverage (Not Table G)**

* **39**   **Handbooks. Resource guides**

100   **General works**
Classify works on specialty and on the specialty and diseases here. Classify works on diseases alone in WJ 140.

101   **Anatomy. Histology. Embryology. Abnormalities**

102   **Physiology. Biochemistry**

140   **Urologic diseases (General)**

141   **Urologic examination (General). Monitoring**
          Classify material on examination of single organ with the organ. Classify works on urinalysis in QY 185.

146   **Urination and urination disorders**

151   **Urinary tract infections**

160   **Neoplasms (General)**

166   **Urologic therapeutics**
          Classify works on the pharmacodynamics of diuretics in QV 160; on the pharmacodynamics of anti-infective agents in QV 243.

168   **Urologic surgery**

190   **Gynecologic urology**
          Classify works that include obstetrical urology here. Classify those on urologic diseases in pregnancy (when treated separately) in WQ 260. Cf. WP 180 Vesicovaginal fistula.

KIDNEY

300   **General works**
          Classify works on kidney functions tests in QY 175; on urinalysis in QY 185.

301   **Anatomy. Histology. Embryology. Physiology. Abnormalities**

302   **Diagnosis. Radiography. Pyelography. Monitoring**

303   **Urinary secretion. Anuria (General)**

340   **Nephrosis**

342   **Kidney failure. Crush syndrome**

343   Proteinuria. Albuminuria. Renal aminoaciduria

344   Hemoglobinuria. Hematuria. Myoglobinuria

348   Uremia

351   Infections
       e.g., Pyelitis, Pyelonephritis

353   Nephritis

356   Kidney calculi. Nephrocalcinosis

358   Neoplasms. Cystic kidney

368   Surgery. Kidney transplantation

378   Artificial kidney. Hemodialysis. Peritoneal dialysis
       *Classify works on hemodialysis and peritoneal dialysis used in treatment of diseases
       of other parts of the body with the disease or part.*

URETER

400   Ureter

BLADDER

500   Bladder. Cystoscopy. Cystoscopic surgery
       Classify works on vesicovaginal fistula in WP 180.

504   Neoplasms

URETHRA

600   Urethra

MALE GENITALIA

700   **General works**
Classify here also works which include both male and female genitalia.

701   **Anatomy. Histology. Embryology**

702   **Physiology**

706   **Neoplasms (General)**

709   **Impotence. Infertility**
Cf. WP 570 for general works on infertility.

710   **Male contraception**
Classify general works on medical aspects of contraceptives in WP 630. Classify works on sociological and religious aspects in HQ 763–766.5. Classify works on contraceptive drugs in QV 177.

712   **Sex differentiation disorders**

750   **Prostate. Seminal vesicles. Ejaculatory ducts**

752   **Diseases of the prostate. Prostatic neoplasms**

768   **Surgery**

780   **Vas deferens. Spermatic cord**

790   **Penis. Foreskin. Circumcision**

800   **Scrotum. Scrotal contents. Epididymis. Tunica vaginalis**

830   **Testis**

834   **Spermatogenesis. Spermatozoa**
Cf. QY 190 Semen (clinical analysis).

840   **Cryptorchidism. Eunuchism and related disorders**

858   **Neoplasms**

Testis – Continued

868   Surgery.   Castration

875   **Testicular hormones and antagonists**
             Include works on related synthetic hormones here.   Classify works on anabolic steroids in WK 150.

WK

ENDOCRINE SYSTEM

Classify general works on the endocrine system and its diseases in WS 330 when related to children; in WY 155 when related to nursing. Classify works on nursing of patients with specific diseases in the WY number also.

WK 1–190	General
WK 200–280	Thyroid Gland
WK 300	Parathyroid Glands
WK 350	Pineal Body
WK 400	Thymus Gland
WK 500–590	Pituitary Gland
WK 700–790	Adrenal Glands
WK 800–885	Islets of Langerhans
WK 900–920	Gonads

GENERAL

* 1   **Societies (Cutter from name of society)**
Includes ephemeral membership lists issued serially or separately. Classify substantial lists with directories. Classify annual reports, journals, etc., in W1.

      Collections (General)
5   **By several authors**
7   **By individual authors**

9   **Addresses. Essays. Lectures (General)**

11   **IIistory (Table G)**
11.1   **General coverage (Not Table G)**

* 13   **Dictionaries. Encyclopedias**

* 15   **Classification. Nomenclature. Terminology**

* 16   **Tables. Statistics**

17   **Atlases. Pictorial works**
Classify atlases limited to a particular part of the system here also.

*NUMBER CAN BE USED FOR BOTH MONOGRAPHS AND SERIALS.

18   **Education**
> *Classify here works about education.*

* 18.2   **Educational materials**
> *Classify here educational materials, e.g., outlines, questions and answers, programmed instruction, catalogs, computer–assisted instruction, etc., regardless of format. Classify textbooks, regardless of format, by subject.*

* 19   **Schools, departments and faculties of endocrinology**

20   **Research (General)**
> *Classify here works about research in general. Classify works about research on a particular subject by subject.*

21   **Endocrinology as a profession. Ethics. Peer review**

* 22   **Directories (Table G)**
* 22.1   **General coverage (Not Table G)**

Laboratories, institutes, etc.
23   **Collective**
24   **Individual (Cutter from name of agency)**

25   **Laboratory manuals. Technique. Experimental studies (General)**

26   **Equipment and supplies**
> *Classify catalogs in W 26.*

26.5   **Medical informatics. Automatic data processing. Computers (General)**
> *Classify works on use for special subjects by subject.*

Hospitals, clinics, dispensaries, etc.
27   **Collective (Table G)**
27.1   **General coverage (Not Table G)**
28   **Individual (Table G)**

* 32   **Laws (Table G)**
* 32.1   **General coverage (Not Table G)**

* 33   **Discussion of law (Table G)**
* 33.1   **General coverage (Not Table G)**

* 39   **Handbooks. Resource guides**

100   **Endocrine glands (General)**
       Classify works on specialty and on the specialty and diseases here. Classify works on diseases alone in WK 140.

102   **Physiology. Biochemistry. Hormones and antagonists (General)**

140   **Endocrine diseases (General)**

148   **Surgery (General)**

150   **Steroid hormones (General or not elsewhere classified)**
       Classify works on hormones of a particular gland with the gland.

170   **Gastrointestinal hormones**
       e.g., Secretin. Enterogastrone

180   **Renal hormones**

185   **Other hormones**
       e.g., Peptide hormones

187   **Synthetic hormones (General or not elsewhere classified)**
       Classify works on specific synthetic hormones with the hormones synthesized.

190   **Hormone therapy**

THYROID GLAND

200   **General works**

201   **Anatomy. Histology. Embryology. Abnormalities**

202   **Physiology. Biochemistry (including iodine metabolism). Thyroid hormones and antagonists**

250   **Hypothyroidism and related disorders (General or not elsewhere classified)**

252   **Cretinism. Myxedema**

259   **Goiter**
        Classify here works on goiter in general and on specific goiters, except exophthalmic goiter which is classed in WK 265.

265   **Hyperthyroidism. Thyrotoxicosis. Exophthalmic goiter**

267   **Medical therapy**

270   **Neoplasms. Cysts**

280   **Surgery**

PARATHYROID GLANDS

300   **Parathyroid glands**

PINEAL BODY

350   **Pineal body**

THYMUS GLAND

400   **Thymus gland**

PITUITARY GLAND

500   **General works**

501   **Anatomy. Histology. Embryology. Abnormalities**

502   **Physiology. Biochemistry**

510   **Anterior pituitary gland (Adenohypophysis)**
        Include here works on the pituitary–adrenal system.

Anterior pituitary gland (Adenohypophysis) – Continued

515   **Hormones and antagonists**
e.g., Corticotropin. Growth hormones
Include works on release and release inhibiting hormones.

520   **Posterior pituitary gland (Neurohypophysis). Hormones and antagonists**
Classify works on antidiuretic vasopressin in QV 160; on oxytocin in QV 173.

550   **Diseases**
e.g., Diabetes insipidus. Pituitary dwarfism. Gigantism. Acromegaly.
Hypopituitarism. Froehlich's syndrome, etc.

585   **Neoplasms**
Include works on the anterior and posterior pituitary glands here also.

590   **Surgery**

ADRENAL GLANDS

700   **General works**

701   **Anatomy. Histology. Embryology. Abnormalities**

702   **Physiology. Biochemistry**

725   **Adrenal medulla. Epinephrine. Norepinephrine and other catecholamines**
Classify works on methyldopa in QV 150 or with the disorder being treated.

750   **Adrenal cortex**
*Classify works on neoplasms in WK 780; on surgery, in WK 790; on the
pituitary–adrenal system, in WK 510.*

755   **Adrenal cortex hormones**
e.g., Cortisone

757   **Synthetic substitutes for cortical hormones**
Classify works on topical glucocorticoids in QV 60.

760   **Diseases of the adrenal cortex**

765   **Adrenal cortex hypofunction**
e.g., Addison's disease

Adrenal cortex
   Diseases of the adrenal cortex – Continued

770   Adrenal cortex hyperfunction
            e.g., Adrenogenital syndrome.   Virilism

780   Neoplasms

790   Surgery

ISLETS OF LANGERHANS

800   General works

801   Anatomy. Histology. Embryology. Abnormalities

810   Diabetes mellitus

815   Therapy

818   Diet

819   Diet lists.   Diabetic cookery

820   Insulin and its modifications

825   Other hypoglycemic agents

830   Diabetic ketoacidosis.   Diabetic coma

835   Complications of diabetes

840   Diabetes as a complication in other conditions
            Classify works on diabetes in pregnancy in WQ 248.

850   Diabetic patients' manuals.   Self care

870   Glycosurias

880   Hyperinsulinism. Hyperglycemia. Hypoglycemia

885   Neoplasms

GONADS

900   Gonads.   Sex hormones (General)
         Cf. WJ 830   Testis; WP 320   Ovary; WJ 875   Androgens; WP 522   Estrogens; WK
         515   Pituitary gonadotropins; WP 530   Corpus luteum hormones.

920   Placental hormones

WL

NERVOUS SYSTEM

Classify general works on the nervous system and its diseases in WS 340 when related to children; in WY 160.5 when related to nursing. Classify works on nursing of patients with specific diseases in WY also.

WL 1–203	General
WL 300–405	Central Nervous System
WL 500–544	Peripheral Nerves
WL 600–610	Autonomic Nervous System
WL 700–710	Sense Organs

GENERAL

* 1   Societies (Cutter from name of society)
      Includes ephemeral membership lists issued serially or separately. Classify substantial lists with directories. Classify annual reports, journals, etc. in W1.

      Collections (General)
5   By several authors
7   By individual authors

9   Addresses. Essays. Lectures (General)

11   History (Table G)
11.1   General coverage (Not Table G)

* 13   Dictionaries. Encyclopedias

* 15   Classification. Nomenclature. Terminology

* 16   Tables. Statistics

17   Atlases. Pictorial works
      Classify atlases limited to a particular part of the system here also.

18   Education
      Classify here works about education.

*NUMBER CAN BE USED FOR BOTH MONOGRAPHS AND SERIALS.

* 18.2   **Educational materials**
Classify here educational materials, e.g., outlines, questions and answers, programmed instruction, catalogs, computer–assisted instruction, etc., regardless of format. Classify textbooks, regardless of format, by subject.

* 19   **Schools, departments, and faculties of neurology**

20   **Research (General)**
Classify here works about research in general. Classify works about research on a particular subject by subject.

21   **Neurology as a profession. Ethics. Peer review**

* 22   **Directories (Table G)**
* 22.1   **General coverage (Not Table G)**

    Laboratories, institutes, etc.
23   **Collective**
24   **Individual (Cutter from name of agency)**

25   **Laboratory manuals. Technique**

26   **Equipment and supplies**
e.g., For electroencephalography
Classify catalogs in W 26.

26.5   **Medical informatics. Automatic data processing. Computers (General)**
Classify works on use for special subjects by subject.

    Hospitals, clinics, dispensaries, etc.
27   **Collective (Table G)**
27.1   **General coverage (Not Table G)**
28   **Individual (Table G)**

30   **Administration of services**
e.g., Services for the epileptic

* 32   **Laws (Table G)**
* 32.1   **General coverage (Not Table G)**

* 33   **Discussion of law (Table G)**
* 33.1   **General coverage (Not Table G)**

* 39   **Handbooks. Resource guides**

*NUMBER CAN BE USED FOR BOTH MONOGRAPHS AND SERIALS.

100   **General works**
Classify works on specialty and on the specialty and diseases here. Classify works on diseases alone in WL 140.

101   **Anatomy. Histology. Embryology. Abnormalities (General)**

102   **Physiology (General)**

102.5   **Neurons**

102.7   **Motor neurons**

102.8   **Synapses**

102.9   **Nerve endings**

103   **Psychophysiology (General)**
Classify works on specific topics by subject. See MeSH tree structure F2 and Index to this Classification.

103.5   **Neuropsychology**

103.7   **Psychoneuroimmunology**

104   **Neurochemistry**

105   **Neuroendocrinology**

106   **Reflexes**
Classify works on conditioned reflexes, etc., in BF 319–319.5.

108   **Physiology of sleep**
Classify works on disorders of sleep WM 188.

140   **Nervous system diseases (General)**

141   **Neurologic examination. Diagnostic principles. Radiography of the brain**
e.g., Ventriculography
Classify works on pediatric neuroradiography in WS 340.

150   **Electroencephalography. Monitoring (General)**

154   **Echoencephalography**

160   **Nervous system neoplasms (General)**

200   **Meninges. Blood–brain barrier**
         Classify works on listeria meningitis in WC 242; on meningococcal meningitis in
         WC 245; on viral meningitis in WC 540.

203   **Cerebrospinal fluid**
         Cf. QY 220 Clinical analysis; WB 377 Spinal, cisternal and ventricular puncture.

CENTRAL NERVOUS SYSTEM

300   **General works (Include works on brain alone)**
         Cf. WL 348 Brain diseases. Classify works on diagnosis in WL 141 General;
         WL 150 Electroencephalography; WL 154 Echoencephalography; WL 405
         Myelography or in a specific number for the disorder.

302   **Cerebrovascular circulation**
         Cf. WG 595.C37 Cerebral arteries.

307   **Cerebrum. Cerebral cortex. Telencephalon**
         Classify here works on basal ganglia, corpus callosum and cerebral ventricles.

310   **Brain stem**

312   **Diencephalon. Thalamus**

314   **Limbic system**

320   **Cerebellum**

330   **Cranial nerves (General or not elsewhere classified)**

335   **Localization of function. Cerebral dominance. Brain mapping**

340   **Neurologic manifestations (General or not elsewhere classified)**
         Cf. WL 390 Movement disorders; WW 460 Neurologic manifestations of eye disease.

Neurologic manifestations – Continued

340.2 **Communication disorders. Speech–language pathology**
Classify here all works on communication disorders except those of psychogenic origins. Classify communication disorders of psychogenic origins in WM 475–475.6.

340.5 **Aphasia**
Classify works on aphasia of psychogenic origin in WM 475.5.

340.6 **Dyslexia**
Classify works on dyslexia of psychogenic origin in WM 475.6.

341 **Consciousness. Unconsciousness**

342 **Headache**

344 **Migraine and other vascular headaches**

346 **Paralysis (General or not elsewhere classified)**

348 **Diseases of the brain**

350 **Congenital (General or not elsewhere classified)**

351 **Inflammatory**
e.g., Abscess. Encephalitis. Encephalomyelitis
Cf. WC 542 Epidemic encephalitis.

354 **Traumatic**
e.g., Concussion. Skull fracture. Brain damage

355 **Cerebrovascular disorders**
e.g., Cerebral hemorrhage

358 **Neoplasms of the brain and of the central nervous system in general**

359 **Degenerative**
e.g., Parkinsonism

360 **Multiple sclerosis**

362 **Kernicterus**

368   **Brain surgery. Neurosurgery (General)**
          Classify works on sympathectomy in WL 610.

370   **Psychosurgery**

385   **Epilepsy**

390   **Movement disorders (General or not elsewhere classified)**
          Classify works on muscular diseases in WE 550–559; on psychomotor disorders in
          WM 197.

400   **Spinal cord. Spinal nerves (General or not elsewhere classified). Nerve roots. Pyramidal tracts**

405   **Myelography**

PERIPHERAL NERVES

500   **General works**
          Cf. WL 330 Cranial nerves; WL 400 Spinal nerves.

544   **Neuritis. Neuralgia**

AUTONOMIC NERVOUS SYSTEM

600   **General works**
          Classify here works on specific autonomic nerve groups, not included below.

610   **Sympathetic nervous system. Parasympathetic nervous system**
          Classify works on cranial nerves in WL 330.

SENSE ORGANS

700   **General works**
          Classify works on specific sense organs with the system involved.

702   **Psychophysics. Sensation (General)**
          Do not confuse with psychophysiology WL 103.

704   **Pain**
Classify works on individual sense organ and/or pain relating to it with the organ.

705   **Perception. Perceptual distortion**
Classify works on psychological aspects of perception in BF 311. Classify works on perceptual distortion and disorders associated with psychoses in WM 204. Classify works on visual perception in WW 105; on auditory perception in WV 272, etc.

710   **Sensation disorders (General or not elsewhere classified)**
Cf. WR 280 for sensory disorders of the skin.

WM

PSYCHIATRY

Classify material on medicolegal psychiatry in W 740; on child psychiatry in WS 350; on adolescent psychiatry in WS 463; on geriatric psychiatry in WT 150; on psychiatric nursing in general and on specific diseases in WY 160. Classify in WM, however, works on specific mental disorders of childhood, adolescence, or old age unless specifically instructed to do otherwise.

* 1   **Societies (Cutter from name of society)**
       Includes ephermeral membership lists issued serially or separately. Classify substantial lists with directories. Classify annual reports, journals, etc., in W1.

       Collections (General)
5   **By several authors**
7   **By individual authors**

9   **Addresses. Essays. Lectures (General)**

11   **History (Table G)**
11.1   **General coverage (Not Table G)**

* 13   **Dictionaries. Encyclopedias**

* 15   **Classification. Nomenclature. Terminology**

* 16   **Tables. Statistics**

17   **Atlases. Pictorial works**

18   **Education**
       Classify here works about education.

* 18.2   **Educational materials**
       Classify here educational materials, e.g., outlines, questions and answers, programmed instruction, catalogs, computer–assisted instruction, etc., regardless of format. Classify textbooks, regardless of format, by subject.

* 19   **Schools and colleges**
       Classify courses of study, catalogs, etc., in W 19.5.

*NUMBER CAN BE USED FOR BOTH MONOGRAPHS AND SERIALS.

19.5	Graduate and continuing education in psychiatry (including fellowships, internships, residencies, etc.)

20   **Research (General)**
Classify here works about research in general. Classify works about research on a particular subject by subject.

21   **Psychiatry, psychoanalysis, etc. as professions. Careers in mental health. Types of practice. Peer review**
Classify works for and about psychiatric aides in WY 160.

* 22   **Directories (Table G)**
* 22.1   **General coverage (Not Table G)**

Laboratories, institutes, etc.
23   **Collective**
24   **Individual (Cutter form name of agency)**

25   **Techniques in experimental psychiatry**

26   **Equipment and supplies**
Classify catalogs in W 26.

26.5   **Medical informatics. Automatic data processing. Computers (General)**
Classify works on use for special subject by subject.

Hospitals, clinics, dispensaries, etc.
Classify works limited to psychiatric hospitals for children in WS 27–28.
27   **Collective (Table G)**
27.1   **General coverage (Not Table G)**
28   **Individual (Table G)**

29   **Community mental health centers. Rehabilitation centers. Halfway houses. Sheltered workshops. Aftercare. Day care (Table G)**
29.1   **General coverage (Not Table G)**

29.5   **Patients. Attitude and compliance. Satisfaction**

30   **Administrative psychiatry**
e.g., Management of hospitals, etc. Supervision of students. Mental health services
Cf. WM 401 for general works on crisis intervention; WA 305 for special population groups.

30.5   **Psychiatric social work**

30.6   Community psychiatry (General)

31   Socioeconomic and environmental factors in mental illness

31.5   Preventive measures in psychiatry

* 32   Laws (Table G)
                e.g., Commitment
                Cf. W 740 Forensic psychiatry.
* 32.1   General coverage (Not Table G)
                Include international law.

* 33   Discussion of law (Table G)
* 33.1   General coverage (Not Table G)

* 34   Handbooks. Resource guides

35   Practices in the care of the mentally ill
                e.g., Ward attendance. Use of restraints. Technique of home care
                Cf. WY 160 Psychiatric nursing.

40   Case histories (General)
                *Classify here case books, biographies and autobiographies of the mentally ill. Classify
                case histories limited to one disease with the disease. Classify works on famous
                persons in WZ 313.*

49   Art and literature as related to psychiatry. Symbolic case histories
                e.g., Electra, Hamlet, Oedipus, Don Juan, etc.

55   Counseling on psychological problems

61   Pastoral care

62   Social relations of the psychiatrist (including relations with patients; relations
                with public, clubs, societies, etc.) Attitude. Ethics

64   Referral and consultation (General)

75   Popular works (General)

90   Psychophysiologic disorders (General) Psychosomatic medicine (General
                works about the profession)
                Classify general works on psychophysiologic sex disorders in WM 611.

*NUMBER CAN BE USED FOR BOTH MONOGRAPHS AND SERIALS.

100   **General works**
> *Classify works on specialty and on the specialty and diseases here. Classify works on diseases alone in WM 140.*

102   **Biological psychiatry**

105   **Clinical psychology. Mental health**
> *Classify popular works in WM 75. Classify works on counseling in WM 55.*

140   **Mental disorders (General)**

141   **Psychiatric examination and diagnosis**

145   **Psychological tests (General or not elsewhere classified)**
> *Classify works on intelligence tests in BF 431–432.5.*

145.5   **Specific tests, A–Z**

.B4	**Bender–Gestalt test**
.C3	**Cattell personality factor questionnaire**
.I5	**Ink blot tests**
.M6	**MMPI**
.N4	**Neuropsychological tests**
.P8	**Projective techniques**
.R7	**Rorschach tests**
.R8	**Rosenzweig picture–frustration study**
.S9	**Szondi test**
.T3	**Thematic apperception test**
.W9	**Word association tests**

165   **Behavioral symptoms (General or not elsewhere classified)**
> *Classify here works on behavioral symptoms for which there are no classification numbers for related disorders. Classify specific symptoms with related disorders, e.g., Anxiety with Anxiety disorders in WM 172; Depression with Depressive disorder in WM 171.*

170   **Neuroses**

171   **Affective symptoms**
> *Include works on depression and depressive disorder here. Cf. WM 207 Manic depressive psychoses.*

172   **Anxiety. Anxiety disorders**

173   **Hysteria and associated disorders**

Neuroses
    Hysteria and associated disorders – Continued

173.5   **Conversion disorder**

173.6   **Dissociative disorders**

173.7   **Amnesia and other memory disorders**

174   **Neurasthenia. Mental fatigue**

175   **Eating disorders associated with neuroses. Anorexia nervosa**
        Cf. WI 143 for eating disorders in general; WS 115–130 for disorders of children and infants.

176   **Obsessive–compulsive neuroses. Compulsive behavior. Obsessive behavior**

178   **Phobic disorders. Hypochondriasis. Sick role**
        Classify works on sick role associated with a particular disease with the disease.

184   **Combat disorders**

188   **Sleep disorders and associated conditions**
        Classify here material on all disorders of sleep regardless of severity. Include popular works. Cf. WL 108 Physiology of sleep.

190   **Personality disorders (General or not elsewhere classified)**
        e.g., Inadequate personality. Passive–dependent personality

193   **Defense mechanisms**
        Cf. WM 173.5 Conversion reaction; WS 350.8.D3 Defense mechanism in children. Classify works on purely psychological aspects of various defense mechanisms in appropriate BF numbers.

193.5   **Special topics, A–Z**

        .A2   **Acting out**
        .D3   **Denial (Psychology)**
        .D5   **Displacement (Psychology)**
        .P3   **Perceptual defense**
        .P7   **Projection**
        .R1   **Rationalization**
        .R2   **Regression**
        .R4   **Repression**
        .S8   **Sublimation. Fantasy**

197   **Psychomotor disorders (General or not elsewhere classified)**
        Classify specific disorders by subject, e.g., Apraxia WL 340.

200   **Psychoses**

202   **Functional**

203   **Schizophrenia and schizophrenic syndromes**

203.5   **Autistic disorder**

204   **Cognition and perceptual disorders associated with psychoses**

205   **Paranoid disorders**

207   **Manic–depressive psychoses and affective syndromes**
        Classify works on reactive depression and on non-psychotic affective symptoms
        in WM 171.

[210]   **[This number not used]**
        Classify works on antisocial personality in WM 190.

220   **Organic (General or not elsewhere classified)**
        e.g., Psychoses associated with infections, convulsive disorders, neurologic
        disorders

270   **Substance–related disorders**
        e.g., Substance dependence.   Substance abuse

274   **Alcohol**

276   **Cannabis**

280   **Cocaine**

284   **Narcotics**

286   **Opium alkaloids**

288   **Heroin**

290   **Nicotine**

300   **Mental retardation.   Down syndrome**
Classify works on mental retardation of children WS 107; on education of the mentally retarded in LC 4601–4640.5.

302   **Case studies.   Biographical accounts**

304   **Evaluation.   Prognosis**

307   **Special problems, A–Z**

      .C6   **Communication**
      .M5   **Mental disorders**
      .S3   **Sex problems (General)**
      .S6   **Social problems (General)**

308   **Rehabilitation and training (General)**

400   **Therapy**
Cf. WL 370 Psychosurgery.

401   **Emergency psychiatric services.   Crisis intervention (including work with victims of rape and other crimes)**
Classify works on community mental health programs in WM 30.

402   **Drug therapy**

405   **Physical therapy (General or not elsewhere classified)**
e.g., Induced hyperthermia

410   **Shock.   Insulin shock therapy**

412   **Electric.   Electronarcosis**

415   **Hypnosis**

420   **Psychotherapy (General or not elsewhere classified)**
Classify works on psychotherapy in childhood in WS 350.2, in adolescence in WS 463, and in old age in WT 150.

420.5   **Special types, A–Z**

      .A2   **Abreaction.   Catharsis**
      .G3   **Gestalt therapy**

Therapy
  Psychotherapy
   Special types, A-Z – Continued

	.I3	Imagery (Psychotherapy)
	.N8	Nondirective therapy
	.P5	Psychotherapy, Brief
	.P7	Psychotherapy, Multiple
	.P8	Psychotherapy, Rational–Emotive

425	Behavior therapy

425.5	Special types, A–Z

	.A9	Aversive therapy
	.B6	Biofeedback (Psychology)
	.C6	Cognitive therapy
	.D4	Desensitization, Psychologic. Implosive therapy
	.R3	Relaxation techniques

426	Self–help groups

428	Socioenvironmental therapy

430	Group psychotherapy

430.5	Special types, A–Z

	.F2	Family therapy
	.H2	Disabled
	.M3	Marital therapy
	.P8	Psychodrama
	.S3	Sensitivity training groups. Encounter groups

Cf. HM 134 for general sociological works.

440	Milieu therapy. Therapeutic community

445	Residential treatment (General)

450	Activity therapy

450.5	Special types, A–Z	
	.A8	Art therapy
	.B5	Bibliotherapy
	.D2	Dance therapy
	.M8	Music therapy
	.O2	Occupational therapy
	.P5	Photography
	.V5	Videotherapy
	.W9	Writing

Therapy – Continued

460   Psychoanalysis.   Psychoanalytic theory

460.5   Special topics associated with psychoanalysis, psychoanalytic therapy or interpretation, A–Z

.B7   Bonding, Human–Pet
.C5   Communication
.C7   Creativeness
.D8   Dreams. Symbolism
.E3   Ego. Self
.E8   Existentialism. Logotherapy
.E9   Extraversion. Introversion
.F8   Free association
.I4   Identification
.I5   Individuation
.L2   Language
.M5   Memory
.M6   Motivation
.O2   Object attachment
.P3   Personality
.P5   Pleasure–pain principle
.P7   Political systems
.R2   Reinforcement
.R3   Religion. Church. Morals. Superego
.S3   Sex
.U6   Unconscious. Id
.W6   Women

460.6   Psychoanalytic therapy

460.7   Psychoanalytic interpretation

475   Communication disorders. Speech–language pathology
Classify works on communication disorders of neurologic origins in WL 340.2.

475.5   Aphasia
Classify works on aphasia of neurologic origin in WL 340.5.

475.6   Dyslexia
Classify works on dyslexia of neurologic origin in WL 340.6.

600   Social behavior disorders (General)
Cf. WS 350.8.S6 for works about children.

610   Paraphilias
e.g., Sadism. Fetishism. Transvestitism. Exhibitionism. Pedophilia

611   **Psychosexual dysfunctions (General or not elsewhere classified)**
        Cf. WJ 712   Sex differentiation disorders;   WP 610   Female sexual adjustment.

WN

RADIOLOGY. DIAGNOSTIC IMAGING

Classify material on ionizing radiation used in the diagnosis and treatment of a specific disease, organ or system with the disease, organ or system. General diagnostic uses of ultrasound and magnetic resonance imaging are included here. Classify material on non-ionizing radiation in WB or other applicable numbers (See Index to this Classification).

WN 1–160	**General**
WN 180–240	**Diagnostic imaging. Radiography**
WN 250–250.5	**Radiotherapy**
WN 300–340	**Radium**
WN 415–665	**Radioactivity (Excluding Roentgen Rays and Radium)**

GENERAL

* 1   **Societies (Cutter from name of society)**
Includes ephemeral membership lists issued serially or separately. Classify substantial lists with directories. Classify annual reports, journals, etc., in W1.

Collections (General)
5   **By several authors**
7   **By individual authors**

9   **Addresses. Essays. Lectures (General)**

11   **History (Table G)**
11.1   **General coverage (Not Table G)**

* 13   **Dictionaries. Encyclopedias**

* 15   **Classification. Nomenclature. Terminology**

* 16   **Tables. Statistics**

17   **Atlases. Pictorial works**
Classify atlases limited to a particular radiological subject here also.

18   **Education**
         Classify here works about education.

* 18.2   **Educational materials**
         Classify here educational materials, e.g., outlines, questions and answers, programmed instruction, catalogs, computer–assisted instruction, etc., regardless of format. Classify textbooks, regardless of format, by subject.

* 19   **Schools and colleges**
         Classify courses of study, catalogs, etc., in W 19.5.

20   **Research (General)**
         Classify here works about research in general. Classify works about research on a particular subject by subject.

21   **Radiology, diagnostic imaging and nuclear medicine as professions. Ethics. Peer review**

* 22   **Directories (Table G)**
* 22.1   **General coverage (Not Table G)**

     Radiological laboratories, institutes, etc.
23   **Collective**
24   **Individual (Cutter from name of agency)**

25   **Laboratory manuals. Technique**

[26]   **[This number not used]**
         Classify works on equipment in WN 150; catalogs of equipment in W 26.

26.5   **Medical informatics. Automatic data processing. Computers (General)**
         Classify works on use for special subjects by subject.

     Hospitals, clinics, etc.
27   **Collective (Table G)**
27.1   **General coverage (Not Table G)**
28   **Individual (Table G)**

* 32   **Laws (Table G)**
* 32.1   **General coverage (Not Table G)**

* 33   **Discussion of law (Table G)**
* 33.1   **General coverage (Not Table G)**

* 39   **Handbooks. Resource guides**

100   **General works. Stereoscopy. Electrokymography**

105   **Ionizing radiation**

110   **Health physics**
         Include here works on the physics of radiation and nuclear medicine.

150   **Equipment and supplies**
         e.g., Film. Screens. Generators. Radiation counters
         Classify works on use of counters, etc., in radiation protection in WN 650. Classify
         catalogs in W 26.

160   **Technology. Contrast media**
         e.g., Positioning
         Classify works on contrast media for particular types of radiography with the specific
         type. Classify works on laboratory techniques in WN 25.

DIAGNOSTIC IMAGING. RADIOGRAPHY

Classify works on diagnosis of a system, region or organ with the specific area.

180   **Diagnostic imaging (General or not elsewhere classified)**

185   **Magnetic resonance imaging**

200   **Radiography (General or not elsewhere classified)**

203   **Radionuclide imaging**

205   **Thermography**

206   **Tomography**

208   **Ultrasonography**

210   **Foreign body localization**

220   **Fluoroscopy**

230   **Dental diagnostic imaging**

240   Pediatric diagnostic imaging

RADIOTHERAPY

250   General works

250.5   Special types, A–Z
           .B7   Brachytherapy
           .R2   Radiotherapy, Computer–assisted
           .R3   Radiotherapy, High–energy
           .X7   X–ray therapy

RADIUM

300   General works

340   Therapeutic use
           e.g., Use of radon seeds, radium needles, etc.

RADIOACTIVITY (EXCLUDING ROENTGEN RAYS AND RADIUM)

Classify here works on specific elements as well as general works. Classify works on medical applications for a specific disease or organ with the disease or organ.

415   General works (On nuclear physics, atomic energy, radioisotopes slanted toward the biological sciences)
           Classify works slanted toward the physical sciences in QC.

420   Radioisotopes. Radioactive elements
           Classify works on medical applications in WN 440–450.

440   Nuclear medicine

445   Diagnosis
           Classify works on radionuclide imaging in WN 203.

450   Therapeutics

600   **Radiobiology. Radiologic health**
Classify here works on general effects of radiation to man, animals, and plant life.

610   **Radiation injuries**
Classify general works on radiation–induced abnormalities in QS 681.

612   **Food contamination**

615   **Air, soil, and water pollution and pollutants (General)**
Classify general works on air pollution in WA 754; on industrial air pollution in WA 450; on soil pollution in WA 785; on water pollution in WA 689.

620   **Injurious effects on man and animals**

630   **Injurious effects on plant life (related to human ecology)**

650   **Radiation protection**
Cf. WA 788 Industrial wastes.

660   **Radiometry**

665   **Radiation dosage**

WO

SURGERY

Note form numbers used also under Anesthesia WO 201–233.1.

WO 1–75	General
WO 100–149	General Surgery
WO 162–198	Surgical Procedure and Armamentarium
WO 200–460	Anesthesia
WO 500–517	Operative Surgery and Surgical Techniques
WO 600–640	Plastic Surgery
WO 660–690	Transplantation
WO 700–820	Traumatic, Industrial, and Emergency Surgery
WO 925–950	Surgery in Special Age Groups

GENERAL

* 1   **Societies (Cutter from name of society)**
    Includes ephemeral membership lists issued serially or separately.   Classify substantial lists with directories.   Classify annual reports, journals, etc., in W1.

    Collections (General)
5   **By authors**
7   **By individual authors**

9   **Addresses.   Essays.   Lectures (General)**

11   **History (Table G)**
11.1   **General coverage (Not Table G)**

* 13   **Dictionaries.   Encyclopedias**

* 15   **Classification.   Nomenclature.   Terminology**

* 16   **Tables.   Statistics.   Collected surgical case reports (General)**

[17]   **[This number not used]**
    Classify atlases in WO 517.

18   **Education**
Classify here works about education.

* 18.2   **Educational materials**
Classify here educational materials, e.g., outlines, questions and answers, programmed instruction, catalogs, computer–assisted instruction, etc., regardless of format. Classify textbooks, regardless of format, by subject.

* 19   **Schools, departments, and faculties of surgery**

20   **Research (General)**
Classify here works about research in general. Classify works about research on a particular subject by subject. Cf. WO 50 Experimental surgery.

21   **Surgery as a profession. Ethics. Peer review**

* 22   **Directories (Table G)**
* 22.1   **General coverage (Not Table G)**

     Laboratories, research institutes, organ banks, etc.
23   **Collective**
24   **Individual (Cutter from name of agency)**

[25]   **[This number not used]**
Classify laboratory manuals in WO 500–512, etc.

[26]   **[This number not used]**
Classify material on surgical instruments and equipment in WO 162; on instruments and equipment used in anesthesia in WO 240; catalogs in W 26.

     Hospitals, clinics, dispensaries, etc.
27   **Collective (Table G)**
27.1   **General coverage (Not Table G)**
28   **Individual (Table G)**

* 32   **Laws (Table G)**
* 32.1   **General coverage (Not Table G)**

* 33   **Discussion of law (Table G)**
* 33.1   **General coverage (Not Table G)**

* 39   **Handbooks. Resource guides**

50   **Experimental surgery (General)**
Classify works on experimental work in a particular area by subject. Classify works about research in WO 20.

*NUMBER CAN BE USED FOR BOTH MONOGRAPHS AND SERIALS.

62   Social relations of the surgeon (including relations with patients, relations with public, clubs, societies, etc.). Attitude

64   Referral and consultation (General)

75   Popular works (General)

GENERAL SURGERY

100   General works
        Cf. WF 980 Thoracic surgery; WI 900 Abdominal surgery; WO 500 Operative surgery.

101   Surgical anatomy

102   Physiology

113   Antisepsis. Sterilization. Asepsis

140   Surgical diseases (General)
        Classify here works that discuss diagnosis, prognosis, treatment. Classify works limited to pathology in WO 142 below.

141   Surgical examination. Surgical diagnosis. Exploratory surgery

142   Surgical pathology (Examination of tissues or organs removed in course of surgery. Examination of biopsy or frozen section material, etc.)
        Cf. WO 140 Surgical diseases.

149   Surgical shock

SURGICAL PROCEDURE AND ARMAMENTARIUM

162   Surgical equipment, instruments and other supplies
        Classify catalogs in W 26. Cf. WO 240 for equipment used in anesthesia.

166   Sutures. Ligatures. Tissue adhesives

167   Surgical dressing. Bandaging technique. Adhesive plaster

Surgical equipment, instruments and other supplies
Surgical dressing. Bandaging technique. Adhesive plaster - Continued

170   Surgical casts

176   Artificial organs
           Classify works on specific organs in the surgery number or lacking that, in the general number for the organ being replaced. Cf. WG 169.5 Artificial heart; WJ 378 Artificial kidney.

178   Principles of surgical care

179   Preoperative care

181   Intraoperative Care

183   Postoperative Care

184   Postoperative complications and treatment

185   Surgical wounds. Surgical wound infection. Wound healing (including healing of non–surgical wounds)

188   Closure of wounds. Drainage

192   Minor surgery. Ambulatory surgery (General)

198   Electrosurgery. Cautery. Laser and electrocoagulation (General)
           Classify works on use in particular fields with the field or the condition, e.g., in ophthalmology WW 168.

ANESTHESIA

200   Surgical anesthesia. Analgesia (General)
           Do not confuse with general anesthesia WO 275.

* 201   Societies (Cutter from name of society)
           Includes ephemeral membership lists issued serially or separately. Classify substantial lists with directories. Classify annual reports, journals, etc., in W1.

           Collections (General)
205   By several authors
207   By individual authors

209   Addresses. Essays. Lectures (General)

*NUMBER CAN BE USED FOR BOTH MONOGRAPHS AND SERIALS.

| 211 | History (Table G) |
| 211.1 | General coverage (Not Table G) |

* 213   **Dictionaries. Encyclopedias**

* 215   **Classification. Nomenclature. Terminology**

218   **Education**
Classify here works about education.

* 218.2   **Educational materials**
Classify here educational materials, e.g., outlines, questions and answers, programmed instruction, catalogs, computer–assisted instruction, etc., regardless of format. Classify textbooks, regardless of format, by subject.

* 219   **Schools, departments, and faculties of anesthesiology**

220   **Research (General)**
Classify here works about research in general. Classify works about research on a particular subject by subject.

221   **Anesthesiology as a profession. Ethics. Peer review**

* 222   **Directories (Table G)**
* 222.1   **General coverage (Not Table G)**

[226]   **[This number not used]**
Classify equipment and supplies for anesthesia in WO 240; catalogs in W 26. Cf. WO 162 Surgical equipment.

* 231   **Handbooks. Resource guides**

* 232   **Laws (Table G)**
* 232.1   **General coverage (Not Table G)**

* 233   **Discussion of law (Table G)**
* 233.1   **General coverage (Not Table G)**

234   **Preanesthetic medication. Preparation of patient**

235   **Choice of anesthesia**
Classify works on choice of anesthesia for patients with cardiac problems in WG 460.

240 **Equipment and supplies**
Classify catalogs in W 26. Cf. WO 162 Surgical equipment.

245 **Accidents. Complications**
e.g., Laryngospasm. Cardiac failure. Vomiting
Classify works written for the cardiologist in WG 460.

250 **Asphyxia. Methods of resuscitation**
Classify here general works on asphyxia and resuscitation. Classify works on first aid in WA 292; on resuscitation of the newborn in WQ 450.

275 **General anesthesia**

277 **Inhalation anesthesia**

280 **Intratracheal anesthesia. Technique of intubation**

285 **Intravenous**

290 **Rectal**

297 **Muscle relaxants and tranquilizing agents in conjunction with anesthesia and analgesia**

300 **Conduction anesthesia**
e.g., Regional anesthesia or local anesthesia

305 **Spinal. Epidural**

340 **Infiltration and topical**

350 **Induced hypothermia, and related topics**

375 **Diagnostic and therapeutic anesthetic procedures**
e.g., Nerve block

440 **Pediatric anesthesia**

445 **Geriatric anesthesia**

450 **Obstetrical anesthesia**

460   Anesthesia in dentistry.   Dental hypnosis

OPERATIVE SURGERY AND SURGICAL TECHNIQUES

500   **General works**
Classify works on abdominal surgery in WI 900; on thoracic surgery in WF 980; on general surgery in WO 100.

505   **Endoscopic surgery**

510   **Cryosurgery**

511   **Laser surgery**

512   **Microsurgery**

517   **Atlases.   Pictorial works**
Classify all types of surgical atlases in this number, except those relating to a particular body system or part.   Classify the latter by system.

PLASTIC SURGERY

600   **General works**
Classify material on plastic surgery of a condition, e.g., burns, with the condition. Classify material on plastic surgery of a region, system or organ with the area covered, e.g., plastic surgery of the nose, in WV 312.

610   **Skin transplantation, tube grafts, etc.**

640   **Prosthesis in plastic surgery**
Cf. WO 176   Artificial organs (General).

TRANSPLANTATION

660   **General works**
Classify works on specific organs in the surgery number or lacking that, in the general number for the organ being replaced.   Classify general works on artificial organs in WO 176.

665   **Tissue preservation**

680   **Immunology**
           Classify works on immunosuppressive agents in QW 920.

690   **Legal, ethical, and religious aspects**
           Classify the text of laws in WO 32.

TRAUMATIC, INDUSTRIAL, AND EMERGENCY SURGERY

700   **General works**

704   **Burns**

800   **Military surgery**

807   **Gunshot wounds**

820   **Blast injuries**

SURGERY IN SPECIAL AGE GROUPS

925   **Pediatric surgery**
           Classify works on pediatric anesthesia in WO 440; on surgery of individual organs in WS 260–360.

950   **Geriatric surgery**
           Classify works on geriatric anesthesia in WO 445

WP

GYNECOLOGY

Classify general works on pediatric gynecology in WS 360; on gynecological nursing and nursing of gynecological diseases in WY 156.7. Classify works on male and female reproductive organs treated together in WJ 700–702; on human reproduction inWQ 205, etc.

WP 1–390	General
WP 400–480	Uterus and Cervix Uteri
WP 505–660	Physiology and Functional Disorders
WP 800–910	Breast

GENERAL

* 1   **Societies (Cutter from name of society)**
Includes ephemeral membership lists issued serially or separately. Classify substantial lists with directories. Classify annual reports, journals, etc., in W1.

Collections (General)
5   **By several authors**
7   **By individual authors**

9   **Addresses. Essays. Lectures (General)**

11   **History (Table G)**
11.1   **General coverage (Not Table G)**

* 13   **Dictionaries. Encyclopedias**

* 15   **Classification. Nomenclature. Terminology**

* 16   **Statistics. Tables**

17   **Atlases. Pictorial works**
Classify here also atlases on specific organs.

18   **Education**
Classify here works about education.

* 18.2 **Educational materials**
Classify here educational materials, e.g., outlines, questions and answers, programmed instruction, catalogs, computer–assisted instruction, etc., regardless of format. Classify textbooks, regardless of format, by subject.

* 19 **Schools, departments, and faculties of gynecology**

20 **Research (General)**
Classify here works about research in general. Classify works about research on a particular subject by subject.

21 **Gynecology as a profession. Ethics. Peer review**

* 22 **Directories (Table G)**
* 22.1   **General coverage (Not Table G)**

    Laboratories, institutes, etc.
23   **Collective**
24   **Individual (Cutter from name of agency)**

25 **Laboratory manuals. Technique**

26 **Equipment and supplies**
Classify catalogs in W 26.

26.5 **Medical informatics. Automatic data processing. Computers (General)**
Classify works on use for special subjects by subject.

    Hospitals, dispensaries, clinics, etc.
27   **Collective (Table G)**
27.1   **General coverage (Not Table G)**
28   **Individual (Table G)**

* 32 **Laws (Table G)**
* 32.1   **General coverage (Not Table G)**

* 33 **Discussion of law (Table G)**
* 33.1   **General coverage (Not Table G)**

34 **Malpractice (Table G)**
34.1   **General coverage (Not Table G)**

* 39 **Handbooks. Resource guides**

*NUMBER CAN BE USED FOR BOTH MONOGRAPHS AND SERIALS.

| 100 | **General works** |
| | *Classify works on specialty and on the specialty and diseases here. Classify works on diseases alone in WP 140.* |

| 101 | **Anatomy** |

| 120 | **Popular works (General)** |

| 140 | **Diseases (General)** |

| 141 | **Examination. Diagnosis. Radiography. Monitoring** |

| 145 | **Neoplasms. Cysts (General)** |
| | *Classify works on neoplasms of specific organs with the organ.* |

| 150 | **Embryology. Congenital abnormalities** |

| 155 | **Pelvis. Pelvic inflammations** |

| 157 | **Gonorrhea in the female** |

| 160 | **Genital tuberculosis** |

| 170 | **Perineal injuries** |

| 180 | **Rectovaginal fistula. Vesicovaginal fistula** |

| 200 | **Vulva** |

| 250 | **Vagina** |

| 255 | **Vaginitis. Leukorrhea** |

| 258 | **Trichomonas vaginitis** |

| 275 | **Adnexa uteri** |

| 300 | **Fallopian tubes** |
| | *Classify works on tubal pregnancy in WQ 220.* |

Adnexa uteri - Continued

320   **Ovary**
Cf. WP 520 Endocrine functions of the ovaries.

322   **Neoplasms. Cysts**

390   **Endometriosis**

UTERUS AND CERVIX UTERI

400   **General works**

440   **Uterine diseases**

451   **Inflammations**

454   **Displacements. Prolapse**

458   **Neoplasms**

459   **Leiomyoma**

460   **Carcinoma. Sarcoma**

465   **Trophoblastic neoplasms**
e.g., Chorioadenoma. Hydatidiform mole

468   **Surgery (General)**

470   **Cervix uteri**

475   **Cervicitis**

480   **Neoplasms**

PHYSIOLOGY AND FUNCTIONAL DISORDERS

505   **Physiology (General)**

520   Endocrine functions of the ovaries

522   Estrogenic hormones, synthetic substitutes, and antagonists

530   Corpus luteum hormones and related compounds
           Classify works on progestational hormones here unless those produced by other organs are discussed exclusively.

540   Ovulation. Ovarian function. Menstrual cycle

550   Menstruation and its disorders

552   Amenorrhea. Hypomenorrhea. Oligomenorrhea

555   Menorrhagia. Metrorrhagia

560   Dysmenorrhea. Premenstrual tension

565   Fertility

570   Infertility (General). Infertility in the female
           Cf. WJ 709 Infertility in the male only.

580   Menopause

610   Problems of the female in sexual adjustment
           e.g., Dyspareunia. Frigidity

630   Contraception
           Classify works on religious and sociological aspects in HQ 763–766.5.

640   Contraceptive devices (General and female)
           Classify works only on male contraceptive devices in WJ 710. Classify works on contraceptive agents (chemical) in QV 177.

650   Gynecological therapy

660   Gynecological surgery
           Classify works on female sexual sterilization here. Classify works on surgery of particular organs with the organ.

BREAST

800   **General works**

815   **Examination. Diagnosis. Radiography**

825   **Functional changes**
           e.g., In pregnancy and lactation

840   **Diseases of the breast**

870   **Neoplasms**

900   **Therapy**
           Classify works on therapy of neoplasms in WP 870.

910   **Surgery**

WQ

OBSTETRICS

Classify works on obstetrical nursing in WY 157.

WQ 1–175	General
WQ 200–260	Pregnancy
WQ 300–330	Labor
WQ 400–450	Obstetrical Surgery
WQ 500–505	Puerperium

GENERAL

* 1   **Societies (Cutter from name of society)**
Includes ephemeral membership lists issued serially or separately. Classify substantial lists with directories. Classify annual reports, journals, etc., in W1.

       Collections (General)
5   **By several authors**
7   **By individual authors**

9   **Addresses. Essays. Lectures (General)**

11   **History (Table G)**
11.1   **General coverage (Not Table G)**

* 13   **Dictionaries. Encyclopedias**

* 15   **Classification. Nomenclature. Terminology**

* 16   **Tables. Statistics**

17   **Atlases. Pictorial works**
Classify atlases limited to a particular part of the system here also.

18   **Education**
Classify here works about education.

* 18.2   **Educational materials**
            *Classify here educational materials, e.g., outlines, questions and answers, programmed
            instruction, catalogs, computer–assisted instruction, etc., regardless of format.
            Classify textbooks, regardless of format, by subject.*

* 19   **Schools, departments, and faculties of obstetrics**

20   **Research (General)**
            *Classify here works about research in general.   Classify works about research on
            a particular subject by subject.*

21   **Obstetrics as a profession.   Ethics.   Peer review**

* 22   **Directories (Table G)**
* 22.1   **General coverage (Not Table G)**

            Clinics, dispensaries, etc.
23   **Collective (Table G)**
23.1   **General coverage (Not Table G)**
24   **Individual (Table G)**

25   **Laboratory manuals.   Technique**

26   **Equipment and supplies**
            Classify catalogs in W 26.

26.5   **Medical informatics.   Automatic data processing.   Computers (General)**
            Classify works on use for special subjects by subject.

            Maternity hospitals
27   **Collective (Table G)**
27.1   **General coverage (Not Table G)**
28   **Individual (Table G)**

* 32   **Laws (Table G)**
* 32.1   **General coverage (Not Table G)**

* 33   **Discussion of law (Table G)**
* 33.1   **General coverage (Not Table G)**

34   **Malpractice (Table G)**
34.1   **General coverage (Not Table G)**

* 39   **Handbooks.   Resource guides**

*NUMBER CAN BE USED FOR BOTH MONOGRAPHS AND SERIALS.

100	General works
150	Popular works on pregnancy and childbirth
152	Natural childbirth
155	Home childbirth
160	Midwifery
165	Manuals for midwives
175	Prenatal care

PREGNANCY

200	General works
202	Diagnosis *Cf. QY 335 Pregnancy tests.*
205	Fertilization. Development of ovum. General physiology of reproduction
206	Sex determination (Diagnostic)
208	Reproduction techniques e.g., Artificial insemination. Embryo transfer. Fertilization in vitro
209	Prenatal diagnosis. Fetal monitoring
210	Fetus. Fetal membranes. Umbilical cord. Perinatology (General) *Classify works on fetal experimentation in general in W 20.5.*
210.5	Fetal anatomy, physiology, and biochemistry
211	Fetal diseases (General or not elsewhere classified)
212	Placenta *Cf. WK 920 Placental hormones.*

215   **Toxemias**
         e.g., Eclampsia

220   **Ectopic pregnancy**

225   **Abortion.   Fetal death**
         Cf. WQ 440   Induced abortion; W 867   Criminal abortion.

235   **Multiple pregnancy**

240   **Pregnancy complications (General or not elsewhere classified)**
         Classify works on pregnancy toxemias in WQ 215.

244   **Cardiovascular complications**

248   **Diabetes**

252   **Hematologic complications**

256   **Infectious diseases**

260   **Urologic complications**

LABOR

300   **General works**

305   **Physiology.   Clinical course**

307   **Presentation**

310   **Dystocia**

320   **Disproportions of the pelvis**

330   **Complications of labor**
         e.g., Postpartum hemorrhage

OBSTETRICAL SURGERY

400   **General works**
Classify works on obstetrical anesthesia in WO 450.

415   **Delivery (including preparatory manipulation)**

425   **Use of forceps**

430   **Cesarean section. Symphysiotomy and similar techniques**

435   **Embryotomy**

440   **Induction of labor. Therapeutic abortion. Techniques of induced abortion**
Classify works on sociological and religious aspects of induced abortion in HQ 767–767.52.

450   **Resuscitation of the newborn**

PUERPERIUM

500   **General works. Postnatal care**

505   **Puerperal infection**

WR

DERMATOLOGY

Classify general works on dermatology in WS 260 when related to children; in WY 154.5 when related to nursing. Classify works on nursing of patients with specific skin diseases in the WY number also.

* 1   **Societies (Cutter from name of society)**
Includes ephemeral membership lists issued serially or separately. Classify substantial lists with directories. Classify annual reports, journals, etc., in W1.

Collections (General)
5   **By several authors**
7   **By individual authors**

9   **Addresses. Essays. Lectures (General)**

11   **History (Table G)**
11.1   **General coverage (Not Table G)**

* 13   **Dictionaries. Encyclopedias**

* 15   **Classification. Nomenclature. Terminology**

* 16   **Tables. Statistics**

17   **Atlases. Pictorial works**
Classify here also atlases on single skin diseases.

18   **Education**
Classify here works about education.

* 18.2   **Educational materials**
Classify here educational materials, e.g., outlines, questions and answers, programmed instruction, catalogs, computer-assisted instruction, etc., regardless of format. Classify textbooks, regardless of format, by subject.

* 19   **Schools, departments, and faculties of dermatology**

20   **Research (General)**
Classify here works about research in general. Classify works about research on a particular subject by subject.

*NUMBER CAN BE USED FOR BOTH MONOGRAPHS AND SERIALS.

21   Dermatology as a profession. Ethics. Peer review

* 22   Directories (Table G)
* 22.1   General coverage (Not Table G)

Laboratories, institutes, etc.
23   Collective
24   Individual (Cutter from name of agency)

25   Laboratory manuals. Technique

26   Equipment and supplies
      Classify catalogs in W 26.

26.5   Medical informatics. Automatic data processing. Computers (General)
      Classify works on use for special subjects by subject.

Hospitals, dispensaries, clinics, etc.
27   Collective (Table G)
27.1   General coverage (Not Table G)
28   Individual (Table G)

* 32   Laws (Table G)
* 32.1   General coverage (Not Table G)

* 33   Discussion of law (Table G)
* 33.1   General coverage (Not Table G)

* 39   Handbooks. Resource guides

100   General works
      *Classify works on specialty and on the specialty and diseases here. Classify works
      on diseases alone in WR 140.*

101   Anatomy. Histology. Embryology

102   Physiology. Chemistry and metabolism of the skin. Sensory functions.
      Skin temperature

105   Pathology

140   Skin diseases (General)

Skin diseases - Continued

141   **Diagnosis. Monitoring**

143   **Skin manifestations**

150   **Erythemas**
           e.g., E. multiforme. E. nodosum

152   **Lupus erythematosus**

160   **Diseases associated with hypersensitivity. Dermatitis**
           Cf. WD 300 for general works on hypersensitivity. Classify works on dermatitis
           herpetiformis in WR 200; on occupational dermatitis in WR 600; on neurodermatitis
           in WR 280.

165   **Drug eruptions**

170   **Urticaria. Angioneurotic edema**
           Classify works on urticaria pigmentosa in WR 267.

175   **Contact dermatitis**
           Cf. WR 600 Occupational dermatitis.

180   **Dermatitis exfoliativa**

190   **Eczema**

200   **Bullous skin diseases of obscure etiology**
           Classify works on erythema multiforme in WR 150.

204   **Papulosquamous dermatoses**
           Classify works on exfoliative dermatitis in WR 180; on seborrhea in WR 415.

205   **Psoriasis**

215   **Lichen planus**

218   **Genetic skin diseases (General or not elsewhere classified)**

220   **Infectious skin diseases (General, bacterial, or not elsewhere classified)**
           Classify works on viral skin infections in WC 570–590; parasitic skin diseases in
           WR 345.

225   **Impetigo. Ecthyma**

Infectious skin diseases - Continued

235   **Furunculosis. Carbuncle**

245   **Cutaneous tuberculosis**
           e.g., Lupus

260   **Scleroderma**

265   **Pigmentation disorders**
           e.g., Lentigo. Vitiligo

267   **Of metabolic origin**
           e.g., Hemochromatosis. Albinism

280   **Neurodermatitis and related sensory disorders**
           Classify works on causalgia in WL 544.

282   **Pruritus. Prurigo**

300   **Dermatomycoses**

310   **Tinea. Tinea pedis**

330   **Tinea capitis**

340   **Maduromycosis**

345   **Parasitic skin diseases (General or not elsewhere classified)**
           Classify works on mucocutaneous leishmaniasis in WR 350.

350   **Tropical diseases of the skin (General or not elsewhere classified)**
           e.g., Leishmaniasis
           Cf. WC 715 Visceral leishmaniasis.

360   **Skin diseases caused by arthropods (General or not elsewhere classified)**

365   **Scabies**

375   **Lice infestations**

390   **Skin appendages**

Skin appendages - Continued

400	Sweat glands. Disorders of the sweat glands
410	Sebaceous glands. Disorders of the sebaceous glands
415	Seborrhea
420	Epidermal cyst
430	Acne. Acneform lesions
450	Hair. Scalp. Diseases of the hair and scalp
455	Hypertrichosis
460	Alopecia
465	Care of the hair
475	Nails. Diseases of the nails
500	Neoplasms. Keratosis (General or not elsewhere classified)

598   **Decubitus ulcer and other skin ulcers**
          Classify works on leg ulcer in WE 850.

600   **Occupational dermatitis**
          Cf. WR 175   Contact dermatitis.

650   **Therapy of skin diseases**

660   **Radiotherapy**

WS

PEDIATRICS

Classify works on diseases of specific body systems in children in WS 260–368. Classify works on anatomy and physiology of the child in QS or QT. Classify pediatric works on topics other than body systems per se with the topic, e.g., surgery of the child in WO 925. Classify works on specific diseases with the disease, e.g., pneumonia in infants in WC 202; schizphrenia in childhood in WM 203, etc. Classify works on diseases limited to the newborn in WS 421; diseases limited to the premature infant in WS 410.

WS 1–141	General
WS 200–463	Diseases of Children
WS 260–368	By System
WS 405–463	By Age Group

GENERAL

* 1   **Societies (Cutter from name of society)**
      Includes ephemeral membership lists issued serially or separately. Classify substantial lists with directories. Classify annual reports, journal, etc., in W1.

      Collections (General)
5   **By several authors**
7   **By individual authors**

9   **Addresses. Essays. Lectures (General)**

11   **History (Table G)**
11.1   **General coverage (Not Table G)**

* 13   **Dictionaries. Encyclopedias**

* 15   **Classification. Nomenclature. Terminology**

* 16   **Tables (development, height, nutrition, weight, etc.) Statistics**

17   **Atlases. Pictorial works**
      Cf. QZ 17 for tissue pathology of disease.

18 **Education**
Classify here works about education.

* 18.2 **Educational materials**
Classify here educational materials, e.g., outlines, questions and answers, programmed instruction, catalogs, computer–assisted instruction, etc., regardless of format. Classify textbooks, regardless of format, by subject.

* 19 **Schools, departments, and faculties of pediatrics**

20 **Research (General)**
Classify here works about research in general. Classify works about research on a particular subject by subject.

21 **Pediatrics as a profession. Ethics. Peer review**

* 22 **Directories (Table G)**
* 22.1 **General coverage (Not Table G)**

Institutes
Classify here works on organizations which provide public or private services for disabled children which include medical, nursing and hygienic aspects, rehabilitation, etc. Cf. WA 320 for public health aspects.
23 **Collective (Table G)**
23.1 **General coverage (Not Table G)**
24 **Individual (Table G)**

25 **Laboratory manuals. Technique**

26 **Equipment and supplies**
e.g., Eating utensils for spastic children
Classify catalogs in W 26.

26.5 **Medical informatics. Automatic data processing. Computers (General)**
Classify works on use for special subjects by subject.

Hospitals, dispensaries, etc. (including psychiatric hospitals for children)
Classify here works on psychiatric hospitals for children only. Classify works on community mental health services for children in WM 30.
27 **Collective (Table G)**
27.1 **General coverage (Not Table G)**
28 **Individual (Table G)**

29 **Hospital staff manuals**

* 32 **Laws (Table G)**
* 32.1 **General coverage (Not Table G)**

*NUMBER CAN BE USED FOR BOTH MONOGRAPHS AND SERIALS.

Laws - Continued

* 33	Discussion of law (Table G)
* 33.1	General coverage (Not Table G)

* 39   Handbooks. Resource guides

100   **General works**
Classify works on specialty and on the specialty and diseases here. Classify works on diseases alone in WS 200.

103   **Normal physical growth and development**

104   **Growth disorders. Failure to thrive**

105   **Normal mental growth and development. Child psychology**
Classify works on psychophysiological aspects in WL, e.g., on physiology of sleep in WL 108; on laterality in WL 335; or with the system involved; on vision and visual perception in WW 103–105; on motor skills in WE 103–104.

105.5   **Special topics, A–Z**

.A8   **Attitudes and adjustments (to death, illness, divorce, etc.)**
.C3   **Child rearing (Psychological aspects)**
           Classify general works including physiological problems with child care in WS 113.
.C7   **Cognition. Fantasy. Imagination**
.C8   **Communication. Verbal behavior**
.D2   **Decision making. Logic. Thinking. Concept formation. Perception (Psychological)**
           Classify works on neurophysiological perception and specific types of perception in WL 705 or with the organ involved.
.D3   **Deprivation (economic, parental, etc.) and security**
.D8   **Dreams**
.E5   **Emotions. Frustrations, etc.**
.E8   **Evaluation of psychological development (General)**
.E9   **External influences (literature, motion pictures, television, war, etc.)**
.F2   **Family relations. Birth order. Only child. Twins. Parent–child relations. Father–child relations. Mother–child relations. Sibling relations, etc.**
.H2   **Disabled child (Psychological problems)**
.H7   **Hospitalized child**
           Cf. WA 310–320 Maternal and child welfare.
.I5   **Interpersonal relations (doctor, peer, stranger, etc.)**
           Cf. WS 105.5.S6 Race relations. Classify works on dentist's relation to the child in WU 480; on nurse's relation to the child in WY 159.

.M2   **Memory**
.M3   **Mental health**
           Classify works on school mental health in WA 352.
.M4   **Morals**
.M5   **Motivation**
.P3   **Personality development**

*NUMBER CAN BE USED FOR BOTH MONOGRAPHS AND SERIALS.

Normal mental growth and development. Child psychology
Special topics, A-Z - Continued

.P5	Play
.S3	Self
.S4	Sex behavior
.S6	Social behavior. Social problems. Race relations

        Cf. WS 105.5.I5 Interpersonal relations.

107   **The retarded child. Down syndrome**
        Classify other material on child psychiatry in WS 350; on education of the mentally retarded in LC 4601-4640.4; on adult mental retardation in WM 300.

107.5   **Special topics when related to the retarded child, A–Z**

.B4	Biochemistry. Genetics
.C2	Case studies. Biographical accounts
.C6	Communication
.D3	Development. Prognosis
.F6	Foster homes
.I4	Institutionalization

        Cf. WS 27–28 Hospitals; WS 105.5.H7 Hospitalized child (General).

.P7	Psychomotor problems
.P8	Psychosocial problems
.R3	Rehabilitation and training (General)
.R4	Relations with doctor, nurse, etc.
.R5	Relations with family. Family adjustment

110   **Learning disorders (physical, mental, and neurologic)**
        Classify works on specific disorders in appropriate numbers, e.g., Aphasia WL 340.5. Classify works for the educator in LC 4704.

113   **Care and training**
        Cf. WS 105.5.C3 for psychological aspects.

115   **Nutritional requirements. Nutrition disorders**

120   **In infancy**

125   **Breast feeding**

130   **In childhood**

135   **Prophylactic immunizations**

141   **Physical examination and diagnosis. Mass screening**
        Classify works on examination and diagnosis of specific age groups in WS 405–460.

DISEASES OF CHILDREN

Classify works on communicable diseases of children, not associated with a system, in the WC schedule.

200   General works

205   Pediatric emergencies

BY SYSTEM

In the numbers for each system, include general works on the diseases of the organs of the system or on special groups of diseases of the system. Classify works on surgery of a single organ here in WS, e.g., Gastrectomy of the child in WS 310. Classify works on surgery of a system with the system, e.g., Neurosurgery of the child in WL 368. Classify works on particular diseases with the disease except for the three disease numbers in WS 312, 322 and 342.

260   Skin

270   Musculoskeletal system

280   Respiratory system

290   Cardiovascular system

300   Hemic and lymphatic system

310   Digestive or gastrointestinal system

312   Diarrheal disorders

320   Urogenital system

322   Enuresis

330   Endocrine system

340   Nervous system

Nervous system - Continued

342   Cerebral palsy

350   Child psychiatry. Child guidance. Psychoses (General)
             Cf. WS 107 The retarded child. Classify works on specific disorders in WM.

350.2   Therapy
             Classify here works on all types of therapy for mental disorders of children. Classify therapy of a particular disorder with the disorder.

350.5   Psychoanalysis

350.6   Behavior disorders. Development disorders. Neuroses (General)
             Classify works on particular neurotic disorders in WM 171-197.

350.8   Special topics in child psychiatry, A-Z

         .A4   Aggression. Violence. Dangerous behavior
         .A8   Attention deficit disorder with hyperactivity
         .D2   Deception
         .D3   Defense mechanisms
         .H9   Hyperkinesis
         .I3   Identity crisis
         .I4   Inhibition
         .P3   Personality disorders
         .R9   Runaway behavior
         .S6   Social behavior disorders
                Classify works on aggression in WS 350.8.A4.

360   Pediatric gynecology (General)

366   Pediatric therapeutics (General)

368   Medical rehabilitation of physically disabled children

BY AGE GROUP

405   Birth injuries

410   Premature infants. Diseases of premature infants
             Classify specific diseases with the disease except those of the premature infants only.

420   Newborn infants. Neonatology

421   **Diseases of newborn infants**
         Classify specific diseases with the disease except those of the newborn only.

430   **Infancy**

440   **Preschool child**

450   **Puberty**

460   **Adolescence (General)**

462   **Adolescent psychology.   Adolescent behavior**

463   **Psychiatric problems of adolescents.   Behavior disorders.   Psychotherapy. Psychoanalysis.   Psychoses.**
         Classify specific mental disorders with the disorder in WM.

WT

GERIATRICS. CHRONIC DISEASE

Classify works on geriatric nursing in WY 152.

WT 1–39	General
WT 100–166	Geriatrics
WT 500	Chronic Disease

GENERAL

* 1   **Societies (Cutter from name of society)**
Includes ephemeral membership lists issued serially or separately. Classify substantial lists with directories. Classify annual reports, journals, etc., in W1.

    Collections (General)
5   **By several authors**
7   **By individual authors**

9   **Addresses. Essays. Lectures (General)**

11   **History (Table G)**
11.1   **General coverage (Not Table G)**

* 13   **Dictionaries. Encyclopedias**

* 15   **Classification. Nomenclature. Terminology**

* 16   **Tables. Statistics**

17   **Atlases. Pictorial works**
Cf. QZ 17 for tissue pathology of disease.

18   **Education**
Classify here works about education.

* 18.2 Educational materials
Classify here educational materials, e.g., outlines, questions and answers, programmed instruction, catalogs, computer–assisted instruction, etc., regardless of format. Classify textbooks, regardless of format, by subject.

* 19 Schools, departments, and faculties of geriatrics

20 Research (General)
Classify here works about research in general. Classify works about research on a particular subject by subject.

21 Geriatrics as a profession. Ethics. Peer review

* 22 Directories (Table G)
* 22.1 General coverage (Not Table G)

Laboratories, institutes, etc.
23 Collective
24 Individual (Cutter from name of agency)

25 Laboratory manuals. Technique

26 Equipment and supplies
Classify catalogs in W 26.

26.5 Medical informatics. Automatic data processing. Computers (General)
Classify works on use for special subjects by subject.

Hospitals, dispensaries, clinics, old age homes, etc.
27 Collective (Table G)
27.1 General coverage (Not Table G)
28 Individual (Table G)

29 Day care centers and programs (Table G)
29.1 General coverage (Not Table G)

30 Surveys. Medicosocial problems of gerontology and chronic disease.

31 Medical care plans. Long term care
Include here works on Medicare. Classify works on nursing care only in WY 152.

* 32 Laws (Table G)
* 32.1 General coverage (Not Table G)

Laws - Continued

* **33**   **Discussion of law (Table G)**
* **33.1**   **General coverage (Not Table G)**

* **39**   **Handbooks.   Resource guides**

GERIATRICS

100   **General works**
Classify works on specific diseases with the disease in other schedules; on nursing of specific diseases in WY 152; on anesthesia in WO 445; on surgery in WO 950.

104   **Anatomical, biochemical and physiological changes in senescence. The aging process.**
Classify works on aging tissue here. Classify works on the aging organ or system with the organ or system.

115   **Nutritional requirements.   Nutrition disorders**

116   **Longevity.   Life expectancy.   Death**
Cf. WS 200 for death of children, and other specific topics related to death, e.g., Attitude to death BF 789.D4, etc.

120   **Popular works (General).   Geriatric hygiene**
Include here autobiographical case histories. Example: Mills. Notings of a nonogenarian. Classify popular works on a particular subject by subject.

141   **Physical examination and diagnosis**

145   **Geriatric psychology.   Mental health**
Classify works on geriatric psychiatry in WT 150.

150   **Geriatric psychiatry.   Mental disorders of senescence**
Classify works on specific disorders with the disorder; on geriatric psychology in WT 145.

155   **Senile dementia.   Alzheimer's disease**
Cf. WM 220 for dementia and presenile dementia.

166   **Therapeutics (General or not elsewhere classified)**

*NUMBER CAN BE USED FOR BOTH MONOGRAPHS AND SERIALS.

CHRONIC DISEASE

500   General works

WU

DENTISTRY. ORAL SURGERY

GENERAL

* 1   **Societies (Cutter from name of society)**
Includes ephemeral membership lists issued serially or separately. Classify substantial lists with directories. Classify annual reports, journals, etc., in W1.

Collections (General)
5   **By several authors**
7   **By individual authors**

9   **Addresses. Essays. Lectures (General)**

11   **History (Table G)**
11.1   **General coverage (Not Table G)**

* 13   **Dictionaries. Encyclopedias**

* 15   **Classification. Nomenclature. Terminology**

* 16   **Tables. Statistics**

17   **Atlases**
Classify atlases limited to a particular part of the system with the part in the form number for atlases where available, e.g., WU 317, WU 417, WU 507, or WU 600.7.

18   **Education**
Classify here works about education.

* 18.2   **Educational materials**
Classify here educational materials, e.g., outlines, questions and answers, programmed instruction, catalogs, computer–assisted instruction, etc., regardless of format. Classify textbooks, regardless of format, by subject.

18.5   **Education of dental assistants, hygienists, and technicians**

* 19   **Schools and colleges**
Classify courses of study, catalogs, etc., in W 19.5.

20   **Graduate and continuing dental education (including fellowships, internships, residencies, etc.)**

20.5   **Dental research (General)**
Classify here works about research in general. Classify works about research on a particular subject by subject.

21   **Dentistry as a profession. Peer review**

* 22   **Directories (Table G)**
* 22.1   **General coverage**

     Laboratories, institutes, etc., including research institutes
23   **Collective**
24   **Individual (Cutter from name of institution)**

24.5   **Banks (Table G)**
24.51   **General coverage (Not Table G)**

25   **Laboratory manuals (General). Technique**
Classify manuals of prosthetic dentistry in WU 500–530.

26   **Equipment and supplies (General)**
Classify catalogs in W 26; works on dental materials in WU 180–190; on orthodontic appliances in WU 426.

26.5   **Medical informatics. Automatic data processing. Computers (General)**
Classify works on use for special subjects by subject.

     Hospitals, clinics, dispensaries, etc.
27   **Collective (Table G)**
27.1   **General coverage (Not Table G)**
28   **Individual (Table G)**

29   **Dental care (including comprehensive dental care). Dental infection control**
Cf. W 260 Dental insurance; WC 195 for general works on infection control; WX 167 for hospital infection control.

30   **Surveys**

* 32   **Laws (Table G)**
* 32.1   **General coverage (Not Table G)**

* 33   **Discussion of law (Table G)**
* 33.1   **General coverage (Not Table G)**

40   **Licensure of dentists and dental hygienists (Table G)**
40.1   **General coverage (Not Table G)**

44   **Malpractice (Table G)**
44.1   **General coverage (Not Table G)**

* 49   **Handbooks. Resource guides**

50   **Dental ethics**

58   **Advertising. Fee–splitting**

61   **Dentist's relation to public, patients and physicians. Attitude**

77   **Dental economics. Practice management**

79   **Group practice. Partnership practice**

80   **Popular works (General)**
Classify works for children in WU 113.6

90   **Auxiliary personnel**
e.g., Duties, professional opportunities, work manuals
Classify works on dental technicians in WU 150.

95   **Dental records**

100   **General works**
Classify works on specialty and on the specialty and diseases here. Classify works on diseases alone in WU 140. Include here works about dentistry written for practitioners of other specialties.

*NUMBER CAN BE USED FOR BOTH MONOGRAPHS AND SERIALS.

101   **Anatomy. Histology. Morphology. Embryology**
Include works on the jaw.

101.5   **Malformations and abnormalities of jaws, mouth, and/or teeth (General)**

102   **Physiology**
e.g., Mastication
Include works on the jaw.

105   **Dental emergencies (General)**

113   **Oral health and hygiene. Preventive and prophylactic dentistry**
Classify here works on school education and prophylactic programs. Cf. WA 350 School dental services. Classify popular works for the adult in WU 80.

113.6   **Works for and about children**
Classify general works on pediatric dentistry in WU 480.

113.7   **Nutrition and oral health (General)**
Cf. WU 270 Caries. Etiology of caries.

140   **Stomatognathic diseases (General). Oral pathology**
Classify works on mouth diseases written for the dentist here; classify works for the gastroenterologist in WI 200; classify works on jaw diseases alone in WU 140.5.

140.5   **Jaw diseases**
Classify here works on temporomandibular joint syndrome also. Cf. WU 600–610 Injuries and surgery of the jaw.

141   **Examination. Diagnosis. Diagnostic methods (General)**
Classify works on X-ray diagnosis in WN 230.

141.5   **Specific diagnostic methods, A–Z**

             .C3   **Cephalometry**
             .O2   **Odontometry**

150   **Dental technology (General) Dental technicians**
Classify works on technology for particular procedures with that procedure.

158   **Oral and dental injuries (General)**
Classify works on maxillofacial injuries and jaw fractures and dislocations in WU 610.

166   **Oral and dental therapeutics**

170   **Dental chemistry (General)**

180   **Dental alloys and metals**

190   **Dental materials (General and those not classed in WU 180)**

210   **Dentition**

220   **Enamel. Dentin**

230   **Dental pulp. Tooth root. Root canals. Dental cementum (Endodontics)**
         Classify works on reimplantation in WU 640.

240   **Periodontium. Alveolar process. Gingiva (Periodontics)**

242   **Periodontitis and related diseases**

250   **Dental deposits**

270   **Caries. Etiology of caries. Effect of fluoridation**

280   **Oral and dental neoplasms**

290   **Oral manifestations**
         Classify works on oral manifestations of specific diseases with the disease.

OPERATIVE DENTISTRY

300   **General works**

317   **Atlases**

350   **Cavities. Cavity treatment**

360   **Inlays**

ORTHODONTICS

400   General works

417   Atlases

426   Orthodontic appliances

440   Occlusion. Malocclusion

SPECIAL GROUPS

460   Dental care for the chronically ill

470   Dental care for the disabled

480   Pediatric dentistry. Dental care for children

490   Geriatric dentistry. Dental care for the aged

PROSTHODONTICS

Classify works on cleft palate prosthesis in WV 440; on maxillofacial and mandibular prosthesis in WU 600.

500   General works. Dental prosthesis (General)

507   Atlases

515   Partial dentures. Bridges. Crowns

530   Complete dentures

ORAL SURGERY

600   **General works**
         Cf. WO 460   Anesthesia in dentistry.   Include here general works on mandibular and maxillofacial prosthesis.

600.7   **Atlases**

605   **Tooth extraction**

610   **Maxillofacial injuries.   Mandibular injuries.   Fractures and dislocations of the jaw**

640   **Dental implantation.   Tooth reimplantation.   Transplantation**

WV

OTOLARYNGOLOGY

Classify works on nursing of patients with ear, nose, or throat diseases in WY 158.5. Note that the numbers WV 1–39 are assigned to works on the specialties otology, rhinology, and laryngology when treated individually as well as in combination. WV 100–190 are for general works only.

WV 1–190	General
WV 200–290	Ear
WV 300–358	Nose and Paranasal Sinuses
WV 400–440	Pharyngeal Region
WV 500–540	Larynx

GENERAL

* 1   **Societies (Cutter from name of society)**
Includes ephemeral membership lists issued serially or separtely.   Classify substantial lists with directories.   Classify annual reports, journals, etc., in W1.

Collections (General)
5   **By several authors**
7   **By individual authors**

9   **Addresses. Essays. Lectures (General)**

11   **History (Table G)**
11.1   **General coverage (Not Table G)**

* 13   **Dictionaries. Encyclopedias**

* 15   **Classification. Nomenclature. Terminology**

* 16   **Tables. Statistics**

17   **Atlases. Pictorial works**
Classify here also atlases on a specific organ.

18   **Education**
Classify here works about education.

*NUMBER CAN BE USED FOR BOTH MONOGRAPHS AND SERIALS.

* **18.2** **Educational materials**
Classify here educational materials, e.g., outlines, questions and answers, programmed instruction, catalogs, computer–assisted instruction, etc., regardless of format. Classify textbooks, regardless of format, by subject.

* **19** **Schools, departments, and faculties of otolaryngology**

20 **Research (General)**
Classify here works about research in general. Classify works about research on a particular subject by subject.

21 **Otolaryngology as a profession. Ethics. Peer review**

* **22** **Directories (Table G)**
* **22.1** **General coverage (Not Table G)**

Laboratories, institutes, etc.
23 **Collective**
24 **Individual (Cutter from name of agency)**

25 **Laboratory manuals. Technique**

26 **Equipment and supplies**
Classify catalogs in W 26.

26.5 **Medical informatics. Automatic data processing. Computers (General)**
Classify works on use for special subjects by subject.

Hospitals, clinics, dispensaries, etc.
27 **Collective (Table G)**
27.1 **General coverage (Not Table G)**
28 **Individual (Table G)**

* **32** **Laws. Estimation of disability for compensation (Table G)**
* **32.1** **General coverage (Not Table G)**

* **33** **Discussion of law (Table G)**
* **33.1** **General coverage (Not Table G)**

* **39** **Handbooks. Resource guides**

100 **General works**
Classify works on specialty and on the specialty and diseases here. Classify works on diseases alone in WV 140.

*NUMBER CAN BE USED FOR BOTH MONOGRAPHS AND SERIALS.

101   **Anatomy. Physiology. Biochemistry. Embryology. Abnormalities**

140   **Otorhinolaryngologic diseases (General)**

150   **ENT signs, symptoms, and diagnosis. Monitoring**

168   **ENT surgery**
        Classify works on surgery of a particular organ with the organ.

180   **Intracranial complications of ENT diseases**

190   **Otorhinolaryngologic neoplasms (General)**

EAR

200   **General works**

201   **Anatomy. Physiology**
        Cf. WV 272 for physiology and testing of hearing.

210   **Examination. Diagnosis**

220   **External ear**

222   **Ear canal. Foreign bodies. Cerumen**

225   **Tympanic membrane**

230   **Middle ear. Eustachian tube. Petrous bone**

232   **Otitis media (including aerotitis)**

233   **Mastoid region**

250   **Labyrinth**

255   **Vestibular apparatus. Equilibrium. Spatial orientation**
        Classify works on motion sickness in WD 630.

Labyrinth - Continued

258   Ménière's disease

265   Otosclerosis

270   Audiology. Hearing. Hearing disorders. Deafness

271   Deafness and other hearing disorders in children

272   Physiology of hearing. Auditory perception. Tinnitus. Function tests

274   Hearing aids

276   Treatment of deafness

280   Deaf–mutism

290   Neoplasms
Classify works on neoplasms of specific parts of the ear with the part.

NOSE AND PARANASAL SINUSES

300   General works
Classify works on nasopharyngeal diseases in WV 410.

301   Anatomy. Physiology. Olfaction

310   External nose

312   Plastic surgery

320   Nasal septum

335   Rhinitis. Hay fever
Cf. WC 510 Common cold.

340   Paranasal sinuses

345   Maxillary

Paranasal sinuses - Continued

350   Frontal

355   Ethmoid

358   Sphenoid

PHARYNGEAL REGION

400   General works
         Classify works on nasopharyngeal diseases in WV 410.

401   Anatomy. Physiology

410   Pharynx. Uvula. Palate
         Classify works relating to respiration and the pharynx in WF 490.

430   Tonsils. Adenoids

440   Cleft lip. Cleft palate

LARYNX

500   General works on larynx, speech, and voice and their organic disorders
         Classify works on neurological speech disorders in WL 340.2–340.6; on psychogenic speech disorders in WM 475–475.6.

501   Anatomy. Physiology. Physiology of speech

505   Laryngoscopy

510   Inflammation

520   Neoplasms

530   Vocal cords

535   Paralysis

540   **Surgery. Laryngectomy. Alaryngeal voice production**
Classify works on artificial larynx here.

WW

OPHTHALMOLOGY

Classify works on ophthalmic nursing in WY 158.

GENERAL

* 1   **Societies (Cutter from name of agency)**
       Includes ephemeral membership lists issued serially or separately. Classify substantial lists with directories. Classify annual reports, journals, etc., in W1.

       Collections (General)
5   **By several authors**
7   **By individual authors**

9   **Addresses. Essays. Lectures (General)**

11   **History of ophthalmology and optometry (Table G)**
11.1   **General coverage (Not Table G)**

* 13   **Dictionaries. Encyclopedias**

* 15   **Classification. Nomenclature. Terminology**

* 16   **Tables. Statistics**
       Classify tables used in optical dispensing calculations in WW 352.

17   **Atlases. Pictorial works**
       Classify here also atlases on a specific part of the eye.

*NUMBER CAN BE USED FOR BOTH MONOGRAPHS AND SERIALS.

18 **Education**
Classify here works about education.

* 18.2 **Educational materials**
Classify here educational materials, e.g., outlines, questions and answers, programmed instruction, catalogs, computer–assisted instruction, etc., regardless of format. Classify textbooks, regardless of format, by subject.

* 19 **Schools and colleges**
Classify courses of study, catalogs, etc., in W 19.5.

20 **Research (General)**
Classify here works about research in general. Classify works about research on a particular subject by subject.

21 **Ophthalmology as a profession. Ethics. Peer review**
Classify works on optometry and opticianry in WW 721.

21.5 **Ophthalmic assistants**

* 22 **Directories (Table G)**
Classify directories of optometrists and/or opticians in WW 722.
* 22.1 **General coverage (Not Table G)**

Laboratories, institutes, eye banks, etc.
23 **Collective**
24 **Individual (Cutter from name of agency)**

25 **Laboratory manuals. Technique**

26 **Equipment and supplies**
Classify catalogs in W 26.

26.5 **Medical informatics. Automatic data processing. Computers (General)**
Classify works on use for special subjects by subject.

Hospitals, clinics, dispensaries, etc.
27 **Collective (Table G)**
27.1 **General coverage (Not Table G)**
28 **Individual (Table G)**

* 32 **Laws. Estimation of disability for compensation (Table G)**
* 32.1 **General coverage (Not Table G)**

* 33 **Discussion of law (Table G)**
* 33.1 **General coverage (Not Table G)**

*NUMBER CAN BE USED FOR BOTH MONOGRAPHS AND SERIALS.

* 39   **Handbooks. Resource guides**

80   **Popular works (General)**

100   **General works**
> *Classify works on specialty and on the specialty and diseases here. Classify works on diseases alone in WW 140.*

EYE

101   **Anatomy. Histology. Embryology. Biochemistry. Abnormalities**

103   **Physiology of the eye. Vision (General)**

105   **Visual perception. Space perception**
> *Cf. WW 150 Color perception.*

109   **Ocular accommodation. Ocular adaptation**

113   **Hygiene. Conservation of vision**
> *Cf. WW 80 Popular works.*

140   **Eye diseases. Vision disorders (General or not elsewhere classified)**

141   **Examination. Diagnostic methods**
> *Classify works on the examination of a part with the part.*

143   **Objective methods**
> e.g., Ophthalmoscopy. Slit lamp microscopy. Tonometry
> *Classify works on electronystagmography in WW 410; on electroretinography in WW 270; on gonioscopy in WW 210; on retinography in WW 300.*

145   **Subjective methods. Evaluation of function**
> e.g., Visual acuity testing. Perimetry

149   **Neoplasms**
> *Classify works on neoplasms of parts of the eye with the part.*

150   **Color perception. Color blindness**
> *Cf. WW 105 Visual perception*

160   **Diseases due to infection, hypersensitivity, etc. (General or not elsewhere classified)**

166   **Ocular therapeutics (Medical)**

168   **Ophthalmological surgery (General)**

170   **Eye bank procedures (including those for specific parts of the eye)**
         Classify material on eye banks in WW 23–24.

PARTS OF THE EYE

202   **Orbit**

205   **Eyelids. Eyebrows**
         Cf. WR 390–465 Skin appendage diseases.

208   **Lacrimal apparatus**

210   **Anterior chamber. Posterior chamber. Aqueous humor (Eyeball)**

212   **Conjunctiva**

215   **Trachoma**

220   **Cornea**

230   **Sclera**

240   **Uvea. Iris. Ciliary body**

245   **Choroid**

250   **Vitreous body**

260   **Crystalline lens. Cataract**

270   **Retina**

276 Blindness. Amblyopia

280 Optic nerve

290 Glaucoma

REFRACTION AND ERRORS OF REFRACTION

300 General works

310 Astigmatism

320 Myopia

CORRECTIVE DEVICES

350 Optical dispensing. Spectacle fitting. Opticianry
   Classify works on optometry and opticianry as specialties in WW 704–722.1.

352 Principles. Calculations. Tables

354 Frames. Eyeglasses
   Classify works on intraocular lenses in WW 358 or if exclusively for cataract therapy, in WW 260.

355 Contact lenses

358 Prosthesis

NEUROMUSCULAR MECHANISM

400 General works

405 Orthoptics (General)

410 Disorders of ocular motility

Disorders of ocular motility - Continued

415   Strabismus

460   Disorders due to diseases of the central nervous system. Neurologic manifestations of eye diseases (General)

PROBLEMS ASSOCIATED WITH EYE DISEASES

475   Eye manifestations of general disease
Classify works on eye manifestations of specific diseases with disease.

480   Medical aspects of reading problems associated with poor vision.

OCCUPATIONAL AND TRAUMATIC OPHTHALMOLOGY

505   Occupational ophthalmology

525   Foreign bodies. Injuries. Toxic injuries

AGE GROUPS

600   Pediatric ophthalmology and optometry
Classify works on particular disorders with the disorder.

620   Geriatric ophthalmology and optometry
Classify works on particular disorders with the disorder.

OPTOMETRY

704   General works. Office management
Classify works on the specific functions of the optometrist in the WW number for the function; on functions of the optician in WW 350-355.

721   Optometry and opticianry as professions. Ethics. Peer review
Classify works on history of the professions in WW 11-11.1.

* 722   Directories (Table G)
* 722.1   General coverage (Not Table G)

*NUMBER CAN BE USED FOR BOTH MONOGRAPHS AND SERIALS.

WX

HOSPITALS AND OTHER HEALTH FACILITIES

WX 1–147	General
WX 150–190	Hospital Administration
WX 200–225	Clinical Departments and Units

GENERAL

* 1　**Societies (Cutter from name of society)**
　　Includes ephemeral membership lists issued serially or separately.　Classify substantial lists with directories.　Classify annual reports, journals, etc., in W1.

* 2　**Serial hospital reports (Table G)**
　　Classify here hospital administrative reports and statistics.　Classify clinical material (e.g., Bulletin of the Johns Hopkins Hospital, Guy's Hospital Reports, etc.) in W1.　Cf. W2 Serials documents for administrative reports and statistics on several hospitals under governmental administration.

　　Collections (General)
5　　**By several authors**
7　　**By individual authors**

9　**Addresses. Essays. Lectures (General)**

11　**General history of hospitals and the hospital movement (Table G)**
　　Cf. WX 27–28　History of individual hospitals or groups of individual hospitals.　Classify history of emergency or ambulance services in WX 215.
11.1　**General coverage (Not Table G)**

* 13　**Dictionaries. Encyclopedias**

* 15　**Classification. Nomenclature. Terminology. Standardization. Accreditation**

* 16　**Tables. Statistics**

17　**Atlases. Pictorial works**

18　**Education**
　　Classify here works about education

*NUMBER CAN BE USED FOR BOTH MONOGRAPHS AND SERIALS.

* **18.2**   **Educational materials**
Classify here educational materials, e.g., outlines, questions and answers, programmed instruction, catalogs, computer–assisted instruction, etc., regardless of format. Classify textbooks, regardless of format, by subject.

* **19**   **Schools, departments, and faculties of hospital administration**

20   **Research (General)**
Classify here works about research in general. Classify works about research on a particular subject by subject.

[21]   **[This number not used]**
Classify hospital administration as a career in WX 155.

* **22**   **Directories (Table G)**
* **22.1**   **General coverage (Not Table G)**

[26]   **[This number not used]**
Classify works on equipment and supplies in WX 147. Classify catalogs in W 26.

26.5   **Medical informatics. Automatic data processing. Computers (General)**
Classify works on use for special subjects by subject.

Hospitals and medical centers. Health facilities (General)
Classify here non–serial hospital reports. Classify serial reports in WX 2; reports of army hospitals in UH 470–475; on those of naval hospitals in VG 410–450. Classify works on special types of hospitals or of specialized departments of general hospitals in the appropriate schedule for the field, e.g., isolation hospitals in WC 27-28; on psychiatric departments of general hospitals in WM 27-28, etc.

27   **Collective (Table G)**
27.1   **General coverage (Not Table G)**
28   **Individual (Table G)**

Hospices and hospice care programs
28.6   **Collective (Table G)**
28.61   **General coverage (Not Table G)**
28.62   **Individual (Table G)**

29   **Day care centers and programs (Table G)**
29.1   **General coverage (Not Table G)**
Cf. WA 310–320 Child day care centers; WT 29–29.1 Geriatric day care centers; WX 205 Hospital outpatient clinics.

* **32**   **Laws (Table G)**
* **32.1**   **General coverage (Not Table G)**

Laws - Continued

* 33   Discussion of law. Jurisprudence (Table G)
* 33.1   General coverage (Not Table G)

* 39   Handbooks. Resource guides

100   General works

140   Health facility planning and construction
            Classify works on special facilities with the specialty.

147   Equipment and supplies
            Classify catalogs in W 26.

HOSPITAL ADMINISTRATION

150   General works

153   Utilization review. Quality of service. Medical audit

155   Hospital administration as a career, e.g., Educational requirements.
            Professional opportunities

157   Financial administration. Business management. Cost accounting

157.4   Multi–institutional systems

157.8   Diagnosis–related groups

158   Hospitalization
            Include here narrative reports on admissions and discharges; also on patient readmissions. Classify works that are largely statistical in WX 16. Classify works on hospitalization insurance in W 160.

158.5   Hospital patients. Attitude and compliance. Satisfaction

159   Hospital personnel administration. Staff manuals. Career literature
            Classify manuals for professional staff only in WX 203.

159.5   Volunteers
            Classify works on professional hospital social work in W 322.

Hospital personnel administration. Staff manuals. Career literature
Continued

159.8   Collective bargaining (Hospitals and hospital personnel)

160   Public relations. Interinstitutional relations. Staff relations. Staff attitudes

161   Hospital shops

162   Patient care planning. Progressive patient care. Long term care
      Classify here works on hospital care only. For general comprehensive works on patient care planning, use W 84.7–84.8. Classify works limited to nursing care in WY; on long term care of geriatric patients in WT 31.

162.5   Patient care team

165   General housekeeping. Maintenance. Laundries. Environmental control

167   Cross infection prevention and control
      Cf. WC 195 for general works on infection control; WU 29 for dental infection control.

168   Hospital food service

173   Medical records. Medical record administrators
      Cf. WB 290 for works on medical history taking in general.

179   Hospital pharmacy service. Hospital medication systems

185   Safety, fire and disaster programs

187   Chaplaincy service

190   Mobile health units

CLINICAL DEPARTMENTS AND UNITS

Classify works on specialty departments in the hospital number for the specialty, e.g., psychiatric wards in WM 27–28.

200   General works
      Include works on services not indexed elsewhere.

203   **Medical personnel. Interns. Staff manuals. Ward manuals and precedent books**

Classify general staff manuals and those for non-professional personnel in WX 159.

205   **Hospital outpatient clinics. Ambulatory care facilities**

Cf. WB 101 for works on general ambulatory care.

207   **Clinical and pathological laboratories**

Classify works on laboratories not connected with hospitals in QY 23–24.

215   **Emergency service. Ambulance service**

Include here works on ambulance and general emergency health services not indexed elsewhere even if they are not connected with hospitals. Classify those connected with occupational medicine in WA 400–495.

218   **Intensive care units. Critical care (General)**

Cf. WB 105 Medical emergencies; WY 154 for works on nursing care. Classify works on critical care in the specialty fields with the specialty, e.g., Cardiac emergencies WG 205; Coronary care units WG 27–28.

223   **Physical therapy department**

225   **Occupational therapy department**

WY

NURSING

GENERAL

* 1 **Societies (Cutter from name of society)**
Includes ephemeral membership lists issued serially or separately. Classify substantial lists with directories. Classify annual reports, journals, etc., in W1.

Collections (General)
5 **By several authors**
7 **By individual authors**

9 **Addresses. Essays. Lectures (General)**

11 **History (Table G)**
11.1 **General coverage (Not Table G)**

* 13 **Dictionaries. Encyclopedias**

* 15 **Classification. Nomenclature. Terminology**

16 **Nursing as a profession. Peer review**
Classify works on specific types of nursing in WY 101–200.

17 **Atlases. Pictorial works**

18 **Education**
Classify here works about education.

* 18.2 **Educational materials**
Classify here educational materials, e.g., outlines, questions and answers, programmed instruction, catalogs, computer-assisted instruction, etc., regardless of format. Classify textbooks, regardless of format, by subject.

*NUMBER CAN BE USED FOR BOTH MONOGRAPHS AND SERIALS.

18.5	Graduate and continuing nursing education (including fellowships, internships, residencies, etc.)

18.8   Practical nursing education

* 19   Schools of nursing
Classify courses of study, catalogs, etc., in W 19.5. Include here works on the history of nursing schools.

20   Organization and administration of nursing schools

20.5   Research (General)
Classify here works about research in general. Classify works about research on a particular subject by subject.

* 21   Licensure. Certification. Registration (Table G)
* 21.1   General coverage (Not Table G)

* 22   Directories (Table G)
* 22.1   General coverage (Not Table G)

26.5   Medical informatics. Automatic data processing. Computers (General)
Classify works on use for special subjects by subject.

29   Employment. Placement agencies
30   Personnel management. Collective bargaining

* 31   Statistics. Surveys

* 32   Laws (Table G)
* 32.1   General coverage (Not Table G)

* 33   Discussion of law. Jurisprudence (Table G)
* 33.1   General coverage (Not Table G)

44   Malpractice. Liability. Liability insurance (Table G)
44.1   General coverage (Not Table G)

* 49   Handbooks. Resource guides

77   Economics of nursing

85   Nursing ethics

NUMBER CAN BE USED FOR BOTH MONOGRAPHS AND SERIALS.

86   Nursing philosophy.   Nursing theory

86.5   Holistic nursing

87   Psychology applied to nursing.   Psychological aspects of nursing.   Relations to patients, physicians, public

90   Referral and consultation (General)

100   General works on nursing procedures
         Classify works on nursing techniques in special fields of medicine in WY 150–164.

100.4   Nursing assessment.   Nursing diagnosis

100.5   Nursing records.   Nursing audit

SPECIAL FIELDS IN NURSING

101   General works.   Primary nursing care
         e.g., Special nursing as a career; types of specialized fields in nursing
         Cf. WY 150   General works on nursing techniques in special fields of medicine.

105   Administrative work.   Supervisory nursing.   Teaching

106   Community health nursing
         Classify works on a particular kind of community nursing with the more specific type, e.g., Public health nursing   WY 108.

107   Transcultural nursing

108   Public health nursing
         e.g., Federal, state, etc.
         Cf. WY 130   Governmental nursing services.

109   Office nursing

113   School nursing

115   Home care services (including visiting nursing and visiting nurse associations, and respite care)

125 **Institutional nursing. Team nursing**
e.g., In hospitals, sanatoriums, etc.
Cf. WY 105 Administrative work.

127 **Private nursing**

128 **Nurse practitioners. Nurse clinicians**

130 **Governmental nursing services**
e.g., Armed Forces. Veterans Administration. Indian Health Service, etc.
Cf. WY 108 Public health nursing; UH 490–495 Army nursing.

137 **Red Cross nursing**

141 **Occupational health nursing**

143 **Transportation nursing**
e.g., On airplanes, ships, trains

145 **Nursing by religious orders**

NURSING TECHNIQUES IN SPECIAL FIELDS OF MEDICINE

Classify background materials on specific subjects prepared for a nursing audience by subject, e.g. surgery for nurses, WO 100; bacteriology for nurses, QW 50.

150 **General works**

150.5 **Rehabilitation nursing**

151 **Nurse anesthetists**

152 **Geriatric and chronic disease nursing. Life support care. Long term care. Terminal care**

152.5 **Cardiovascular nursing. Hemic and lymphatic disease nursing**

153 **Communicable disease nursing**

153.5 **AIDS/HIV nursing**

154   Emergency nursing. Critical care. Intensive care. Recovery room care.
           Postanesthesia nursing

154.5   Dermatological nursing

155   Endocrine disease nursing

156   Oncologic nursing

156.5   Gastroenterologic nursing

156.7   Gynecological nursing

157   Obstetrical nursing

157.3   Maternity nursing. Maternal–child nursing. Neonatal nursing. Perinatal
           nursing
           *Classify here works on care of the mother and child shortly before and after the
           child is born.*

157.6   Nursing of diseases of the musculoskeletal system. Orthopedic nursing

158   Ophthalmic nursing

158.5   Otolaryngological nursing

159   Pediatric nursing. Adolescent nursing
           *Classify works on pediatric and adolescent nursing in special fields by type, e.g., on
           pediatric surgical nursing in WY 161.*

160   Psychiatric nursing
           *Include works on psychiatric aides and ward attendants here. Classify works on
           supervision of ward attendance in WM 35.*

160.5   Neurological nursing

161   Surgical nursing. Perioperative nursing

162   Operating room techniques

163   Nursing of diseases of the respiratory system

164   Urologic nursing

OTHER NURSING SERVICES

191   Male nurses

193   Nurses' aides, ward attendants and orderlies
           Classify ward attendants for psychiatric institutions in WY 160.

195   Practical nursing

200   Home nursing

BY COUNTRY

300   Nursing by country (Table G)

WZ

HISTORY OF MEDICINE

Classify history of a particular subject with the subject, e.g., History of surgery WO 11.

WZ 1–40   General
WZ 51–80.5   History, By Period, Locality, etc.
WZ 100–150   Biography
WZ 220–225   Manuscripts
WZ 230–260   Early Printed Books
WZ 270   Americana
WZ 290–294   Modern Editions and Criticism of Early Works
WZ 305–350   Miscellany Relating to Medicine

GENERAL

* 1   **Societies (Cutter from name of society)**
         Includes ephemeral membership lists issued serially or separately. Classify substantial lists with directories. Classify annual reports, journals, etc. in W1.

         Collections (General)
5   **By several authors**
7   **By individual authors**

9   **Addresses. Essays. Lectures (General)**

[11]   **[This number not used]**

* 13   **Dictionaries. Encyclopedias**

17   **Atlases. Pictorial works**

18   **Education**
         Classify here works about education.

* 18.2   **Educational materials**
         Classify here educational materials, e.g., outlines, questions and answers, programmed instruction, catalogs, computer-assisted instruction, etc., regardless of format. Classify textbooks, regardless of format, by subject.

*NUMBER CAN BE USED FOR BOTH MONOGRAPHS AND SERIALS.

* 22   Directories (Table G)
* 22.1   General coverage (Not Table G)

  23   Institutes (Cutter from name of institute)

              Museums
  27   Collective
  28   Individual (Cutter from name of museum)

  30   Chronologies

* 39   Handbooks.   Resource guides

  40   General works

HISTORY, BY PERIOD, LOCALITY, ETC.

Except in WZ 51 (which see) prefer classification by locality if applicable.

  51   **Ancient (to 476 A.D.)**
              *Include works on countries of the western world.   Classify those on history of medicine
              in other countries by locality in WZ 70.*

  54   **Medieval (to 1453 A.D.)**

  55   **Modern (1454 A.D.–   )**

  56   **Early modern (to 1800 A.D.)**

  59   **Late modern (1801 A.D.–   )**

  60   19th century

  64   20th century

  70   History (By locality) (Table G)

  80   History (Special groups, general or not elsewhere classified)

History - Continued

80.5   Specific groups, A–Z

.A8   Arabic and Islamic groups
.B5   Blacks
.H6   Hindu
.I3   Indians, North American
.J3   Jews
.O6   Asian
.W5   Women

BIOGRAPHY

100   **Individual biography (Cutter from name of biographee)**
Classify here biographies and bibliographies of persons in the medical field, the preclinical sciences and other related fields. Cf. WZ 294 Modern criticism and bibliographies of early works. Include here works about two persons or a family, e.g., the Mayos.

* 112   **Collective biography (General or not specified below)**
Classify here collective biographies in the field of medicine and the preclinical sciences. Classify collective biographies of persons in other fields in the appropriate LC schedule.

* 112.5   **By specialty, A–Z**
Classify biography of individuals in WZ 100 regardless of specialty.

.C2   Cardiologists
.D3   Dentists
.I5   Immunologists
.M4   Military physicians and surgeons
.N4   Neurologists, neurosurgeons, etc.
.N8   Nurses
.O5   Oncologists
.O7   Ophthalmologists, optometrists, etc.
.O8   Otolaryngologists
.P2   Pathologists
.P4   Pharmacists
.P5   Physiologists
.P6   Psychiatrists
.S8   Surgeons
           Cf. WZ 112.5.M4 above.

Collective biography (By period)
Prefer specialty numbers above or if not applicable locality number below.

* 121   **Ancient (to 476 A.D.)**
* 124   **Medieval (to 1453 A.D.)**
* 126   **Early modern (to 1800 A.D.)**

*NUMBER CAN BE USED FOR BOTH MONOGRAPHS AND SERIALS.

Collective biography (By period) - Continued

*	129	Late modern (1801 A.D.–)
*	132	19th century
*	134	20th century

* 140   **Collective biography (By locality) (Table G)**

* 150   **Collective biography (Special groups)**
            e.g., Women

MANUSCRIPTS

220   **Early Western manuscripts**
            Note that at NLM western manuscripts produced before 1601 are classified in WZ 220, those produced after 1601 are classified as MS B (Manuscripts Books), MS C (Manuscripts Collections), or MS F (Manuscripts Oversize books).

225   **Other early manuscripts**

EARLY PRINTED BOOKS

Works published before 1801 (or later if considered Americana) are not classed by subject; instead, they are arranged alphabetically by author under classification number for period during which they were printed.

230   **Incunabula**
            pre–1501

240   **XVI century**

250   **XVII century**

260   **XVIII century**

For 19th century publications see separate schedule below.

AMERICANA

270   **Americana**
The closing dates given in the following table (based on the American Imprints Inventory for the U.S.) will be used to determine inclusion in this class.

North and South America (except U.S.), 1820

United States

     Alabama, 1840

     Alaska, 1890

     Arizona, 1890

     Arkansas, 1870

     California, 1875

     Colorado, 1876

     Connecticut, 1820

     Delaware, 1820

     District of Columbia, 1820

     Florida, 1860

     Georgia, 1820

     Hawaii, 1860

     Idaho, 1890

     Illinois (except Chicago), 1850

       Chicago, 1871

     Indiana, 1850

Iowa, 1860

Kansas, 1875

Kentucky, 1830

Louisiana, 1820

Maine, 1820

Maryland, 1820

Massachusetts, 1820

Michigan, 1850

Minnesota, 1865

Mississippi, 1840

Missouri, 1850

Montana, 1890

Nebraska, 1875

Nevada, 1890

New Hampshire, 1820

New Jersey, 1820

New Mexico, 1875

New York (except N.Y. City, Brooklyn, and Hudson River towns), 1850

New York City, 1820

    Brooklyn, 1825

    Hudson River towns, e.g., Poughkeepsie, Hudson, Troy, Albany, 1830

North Carolina, 1820

North Dakota, 1890

Ohio, 1840

Oklahoma, 1870

Oregon, 1875

Pennsylvania (except Philadelphia), 1830

    Philadelphia, 1820

Rhode Island, 1820

South Carolina, 1820

South Dakota, 1890

Tennessee, 1840

Texas, 1860

Utah, 1890

Vermont, 1820

Virginia, 1820

Washington, 1875

West Virginia, 1830

Wisconsin, 1850

Wyoming, 1890

MODERN EDITIONS AND CRITICISM OF EARLY WORKS

290   **Modern editions of early works**
Classify here 1801–   editions of works originally published before 1801, except for Americana (Cf. WZ 270). Classify by subject editions of Americana published after the closing date for the particular area, e.g., an 1825 edition of a workwith a New York City imprint, originally published before 1820.

* 292   **Modern collections of early works**
Classify here collections (including those serially issued) which contain pre–1801 works of three or more authors. Classify works of only two authors in WZ 290 with the first author.

294   **Modern criticism of early works and bibliographies of single titles**
Classify here studies, commentaries, etc, of pre–1801 works including Americana unless they are largely the biography of one or two authors, in which case classify them in WZ 100. Classify in WZ 290 works that include the original text unless itis decidedly subordinate to the commentary. Classify here a bibliography of a single work. Cf. WZ 100 for bibliography of a single author's works.

MISCELLANY RELATING TO MEDICINE

305   **Anecdotes. Humor. Light verse**

305.5   **Surgery. Hospitalization**

308   **Curiosities**

309   **Folklore. Proverbs. Superstitions**

310   **Quacks. Quackery**
Classify here works the subject of which the author considers quackery. Works on special systems of therapeutics are classed in WB 890–962.

313   **Biographical clinics (Diagnosis of diseases of famous persons, derived from records, memoirs, letters, portraits, etc.)**

320   **Body snatching. Resurrectionists**

330   **Medicine etc., as depicted in art and literature (critical studies) e.g., Medicine in the works of Rabelais**
        Cf. WM 49 Art and literature as related to psychiatry.

332   **Anniversaries and special events**
        Classify here general works only. Classify material on specific events by subject.

334   **Emblems, insignia, etc.**

336   **Caricatures. Cartoons**

340   **Numismatics, philately, bookplates, etc.**

345   **Medical writing and publishing. Historiography**

348   **Medical illustration (General)**

350   **Literary and artistic works by physicians and other association items**
        Cf. WZ 330 Medicine in art and literature.

19TH CENTURY SCHEDULE

Classify here works published between 1801–1913.

QS   Anatomy

QS 22   Directories (Table G)

QSA   Histology

QSB   Embryology

QT   Physiology

QT 22   Directories (Table G)

QTA   Hygiene

QU   Biochemistry

QU 22   Directories (Table G)

QV   Pharmacology. Pharmacy. Materia medica

QV 22   Directories (Table G)

QVA   Pharmacopoeias (Official)

QVB   Toxicology

QW   Microbiology

QW 22   Directories (Table G)

QWA   Immunology

QX   Parasitology

QX 22   Directories (Table G)

QY   Clinical pathology

[QY 22]   [Directories. Use QZ 22]

QZ   Pathology

QZ 22   Directories (Table G)

QZA   Neoplasms

W   Medicine (General)

W1   Serials. Periodicals

W2   Documents

W3   Congresses
          NLM no longer assigns W3 to newly acquired publications.

W4   Dissertations

W4A   American dissertations

W5   Collections by several authors

W6   Pamphlet volumes

W 22   Directories (Table G)

W 600   Medical jurisprudence

WA   Public health

WA 22   Directories (Table G)

Public Health - Continued

WAA	Sanitation and sanitary control
WB	Practice of medicine
WB 22	Directories (Table G)
WBA	Popular medicine
WBB	Diagnosis
WBC	Therapeutics (General)
WBD	Dietetics
WBE	Electric stimulation therapy
WBF	Hydrotherapy
WBG	Massage
WBH	Climatology. Geography of disease
WBI	Health resorts
WBJ	Special systems (General)
WBK	Homeopathy
WBL	Osteopathic medicine
WC	Communicable diseases (General)
WC 22	Directories (Table G)
WCA	Sexually transmitted diseases
WCB	Cholera
WCC	Diphtheria

Communicable Diseases - Continued

WCD   Influenza

WCE   Leprosy

WCF   Malaria

WCG   Plague

WCH   Smallpox

WCI   Typhoid fever

WCJ   Typhus fever

WCK   Yellow fever

WDA   Deficiency diseases. Metabolic diseases (including obesity and disorders of acid–base balance)

WDB   Hypersensitivity

WDC   Animal poisons. Plant poisons

WDD   Diseases due to physical agents

WE   Musculoskeletal system

WE 22   Directories (Table G)

WEA   Fractures. Dislocations. Sprains

WF   Respiratory system

WF 22   Directories (Table G)

WFA   Tuberculosis

WG   Cardiovascular system

Cardiovascular Diseases - - Continued

WG 22   Directories (Table G)

WH   Hemic and lymphatic systems

WH 22   Directories (Table G)

WI   Digestive system

WI 22   Directories (Table G)

WIA   Stomach

WIB   Anus and rectum

WIC   Liver

WJ   Urogenital system

WJ 22   Directories (Table G)

WJA   Male genitalia

WK   Endocrine system

WK 22   Directories (Table G)

WKA   Diabetes

WL   Nervous system

WL 22   Directories (Table G)

WLA   Epilepsies

WM   Psychiatry

WM 22   Directories (Table G)

WMA   Substance–related disorders

WN   Radiology

WN 22   Directories (Table G)

WO   Surgery

WO 22   Directories (Table G)

WOA   Anesthesia

WP   Gynecology

WP 22   Directories (Table G)

WPA   Breast

WQ   Obstetrics

WQ 22   Directories (Table G)

WR   Dermatology

WR 22   Directories (Table G)

WS   Pediatrics

WS 22   Directories (Table G)

WT   Geriatrics. Chronic disease

WT 22   Directories (Table G)

WU   Dentistry. Oral surgery

WU 22   Directories (Table G)

WV   Otolaryngology. Nose

WV 22   Directories (Table G)

Otolaryngology. Nose - Continued

WVA   Ear

WVB   Throat. Larynx

WW   Ophthalmology

WW 22   Directories (Table G)

WX   Hospitals

WX 2   Serial reports of hospitals (Table G)

WX 22   Directories (Table G)

WY   Nursing

WY 22   Directories (Table G)

History of medicine
Use schedule in full, as for twentieth century.

INTRODUCTION TO THE
INDEX TO THE CLASSIFICATION

The Index to the *National Library of Medicine Classification* consists primarily of entries from the current *Medical Subject Headings* (MeSH) and some non-MeSH terms when no appropriate MeSH term is available to express a concept. All MeSH entries in the Index were updated to be consistent with the 1999 edition of MeSH. The index terms are arranged in alphabetical order with Roman numerals filed as letters in this arrangement. Arabic numerals are found at the end of the Index following the letter Z.

The classification numbers assigned to the index terms are usually general numbers for the concept represented or numbers reflecting a medical view when that is more appropriate. In this edition see references no longer contain a classification notation.

Indented terms represent more specific aspects of the subject or aspects of the subject to which a number different from the general number has been assigned. The indented terms are often elliptical and should be interpreted broadly. For example, when "Organic chemistry" is used as a term indented under the name of a chemical, the number following is to be selected if the principal focus of the work being classified is the organic chemistry of the chemical. Some subheadings refer the user to another heading. General references or see also references are listed at the end of the alphabetical sequence of the indented terms under the index term.

Example:

> Electrodes   QD 571
> > Biomedical engineering   QT 36
> > In electric stimulation therapy   WB 495
> > Used for special purposes, by subjects, e.g., in
> > > Urinalysis   QY 185
> >
> > See also Microelectrodes   QT 36, etc.

Library of Congress numbers are assigned to subjects that fall outside the scope of the *NLM Classification*. When a concept represented in MeSH has no exact equivalent in LC's schedules a number was selected that fitted the concept most closely. Since NLM rarely uses LC's K (Law) schedules the numbers provided for index terms relating to laws are for the subject rather than the law.

How to use the Index

1. The Index is not a substitute for the main schedules. A user should always refer to the schedules for confirmation of the proper application of the number and its relationship to other numbers.

2. Many headings are assigned a range of numbers rather than a specific number. The schedules of the *NLM Classification* or the *Library of Congress Classification* are the only source of the meaning of specific numbers within the range.

3. The number assigned to a heading in this Index should not be used unless it represents the principal subject of the material being cataloged.

4. The Index represents only those MeSH terms that are linked to an NLM or LC classification notation. The Index does not include all MeSH headings found in the *Medical Subject Headings Annotated Alphabetic List* and it is not a substitute for the *Annotated Alphabetic List*.

When assigning MeSH headings to a work the *Annotated Alphabetic List* must always be consulted. The Index does not provide annotations nor does it show relationships between headings; these are found in the *Annotated Alphabetic List* and the *Tree Structures*, respectively.

5. The number of indented terms under an index term varies greatly. The choice was dependent upon the needs that arose in the past. Therefore, the list is in no way exhaustive of the possibilities that can occur.

6. The Index contains over ten thousand index terms to which classification notations are assigned. Many terms are found only in the index and will not appear in the schedules. They refer to a number in the schedule where only a broader term or a related term appears.

7. Cross References:
There are several types of cross references used in the index.
7.1 *See* References Pointing to a Single Index Term
A *see* reference points to a single index term or concept when any or all numbers assigned to the index term or concept apply also to the reference term.

    Acquired Immunity see Immunity

7.2 See References Pointing to Multiple Index Terms
A *see* reference points to multiple index terms or concepts when no one index term or concept represents the entire concept of the reference term.

    Abrasions see Dermabrasion; Tooth Abrasion; Wounds and Injuries

7.3 *See* References Under Index Terms
See references that are indented under index terms link the concept to a more specific index term.

    Health
        Developing countries   WA 395
        [etc.]
        Mental see Mental Health   WM 105, etc.
        Oral see Oral Health   WU 113
        Public see Public Health   WA, etc.
        [etc.]

7.4 General References Under Index Terms
General references following all indented terms or concepts relate to the main index term or concept. Examples of general references are: "Used for special purposes, by subject " " Specific types of [topic], by subject," etc.

    Disasters   HC 79.D45
        First aid   WA 292
        [etc.]
        Hospital programs see Disaster Planning   WX 185
        [etc.]
        Specific types of disaster, by subject
        See also Civil Defense   UA 926-929, etc.

7.5 *See also* References Under Indented Terms
A *See also* reference provided under an indented term relates only to the indented term. When the *See also* reference is related to the main index term only it follows all indented terms and general references. The latter is represented in the Disasters example above (See also Civil Defense   UA 926-929, etc.). The former is represented here.

    Advertising
        Alcoholic beverages   HF 6161.L46
        [etc.]
        Pharmaceutical   QV 736
            See also Drug Labeling   QV 835
        Tobacco   HF 6161.T6
        Other special subjects, by business in HF 6161
            or other appropriate number

7.6 *See also* References to General Terms

See also references lead the user from one index term to a more general index term under which are listed indented terms that apply equally to both headings.

Accidents, Home   WA 288
 See also special topics under Accidents

Accidents
 First aid   WA 292
 In anesthesia   WO 288
 Medicolegal aspects
  Cause of death   W 843
  Disability evaluation   W 900-925
 See also Insurance, Accident   W 100-250, etc.

Note when "etc." follows a number in any type of reference, it indicates that in addition to the numbers given in the reference, there are other numbers which also represent the index term. The user will find these other numbers listed under the main entry for the index term.

8. Drugs, etc.:

The numbers provided after index terms for drugs, chemicals and biological agents represent their biochemical, pharmacological or chemical properties. The index rarely gives a number for these agents when the material being cataloged discusses their use in the therapy of a particular disease or in a particular study. In such cases the material is classified with the disease or the subject of the study.

A

A Fibers see Nerve Fibers, Myelinated
Abate see Temefos
Abattoirs   WA 707
Abbreviations
    Chemistry   QD 7
    General   P 365–365.5
    Library symbols (U.S.)   Z 881
    Medical   W 13
        By specialties (Form number 13 in any NLM
        schedule where applicable)
    Organizations (General)   AS 8
    Periodical titles   Z 6945.A2
    Science (General)   Q 179
    Particular languages, by language in appropriate
    LC schedule
Abdomen   WI 900–970
    Radiography see Radiography, Abdominal   WI
    900
    Surgery   WI 900–970
Abdomen, Acute   WI 900
    Child   WI 900
    Infant   WI 900
Abdominal Cramps see Colic
Abdominal Injuries   WI 900
Abdominal Muscles   WI 900
Abdominal Neoplasms   WI 970
Abdominal Pain   WI 147
Abdominal Wall see Abdominal Muscles
Abducens Nerve   WL 330
Abiogenesis see Biogenesis
Abnormal Reflex see Reflex, Abnormal
Abnormalities
    Congenital   QS 675–681
        Autosome see Autosome Abnormalities   QS
        677
        Bone   WE 250
        Brain   WL 350
        Cardiovascular see Cardiovascular
        Abnormalities   WG 220
        Chromosome see Chromosome Abnormalities
        QS 677
        Digestive system see Digestive System
        Abnormalities   WI 101
        Embryological   QS 675–681
        Etiology   QS 675
        Foot   WE 883
        Gynecological
            General   WP 150
            Pelvic   WQ 320
        Heart see Heart Defects, Congenital   WG 220
        Intestines   WI 412
        Jaw see Jaw Abnormalities   WU 101.5
        Maxillofacial see Maxillofacial Abnormalities
        WE 705, etc.
        Medical curiosities   WZ 308
        Mouth see Mouth Abnormalities   WU 101.5
        Musculoskeletal see Musculoskeletal
        Abnormalities   WE 101
        Nervous system see Nervous System
        Abnormalities   WL 101
        Otolaryngology   WV 101

        Respiratory system see Respiratory System
        Abnormalities   WF 101
        Sex chromosome see Sex Chromosome
        Abnormalities   QS 677
        Skin see Skin Abnormalities   WR 218
        Stomatognathic system see Stomatognathic
        System Abnormalities   WU 101.5
        Tooth see Tooth Abnormalities   WU 101.5
        Urogenital system see Urogenital
        Abnormalities   WJ 101
        Vertebrae   WE 730–735
        Veterinary   SF 769
    Developmental   QZ 45
    See also names of other organs affected or of
    specific abnormalities
Abnormalities, Drug-Induced   QS 679
Abnormalities, Multiple   QS 675
Abnormalities, Radiation-Induced   QS 681
Abomasum   QL 862
Aborigines
    Indians   E 51–99
    Eskimos   E 99.E7
    Special topics, by subject
    See also Australoid Race   GN 662–671
Abortifacient Agents   QV 175
Abortifacient Agents, Non-Steroidal   QV 175
Abortifacient Agents, Steroidal   QV 175
Abortion, Criminal   W 867
Abortion, Habitual   WQ 225
Abortion, Illegal see Abortion, Criminal
Abortion, Incomplete   WQ 225
Abortion, Induced
    Religious and social aspects   HQ 767–767.52
    Technique   WQ 440
Abortion, Legal   WQ 440
    See also Family Planning   HQ 763.5–767.7
Abortion, Missed   WQ 225
Abortion on Demand see Abortion, Legal
Abortion, Septic   WQ 256
    Veterinary   SF 887
Abortion, Spontaneous   WQ 225
    Drugs provoking see Abortifacient Agents   QV
    175
    Medicolegal aspects   W 867
    Religious and social aspects   HQ 767–767.52
Abortion, Therapeutic   WQ 440
Abortion, Threatened   WQ 225
Abortion, Veterinary   SF 887
Abrasions see Dermabrasion; Tooth Abrasion;
    Wounds and Injuries
Abreaction   WM 420.5.A2
Abruptio Placentae   WQ 212
Abscess   WC 195
    Bone   WE 251
    Cerebral see Brain Abscess   WL 351
    General (requiring surgery)   WO 140
    Liver see Liver Abscess   WI 730
    Lung see Lung Abscess   WF 651
    Pelvic   WP 155
    Periapical see Periapical Abscess   WU 230
    Puerperal   WQ 505
    Subphrenic see Subphrenic Abscess   WI 575
    Surgery   WO 140

Other localities, by site

Abscess, Amebic, Hepatic see Liver Abscess, Amebic

Abscess, Cerebral see Brain Abscess

Abscess, Hepatic see Liver Abscess

Abscess, Hepatic, Amebic see Liver Abscess, Amebic

Abscess, Liver, Amebic see Liver Abscess, Amebic

Abscess, Periapical see Periapical Abscess

Abscess, Pulmonary see Lung Abscess

Abscess, Subphrenic see Subphrenic Abscess

Absence Seizures see Epilepsy, Absence

Absenteeism
    Workplace   HD 5115-5115.2
    School   WA 350

Absorption
    Immunochemistry   QW 504.5
    Intestinal see Intestinal Absorption   WI 402
    Of drugs   QV 38
    Of foods   WI 102
    Of gases   QC 162
    Skin see Skin Absorption   WR 102
    Of other substances, with the substance

Absorption, Intestinal see Intestinal Absorption

Absorption, Skin see Skin Absorption

Abstinence Syndrome, Neonatal see Neonatal Abstinence Syndrome

Abstracting and Indexing   Z 695.9-695.92

Abstracts
    Of subjects represented in NLM's classification, appropriate classification number preceded by the letter Z
    Of other subjects, LC's Z schedule

Abuse of Health Services see Health Services Misuse

Abuse Reporting see Mandatory Reporting

Academies and Institutes   AS
    (Form numbers 23-24 in any NLM schedule where applicable)
    For other particular purposes, by subject

Acanthocephala   QX 200

Acantholysis Bullosa see Epidermolysis Bullosa

Acanthosis Nigricans   WR 265

Acari   QX 473

Acariasis see Mite Infestations

Acarina see Acari

Acarus see Mites

Acceleration   WD 720

Accelography see Kinetocardiography

Acceptability of Health Care see Patient Acceptance of Health Care

Access to Health Care see Health Services Accessibility

Accessibility of Health Services see Health Services Accessibility

Accessory Cells, Immunologic see Antigen-Presenting Cells

Accessory Nerve   WL 330

Accident Insurance see Insurance, Accident

Accident Prevention   WA 250-288
    In hospitals   WX 185
    In workplace see Accidents, Occupational   WA 485-491
    Radiation injuries   WN 650

See also specific types of accidents, e.g., Prevention & control under Accidents, Traffic WA 275; Protective devices   WA 260, etc.

Accident Services see Ambulances; Emergency Health Services; Insurance, Accident; Occupational Health Services

Accidental Falls
    In the home   WA 288

Accidents
    First aid   WA 292
    In anesthesia   WO 245
    Medicolegal aspects
        Cause of death   W 843
        Disability evaluation   W 900-925
    See also Insurance, Accident   W 100-250, etc.

Accidents, Aviation   WD 740
    See also special topics under Accidents

Accidents, Home   WA 288
    See also special topics under Accidents

Accidents, Industrial see Accidents, Occupational

Accidents, Occupational   WA 485-491, etc.
    Of the eye   WW 505-525
    See also special topics under Accidents

Accidents, Radiation
    In industry   WA 470

Accidents, Traffic   WA 275
    Prevention & control   WA 275
    See also special topics under Accidents

Acclimatization   QT 145
    Cold climate   QT 160
    Hot climate   QT 150
    See also Desert climate   QT 150, etc.; Tropical climate   QT 150, etc.

Accommodation, Ocular   WW 109

Accountable Health Plans see Managed Competition

Accounting
    Dental administration   WU 77
    Hospital administration   WX 157
    Medical administration   W 80
    Nursing administration   WY 77
    Pharmacy administration   QV 736
    In other specific fields, by subject

Accounts Payable and Receivable see Accounting

Accreditation
    Dentists   WU 40
    Hospitals   WX 15
        Special (Form numbers 27-28 in any NLM schedule where applicable)
    Physicians   W 40
    Schools (Form numbers 18 or other appropriate education number in any NLM schedule where applicable)
    Other institutes, etc. (Form numbers 23-24 in any NLM schedule where applicable)
    Other professionals (Form number 21 in any NLM schedule where applicable)

Acculturation   GN 366-367
    Of particular customs, by subject
    Of particular peoples, by race or country

ACE Inhibitors see Angiotensin-Converting Enzyme Inhibitors

Acephen see Meclofenoxate

Acetabularia   QK 569.D33

Acetabulum   WE 750
Acetaldehyde   QU 99
  In alcohol metabolism   QV 84
  Organic chemistry   QD 305.A6
  Special topics, by subject, e.g., in experiments
    on muscle contraction   WE 500
Acetanilides   QV 95
Acetarsone see Arsenic
Acetates   QU 90
  Organic chemistry   QD 305.A2
Acetic Acids   QU 90
  Organic chemistry   QD 305.A2
Acetoacetates   QU 90
  Organic chemistry   QD 305.A2
Acetobacter   QW 131
Acetonchloroform see Chlorobutanol
Acetone
  In urine   QY 185
  Organic chemistry   QD 305.K2
Acetone Bodies see Ketone Bodies
Acetophenetidin see Phenacetin
Acetyl Carnitine see Acetylcarnitine
Acetyl Glyceryl Ether Phosphorylcholine see
  Platelet Activating Factor
Acetylbenzoylaconine see Aconitine
Acetylcarnitine   QU 187
Acetylcholine   QV 122
Acetylcholine Antagonists see Cholinergic
  Antagonists
Acetylcholine Receptors see Receptors, Cholinergic
Acetylcholinesterase   QU 136
Acetylcholinesterase Inhibitors see Cholinesterase
  Inhibitors
Acetylene
  Organic chemistry   QD 305.H8
  Plant and soil microbiology   QW 60
  Toxicology   QV 633
Acetylformaldehyde see Pyruvaldehyde
Acetylmuramyl-Alanyl-Isoglutamine   QW 800
  Biochemistry   QU 68
Acetylsalicylic Acid see Aspirin
Achalasia, Esophageal see Esophageal Achalasia
Achievement   BF 637.S8
  For infants or children
    Measurement   WS 105.5.E8
    Motivation   WS 105.5.M5
  Motivation   BF 501-505
  Personality development   BF 698.9.A3
  Success   BF 1611-1618
  See also Educational Measurement   LB
    3050-3060.87
Achilles Tendon   WE 880
Achlorhydria   WI 308
Achondroplasia   WE 250
Achromobacter see Alcaligenes
Achromobacteriaceae see Gram-Negative Aerobic
  Bacteria
Achylia Gastrica see Achlorhydria
Acid Aspiration Syndrome see Pneumonia,
  Aspiration
Acid-Base Equilibrium   QU 105
Acid-Base Imbalance   WD 220
Acid Etching, Dental   WU 190

Acid Phosphatase   QU 136
Acid Seromucoid see Orosomucoid
Acidosis   WD 222
  Veterinary   SF 910.W38
Acidosis, Diabetic see Diabetic Ketoacidosis
Acidosis, Renal Tubular   WJ 301
Acidosis, Respiratory   WF 140
Acids
  Inorganic chemistry   QD 167
  Organic chemistry
    Aliphatic compounds   QD 305.A2
    Aromatic compounds   QD 341.A2
  Toxicology
    Inorganic   QV 612
    Organic   QV 632
  See also names of specific acids
Aciphenochinolium see Cinchophen
Aclacinomycin A see Aclarubicin
Aclarubicin   QV 269
Acne see Acne Vulgaris
Acne Rosacea   WR 430
Acne Vulgaris   WR 430
Acneform Lesions see Acne
Acneiform Eruptions   WR 430
Acomys see Muridae
Aconite
  Toxicology   QV 628
Aconitine
  Toxicology   QV 628
Acosta's Disease see Altitude Sickness
Acoustic Evoked Brain Stem Potentials see Evoked
  Potentials, Auditory, Brain Stem
Acoustic Impedance Tests   WV 272
Acoustic Nerve   WL 330
  Physiology of hearing   WV 272
  See also Cochlear Nerve   WL 330; Vestibular
    Nerve   WL 330
Acoustic Nerve Diseases   WL 330
  See also Neuroma, Acoustic   WV 250
Acoustic Neuroma see Neuroma, Acoustic
Acoustic Sense see Hearing
Acoustic Trauma see Hearing Loss, Noise-Induced
Acoustics
  Noise abatement
    General   WA 776
    Housing   WA 795
    Industrial   WA 470
    Public buildings   WA 799
  Physics   QC 221-246
  Sound recording industry   TS 2301.S6
  See also Hearing   WV 270-280
    Noise   WA 776, etc.
Acoustics, Speech see Speech Acoustics
Acquired Immunity see Immunity
Acquired Immunodeficiency Syndrome   WC
  503-503.7
  General works   WC 503
  Complications   WC 503.5
  Diagnosis   WC 503.1
  Epidemiology   WC 503.4
  Etiology. Transmission   WC 503.3
  Nursing   WY 153.5
  Prevention & control   WC 503.6

**ALWAYS CONSULT MAIN SCHEDULES. USE NUMBER ASSIGNED ONLY WHEN
SUBJECT REPRESENTS MAJOR EMPHASIS OF WORK BEING CLASSIFIED**

Psychosocial aspects   WC 503.7
Therapy   WC 503.2
Acridines
   Dyes
      As a disinfectant   QV 235
      As a stain, etc.   QV 240
      In amino acid biochemistry   QU 65
      Organic chemistry   QD 401
Acrocephalosyndactylia   WE 250
Acrocephaly see Craniosynostoses
Acrodermatitis   WR 218
Acrolein
   Toxicology   QV 627
Acromegaly   WK 550
Acromelalgia see Erythromelalgia
Acromioclavicular Joint   WE 810
Acronine   QV 269
Acronycine see Acronine
Acronyms
   Medical   W 13
      By specialties (Form number 13 in any NLM
      schedule where applicable)
Acrosin   QU 136
Acrosomal proteinase see Acrosin
Acrylamides   QU 62
   Organic chemistry   QD 305.A7
Acrylates
   Chemical technology   TP 1180.A35
   In dentistry   WU 90
   In orthopedics   WE 190
   Pharmacology   QV 50
   Used in particular procedure, with the procedure
Acrylic Resins
   Chemical technology   TP 1180.A35
   In dentistry   WU 190
   Pharmacology   QV 50
   Used for special purposes, by subject, e.g., in
      orthopedic surgery   WE 190
   See also Bone Cements   WE 190
ACTH see Corticotropin
ACTH-Releasing Factor see
   Corticotropin-Releasing Hormone
Actihaemyl   QV 370
Actin-Binding Proteins see Microfilament Proteins
Acting Out   WM 193.5.A2
   Adolescence   WS 463
   Child   WS 350.8.D3
   Infant   WS 350.8.D3
Actinic Rays see Ultraviolet Rays
Actinides see Metals, Actinoid
Actinium   WN 420
   Nuclear physics   QC 796.A2
Actinoids see Metals, Actinoid
Actinomyces   QW 125.5.A2
Actinomyces Infections see Actinomycosis
Actinomycetaceae   QW 125.5.A2
Actinomycetales   QW 125–125.5
Actinomycetales Infections   WC 302
Actinomycete Infections see Actinomycetales
   Infections
Actinomycetes see Bacteria; names of specific
   organisms or groups, e.g., Coryneform group
Actinomycin see Dactinomycin

Actinomycosis   WC 302
Actinomycosis, Cervicofacial   WC 302
Actinon see Radon
Actinotherapy see Ultraviolet Therapy
Action Potentials   WL 102
   Muscles   WE 102
   Other sites: classify in physiology number for the
      site or the general number if no physiology
      number exists.
Activation Analysis   QD 606
Activator Appliances   WU 426
Active Immunity see Immunity, Active
Active Site see Binding Sites
Active Transport see Biological Transport, Active
Activities of Daily Living
   Aged   WT 120
   Disabled   HV 3011
      Homemaking   HV 3011
   Orthopedic devices for   WE 172
      Catalogs for   WE 26
   Special disabilities or diseases, by subject
   Special types of activity not limited to a special
      group of people, by activity
Activity Cycles   QT 167
Activity Therapy
   In psychotherapy   WM 450
   In therapy of physical diseases   WB 555
Actuarial Analysis   HG 8779–8793
   Related to specific service plans, by subject, e.g.,
      Psychiatric insurance   W 270
Acuity, Visual see Visual Acuity
Acupoints see Acupuncture Points
Acupressure   WB 537
Acupuncture   WB 369
   Veterinary   SF 914.5
Acupuncture Anesthesia   WB 369
Acupuncture Points   WB 369
Acupuncture Therapy   WB 369
Acute Abdomen see Abdomen, Acute
Acute Disease   WB 105
   Child   WS 200
   Infant   WS 200
Acute-Phase Proteins   WH 400
Acute Phase Reactants see Acute Phase Proteins
Acute-Phase Reaction   QZ 150
   Localized, by site
Acute-Phase State see Acute-Phase Reaction
Acycloguanosine see Acyclovir
Acyclovir   QV 268.5
Acyltransferases   QU 141
   Deficiency   WD 105
Adamantinoma see Ameloblastoma
Adams-Stokes Syndrome   WG 330
Adaptation, Biological   QH 546
Adaptation, Ocular   WW 109
Adaptation, Physiological   QT 140
   Aviation   WD 710
   Space flight   WD 752
Adaptation, Psychological   BF 335
   Adolescence   WS 462
   Aviation   WD 730
   Child   WS 105.5.A8
   Infant   WS 105.5.A8

**ALWAYS CONSULT MAIN SCHEDULES. USE NUMBER ASSIGNED ONLY WHEN
SUBJECT REPRESENTS MAJOR EMPHASIS OF WORK BEING CLASSIFIED**

I-4

Space flight   WD 754
Other specific subjects, by subject
Adaptation Syndrome see Stress
Addictive Behavior see Behavior, Addictive
Addison's Anemia see Anemia, Pernicious
Addison's Disease   WK 765
Addresses see Form number 9 in any NLM schedule
  where applicable
Adenine
  In nucleic acids   QU 58
  Organic chemistry   QD 401
Adenine Arabinoside see Vidarabine
Adenine Nucleotides
  Biochemistry   QU 57
  Pharmacology   QV 185
Adenitis see Lymphadenitis
Adenocarcinoma   QZ 365
  Localized, by site
Adenocarcinoma, Bronchiolo-Alveolar   WF 658
Adenocarcinoma, Renal Cell see Carcinoma, Renal
  Cell
Adenofibroma   QZ 310
  Localized, by site
Adenohypophysis see Pituitary Gland, Anterior
Adenoidectomy   WV 430
Adenoids   WV 430
Adenolymphoma   WI 230
Adenoma   QZ 365
Adenoma, Acidophil   WK 585
Adenoma, Chromophobe   WK 585
Adenoma, Eosinophilic see Adenoma, Acidophil
Adenoma, Islet Cell   WK 885
Adenoma, Prolactin-Secreting, Pituitary see
  Prolactinoma
Adenoma, Prostatic see Prostatic Hyperplasia
Adenoma, Sweat Gland   WR 500
  Localized, by site
Adenoma, Virilizing   WK 780
Adenomatous Polyposis Coli   WI 520
Adenomyosis see Endometriosis
Adenosine   QU 57
  Pharmacology   QV 185
Adenosine Aminohydrolase see Adenosine
  Deaminase
Adenosine Cyclic Monophosphate see Cyclic AMP
Adenosine Cyclic 2',3'-Monophosphate see Cyclic
  AMP
Adenosine Cyclic 3',5'-Monophosphate see Cyclic
  AMP
Adenosine Deaminase   QU 136
Adenosine Diphosphate   QU 57
  Pharmacology   QV 185
Adenosine Diphosphate Ribose   QU 57
Adenosine Diphosphoribose see Adenosine
  Diphosphate Ribose
Adenosine Phosphates see Adenine Nucleotides
Adenosine Pyrophosphate see Adenosine
  Diphosphate
Adenosine Receptors see Receptors, Purinergic P1
Adenosine Triphosphate   QU 57
  In general metabolism   QU 120
  Pharmacology   QV 185
Adenosinetriphosphatase   QU 136

Adenosinetriphosphatase, Calcium see
  Ca(2+)-Transporting ATPase
Adenosinetriphosphatase, Calcium, Magnesium see
  Ca(2+) Mg(2+)-ATPase
Adenosinetriphosphatase F1 see H(+)-Transporting
  ATP Synthase
Adenosinetriphosphatase, Magnesium see Ca(2+)
  Mg(2+)-ATPase
Adenosinetriphosphatase, Sodium, Potassium see
  Na(+)-K(+)-Exchanging ATPase
Adenosis of Breast see Fibrocystic Disease of Breast
Adenoviridae   QW 165.5.A3
Adenoviridae Infections   WC 500
Adenovirus Infections see Adenoviridae Infections
Adenyl Cyclase see Adenylate Cyclase
Adenylate Cyclase   QU 139
Adenylpyrophosphate see Adenosine Triphosphate
Adhesion, Bacterial see Bacterial Adhesion
Adhesions
  Abdominal   WI 900
  Gynecologic   WP 140
  Localized, by site
Adhesive Plaster see Bandages
Adhesiveness   QC 183
  Chemical technology   TP 967-970
Adhesives   TP 967-970
Adipocere see Postmortem Changes
Adipose Tissue   QS 532.5.A3
Adiposis Dolorosa   WD 214
Adjustment Disorders   WM 171
  Psychotic see Affective Disorders, Psychotic
  WM 207
Adjustment, Social see Social Adjustment
Adjuvants, Anesthesia   QV 81
Adjuvants, Immunologic   QW 800
Adjuvants, Pharmaceutic   QV 38
ADL see Activities of Daily Living
Administration see Organization and Administration
Administration, Cutaneous   WB 340
Administration, Health see Public Health
  Administration
Administration, Inhalation   WB 342
Administration, Intranasal   WB 342
Administration, Intravesical   WB 340
Administration of Medicine see Administrative
  methods   WB 340-356 under Drugs
Administration, Oral   WB 350
Administration, Rectal   WB 344
Administration Research, Nursing see Nursing
  Administration Research
Administration Schedule, Drug see Drug
  Administration Schedule
Administration, Topical   WB 340
Administrative Personnel
  Business administration   HF 5549-5549.5
  Hospital administration   WX 155
  Industrial management   HD 28-70
  Nursing administration   WY 105
  Public health administration   WA 525-546
  See also names of particular types of
    administrators, e.g., Medical record
    administrators   WX 173
Administrative Work see Organization and
  Administration

**ALWAYS CONSULT MAIN SCHEDULES. USE NUMBER ASSIGNED ONLY WHEN
SUBJECT REPRESENTS MAJOR EMPHASIS OF WORK BEING CLASSIFIED**

Administrators see Administrative Personnel

Admission Tests, Routine see Diagnostic Tests, Routine

Admitting Department, Hospital   WX 158
   Of specialty hospitals (Form number 27–28 in any NLM schedule where applicable)

Adnexa Uteri   WP 275–322

Adnexal Diseases   WP 275–322

Adnexitis   WP 275
   Pelvic inflammations   WP 155–157

Adolescence   WS 460–463
   Pregnancy see Pregnancy in Adolescence   WS 462, etc.

Adolescent Behavior   WS 462

Adolescent Health Services   WA 330

Adolescent, Hospitalized   WS 460–463

Adolescent, Institutionalized   WS 460–463

Adolescent Medicine   WS 460

Adolescent Pregnancy see Pregnancy in Adolescence

Adolescent Psychiatry   WS 463
   As a career   WS 463

Adolescent Psychology   WS 462

Adoption
   Psychological aspects   WS 105.5.F2
   Sociological aspects   HV 874.8–875.7

Adoptive Cell Transfer see Immunotherapy, Adoptive

Adoptive Cellular Immunotherapy see Immunotherapy, Adoptive

ADP see Adenosine Diphosphate

ADP Receptors see Receptors, Purinergic P2

ADP Ribose see Adenosine Diphosphate Ribose

ADP–Ribosyltransferase (Polymerizing) see NAD+ ADP–Ribosyltransferase

Adrenal Cortex   WK 750–770

Adrenal Cortex Diseases   WK 760

Adrenal Cortex Function Tests   WK 750

Adrenal Cortex Hormones   WK 755
   Synthetic   WK 757

Adrenal Cortex Hyperfunction see Adrenal Gland Hyperfunction

Adrenal Cortex Hypofunction see Adrenal Gland Hypofunction

Adrenal Cortex Neoplasms   WK 780

Adrenal Gland Diseases   WK 700–790

Adrenal Gland Hyperfunction   WK 770

Adrenal Gland Hypofunction   WK 765

Adrenal Gland Neoplasms   WK 780

Adrenal Glands   WK 700–790

Adrenal Hyperplasia, Congenital   WK 700

Adrenal Insufficiency see Adrenal Gland Hypofunction

Adrenal Medulla   WK 725

Adrenalectomy   WK 790

Adrenalin see Epinephrine

Adrenaline see Epinephrine

Adrenergic Agents   QV 129–132

Adrenergic Agonists   QV 129

Adrenergic alpha–Agonists   QV 129

Adrenergic alpha–Antagonists   QV 132

Adrenergic alpha–Receptor Agonists see Adrenergic alpha–Agonists

Adrenergic alpha Receptor Blockaders see Adrenergic alpha–Antagonists

Adrenergic alpha–Receptors see Receptors, Adrenergic, alpha

Adrenergic Antagonists   QV 132

Adrenergic beta–Agonists   QV 129

Adrenergic beta–Antagonists   QV 132

Adrenergic beta–Receptor Agonists see Adrenergic beta–Agonists

Adrenergic beta–Receptor Blockaders see Adrenergic beta–Antagonists

Adrenergic beta–Receptors see Receptors, Adrenergic, beta

Adrenergic–Blocking Agents see Adrenergic Antagonists

Adrenergic Neuron Agents see Adrenergic Agents

Adrenergic Receptor Agonists see Adrenergic Agonists

Adrenergic Receptors see Receptors, Adrenergic

Adrenoceptors see Receptors, Adrenergic

Adrenochrome   QV 77.7

Adrenocorticotropic Hormone see Corticotropin

Adrenocorticotropin see Corticotropin

Adrenogenital Syndrome see Adrenal Hyperplasia, Congenital

Adrenoleukodystrophy   WD 205.5.L5

Adrenoleukodystrophy, Neonatal see Peroxisomal Disorders

Adrenolytics see Adrenergic Agents

Adrenomimetics see Adrenergic Agents

Adrenomyeloneuropathy see Adrenoleukodystrophy

Adriamycin see Doxorubicin

Adsorbents see Dermatologic Agents; Gastrointestinal Agents; Powders

Adsorption
   Immunochemistry   QW 504.5
   Of drugs   QV 38
   Of gases   QC 162
      Chemical engineering   TP 156.A35
   Of matter   QC 182
   Of solutions   QD 547
   Virology   QW 160
   Of other substances, with the substance

Adult
   Developmental psychology   BF 724.5–724.85
      Middle age   BF 724.6–724.65
   Other particular topics, by subject
   See also Aging   WT 104

Adult Respiratory Distress Syndrome see Respiratory Distress Syndrome, Adult

Adult T–Cell Leukemia–Lymphoma Virus I see HTLV–I

Adulteration of Drugs see Drug Contamination; Legislation, Drug

Adulteration of food see Food Contamination

Advance Directives   W 85.5

Advertising
   Alcoholic beverages   HF 6161.L46
   Cigarette   HF 6161.T6
   Dental   WU 58
   Medical   W 58
   Pharmaceutical   QV 736

See also Drug Labeling QV 835
Tobacco HF 6161.T6
Other special subjects, by business in HF 6161
  or other appropriate number
Aedes QX 525
Aerobacter see Enterobacter
Aerobic Exercise see Exercise
Aerobiosis QU 120
Aeroembolism see Embolism, Air
Aerophagy WI 150
Aerophobia see Phobic Disorders
Aeroplanes see Aircraft
Aerosols
  Disinfectant QV 220
  Dosage form QV 785
  Pollutant see Air Pollutants WA 450; WA 754
  Used in inhalation therapy WB 342
Aerospace Medicine WD 700–758
  Aviation medicine WD 700–745
    Psychological aspects WD 730
  General WD 700–745
  Space medicine WD 750–758
    Psychological aspects WD 754
Aerotherapy see Therapy WB 460 under Air
AET WN 650
Affect BF 511–568
  Adolescence WS 462
  Child WS 105.5.E5
  Infant WS 105.5.E5
Affective Disorders see Mood Disorders
Affective Disorders, Psychotic WM 207
Affective Disturbances see Affective Symptoms
Affective Psychosis, Bipolar see Bipolar Disorder
Affective Symptoms
  Adolescence WS 463
  Child WS 350.6
  Infant WS 350.6
  Neurotic WM 171
  Psychotic WM 207
Affinity, Antibody see Antibody Affinity
Afibrinogenemia WH 322
Aflatoxins QW 630
AFP see alpha Fetoproteins
African Americans see Blacks
African Green Monkey see Cercopithecus aethiops
African Lymphoma see Burkitt Lymphoma
African Swine Fever SF 977.A4
African Swine Fever Virus QW 165.5.I6
Afterbirth see Fetal Membranes; Placenta
Afterbrain see Cerebellum; Pons
Aftercare
  Child WS 366
  Infant WS 366
  Of the mentally ill WM 29
  Of the physically ill and disabled WB 325
  Of particular diseases, with the disease
  See also Nursing Care WY 100; Postoperative
    Care WO 183; Perioperative Nursing WY
    161
Afterimage WW 105
Agammaglobulinemia WH 400
Agar QU 83
  Cathartic QV 75

Culture medium QY 26
Agaric, Fly see Mushrooms
Agaricaceae see Agaricales
Agaricales QW 180.5.B2
  Poisoning WD 520
Age Determination by Skeleton GN 70
Age Determination by Teeth GN 209
  Animal SF 869
Age Factors
  As a cause of disease QZ 53
  Demography HB 1531–1737
  Related to other particular subjects, by subject
  See also Gestational Age WQ 210.5
Age-Related Osteoporosis see Osteoporosis
Aged WT
  Anesthesia WO 445
  Dentistry see Geriatric Dentistry WU 490
  Mental health WT 145
  Nursing see Geriatric Nursing WY 152
  Nutritional requirements; Nutrition Disorders
    WT 115
  Physical examination and diagnosis WT 141
  Psychiatry see Geriatric Psychiatry WT 150
    See also Dementia, Senile WT 155
  Psychology WT 145
  Social problems; Surveys WT 30
  Surgery WO 950
  Therapeutics (General) WT 166
  See also Geriatrics
Aged Abuse see Elder Abuse
Aged, 80 and over WT
  See special topics under Aged
AGEPC see Platelet Activating Factor
Agglutination QW 640
  Diagnostic reactions QY 265
  See also Hemagglutination QW 640
Agglutination Tests QY 265
Agglutinins QW 640
  Plant QW 640
Agglutinins, Plant see Lectins
Aggression
  Animals QL 758.5
  Psychology
    Adolescence WS 462
    Adult BF 575.A3
    Child WS 105.5.S6
    Infant WS 105.5.S6
  Social behavior disorder
    Adolescence WS 463
    Adult WM 600
    Child WS 350.8.A4
    Infant WS 350.8.A4
    See also Violence HM
Aggressiveness see Aggression
Aging WT 104
  Psychological changes WT 145
Aging, Premature
  Child WS 104
  Infant WS 104
    See also Progeria WS 104
  Adult (General, not associated with specific
    disease, life style, or pathological process)
    WT 104

**ALWAYS CONSULT MAIN SCHEDULES. USE NUMBER ASSIGNED ONLY WHEN
SUBJECT REPRESENTS MAJOR EMPHASIS OF WORK BEING CLASSIFIED**

Adult in association with general pathological
processes   QZ 45
In association with specific diseases or
behaviors, with the disease or behavior
Genetics   QZ 45
See also Werner Syndrome   QZ 45
Agkistrodon rhodostoma Venom Protease see
Ancrod
Agkistrodon Serine Proteinase see Ancrod
Agnosia   WL 340
Agonistic Behavior   QL 758.5
Agoraphobia   WM 178
Agrammatism see Aphasia, Broca
Agranulocytosis   WH 200
Agraphia   WL 340
Agricultural Chemistry see Chemistry, Agricultural
Agricultural Workers' Diseases   WA 400
See also Farmer's Lung   WF 652
Agriculture   S
General works   S 491–494.5
AH 5158 see Labetalol
AHG–CDC Tests see Cytotoxicity Tests,
Immunologic
Aid to Families with Dependent Children   HV
697–700
Public health aspects   WA 320
Aid to the Blind see Social Security
Aid to the Totally Disabled see Social Security
AIDS see Acquired Immunodeficiency Syndrome
AIDS Antibodies see HIV Antibodies
AIDS–Associated Enteropathy see HIV
Enteropathy
AIDS–Associated Nephropathy   WC 503.5
AIDS Dementia Complex   WC 503.5
AIDS Drugs see Anti–HIV Agents
AIDS Encephalopathy see AIDS Dementia
Complex
AIDS Enteropathy see HIV Enteropathy
AIDS–Related Complex   WC 503–503.7
AIDS–Related Opportunistic Infections
General   WC 503.5
See also names of specific infections
AIDS Seroconversion see HIV Seropositivity
AIDS Serodiagnosis   QY 265
AIDS Serology see AIDS Serodiagnosis
AIDS Seropositivity see HIV Seropositivity
AIDS Virus see HIV–1
AIDS Wasting Syndrome see HIV Wasting
Syndrome
Ainhum   WE 835
Air
Industrial hygiene   WA 450
Public health aspects   WA 750–776
Relation to personal health   QT 230
Therapy
Pharmacology   QV 310
Physical medicine   WB 460
See also Atmosphere   WA 750–776, etc.
Air Bladder see Air Sacs
Air Conditioning   WA 774
Air Defense see Aviation; Civil Defense; Military
Science

Air Ionization
Physics
Electricity   QC 702
Meteorology   QC 969
Physiology   QT 162.A5
Public health hazard   WA 750
Therapeutic use   WB 460
For other uses, by subject
Air Microbiology   QW 82
Air Movements   QC 880.4.A8
Clinical aspects of disease caused by
Aviation problems   WD 720
Extraterritorial environment   WD 758
General works   WD 600
Motion sickness   WD 630
Vibration disorders   WD 640
Etiology of disease   QZ 57
Spread of pesticides   WA 240
Wind (General)   QC 930.5–959
Air Pollutants   WA 754
See also names of specific pollutants
Air Pollutants, Environmental   WA 754
Air Pollutants, Occupational   WA 450
Air Pollutants, Radioactive   WN 615
Air Pollution   WA 754
In industry   WA 450
Legislation   WA 32–33
Air Pollution, Indoor   WA 754
Air Pollution, Radioactive   WN 615
See also Air Pollutants, Radioactive   WN 615;
Radioactive Pollutants   WN 615, etc.; names
of specific pollutants
Air Pollution, Tobacco Smoke see Tobacco Smoke
Pollution
Air Pressure
High altitude   WD 710
Underwater   WD 650
Air Quality, Indoor see Air Pollution, Indoor
Air Radiography see Pneumoradiography
Air Raid Protection see Civil Defense
Air Sacs   QL 855
Air Swallowing see Aerophagy
Air Travel, Accidents see Accidents, Aviation
Aircraft
As ambulances   WX 215
Industrial diseases of aircraft construction and
maintenance workers   WA 400–495
Noise effects
On aviators and passengers   WD 735
On animals and humans on the ground   WA
776
Nursing service   WY 143
Pollution   WA 754
Relation to aviation and space medicine   WD
700–758
Sanitation   WA 810
Speed effects   WD 720
See also Aviation   WD 705, etc.
Airsickness see Motion Sickness
Airway Obstruction   WF 140
In anesthesia   WO 250
Airway Resistance   WF 102
Tests   WF 141

**ALWAYS CONSULT MAIN SCHEDULES.   USE NUMBER ASSIGNED ONLY WHEN
SUBJECT REPRESENTS MAJOR EMPHASIS OF WORK BEING CLASSIFIED**

Akamushi Disease see Scrub Typhus
Akinetic Mutism   WL 348
Akinetic Petit Mal see Epilepsy, Absence
Alalia see Speech Disorders
Alanine Transaminase   QU 141
Alarm Reaction see Stress
Alaryngeal Speech see Speech, Alaryngeal
Albers-Schoenberg Disease see Osteopetrosis
Albinism   WR 267
Albright's Disease see Fibrous Dysplasia of Bone
Albumins   QU 55
    Serum see Serum Albumin   WH 400, etc.
Albuminuria   WJ 343
Alcaligenes   QW 131
Alchemy   QD 23.3–26.5
    Therapeutics   WB 890
Alcohol Abuse see Alcoholism
Alcohol Amnestic Disorder   WM 274
Alcohol Consumption see Alcohol Drinking
Alcohol Dehydrogenase   QU 140
Alcohol Drinking   WM 274
    Adolescents and children
        Psychiatric problem   WM 274
        School problem   WA 352
        Sociological problem   HV 5006–5722
        Traffic accidents   WA 275
Alcohol, Ethyl see Ethanol
Alcohol, Methyl see Methanol
Alcohol Oxidoreductases   QU 140
Alcohol, Propyl see 1-Propanol
Alcohol-Related Disorders   WM 274
Alcohol Withdrawal Delirium   WM 274
Alcoholic Beverages
    As dietary supplement in health or disease   WB 444
    Chemical technology   TP 500–617
    See also Alcoholism   WM 274; Alcohol, Ethyl QV 84, etc.
Alcoholic Cardiomyopathy see Cardiomyopathy, Alcoholic
Alcoholic Cirrhosis see Liver Cirrhosis, Alcoholic
Alcoholic Fatty Liver see Fatty Liver, Alcoholic
Alcoholic Hepatitis see Hepatitis, Alcoholic
Alcoholic Intoxication   QV 84
    Associated with traffic accidents   WA 275
    In forensic medicine   W 780
Alcoholic Liver Diseases see Liver Diseases, Alcoholic
Alcoholic Pancreatitis see Pancreatitis, Alcoholic
Alcoholism   WM 274
    Classify like material on Alcohol drinking
    See also Fatty liver, Alcoholic   WI 700;
      Hepatitis, Alcoholic   WI 715; Liver Cirrhosis,
      Alcoholic   WI 725; Psychoses, Alcoholic
      WM 274; Skid Row Alcoholics   WM 274, etc.
Alcohols   QV 82–84
    Organic chemistry
        Aliphatic compounds   QD 305.A4
        Aromatic compounds   QD 341.A4
Alcohols, Sugar see Sugar Alcohols
Aldehyde Dehydrogenase   QU 140
Aldehyde Reductase   QU 140
Aldehydes   QU 99

    In alcohol metabolism   QV 84
    Organic chemistry
        Aliphatic compounds   QD 305.A6
        Aromatic compounds   QD 341.A6
    Used for particular experiments, by main topic
      of the work, e.g. as a fixative in histological
      experiments   QS 525–530
Aldicarb
    Agriculture   SB 952.C3
    Public health   WA 240
Aldolase see Fructose–Bisphosphate Aldolase
Aldose Reductase see Aldehyde Reductase
Aldosterone   WK 755
    Deficiency   WK 760
        As a cause of a particular disorder, with the
        disorder
Aldosterone Antagonists   WK 755
Aldosteronism see Hyperaldosteronism
Aleutian Disease Virus see Aleutian Mink Disease
    Virus
Aleutian Mink Disease   SF 997.5.M5
Aleutian Mink Disease Parvovirus see Aleutian Mink
    Disease Virus
Aleutian Mink Disease Virus   QW 165.5.P3
Aleuts see Eskimos
Alexia see Dyslexia, Acquired
Alexin see Complement
Alexithymia see Affective Symptoms
Algae   QK 564–580.5
Algae, Blue–Green see Cyanobacteria
Alginates
    Biochemistry   QU 83
    Phytochemistry   QK 898.A3
    Used in dentistry   WU 190
    Used in surgical dressings   WO 167
Algodystrophic Syndrome see Reflex Sympathetic
    Dystrophy
Algolagnia see Paraphilias
Algor Mortis see Postmortem Changes
Algorithms
    For computers (General)   QA 76.9.A43
    In particular fields (Form number 26.5 in any
      NLM schedule where applicable)
    Applied to special topics, by subject
Alienation, Social see Social Alienation
Alienists see Biography   WZ 112.5.P6, etc. under
    Psychiatry; Directories   WM 22 under
    Psychiatry
Alimentary Tract see Digestive System
Alimentation (Therapeutics) see Diet Therapy
Aliphatic Compounds see Anti-Infective Agents,
    Local; Formaldehyde; Nitrofurans; Hydrocarbons
    or Aliphatic compounds under Chemistry,
    Organic
Alkalemia see Alkalosis
Alkali Disease see Tularemia
Alkalies
    Pharmacology   QV 275
    Toxicology   QV 612
Alkaline Earth Metals see Metals, Alkaline earth
Alkaline Phosphatase   QU 136
Alkaloids
    As a therapeutic system   WB 890

Organic Chemistry   QD 421.A1–421.7
    Toxicology   QV 628
Alkalosis   WD 226
Alkalosis, Respiratory   WF 140
Alkanes
    Microbial chemistry   QW 52
    Organic chemistry   QD 305.H6
Alkanesulfonates   QU 98
    Organic chemistry   QD 305.S3
Alkenes
    Microbial chemistry   QW 52
    Organic chemistry   QD 305.H7
Alkyl Sulfonates see Alkanesulfonates
Alkylating Agents   QV 269
Alkylation   QD 281.A5
Alkynes
    Organic chemistry   QD 305.H8
ALL, Childhood see Leukemia, Lymphocytic, Acute, L1
Allantiasis see Botulism
Allantoin
    In amino acid metabolism   QU 65
Allantois
    Embryology   QS 645
Alleles   QH 447
Allergen Bronchial Provocation Tests see Bronchial Provocation Tests
Allergen Immunotherapy see Desensitization, Immunologic
Allergens   QW 900
Allergic Angiitis see Churg–Strauss Syndrome
Allergic Conjunctivitis see Conjunctivitis, Allergic
Allergic Cutaneous Angiitis see Vasculitis, Allergic Cutaneous
Allergic Cutaneous Vasculitis see Vasculitis, Allergic Cutaneous
Allergic Diseases see Hypersensitivity
Allergic Granulomatous Angiitis see Churg–Strauss Syndrome
Allergy see Hypersensitivity
Allergy and Immunology   QW 501–949
    Animals   SF 757.2
      Individual, by animal in   QL or SF
    Biography of immunologists
      Collective   WZ 112.5.I5
      Individual   WZ 100
    Directories   QW 522
    Military bacteriology, etc.   UH 450–455
    Nursing texts   QW 504, etc.
    Transplantation see Transplantation Immunology WO 680
    Associated with a particular disease, with the disease
Allergy (Specialty) see Allergy and Immunology
Allied Health Occupations   W 21.5
Allied Health Personnel   W 21.5
    Directories
      General   W 22
      Special types of personnel, in the directory number for the specialty involved
    Education   W 18
Alligators and Crocodiles   QL 666.C925
    Diseases   SF 997.5.R4

Allium
    As a medicinal plant   QV 766
    Botany   QK 495.L72
    As a dietary supplement in health and disease WB 430
Allium cepa see Onions
Allium porrum see Onions
Allium sativum see Garlic
Alloantibodies see Isoantibodies
Alloantigens see Isoantigens
Allograft see Transplantation, Homologous
Allograft Dressings see Biological Dressings
Allosteric Regulation   QU 34
    Special topics, by subject
Allosteric Site   QU 34
Allotypes, Immunoglobulin see Immunoglobulin Allotypes
Allotypic Antibodies see Immunoglobulin Allotypes
Allowing to Die see Euthanasia, Passive
Alloxan Diabetes see Diabetes Mellitus, Experimental
Alloys
    Analysis   QD 133–137
    Dental applications   WU 180
    Particular applications, by subject, e.g. used in orthopedics,   WE 26, WE 172, etc.
Allspice see Rosales
Almanacs   AY 30–1730
Aloe
    As a medicinal plant   QV 766
    As a cathartic   QV 75
Alopecia   WR 460
Alopecia, Androgenetic see Alopecia
Alopecia, Male Pattern see Alopecia
Alpacas see Camelids, New World
Alpers Syndrome see Cerebral Sclerosis, Diffuse
alpha–Adrenergic Blocking Agents see Adrenergic alpha–Antagonists
alpha Adrenergic Receptor Agonists see Adrenergic alpha–Agonists
alpha–Adrenergic Receptor Blockaders see Adrenergic alpha–Antagonists
alpha–Adrenergic Receptors see Receptors, Adrenergic, alpha
alpha–Aminotoluene see Benzylamines
alpha–Blockers, Adrenergic see Adrenergic alpha–Antagonists
alpha–Cell Tumor see Glucagonoma
alpha–Fetoproteins   WQ 210.5
alpha–Glucosidases   QU 136
alpha–Heparin see Heparin
alpha–Hypophamine see Oxytocin
alpha Immunoglobulins see Immunoglobulins, alpha–Chain
Alpha Particles   WN 110
    In nuclear physics (General)   QC 793.5.A22–793.5.A229
    Specific topics, by subject, e.g., of radioisotopes WN 420
Alpha Rays see Alpha Particles
Alpha Rhythm   WL 150
alpha–Trichosanthin see Trichosanthin
alpha 1-Acid Glycoprotein see Orosomucoid

ALWAYS CONSULT MAIN SCHEDULES. USE NUMBER ASSIGNED ONLY WHEN SUBJECT REPRESENTS MAJOR EMPHASIS OF WORK BEING CLASSIFIED

alpha 1–Acid Seromucoid see Orosomucoid
alpha 1–Antitrypsin   WH 400
    As an enzyme inhibitor   QU 143
alpha 1–Protease Inhibitor see alpha 1–Antitrypsin
alpha 1–Proteinase Inhibitor see alpha 1–Antitrypsin
Alphamethyldopa see Methyldopa
Alport's Syndrome see Nephritis, Hereditary
Alprenolol   QV 132
Alprostadil   QU 90
Alteplase see Tissue Plasminogen Activator
Alternative Medicine   WB 890–962
    Cupping   WB 371
    Directories   WB 22
    Veterinary   SF 745.5
Alternatives to Animal Testing see Animal Testing
    Alternatives
Altitude
    Physiological effects   WD 710–715
Altitude Sickness   WD 715
Altruism   BJ 1474
    Special topics, by subject
Aluminosis see Pneumoconiosis
Aluminum
    Inorganic chemistry   QD 181.A4
    Pharmacology   QV 65
Aluminum Hydroxide
    As an antacid   QV 69
Aluminum Hydroxide Gel see Aluminum Hydroxide
Aluminum Silicates
    Inorganic chemistry   QD 181.S6
    Pharmacology   QV 65
Aluminum Sucrose Sulfate see Sucralfate
Alveolar Abscess, Apical see Periapical Abscess
Alveolar Bone Loss   WU 240
Alveolar Echinococcis, Hepatic see Echinococcosis,
    Hepatic
Alveolar Lavage Fluid see Bronchoalveolar Lavage
    Fluid
Alveolar Nerve, Inferior see Mandibular Nerve
Alveolar Process   WU 240
Alveolar Resorption see Alveolar Bone Loss
Alveolar Ridge Augmentation   WU 600
Alveolitis, Fibrosing see Pulmonary Fibrosis
Alzheimer Disease   WT 155
Amalgam Filling see Dental Amalgam
Amanita   QW 180.5.B2
Amanitz see Agaricales
Amaurosis see Blindness
Amaurotic Familial Idiocy see Lipoidosis
Ambidexterity see Laterality
Amblyopia   WW 276
    Toxic   WW 276
Amblystoma see Ambystoma
Amboceptor see Bacteriolysis; Hemolysins
Ambulances   WX 215
    Military   UH 500–505
Ambulatory Care
    General   WB 101
    Child   WS 200
        Clinics   WS 27–28
    In hospitals   WX 205
    Infant   WS 200
        Clinics   WS 27–28

    Nursing   WY 150
        Pediatric nursing   WY 159
    Of a patient with a particular disease, with the
    disease
Ambulatory Care Facilities   WX 205
Ambulatory Care Facilities, Hospital see Outpatient
    Clinics, Hospital
Ambulatory Care Information Systems   WX 26.5
Ambulatory Electrocardiography see
    Electrocardiography, Ambulatory
Ambulatory Surgical Procedures   WO 192
    Of particular parts, by subject
Ambystoma   QL 668.C23
    As laboratory animals   QY 60.A6
Ambystoma mexicanum   QL 668.C23
    As laboratory animals   QY 60.A6
    Diseases   SF 997.5.A45
Ameba see Amoeba
Amebiasis   WC 285
Amebiasis, Hepatic see Liver Abscess, Amebic
Amebiasis, Intestinal see Dysentery, Amebic
Amebic Dysentery see Dysentery, Amebic
Amebicides   QV 255
Ameboma see Amebiasis
Ameloblastoma   WU 280
Amenorrhea   WP 552
Americana see Books
Americium   WN 420
    Nuclear physics   QC 796.A5
    See also special topics under Radioisotopes
Amerinds, Central American see Indians, Central
    American
Amerinds, North American see Indians, North
    American
Amerinds, South American see Indians, South
    American
Amethocaine see Tetracaine
Amethopterin see Methotrexate
Ametropia see Refractive Errors
Amidases see Amidohydrolases
Amidazine see Ethionamide
Amides   QU 62
    Organic chemistry
        Aliphatic compounds   QD 305.A7
        Aromatic compounds   QD 341.A7
Amidines   QU 61
    Organic chemistry   QD 305.A8
Amidohydrolases   QU 136
Amidone see Methadone
Amidophenazon see Aminopyrine
Amidotrezoate see Diatrizoate
Amifostine
    As a radiation–protective agent   WN 650
Amiloride   QV 160
Amine Oxidase (Copper–Containing)   QU 140
Amines   QU 61
    Organic chemistry
        Aliphatic compounds   QD 305.A8
        Aromatic compounds   QD 341.A8
Amines, Biogenic see Biogenic Amines
Amines, Sympathomimetic see Sympathomimetics
Amino Acid Decarboxylases, Aromatic see
    Aromatic–L–Amino–Acid Decarboxylases

Amino Acid Metabolism, Inborn Errors   WD 205.5.A5

Amino Acid Oxidoreductases   QU 140

Amino Acid Sequence   QU 60

Amino Acids   QU 60

Amino Acids, Branched-Chain   QU 60

Amino Acids, Essential   QU 60

Amino Acids, Sulfur   QU 60

Amino Acyl tRNA see RNA, Transfer, Amino Acyl

Amino Alcohols
    Organic chemistry   QD 305.A4
    Pharmacology   QV 82

Amino Sugars   QU 75

Aminoaciduria, Renal   WJ 343

Aminobenzoic Acids   QU 195

Aminobutyrate Aminotransferase see
    4-Aminobutyrate Transaminase

Aminobutyric Acids   QU 60

Aminocaproic Acids   QU 60

Aminocaproic Lactam see Caprolactam

Aminoethanols see Ethanolamines

Aminoform see Methenamine

Aminoglycoside Antibiotics see Antibiotics,
    Aminoglycoside

Aminoglycosides   QU 75

Aminohippuric Acids   QU 62
    Organic chemistry   QD 341.A7

Aminohydrolases   QU 136

Aminophenazone see Aminopyrine

Aminophenurobutane see Carbutamide

Aminopropanols see Propanolamines

Aminopropionitrile
    Organic chemistry
        Aliphatic compounds   QD 305.N7
    In plant poisoning   WD 500

Aminopyrine   QV 95

Aminosalicylic Acids   QV 268

Aminotransferases see Transaminases

Amiodarone   QV 150

Ammoidin see Methoxsalen

Ammonia
    Detergent use QV 233
    In nitrogen fixation
        Biochemistry (General)   QU 70
        Phytochemistry   QK 898.N6
        Plant and soil   QW 60
    Inorganic chemistry   QD 181.N1

Ammonia-Lyases   QU 139

Ammonium Chloride
    Inorganic chemistry   QD 181.N1
    Pharmacology   QV 280

Ammonium Compounds
    Chemical technology   TP 223
    Detergent use   QV 233
    Organic chemistry   QD 305.A8
    Quaternary see Tetraethylammonium Compounds
        QV 132
    See also names of specific compounds

Ammotherapy   WB 525

Amnesia   WM 173.7

Amniocentesis   WQ 209

Amnion
    Animal embryology   QL 975

Human embryology   QS 645
    Obstetrics   WQ 210.5

Amniotic Fluid
    Animal embryology   QL 975
    Human embryology   QS 645
    Obstetrics   WQ 210.5
    See also Embolism, Amniotic Fluid   WQ 244

Amniotic Membrane Dressings see Biological
    Dressings

Amoeba   QX 55

Amoebiasis see Amebiasis

Amoxapine   QV 77.5

Amoxicillin   QV 354

Amphetamines   QV 102
    Dependence   WM 270

Amphibia   QL 640-669.3
    As laboratory animals   QY 60.A6

Amphibian Venoms   WD 400

Amphiuma see Urodela

Ampholines see Ampholyte Mixtures

Ampholyte Mixtures   QV 786

Ampicillin   QV 354

Ampicillin Pivaloyl Ester see Pivampicillin

Ampulla of Vater see Vater's Ampulla

Amputation   WE 170

Amputation Stumps   WE 172

Amputees   WE 172
    Psychology   BF 727.P57
        Child psychology   WS 105.5.H2
    Rehabilitation
        General and medical aspects   WE 172
        Of children   WS 368
        Of disabled soldiers   UB 360-366
        Sociological aspects
            Disabled workers   HD 7255-7256
            Vocational rehabilitation   HV 3018-3019

Amygdala see Amygdaloid Body

Amygdalin   QV 269

Amygdaloid Body   WL 314

Amygdaloside see Amygdalin

Amyl Nitrate   QV 156

Amylases   QU 136
    Pancreatic   WI 802

Amyloid P Component   WH 400

Amyloidosis   WD 205.5.A6

Amyoplasia Congenita see Arthrogryposis

Amyotonia Congenita see Neuromuscular Diseases

Amyotrophic Lateral Sclerosis   WE 550

Anabolic Steroids   WK 150
    See also Metabolism   QU 120, etc.; names of
        anabolic steroids that are also synthetic
        androgens, e.g. Methandrostenolone   WJ 875

Anabolism see Metabolism

Anaerobic Bacteria see Bacteria, Anaerobic

Anaerobiosis   QU 120

Anal Drug Administration see Administration,
    Rectal

Anal Fissure see Fissure in Ano

Anal Fistula see Rectal Fistula

Anal Gland see Anus

Anal Sphincter see Anus

Anal Stage see Psychosexual Development

Anal Ulcer see Fissure in Ano

Analeptics see Central Nervous System Stimulants
Analgesia   WO 200
    In labor see Anesthesia Obstetrical   WO 450
    Muscle relaxants with   WO 297
    Preanesthetic medication   WO 234
    Veterinary   SF 914
Analgesia, Epidural   WO 305
Analgesia in Labor see Anesthesia, Obstetrical
Analgesia Tests see Pain Measurement
Analgesic Cutaneous Electrostimulation see
    Transcutaneous Electric Nerve Stimulation
Analgesics   QV 95
Analgesics, Addictive see Analgesics, Opioid
Analgesics, Anti-Inflammatory see
    Anti-Inflammatory Agents, Non-Steroidal
Analgesics, Narcotic see Analgesics, Opioid
Analgesics, Non-Narcotic   QV 95
Analgesics, Opioid   QV 89-92
    In preanesthetic medication   WO 234
Analgin see Dipyrone
Analogue Pain Scale see Pain Measurement
Analysis see Chemistry, Analytical; names of
    substances being analyzed
Analysis of Variance   QA 279
    Particular variables, by subject
Analytical Psychology see Psychoanalysis
Analyzers, Neural see Neural Analyzers
Anankastic Personality see Compulsive Personality
    Disorder
Anaphylatoxins   QU 68
    In complement activation   QW 680
Anaphylaxis   QW 900
Anaplasma   QW 150
Anaplasmosis   WC 600
    Veterinary   SF 967.A6
Anarthria see Speech Disorders
Anastomosis, Arteriovenous see Arteriovenous
    Anastomosis
Anastomosis, Surgical
    In surgery for a particular condition, with the
    condition
Anatomic Models see Models, Anatomic
Anatomists see Biography   WZ 112, etc., and
    Directories   QS 22 under Anatomy
Anatomy   QS
    Adrenal glands   WK 701
    Bacterial   QW 51
    Cardiovascular system   WG 101
    Directories   QS 22
    Domestic animals   SF 761-767
    Ear   WV 201
    Eye   WW 101
    Fetus   WQ 210.5
    Gastrointestinal system   WI 101
    Gynecology   WP 101
    Heart   WG 201
    Islands of Langerhans   WK 801
    Kidney   WJ 301
    Larynx   WV 501
    Male genitalia   WJ 701
    Musculoskeletal system   WE 101
    Nervous system   WL 101
    Nose   WV 301

Nursing texts   QS 4, etc.
Otolaryngology   WV 101
Pathological (General)   QZ
Pharyngeal region   WV 401
Pituitary gland   WK 501
Respiratory system   WF 101
Skin   WR 101
Stomach   WI 301
Surgical   WO 101
Tooth   WU 101
Thyroid gland   WK 201
Urogenital system   WJ 101
Wild animals   QL 801-950.9
    See also names of specific animals
Other organs or systems, in the general number
    for the organ or system
Anatomy, Artistic   NC 760 783.8
Anatomy, Comparative
    Animals only   QL 801-950.9
    Human and animals   QS 124
Anatomy, Cross-Sectional   QS 4
    See also special organs or systems under Anatomy
Anatomy, Regional   QS 4
    For surgeons   WO 101
Anatomy, Sectional see Anatomy, Cross-Sectional
Anatomy, Veterinary   SF 761-767
    See also Anatomy, Comparative   QL 801-950.9,
    etc.
Anatoxins see Toxoids
Anavar see Oxandrolone
Anchored PCR see Polymerase Chain Reaction
Ancillary Information Systems see Information
    Systems
Ancillary Services, Hospital   WX 162
    Specific topics, by subject
Ancrod
    As an anticoagulant   QV 193
    Biochemistry   QU 136
Ancylostoma   QX 243
Ancylostoma caninum see Ancylostoma
Ancylostoma duodenale see Ancylostoma
Ancylostomatoidea   QX 243
Ancylostomiasis   WC 890
Andresen Appliance see Activator Appliances
Androblastoma   WP 322
Androgen Analogs see Androgens, Synthetic
Androgen Antagonists   WJ 875
Androgens   WJ 875
Androgens, Synthetic   WJ 875
Andrology see Urology
Androstenedione   WJ 875
Anecdotes   PN 6259-6268
    Medicine, medical specialties and related fields
    WZ 305-305.5
Anemia   WH 155-175
    Cooley's see Thalassemia   WH 170
    Erythroblastic see Thalassemia   WH 170
    Megaloblastic see Anemia, Macrocytic   WH 165
    Miners' see Hookworm Infections   WC 890, etc.
    Osteosclerotic see Anemia, Myelophthisic   WH
    175
    Pregnancy   WQ 252
    Tunnel see Ancylostomiasis   WC 890

Specific named types not listed here, see for
    example: Hemoglobinuria   WJ 344
    Veterinary (General)   SF 769.5
Anemia, Addison's see Anemia, Pernicious
Anemia, Aplastic   WH 175
Anemia, Diamond–Blackfan see Fanconi's Anemia
Anemia, Fanconi see Fanconi's Anemia
Anemia, Hemolytic   WH 170
    See also Favism   WD 515; Hemoglobinuria
    WJ 344 and other special topics
Anemia, Hemolytic, Acquired see Anemia,
    Hemolytic
Anemia, Hemolytic, Autoimmune   WH 170
Anemia, Hemolytic, Congenital   WH 170
Anemia, Hemolytic, Idiopathic Acquired see
    Anemia, Hemolytic, Autoimmune
Anemia, Hypochromic   WH 160
Anemia, Hypoplastic see Anemia, Aplastic
Anemia, Hypoplastic, Congenital see Fanconi's
    Anemia
Anemia, Iron–Deficiency   WH 160
Anemia, Leukoerythroblastic see Anemia,
    Myelophthisic
Anemia, Macrocytic   WH 165
Anemia, Megaloblastic   WH 165
Anemia, Microangiopathic see Anemia, Hemolytic
Anemia, Myelophthisic   WH 175
Anemia, Neonatal   WS 421
Anemia, Pernicious   WH 165
Anemia, Sickle Cell   WH 170
Anemia, Splenic see Hypersplenism
Anencephaly   QS 675
Anesthesia   WO 200–460
    Adverse effects   WO 245
    Aged   WO445
    Cardiac problems   WG 460
        Written for the anesthesiologist   WO 245
    Child   WO 440
    Choice of   WO 235
    Drugs producing see Anesthetics   QV 81, etc.;
        Anesthetics, Local   QV 110–115
    In pregnancy see Anesthesia, Obstetrical   WO
        450
    Infant   WO 440
    Nurses administering see Nurse anesthetists   WY
        151
    Of laboratory animals   QY 58
    Veterinary   SF 914
    See also the specialty Anesthesiology   WO
        200–222
Anesthesia Adjuvants see Adjuvants, Anesthesia
Anesthesia Assistants see Physician Assistants
Anesthesia, Caudal   WO 305
Anesthesia, Closed–Circuit   WO 277
Anesthesia, Conduction   WO 300–340
Anesthesia, Dental   WO 460
Anesthesia Department, Hospital   WO 27–28
Anesthesia, Electric see Electronarcosis
Anesthesia, Epidural   WO 305
Anesthesia, Extradural see Anesthesia, Epidural
Anesthesia, General   WO 275
Anesthesia, Inhalation   WO 277
Anesthesia, Intratracheal   WO 280

Anesthesia, Intravenous   WO 285
Anesthesia, Local   WO 300
    Infiltration anesthesia   WO 340
    Surface anesthesia   WO 340
    Topical anesthesia   WO 340
Anesthesia, Obstetrical   WO 450
Anesthesia, Peridural see Anesthesia, Epidural
Anesthesia, Rebreathing see Anesthesia,
    Closed–Circuit
Anesthesia Recovery Period   WO 183
Anesthesia, Rectal   WO 290
Anesthesia, Refrigeration see Hypothermia, Induced
Anesthesia, Regional see Anesthesia, Conduction
Anesthesia, Sacral Epidural see Anesthesia, Caudal
Anesthesia, Spinal   WO 305
Anesthesiology   WO 200–460
    For children and other special groups see Infant
        or Child, etc. under Anesthesia
Anesthetics   QV 81
    Diagnostic use   WO 375
    Therapeutic use   WO 375
    Topical see Anesthetics, Local   QV 115
    See also Analgesics   QV 95, etc.
Anesthetics, Combined
    For general anesthesia   QV 81
Anesthetics, Conduction Blocking see Anesthetics,
    Local
Anesthetics, Local   QV 110–115
    Synthetic   QV 115
Anestrus   SF 105
Aneuploidy   QH 461
Aneurin see Thiamine
Aneurysm   WG 580
    Aortic see Aortic Aneurysm   WG 410
    Arteriovenous see Arteriovenous Fistula   WG
        590
    Cardiac see Heart Aneurysm   WG 300
    Cerebral see Cerebral Aneurysm   WL 354–355
    See also Bone Cyst
Aneurysm, Arteriovenous see Arteriovenous Fistula
Aneurysm, Bacterial see Aneurysm, Infected
Aneurysm, Infected   WG 580
Aneurysm, Mycotic see Aneurysm, Infected
ANF see Atrial Natriuretic Factor
Angel Dust Abuse see Phencyclidine Abuse
Anger   BF 575.A5
    Adolescence   WS 462
    Child   WS 105.5.E5
    Infant   WS 105.5.E5
Angiitis see Vasculitis
Angiitis, Allergic Cutaneous see Vasculitis, Allergic
    Cutaneous
Angiitis, Allergic Granulomatous see Churg–Strauss
    Syndrome
Angina Pectoris   WG 298
Angina Pectoris, Variant   WG 298
Angina, Preinfarction see Angina, Unstable
Angina, Unstable   WG 298
Angiocardiography   WG 141.5.A3
Angioedema see Angioneurotic Edema
Angiogenesis Factor
    As a growth substance   QU 107
    In mitosis   QH 605.2

**ALWAYS CONSULT MAIN SCHEDULES. USE NUMBER ASSIGNED ONLY WHEN
SUBJECT REPRESENTS MAJOR EMPHASIS OF WORK BEING CLASSIFIED**

Angiogenesis, Pathologic see Neovascularization, Pathologic

Angiogenesis, Physiologic see Neovascularization, Physiologic

Angiography   WG 500
   Cerebral   WL 141
   Veterinary   SF 757.8
   Other specific organ or system, by site

Angiography, Cerebral see Cerebral Angiography

Angiohemophilia see von Willebrand Disease

Angioid Streaks   WW 270
   As a manifestation of diseases   WW 475

Angioimmunoblastic Lymphadenopathy see Immunoblastic Lymphadenopathy

Angiokeratoma   WR 500

Angioma see Hemangioma

Angiomatosis   QZ 340
   Localized, by site, in the neoplasm number if available

Angioneurotic Edema   WR 170

Angioplasty   WG 166.5.A3
   In the treatment of a particular disease, with the disease
   See also Endarterectomy   WG 170

Angioplasty, Balloon   WG 166.5.B2
   In the treatment of arterial occlusive diseases WG 510

Angioplasty, Balloon, Coronary see Angioplasty, Transluminal, Percutaneous Coronary

Angioplasty, Coronary Balloon see Angioplasty, Transluminal, Percutaneous Coronary

Angioplasty, Laser   WG 166.5.A5

Angioplasty, Transluminal see Angioplasty, Balloon

Angioplasty, Transluminal, Percutaneous Coronary WG 300

Angiotensin see Angiotensin II

Angiotensin Binding Sites see Receptors, Angiotensin

Angiotensin-Converting Enzyme Inhibitors
   As antihypertensive agents   QV 150
   As protease inhitors   QU 136

Angiotensin-Forming Enzyme see Renin

Angiotensin II   QU 68

Angiotensin Receptors see Receptors, Angiotensin

Angiotensinogen   QU 68

Angiotensinogenase see Renin

Angiotensins   QU 68

Angor Pectoris see Angina Pectoris

Anguilluliasis see Strongyloidiasis

Anhidrosis see Hypohidrosis

Anhidrotic Ectodermal Dysplasia see Ectodermal Dysplasia

Anhydrides
   Organic chemistry
      Aliphatic compounds   QD 305.A2
      Aromatic compounds   QD 341.A2
   Used for special purposes, by subject, e.g., for radiolabeling of proteins   QU 55

Aniline Compounds
   Organic chemistry   QD 341.A8
   Toxicology   QV 632

Animal-Borne Diseases see Zoonoses

Animal Care Committees see Animal Welfare

Animal Communication
   General   QL 776

Animal Culture see Animal Husbandry

Animal Diseases   SF 600-1100
   See also Zoonoses   WC 950

Animal Feed   SF 95-99

Animal Hospitals see Hospitals, Animal

Animal-Human Bonding see Bonding, Human-Pet

Animal Husbandry   SF 1-597
   Waste disposal   WA 778-785

Animal Identification Systems   QL 60.5

Animal Magnetism see Hypnosis; Mental Healing

Animal Nutrition   SF 95-99

Animal Parasites see Parasites

Animal Poisons see Animals, Poisonous; Fishes, Poisonous

Animal Structures
   Domestic animals   SF 761-767
   Wild animals   QL 801-950.9
   See also names of specific animals, groups of animals, or specific animal organ or structure

Animal Testing Alternatives   W 20.55.A5
   Special topics, by subject

Animal Viruses see Viruses

Animal Vocalization see Vocalization, Animal

Animal Welfare
   Laboratory animals   QY 54
   Other Animals   HV 4701-4959

Animals
   Bites see Bites and stings and entries under it WD 400-430, etc.
   Clinical use see Animals, Laboratory   QY 50-60, etc.
   Inoculation see Veterinary   SF 757.2 under Vaccination
   Laboratory see Animals, Laboratory   QY 50-60, etc.
   Microbiology   QW 70
   Quarantine   SF 740
      General works   SF 740
      By country   SF 621-723
   Wounds by   WO 700
   See also Animal Structures; Animals, Domestic; Animals, Laboratory; Animals, Wild

Animals, Domestic   SF
   Anatomy and physiology   SF 761-768.2
   Culture   SF 1-597
   Diseases   SF 600-1100
   Laboratory see Animals, Laboratory   QY 50-60
   See also Animals

Animals, Infancy of see Animals, Newborn

Animals, Laboratory   QY 50-60
   Domestic
      Anatomy and physiology   SF 761-768.2
      Care and breeding   QY 54
      Diseases   SF 996.5
      See also names of specific animals or groups of animals
   Wild
      Anatomy   QL 801-950.9
      Care and breeding   QY 54
      Diseases   SF 996.5
      Physiology   QP

See also names of specific animals or groups
of animals

Animals, Newborn
  Animal behavior   QL 751
  Developmental behavior   QL 763–763.2
  Popular works   QL 50
Animals, Nondomestic see Animals, Wild
Animals, Poisonous   WD 400–430
Animals, Suckling
  As laboratory animals   QY 60.M2
  Diseases   SF 600–1100
  Domestic   SF
  Wild   QL 700–739.8
Animals, Transgenic
  As laboratory animals   QY 50
  Genetics   QH 442.6
Animals, Wild
  Anatomy   QL 801–950.9
  Diseases   SF 996.35–996.45
  Laboratory see Animals, Laboratory
  Physiology   QP
Animals, Zoo   QL 77.5
  Diseases   SF 996
  See also names of individual animals
Anion Gap see Acid–Base Equilibrium
Anion Transport Protein, Erythrocyte see Band 3
  Protein
Anions   QV 280–285
Aniseikonia   WW 300
Anisoles
  Organic chemistry   QD 341.E7
  Toxicology   QV 632
Anisometropia   WW 300
Ankle   WE 880–883
Ankle Injuries   WE 880
Ankle Joint   WE 880
Ankylosis   WE 346
  Veterinary   SF 901
  Localized, by site
Annelida   QX 451
Anniversaries and Special Events
  Medical, dental, pharmaceutical, etc. (General)
    WZ 332
  Specific occasions, by subject
Anniversary Reaction see Adjustment Disorders
Annual Implementation Plans see Regional Health
  Planning
Anoci–Association see Preanesthetic Medication
Anode see Electrodes
Anodontia   WU 101.5
Anodynes see Analgesics
Anomalies see Abnormalities
Anomie   HM
Anonyms and Pseudonyms   Z 1041–1121
Anopheles   QX 515
Anoplura   QX 502
Anorectics see Appetite Depressants
Anorexia   WI 143
  See also Anorexia Nervosa   WM 175
Anorexia Nervosa   WM 175
Anosmia   WV 301
ANOVA see Analysis of Variance
Anovulation   WP 540

Anoxemia   WF 143
  Associated with high altitude   WD 715
  Associated with high atmospheric pressure   WD
    655
Anoxia   WF 143
  Altitude see Altitude Sickness   WD 715
  Cerebral see Cerebral Anoxia   WL 355
  Fetal see Fetal Anoxia   WQ 211
  Submarine medicine   WD 655
Anoxia, Cellular see Cell Hypoxia
Anoxia, Fetal see Fetal Anoxia
ANP see Atrial Natriuretic Factor
Ant Venoms   WD 430
Antacids   QV 69
Antagonism of Drugs see Drug Antagonism
Antagonists see Names of substances affected, e.g.,
  Hormone Antagonists
Anterior Chamber   WW 210
Anterior Chamber Epithelium see Endothelium,
  Corneal
Anterior Corneal Epithelium see Epithelium,
  Corneal
Anterior Cruciate Ligament   WE 870
Anterior Eye Segment   WW 210
Anterior Lobe Hormones see Pituitary Hormones,
  Anterior
Anterior Perforated Substance see Olfactory
  Pathways
Anthelmintics   QV 253
Anthemorrhagics see Hemostatics
Anthocyanins   QU 75
Anthracenediones see Anthraquinones
Anthracenes
  As carcinogens   QZ 202
  As cathartics   QV 75
Anthracosilicosis   WF 654
Anthracosis see Anthracosilicosis; Pneumoconiosis
Anthracycline Antibiotics see Antibiotics,
  Anthracycline
Anthralin
  Pharmacology   QV 60
Anthraquinones   QV 240
  Organic chemistry   QD 393
Anthrax   WC 305
  Veterinary   SF 787
Anthropoidea see Haplorhini
Anthropology   GN
  Criminal   HV 6035–6197
  Medical   GN 296–296.5
  Parapsychology   BF 1045.A65
  Psychological   GN 502–517
Anthropology, Cultural   GN 307–673
  See also Ethnopsychology   GN 270–279
Anthropology, Physical   GN 50.2–298
  Miscegenation   GN 254
    In marriage   HQ 1031
Anthropometry   GN 51–59
  Criminal see Anthropology   HV 6035–6197, etc.
Anthroposophy
  Philosophy   BP 595–597
  Alternative medicine   WB 903
Anti–AIDS Agents see Anti–HIV Agents
Anti–Allergic Agents   QV 157

Anti-Antibodies see Antibodies, Anti-Idiotypic
Anti-Anxiety Agents   QV 77.9
Anti-Anxiety Agents, Benzodiazepine   QV 77.9
Anti-Arrhythmia Agents   QV 150
Anti-Asthmatic Agents   QV 120
Anti-DNA Antibodies see Antibodies, Antinuclear
Anti-HIV Agents   QV 268.5
Anti-HIV Positive see HIV Seropositivity
Anti-Human Globulin Complement-Dependent
    Cytotoxicity Tests see Cytotoxicity Tests,
    Immunologic
Anti-Human Globulin Consumption Test see
    Coombs' Test
Anti-Idiotype Antibodies see Antibodies,
    Anti-Idiotypic
Anti-Infective Agents   QV 250–268.5
Anti-Infective Agents, Local   QV 220–239
    Oxidizing antiseptics   QV 229
Anti-Infective Agents, Quinolone   QV 250
Anti-Infective Agents, Urinary   QV 243
Anti-Inflammatory Agents   QV 247
Anti-Inflammatory Agents, Gold see Antirheumatic
    Agents, Gold
Anti-Inflammatory Agents, Non-Steroidal   QV 95
Anti-Inflammatory Agents, Steroidal   QV 247
Anti-Inflammatory Agents, Topical   QV 60
Anti-Obesity Agents   QV 126
    As appetite depressants   QV 129
Anti-Rheumatic Agents, Non-Steroidal see
    Anti-Inflammatory Agents, Non-Steroidal
Anti-Rheumatic Agents, Steroidal see
    Anti-Inflammatory Agents, Steroidal
Anti-Ulcer Agents   QV 69
Antiadrenergic Agents see Adrenergic Antagonists
Antiaggregants, Platelet see Platelet Aggregation
    Inhibitors
Antiandrogens see Androgen Antagonists
Antibiotic Prophylaxis
    General   QV 350
    In surgery   WO 178–188
    For prevention of specific disease, class with the
        disease; for use of specific antibiotic, class with
        the drug
Antibiotic Resistance see Drug Resistance, Microbial
Antibiotics   QV 350–360
    See also specific types of antibiotics
Antibiotics, Aminoglycoside   QV 350
Antibiotics, Anthracycline   QV 269
Antibiotics, Antifungal   QV 252
Antibiotics, Antineoplastic
    Pharmacology   QV 269
    Therapeutic use   QZ 267
Antibiotics, Antitubercular
    Pharmacology   QV 268
    Therapeutic use   WF 360
Antibiotics, beta-Lactam see Antibiotics, Lactam
Antibiotics, Glycoside see Antibiotics,
    Aminoglycoside
Antibiotics, Lactam   QV 350
Antibiotics, Macrolide   QV 350
Antibodies   QW 575
    See also Antigen–Antibody reactions   QW 570
Antibodies, Allotypic see Immunoglobulin Allotypes

Antibodies, Anti-DNA see Antibodies, Antinuclear
Antibodies, Anti-Idiotypic   QW 575
Antibodies, Antinuclear   QW 575
Antibodies, Bacterial   QW 575
Antibodies, Heterogenetic see Antibodies,
    Heterophile
Antibodies, Heterophile   QW 575
Antibodies, Heterotypic see Antibodies, Heterophile
Antibodies, Monoclonal   QW 575.5.A6
Antibodies, Neoplasm   QW 575
    Neoplastic pathogenesis   QZ 202
Antibodies, Viral   QW 575
Antibodies, Xenogeneic see Antibodies, Heterophile
Antibody Affinity   QW 570
Antibody Avidity see Antibody Affinity
Antibody Binding Sites see Binding Sites, Antibody
Antibody Deficiency Syndrome see Immunologic
    Deficiency Syndromes
Antibody-Dependent Cell Cytotoxicity   QW 568
Antibody Diversity   QW 575
    Immunogenetic aspects   QW 541
Antibody Enzyme Technique, Unlabeled see
    Immunoenzyme Techniques
Antibody Formation   QW 575
Antibody-Producing Cells   QW 575
Antibody-Secreting Cells see Antibody-Producing
    Cells
Antibody Specificity   QW 570
Antibody-Toxin Conjugates see Immunotoxins
Antibody-Toxin Hybrids see Immunotoxins
Anticancer Drug Combinations see Antineoplastic
    Agents, Combined
Anticancer Drug Sensitivity Tests see Drug
    Screening Assays, Antitumor
Anticestodal Agents   QV 253
Anticholesteremic Agents   QU 95
Anticholinergic Agents see Cholinergic Antagonists
Anticholinesterase Agents see Cholinesterase
    Inhibitors
Anticoagulants   QV 193
Anticonvulsants   QV 85
Antidepressants see Antidepressive Agents
Antidepressive Agents   QV 77.5
Antidiabetics see Hypoglycemic Agents; Insulin
Antidiarrheals   QV 71
Antidiuretic Hormones see Vasopressins
Antidiuretics see Vasopressins
Antidotes   QV 601
    Lists   QV 605
    For a particular poison, with the poison
Antidromic Potentials see Evoked Potentials
Antiemetics   QV 73
Antiepileptic Agents see Anticonvulsants
Antiestrogens see Estrogen Antagonists
Antifibrillatory Agents see Anti-Arrhythmia Agents
Antifibrinolysins see Antifibrinolytic Agents
Antifibrinolytic Agents   QV 195
Antifungal Agents   QV 252
    See also Antibiotics, Antifungal   QV 252;
        Fungicides, Industrial   SB 951.3
Antigamma Globulin Antibodies see Antibodies,
    Anti-Idiotypic
Antigen–Antibody Complex   QW 570

Antigen–Antibody Reactions   QW 570
Antigen Bronchial Provocation Tests see Bronchial
   Provocation Tests
Antigen–Presenting Cells   QW 568
Antigen Receptors see Receptors, Antigen
Antigen Receptors, T–Cell see Receptors, Antigen,
   T–Cell
Antigenic Determinants see Epitopes
Antigenic Specificity see Epitopes
Antigens   QW 573
   In histocompatibility   WO 680
Antigens, Bacterial   QW 573
Antigens, Carbohydrate, Tumor–Associated see
   Antigens, Tumor–Associated, Carbohydrate
Antigens, CD   QW 573
Antigens, CD25 see Receptors, Interleukin–2
Antigens, CD4   QW 573
Antigens, Differentiation   QW 573
Antigens, Differentiation, B–Cell see Antigens,
   Differentiation, B–Lymphocyte
Antigens, Differentiation, B–Lymphocyte   QW 573
Antigens, Fungal   QW 573
Antigens, Helminth   QW 573
Antigens, HLA–D see HLA–D Antigens
Antigens, Immune Response see Histocompatibility
   Antigens Class II
Antigens, Neoplasm   QW 573
   Neoplasm etiology   QZ 202
   Neoplasm research   QZ 206
Antigens, Neoplasm, Viral see Antigens, Viral,
   Tumor
Antigens, Surface   QW 573
Antigens, Synthetic see Vaccines, Synthetic
Antigens, Tumor–Associated, Carbohydrate   QW
   573
Antigens, Viral   QW 573
Antigens, Viral, Tumor   QW 573
   Neoplasm etiology   QZ 202
Antiglobulin Consumption Test see Coombs' Test
Antiglobulin Test see Coombs' Test
Antiglobulins see Antibodies, Anti–Idiotypic
Antigout Agents see Gout Suppressants
Antihistamines, Classical see Histamine H1
   Antagonists
Antihistaminics, Classical see Histamine H1
   Antagonists
Antihistaminics, H1 see Histamine H1 Antagonists
Antihistaminics, H2 see Histamine H2 Antagonists
Antihypertensive Agents   QV 150
Antileprotic Agents see Leprostatic Agents
Antilipemic Agents   QU 85
Antiluetics see Syphilis
Antilymphoblast Globulins see Antilymphocyte
   Serum
Antilymphocyte Antibodies see Antilymphocyte
   Serum
Antilymphocyte Globulin see Antilymphocyte
   Serum
Antilymphocyte Serum   QW 815
   Immunosuppressive agent   QW 920
Antimalarials   QV 256–258
Antimetabolites   QV 38
   See also names of specific antimetabolites

Antimetabolites, Antineoplastic   QV 269
   Therapeutic use   QZ 267
Antimitotic Agents see Antineoplastic Agents
Antimony   QV 295
Antimony Potassium Tartrate   QV 253
   As an emetic   QV 73
Antimuscarinic Agents see Muscarinic Antagonists
Antimycin A   QV 252
Antineoplastic Agents   QV 269
   Therapeutic use   QZ 267
   See also Antibiotics, Antineoplastic   QV 269
Antineoplastic Agents, Combined   QV 269
   Therapeutic use   QZ 267
Antineoplastic Agents, Phytogenic   QV 269
   Therapeutic use   QZ 267
Antineoplastic Drug Combinations see
   Antineoplastic Agents, Combined
Antineoplastic Drug Resistance see Drug Resistance,
   Neoplasm
Antineoplastics, Botanical see Antineoplastic Agents,
   Phytogenic
Antinociceptive Agents see Analgesics
Antinuclear Antibodies see Antibodies, Antinuclear
Antinuclear Antibody Test, Fluorescent see
   Fluorescent Antibody Technique
Antinuclear Factors see Antibodies, Antinuclear
Antioncogenes see Genes, Suppressor, Tumor
Antioxidants
   As a pharmaceutic aid   QV 800
   In food preservation   WA 710–712
Antiparasitic Agents   QV 250
Antiparkinson Agents   QV 80
   See also Levodopa   WK 725
Antiperspirants see Astringents
Antiplasmins see Antifibrinolytic Agents
Antiplatelet Agents see Platelet Aggregation
   Inhibitors
Antiprotozoal Agents   QV 254–258
Antipruritics   QV 60
Antipsychotic Agents   QV 77.9
Antipsychotic Agents, Butyrophenone   QV 77.9
Antipsychotic Agents, Phenothiazine   QV 77.9
Antipyretics see Analgesics, Non–Narcotic
Antirejection Therapy see Immunosuppression
Antireticular Cytotoxic Serum see Immune Sera
Antirheumatic Agents   QV 247
Antirheumatic Agents, Gold   QV 247
Antisense DNA see DNA, Antisense
Antisense Elements (Genetics)   QU 57
Antisense Oligonucleotides see Oligonucleotides,
   Antisense
Antisense Probes see Antisense Elements (Genetics)
Antisense RNA see RNA, Antisense
Antisepsis
   Dental   WU 300
   In labor   WQ 400
   Public health aspects   WA 240
   Surgical   WO 113
Antiseptics see Anti–infective Agents, Local
Antiseptics, Urinary see Anti–Infective Agents,
   Urinary
Antisera see Immune Sera
Antiserotonergic Agents see Serotonin Antagonists

**ALWAYS CONSULT MAIN SCHEDULES. USE NUMBER ASSIGNED ONLY WHEN
SUBJECT REPRESENTS MAJOR EMPHASIS OF WORK BEING CLASSIFIED**

Antisickling Agents   QV 180
Antisocial Personality Disorder   WM 190
    Child   WS 350.8.P3
    Infant   WS 350.8.P3
Antispasmodics see Parasympatholytics
Antisyphilitics see Syphilis
Antithrombin II see Antithrombin III
Antithrombin III   QV 193
Antithrombins   QV 193
Antithrombotic Agents see Fibrinolytic Agents
Antithyroid Agents   WK 202
Antitoxins
    Immunology
        Immunizing agent   QW 805
        Pharmacology   QW 630
    Used for particular diseases, with the disease
    See also names of specific antitoxins
Antitrichomonal Agents   QV 254
Antitrust Laws
    (Form number 32-33 in any NLM schedule where
    applicable)
Antitrust Liability see Antitrust Laws
Antitubercular Agents
    Pharmacology   QV 268
    Therapeutic use   WF 360
    See also Antibiotics, Antitubercular   QV 268
Antitumor Drug Screening Assays see Drug
    Screening Assays, Antitumor
Antitussive Agents   QV 76
Antivenins
    Immunology
        Immunizing agent   QW 805
        Pharmacology   QW 630
    Therapy   WD 400-430
Antiviral Agents   QV 268.5
Antivivisection see Vivisection
Antrum of Highmore see Maxillary Sinus
Antrum, Pyloric see Pyloric Antrum
Ants   QX 565
Anura   QL 668.E2-668.E275
    As laboratory animals   QY 60.A6
    Diseases   SF 997.5.A45
Anuria   WJ 303
Anus   WI 600-650
Anus, Artificial see Colostomy
Anus Diseases   WI 600
Anus Neoplasms   WI 610
Anus Prolapse see Rectal Prolapse
Anxiety   WM 172
    Adolescence   WS 463
    Child   WS 350.6
    Infant   WS 350.6
    Neuroses see Neuroses, Anxiety   WM 172
Anxiety Disorders   WM 172
Anxiety Neuroses see Anxiety Disorders
Anxiety States, Neurotic see Anxiety Disorders
Anxiolytic Agents see Anti-Anxiety Agents
Anxiolytics, Benzodiazepine see Anti-Anxiety
    Agents, Benzodiazepine
Aorta   WG 410
Aorta, Abdominal   WG 410
Aorta, Ascending see Aorta
Aorta, Descending see Aorta, Thoracic

Aorta, Thoracic   WG 410
Aortic Aneurysm   WG 410
Aortic Arch see Aorta, Thoracic
Aortic Arch Syndromes   WG 410
Aortic Bodies   WL 600
Aortic Coarctation   WG 220
Aortic Incompetence see Aortic Valve Insufficiency
Aortic Regurgitation see Aortic Valve Insufficiency
Aortic Stenosis see Aortic Valve Stenosis
Aortic Stenosis, Supravalvular see Aortic Valve
    Stenosis
Aortic Valve   WG 265
Aortic Valve Incompetence see Aortic Valve
    Insufficiency
Aortic Valve Insufficiency   WG 265
Aortic Valve Stenosis   WG 265
Aorticopulmonary Septal Defect see
    Aortopulmonary Septal Defect
Aortitis   WG 410
Aortitis Syndrome see Aortic Arch Syndromes
Aortitis, Syphilitic see Syphilis, Cardiovascular
Aortocoronary Bypass see Coronary Artery Bypass
Aortography   WG 410
Aortopulmonary Septal Defect   WG 220
Aotus trivirgatus   QL 737.P925
    Diseases   SF 997.5.P7
    As laboratory animals   QY 60.P7
Apazone   QV 95
Ape, Barbary see Macaca
Ape, Black see Macaca
Ape, Celebes see Macaca
Apert Syndrome see Acrocephalosyndactylia
Apes see Pongidae
Apex Cardiography see Kinetocardiography
Aphakia   WW 260
Aphakia, Postcataract   WW 260
Aphaniptera see Fleas
Aphasia
    Neurologic   WL 340.5
    Psychogenic   WM 475.5
Aphasia, Acquired see Aphasia
Aphasia, Acquired Epileptic see Landau-Kleffner
    Syndrome
Aphasia, Broca   WL 340.5
    Psychogenic   WM 475.5
Aphasia, Childhood   WL 340.5
    Psychogenic   WM 475.5
Aphasia, Epileptic, Acquired see Landau-Kleffner
    Syndrome
Aphasia, Expressive see Aphasia, Broca
Aphasia, Motor see Aphasia, Broca
Aphasia, Nonfluent see Aphasia, Broca
Aphasia Tests see Neuropsychological Tests
Aphemia see Aphasia
Apheresis see Blood Component Removal
Aphids   QX 503
    As vectors of plant virus diseases   SB 736
Aphonia
    Neurologic origin   WL 340.2
    Psychogenic origin   WM 475
Aphorisms and Proverbs   PN 6269-6278
    Medicine and related fields   WZ 309
Aphrodisiacs   QV 170

Aphthae see Stomatitis, Aphthous; Moniliasis, Oral
Aphthovirus   QW 168.5.P4
Apicoectomy   WU 230
Apis see Bees
Apis Venoms see Bee Venoms
Aplastic Anemia see Anemia, Aplastic
Aplysia   QX 675
Apnea   WF 143
Apnea, Central see Sleep Apnea Syndromes
Apnea, Obstructive see Sleep Apnea Syndromes
Apnea, Sleep see Sleep Apnea Syndromes
Apocrine Glands   WR 400
Apodemus see Muridae
Apomorphine   QV 73
Apoplexy see Cerebrovascular Disorders
Apoptosis   QH 671
Apothecaries see Pharmacies
Apparatus see Equipment and Supplies
Apparatus and Instruments see Equipment and
   Supplies
Appendectomy   WI 535
Appendiceal Neoplasms   WI 535
Appendicitis   WI 535
Appendix   WI 535
Appetite   WI 102
Appetite Depressants   QV 129
Appetite Disorders see Eating Disorders
Appetite Regulation   WI 102
Appetite Stimulants   QV 100
   Used for a specific disorder, with the disorder
Appetite Suppressants see Appetite Depressants
Appetitive Behavior   BF 685
   Animal aspects   QL 758-785
   Sex psychology   BF 692
Apple see Rosales
Appointments and Schedules
   In hospitals   WX 159
   Practice management
      Dental   WU 77
      Medical   W 80
      Nursing, by type, e.g. Private duty nursing
         WY 127
Appropriateness Review see Regional Health
   Planning
Apraxia   WL 340
Apricot see Rosales
Aprotinin   QU 143
Aptitude Tests   BF 431-433
   In special fields, in the career number for the
      field, e.g., for dentistry   WU 21
APUD Cells   WL 102
Apudoma   QZ 200-380
   Localized, by site
Aqueous Humor   WW 210
Ara-A see Vidarabine
Ara-C see Cytarabine
Arabic Physicians see Physicians
Arabinofuranosyladenine see Vidarabine
Arabinofuranosylcytosine see Cytarabine
Arabinofuranosylnucleotides see Arabinonucleotides
Arabinonucleotides   QU 57
Arabinosyladenine see Vidarabine
Arabinosylcytosine see Cytarabine

Arachis see Peanuts
Arachnid Venoms see Spider Venoms
Arachnida   QX 467-483
Arachnidism   WD 420
Arachnoid   WL 200
Arachnoiditis   WL 200
Araneid Venoms see Spider Venoms
Arbovirus, Group B see Flavivirus
Arbovirus Infections   WC 524-532
   General works   WC 524
   See also Encephalitis, Epidemic   WC 542
Arboviruses   QW 168.5.A7
Archaea
   Anatomy and morphology   QW 51
   General works   QW 50
   Physiology, chemistry, and metabolism   QW 52
Archaebacteria see Archaea
Archaeobacteria see Archaea
Archaeology
   General   CC (entire schedule)
   Individual countries   D-F
   Prehistoric   GN 700-890
Architectural Accessibility
   In health facilities   WX 140
   Public health aspects   WA 795-799
   See also specific types of buildings, e.g., Drug
      Treatment Centers   WM 29-29.1, etc.
Architecture   NA
   Public health aspects   WA 795-799
   See also Design and Construction, Hospital   WX
      140; Housing   WA 795, etc; types of particular
      buildings, e.g., Laboratories, Dental   WU
      23-24
Archives   CD 931-4280
   Cataloging   Z 695.2
Arctic Regions
   Physiological effects and adaptation   QT 160
Arcus Senilis   WW 220
ARDS, Human see Respiratory Distress Syndrome,
   Adult
Area Health Education Centers   W 19
Areawide Planning see Regional Health Planning
Areca
   As medicinal plant   QV 766
   Botany   QK 495.P17
   Culture   SB 317.P3
Arenaviridae   QW 168.5.A8
Arenaviridae Infections   WC 501
Arenavirus Infections see Arenaviridae Infections
Argentaffin Cells see Enterochromaffin Cells
Argentaffin System see Chromaffin System
Argentaffinoma see Carcinoid Tumor
Arginase   QU 136
Arginine   QU 60
Arginine Vasopressin see Argipressin
Argipressin   WK 520
   As an antidiuretic   QV 160
Argon
   Inorganic chemistry   QD 181.A6
   Pharmacology   QV 310
Argyria   WR 265
Arizona Bacteria see Salmonella arizonae
Arm   WE 805

ALWAYS CONSULT MAIN SCHEDULES. USE NUMBER ASSIGNED ONLY WHEN
SUBJECT REPRESENTS MAJOR EMPHASIS OF WORK BEING CLASSIFIED

Artificial see Artificial Limbs   WE 172
Upper arm   WE 810
See also Forearm   WE 820
Arm Bones see Bones of Upper Extremity
Arm Ergometry Test see Exercise Test
Arm Injuries   WE 805
See also Forearm Injuries   WE 820
Armadillos   QL 737.E23
As laboratory animals   QY 60.M2
Armed Forces Personnel see Military Personnel
Armpit see Axilla
Arnold–Chiari Deformity   WL 101
Aroclors
As air pollutants   WA 754, etc.
As water pollutants   WA 689
Organic chemistry   QD 341.H9
Toxicology (General)   QV 633
Aromatase   QU 140
Aromatherapy   WB 925
Used for special purposes, by subject
Aromatic Amino Acid Decarboxylases see
Aromatic-L-Amino-Acid Decarboxylases
Aromatic Compounds see Anti-Infective Agents,
Local; Cresols; Phenols   QV 223, etc. and other
compounds by name; Hydrocarbons; Polycyclic
Hydrocarbons; Aromatic Compounds   QD
330–341 under Chemistry, Organic
Aromatic-L-Amino-Acid Decarboxylases   QU
139
Arousal   WL 103
Behaviorism   BF 199
Child   WS 105.5.C7
Infant   WS 105.5.C7
Arrhenoblastoma see Androblastoma
Arrhythmia   WG 330
Arrhythmia, Sinus   WG 330
Arrhythmogenic Right Ventricular Cardiomyopathy
see Arrhythmogenic Right Ventricular Dysplasia
Arrhythmogenic Right Ventricular Dysplasia   WG
330
Arsenic   QV 294
Arsenic Compounds see Arsenicals
Arsenicals   QU 143
As amebicides   QV 255
As antisyphilitic agents   QV 262
Arson see Firesetting Behavior
Arsphenamine   QV 262
Art   N
Accidents in professional work   WA 487.5.A78
Anatomy see Anatomy, Artistic   NC 760–783.8
By physicians   WZ 350
Child study   WS 105.5.E8
In psychotherapy see Art Therapy   WM
450.5.A8
Related to medicine see Medicine in Art   WZ
330, etc.
Related to psychiatry   WM 49
See also Medical Illustration   WZ 348
Art Therapy   WM 450.5.A8
Adolescence   WS 463
Child   WS 350.2
Artemia   QX 463
Arterenol see Norepinephrine

Arterial Catheterization, Peripheral see
Catheterization, Peripheral
Arterial Lines see Catheters, Indwelling
Arterial Obstructive Diseases see Arterial Occlusive
Diseases
Arterial Occlusive Diseases   WG 510
Arteries   WG 510–595
Coronary see Coronary Vessels   WG 300
See also Aorta   WG 410
Arteriography see Angiography
Arteriosclerosis   WG 550
Cerebral see Cerebral Arteriosclerosis   WL 355
Veterinary   SF 811
Arteriosclerosis, Coronary see Coronary
Arteriosclerosis
Arteriosclerosis Obliterans   WG 550
Arteriosclerotic Dementia see Dementia, Vascular
Arteriosclerotic Heart Disease see Coronary Disease
Arteriovenous Anastomosis   WG 590
Arteriovenous Aneurysm see Arteriovenous Fistula
Arteriovenous Fistula   WG 590
Congenital see Arteriovenous Malformations
WG 500
Arteriovenous Hemofiltration see Hemofiltration
Arteriovenous Malformations   WG 500
Cerebral see Cerebral Arteriovenous
malformations   WL 355
Arteriovenous Malformations, Cerebral see Cerebral
Arteriovenous Malformations
Arteriovenous Shunt, Surgical   WG 170
Arteritis   WG 515
Coronary   WG 300
See also Endarteritis   WG 515; Periarteritis
Nodossa   WG 518; Temporal Arteritis   WG
510
Arteritis, Temporal see Temporal Arteritis
Arthritis   WE 344–348
Arthritis, Bacterial see Arthritis, Infectious
Arthritis, Degenerative see Osteoarthritis
Arthritis, Infectious   WE 344
Arthritis, Juvenile Chronic see Arthritis, Juvenile
Rheumatoid
Arthritis, Juvenile Rheumatoid   WE 346
Arthritis, Rheumatic, Acute see Rheumatic Fever
Arthritis, Rheumatoid   WE 346
Arthritis, Septic see Arthritis, Infectious
Arthritis, Viral see Arthritis, Infectious
Arthrodesis   WE 312
Localized, by site
Arthrography   WE 300
Arthrogryposis   WE 300
Arthromyodysplasia, Congenital see Arthrogryposis
Arthropathy, Neurogenic   WE 344
Arthroplasty   WE 312
Localized, by site
Arthroplasty, Replacement   WE 312
Localized, by site
Arthroplasty, Replacement, Hip   WE 860
Arthroplasty, Replacement, Knee   WE 870
See also Knee Prosthesis   WE 870
Arthropod-Borne Viruses see Arboviruses
Arthropod Vectors   QX 460
See also Insect vectors   QX 650

Arthropod Venoms   WD 400–430
Arthropods   QX 460–570
   Bites, stings and poisoning   WD 400–430
   Cause of skin diseases   WR 360–375
   Non–medical
      Paleozoology   QE 815–832
      Zoology   QL 434–599.82
   See also specific arthropods
Arthroscopy   WE 304
Arthus Phenomenon see Arthus Reaction
Arthus Reaction   QW 900
Artic Regions see Cold Climate
Articular Disk, Temporomandibular see
   Temporomandibular Joint Disk
Articulation see Speech
Articulation Disorders
   Neurologic   WL 340.2
   Psychologic   WM 475
Articulators see Dental Articulators
Artificial Eye see Eye, Artificial
Artificial Fats see Fat Substitutes
Artificial Fever see Hyperthermia, Induced
Artificial Heart see Heart, Artificial
Artificial Hibernation see Hibernation, Artificial
Artificial Insemination see Insemination, Artificial
Artificial Intelligence   Q 334–341
   In medicine (General)   W 26.55.A7
   In other special fields (Form number 26.5 in any
     NLM schedule where applicable)
   Used for special purposes, by subject
Artificial Kidney see Kidney, Artificial
Artificial Limbs   WE 172
Artificial Liver see Liver, Artificial
Artificial Organs   WO 176
   Banks   WO 23–24
   See also names of specific artificial organs
Artificial Pancreas see Pancreas, Artificial
Artificial Pneumothorax see Pneumothorax,
   Artificial
Artificial Respiration see Respiration, Artificial
Artificial Sweeteners see Sweetening Agents
Artificial Tears see Ophthalmic Solutions
Artificial Teeth see Dental Prosthesis; Denture,
   Partial; Denture, Complete; Tooth, Artificial
Artificial Ventricle see Heart–Assist Devices
Artiodactyla
   Diseases   SF 997.5.U5
   Wild   QL 737.U5–737.U595
Artistic Anatomy see Anatomy, Artistic
Arvicolinae see Microtinae
Arvicolines see Microtinae
Arvin see Ancrod
Arylsulfonates   QU 98
   Organic chemistry   QD 341.S3
As If Personality see Personality Disorders
Asbestos
   As a mineral   TN 930
   As air pollutant   WA 754
   In industry   WA 450
   Industrial wastes   WA 788
   Toxicology   QV 610
Asbestosis   WF 654
Ascariasis   WC 870

Veterinary   SF 810.A5
Ascaridiasis   WC 870
Ascaridoidea   QX 277
Ascaris   QX 277
Ascaroidea see Ascaridoidea
Aschelminthes see Helminths
Ascites   WI 575
Ascites Shunt, Peritoneovenous see Peritoneovenous
   Shunt
Ascitic Fluid   WI 575
   Clinical analysis   QY 210
Ascomycota   QW 180.5.A8
Ascorbic Acid   QU 210
Ascorbic Acid Deficiency   WD 140
Asepsis
   Dental   WU 300
   Surgical   WO 113
Asialia see Xerostomia
Asialoglycoproteins   QU 55
Asian Americans   E 184.O6
   Specific topics, by subject
   See also special topics under Ethnic Groups
Asiatic Race see Mongoloid Race
Asjike see Beriberi
ASPA Cement see Glass Ionomer Cements
Asparaginase   QV 269
   Enzymology   QU 136
Asparagine   QU 60
Aspartame   WA 712
   Peptides   QU 68
Aspartate Aminotransferase Isoenzymes see
   Aspartate Transaminase
Aspartate Aminotransferase Isozymes see Aspartate
   Transaminase
Aspartate Transaminase   QU 141
Aspartic Acid   QU 60
Aspartic Proteinases   QU 136
Aspartyl Proteinases see Aspartic Proteinases
Aspartylphenylalanine Methyl Ester see Aspartame
Aspergillosis   WC 450
   Veterinary   SF 809.A86
Aspergillus   QW 180.5.D38
Aspergillus flavus   QW 180.5.D38
Asphyxia   WO 250
   First aid   WA 292
Asphyxia Neonatorum   WQ 450
Aspiculariasis see Oxyuriasis
Aspidium   QV 253
Aspiration Biopsy see Biopsy, Needle
Aspiration Lipectomy see Lipectomy
Aspiration, Mechanical see Suction
Aspiration of Gastric Contents see Pneumonia,
   Aspiration
Aspiration, Pneumatic see Suction
Aspiration Pneumonia see Pneumonia, Aspiration
Aspirin   QV 95
Aspirin–Like Agents see Anti–Inflammatory Agents,
   Non–Steroidal
Assassin Bugs see Reduviidae
Assay see Biological Assay
Assertiveness
   Psychology
      Adolescence   WS 462

**ALWAYS CONSULT MAIN SCHEDULES. USE NUMBER ASSIGNED ONLY WHEN
SUBJECT REPRESENTS MAJOR EMPHASIS OF WORK BEING CLASSIFIED**

Adult   BF 575.A85
Child   WS 105.5.S6
Infant   WS 105.5.S6
Social behavior disorders
Adolescence   WS 463
Adult   WM 600
Child   WS 350.8.S6
Assessment, Educational see Educational
Measurement
Assessment of Health Care Needs see Needs
Assessment
Assimilation see Acculturation
Assimilation of Food see Metabolism
Assisted Circulation   WG 168
Associateship Practice, Dental see Partnership
Practice, Dental
Association
Free see Free Association   WM 460.5.F8
Of ideas (psychology)   BF 365–395
Word tests see Word Association Tests   WM
145.5.W9, etc.
Association, Free see Free Association
Association Learning   BF 319.5.P34
Astasia-Abasia see Conversion Disorder
Asthenia   WB 146
Neurocirculatory see Neurocirculatory Asthenia
WG 320
See also Neurasthenia   WM 174
Asthma
Bronchial   WF 553
Cardiac see Dyspnea, Paroxysmal   WG 370
Asthma, Bronchial see Asthma
Asthma, Cardiac see Dyspnea, Paroxysmal
Asthma, Exercise-Induced   WF 553
Asthmatic Crisis see Status Asthmaticus
Asthmatic Shock see Status Asthmaticus
Astigmatism   WW 310
Astralophocaena see Porpoises
Astringents   QV 65
Astrocytes   WL 102.5
Astrocytoma   QZ 380
Localized, by site
Astrology   BF 1651–1729
And birth control   BF 1729.B4
And medicine   BF 1718
And sex   BF 1729.S4
Astronauts, Physical Standards see Standards   WD
752 under Space flight
Astronomy   QB
General works   QB 42–43.2
Asylums, Insane see Hospitals, Psychiatric
Asystole see Heart Arrest
Atabrine see Quinacrine
Ataractics see Tranquilizing Agents
Ataxia   WL 390
See also Cerebellar Ataxia   WL 320
Ataxia, Cerebellar see Cerebellar Ataxia
Ataxia, Locomotor see Tables Dorsalis
Atelectasis   WF 645
Atelectasis, Congestive see Respiratory Distress
Syndrome, Adult
Ateles see Cebidae
Atelinae see Cebidae

Atenolol   QV 132
Atheroma see Atherosclerosis
Atherosclerosis   WG 550
Atherosclerosis, Coronary see Coronary
Arteriosclerosis
Athetosis   WL 390
Athlete's Foot see Tinea Pedis
Athletic Equipment see Sports Equipment
Athletic Injuries   QT 261
First aid   WA 292
In a particular sport activity, with the activity
Athletics see Sports
Athymic Mice see Mice, Nude
Atlanto-Axial Joint   WE 725
Atlanto-Occipital Joint   WE 708
Atlas   WE 725
Atlases   G
(Form number 17 in any NLM schedule where
applicable)
Embryology   QS 617
Forensic medicine and dentistry   W 617
Histology   QS 517
Immunology   QW 517
Operative dentistry   WU 317
Oral surgery   WU 600.7
Orthodontics   WU 417
Pharmacy and pharmaceutics   QV 717
Prosthodontics   WU 507
Surgery   WO 517
Atloido-Occipital Joint see Atlanto-Occipital Joint
ATLV see HTLV-I
Atmosphere   QC 851–999
Control   WA 750–776
In industry   WA 450
See also Environment, Controlled   WA 750,
etc.
Pollutants see Air pollutants   WA 754, etc.
Relation to disease see Climate   WB 700
Atmospheric Pressure
High altitude   WD 710
In industry   WA 450
Meteorology   QC 885–896
Underwater   WD 650
Atomic Absorption see Spectrophotometry, Atomic
Absorption
Atomic Energy see Nuclear Energy
Atomic Medicine see Nuclear Medicine
Atomic Warfare see Nuclear Warfare
Atomizers see Nebulizers and Vaporizers
Atopic Hypersensitivity see Hypersensitivity,
Immediate
Atopy see Hypersensitivity, Immediate
ATP see Adenosine Triphosphate
ATP Receptors see Receptors, Purinergic P2
ATPase see Adenosinetriphosphatase
ATPase, Calcium see Ca(2+)-Transporting ATPase
ATPase, Calcium Magnesium see Ca(2+)
Mg(2+)-ATPase
ATPase, F0 see H(+)-Transporting ATP Synthase
ATPase, F1 see H(+)-Transporting ATP Synthase
ATPase, Magnesium see Ca(2+) Mg(2+)-ATPase
ATPase, Sodium, Potassium see
Na(+)-K(+)-Exchanging ATPase

**ALWAYS CONSULT MAIN SCHEDULES. USE NUMBER ASSIGNED ONLY WHEN
SUBJECT REPRESENTS MAJOR EMPHASIS OF WORK BEING CLASSIFIED**

Atractylic Acid see Atractyloside
Atractyloside   QU 75
Atracurium   QV 140
Atracurium Besylate see Atracurium
Atracurium Dibesylate see Atracurium
Atrial Fibrillation   WG 330
Atrial Flutter   WG 330
Atrial Natriuretic Factor   QU 68
Atrial Natriuretic Peptides see Atrial Natriuretic
   Factor
Atriopeptins see Atrial Natriuretic Factor
Atrioventricular Block see Heart Block
Atrioventricular Bundle see Bundle of His
Atrioventricular Node   WG 201-202
Atrocities see Violence
Atropa Belladonna see Belladonna
Atrophy
   Manifestation of disease   QZ 180
Atropine   QV 134
Atropine Derivatives   QV 134
Attendants see Nurses' Aides; Psychiatric Aides;
   Allied Health Personnel
Attention   BF 321-323
   Child   WS 105.5.C7
   Infant   WS 105.5.C7
   Vigilance   BF 323.V5
Attention Deficit and Disruptive Behavior Disorders
   WS 350.6
   Adult   WM 190
   See also Conduct Disorder   WS 350.6, etc.
Attention Deficit Disorder with Hyperactivity   WS
   350.8.A8
   Adult   WM 190
Attention Deficit Hyperactivity Disorder see
   Attention Deficit Disorder with Hyperactivity
Attitude   BF 327
   Adolescence   WS 462
   Child   WS 105.5.A8
   Infant   WS 105.5.A8
   Of patients   W 85
      In hospitals   WX 158.5
      In mental hospitals   WM 29.5
   Toward health insurance   W 275
   To specific topics, by subject
Attitude of Health Personnel
   Allied health personnel   W 21.5
   Dentists   WU 61
   Hospital staff   WX 160
   Nurses   WY 87
   Physicians   W 62
   Psychiatrists   WM 62
   Special areas, with the area
Attitude to Computers   QA 76.9.P75
Attitude to Death   BF 789.D4
   Child   WS 105.5.A8
   Pastoral care   WM 61
   Speculative philosophy   BD 443.8-445
Attitude to Health   W 85
   Other specific subjects, by subject
Audiology   WV 270-280
   See also Hearing   WV 270-280
Audiometry   WV 272
Audiometry, Electroencephalic Response see

Audiometry, Evoked Response
Audiometry, Evoked Response   WV 272
Audiometry, Impedance see Acoustic Impedance
   Tests
Audiometry, Speech   WV 272
Audiovisual Aids
   (Form number 18.2 in any NLM schedule where
   applicable)
   Special topics, by subject
Audition, Limits of see Auditory Threshold
Auditory Brain Stem Evoked Responses see Evoked
   Potentials, Auditory, Brain Stem
Auditory Canal, External see Ear Canal
Auditory Cortex   WL 307
Auditory Diseases, Central   WV 270
Auditory Evoked Potentials see Evoked Potentials,
   Auditory
Auditory Evoked Response see Evoked Potentials,
   Auditory
Auditory Fatigue   WV 272
Auditory Localization see Sound Localization
Auditory Nerve see Acoustic Nerve
Auditory Ossicles see Ear Ossicles
Auditory Pathways   WV 272
Auditory Perception   WV 272
   Infant or Child and other groups   WV 272
   Paracusis   WV 272
Auditory Perceptual Disorders   WV 270
Auditory Prosthesis see Cochlear Implants
Auditory Threshold   WV 272
   Infant or Child and other groups   WV 272
Auditory Tube see Eustachian Tube
Auerbach's Plexus see Myenteric Plexus
Aujeszky's Disease see Pseudorabies
Aujeszky's Disease Virus see Herpesvirus 1, Suid
Aural Vertigo see Ménière's Disease
Auramine O see Benzophenoneidum
Auranofin   QV 247
Aureolic Acid see Plicamycin
Aureomycin see Chlortetracycline
Auricle, Ear see Ear, External
Auricular Fibrillation see Atrial Fibrillation
Auricular Flutter see Atrial Flutter
Auriculin see Atrial Natriuretic Factor
Auriculo-Ventricular Dissociation see Heart Block
Auriculoventricular Bundle see Heart Conduction
   System
Aurothioglucose   QV 247
Auscultation   WB 278
   Heart see Heart Auscultation   WG 141.5.A9
   Used for special purposes, by subject
Australia Antigen see Hepatitis B Antigens
Australoid Race
   Anthropology   GN 662-671
   See also applicable special topics under Ethnic
   groups
Authoritarianism
   Psychology   BF 698.35.A87
   Social psychology   HM
Autism, Infantile see Autistic Disorder
Autistic Disorder   WM 203.5
Autoanalysis   Q 183.9
   Analysis in a special field, in the technique number

**ALWAYS CONSULT MAIN SCHEDULES. USE NUMBER ASSIGNED ONLY WHEN
SUBJECT REPRESENTS MAJOR EMPHASIS OF WORK BEING CLASSIFIED**

for the field, e.g. QY 25 for clinical analysis
   Special topics, by subject
Autoantibodies   QW 575
   As a cause of autoimmune diseases   WD 305
Autobiography   CT
   As a literary form   CT 25
   Of mentally ill   WM 40
   Of physicians   WZ 100
   Of specialists in dentistry, nursing, pharmacy, psychology, science, etc.   WZ 100
   Of patients with a particular disease, with the disease
Autoeroticism see Paraphilias
Autogenic Training
   Parapsychology   BF 1156.S8
   Psychiatry   WM 415
Autograft see Transplantation, Autologous
Autohemolysis see Hemolysis
Autoimmune Diseases   WD 305
Autoimmune Hepatitis see Hepatitis, Autoimmune
Autoimmunity   QW 545
Autolysis   QZ 180
Automated Multiphasic Health Testing see Multiphasic Screening
Automatic Data Processing
   In medicine (General)   W 26.55.A9
   In other special fields (Form number 26.5 in any NLM schedule where applicable)
   Space medicine   WD 751.6
   Used for special purposes, by subject
Automation   T 59.5
   Used for special purposes, by subject, e.g., of clinical laboratory procedures   QY 23
Automation, Office see Office Automation
Automatism
   Parapsychology (General)   BF 1321
   Psychiatry   WM 197
   Other special topics by subject, e.g., Automatic writing   BF 1343
Automobile Accidents see Accidents, Traffic
Automobile Driver Examination   WA 275
Automobile Driving
   Public health aspects   WA 275
Automobile Exhaust see Vehicle Emissions
Automobiles   TL 1–390
   Human engineering in design   TL 250
   Noise hazard   WA 776
   Sanitary conditions of buses and other public carriers   WA 810
   Sanitary disposal   WA 778
Autonomic Agents   QV 120–137
Autonomic Denervation   WL 600
Autonomic Ganglia see Ganglia, Autonomic
Autonomic Nerve Block   WO 375
Autonomic Nervous System   WL 600–610
Autonomic Nervous System Diseases   WL 600
Autonomous Replication see DNA Replication
Autopsy   QZ 35
   Medicolegal   W 825
   Veterinary   SF 769
   See also names of particular conditions requiring autopsy, e.g., Substance-Related Disorders   WM 270–290

Autoradiography
   Biochemistry
     General   QU 4
     Techniques   QU 25
   Biology   QH 324.9.A9
   Cytological techniques   QH 585–585.5
     Clinical pathology   QY 95
   Diagnosis (General)   WN 445
   Histological technique   QS 525
   Used for special purposes, by subject
Autoregulation see Homeostasis
Autosexuality see Narcissism
Autosome Abnormalities see Chromosome Abnormalities
Autosuggestion
   Parapsychology   BF 1156.S8
   Psychiatry   WM 415
Autotransplant see Transplantation, Autologous
AV Node see Atrioventricular Node
Availability Equivalency see Biological Availability
Availability of Health Services see Health Services Accessibility
Aversive Therapy   WM 425.5.A9
Avertin see Alcohol, Ethyl
Avian Hypersensitivity Pneumonitis see Bird Fancier's Lung
Avian Infectious Bronchitis Virus see Infectious Bronchitis Virus, Avian
Avian Leukosis   SF 995.6.L4
Avian Orthomyxovirus Type A see Influenza A Virus, Avian
Avian Sarcoma Virus B77 see Sarcoma Viruses, Avian
Aviation   TL
   Air defense   UG 730, etc.
   Standards
     Physical   WD 705
     Psychological   WD 730
   See also Aircraft   WD 700, etc.; Space Flight   WD 750–758
Aviation Accidents see Accidents, Aviation
Aviation Dentistry see Dentistry; Aerospace Medicine; Military Dentistry
Aviation Medicine see Aerospace Medicine
Aviation Nursing see Aviation   WY 143 under Nursing
Aviation, Physical Standards see Standards   WD 705 under Aviation
Avidin   QU 55
Avidity, Antibody see Antibody Affinity
Avitaminosis   WD 105–155
   Pathogenesis of disease in general   QZ 109
   Veterinary   SF 855.V58
   See also names of specific vitamin deficiencies
Avoidance Learning   BF 319.5.A9
Awareness   BF 321
Axenic Animals see Germ-Free Life
Axilla   WE 812
Axillary Artery   WG 595.A9
Axillary Vein   WG 625.A9
Axis   WE 725
Axolotl see Ambystoma
Axolotl, Mexican see Ambystoma mexicanum

ALWAYS CONSULT MAIN SCHEDULES. USE NUMBER ASSIGNED ONLY WHEN SUBJECT REPRESENTS MAJOR EMPHASIS OF WORK BEING CLASSIFIED

Axons   WL 102.5
Ayerza's Syndrome see Hypertension, Pulmonary
Ayurvedic Medicine see Medicine, Ayurvedic
Azacyclopropanes see Aziridines
Azapropazone see Apazone
Azaserine   QU 60
   As antifungal agent   QV 252
   Cancer chemotherapy   QZ 267
   Immunosuppression   QW 920
Azathioprine   QV 269
   Cancer chemotherapy   QZ 267
   Immunosuppression   QW 920
Azeserine see Azaserine
Azides   QU 54
   Organic chemistry
      Aliphatic compounds   QD 305.N84
Azidothymidine see Zidovudine
Aziridines
   Organic chemistry   QD 401
   As carcinogens   QZ 202
Azirines
   Organic chemistry   QD 401
Azo Compounds   QV 235
   Organic chemistry
      Aliphatic compounds   QD 305.A9
      Aromatic compounds   QD 341.A9
Azoles
   Organic chemistry   QD 401
Azotemia see Uremia
Azotobacter   QW 131
AZT (Antiviral) see Zidovudine
Aztreonam   QV 350
Azygos Vein   WG 625.A99

B

B-Cell Differentiation Antigens see Antigens,
   Differentiation, B-Lymphocyte
B-Cells see B-Lymphocytes
B-K Mole Syndrome see Dysplastic Nevus
   Syndrome
B-Lymphocyte Differentiation Antigens see
   Antigens, Differentiation, B-Lymphocyte
B-Lymphocytes   WH 200
Babesiasis see Babesiosis
Babesiosis   SF 791
Baboon, Gelada see Theropithecus
Baboons see Papio
Baboons, Savanna see Papio
Bacillaceae   QW 127
Bacillary Dysentery see Dysentery, Bacillary
Bacillus   QW 127.5.B2
Bacillus anthracis   QW 127.5.B2
Bacillus megaterium   QW 127.5.B2
Bacillus stearothermophilus   QW 127.5.B2
Bacillus subtilis   QW 127.5.B2
Bacillus thuringiensis   QW 127.5.B2
Bacitracin   QV 350
Back   WE 720–755
Back Injuries   WE 720–755
Back Pain   WE 720
   See also Low back pain   WE 755
Backache see Back Pain

Background Radiation   WN 105
Baclofen
   Biochemistry   QU 60
   As a central muscle relaxant   QV 140
Baclophen see Baclofen
Bacteremia see Septicemia   WC 240
Bacteria   QW
   Actinomycetes   QW 115, etc.
   Anatomy and morphology   QW 51
   As cause of disease   QZ 65
   Budding and/or appendaged see Budding and
      Appendaged Bacteria   QW 153
   General works   QW 50
   Gliding see Gliding Bacteria   QW 128
   Gram-positive see Gram-Positive Bacteria   QW
      142–142.5
   Invasiveness   QW 730
   Metabolism   QW 52
   Physiology see Bacterial Physiology   QW 52
   Sheathed   QW 153
   Spiral and curved see Spiral and Curved Bacteria
      QW 154
   See also Gram-Negative Facultatively Anaerobic
     Rods   QW 137–141; Gram-Positive
     Asporogenous Rods   QW 142.5.A8;
     Gram-Positive Cocci   QW 142.5.C6
Bacteria, Anaerobic   QW 52
Bacterial Adhesion   QW 52
Bacterial Antibodies see Antibodies, Bacterial
Bacterial Antigens see Antigens, Bacterial
Bacterial Conjugation see Conjugation, Genetic
Bacterial DNA see DNA, Bacterial
Bacterial Drug Resistance see Drug Resistance,
   Microbial
Bacterial Gene Expression Regulation see Gene
   Expression Regulation, Bacterial
Bacterial Gene Products see Bacterial Proteins
Bacterial Gene Proteins see Bacterial Proteins
Bacterial Genetics see Genetics, Microbial
Bacterial Infections   WC 200–425
   Child   WC 200–425
   Enteric   WC 260–290
   In plants   SB 734
   Infant   WC 200–425
   Of the kidney   WJ 351
   Veterinary   SF 780.3
   Specific infection see name of infection
   Other particular organ affected, by organ or
     region
Bacterial Outer Membrane Proteins   QW 52
Bacterial Physiology   QW 52
Bacterial Pili see Pili, Sex
Bacterial Polysaccharides see Polysaccharides,
   Bacterial
Bacterial Proteins   QW 52
   Therapeutic use, with the disease being treated
Bacterial RNA see RNA, Bacterial
Bacterial Sensitivity Tests see Microbial Sensitivity
   Tests
Bacterial Spores see Spores, Bacterial
Bacterial Toxins   QW 630.5.B2
Bacterial Vaccines   WC 200
   Pyrogenic   WB 469 or with disease being treated

**ALWAYS CONSULT MAIN SCHEDULES. USE NUMBER ASSIGNED ONLY WHEN
SUBJECT REPRESENTS MAJOR EMPHASIS OF WORK BEING CLASSIFIED**

For specific diseases, with the diseases
Bacterial Warfare see Biological Warfare
Bactericidal Action of Antibodies see Bacteriolysis
Bacteriocins   QV 350
Bacteriodaceae   QW 133
Bacteriological Techniques   QW 25
   Clinical pathology   QY 100
   Veterinary   QW 70
Bacteriologists, Directories see Directories   QW 22
   under Bacteriology
Bacteriology   QW 1-155
   General works   QW 50
   Clinical see Bacteriological Techniques   QY 100
   Dental   QW 65
   Directories   QW 22
   Industrial   QW 75
   Nursing texts   QW 50, etc.
   Of air see Air Microbiology   QW 82
   Of food see Food Microbiology   QW 85
   Of milk   QW 85
   Of plants   QW 60
   Of sewage   QW 80
   Of soil see Soil Microbiology   QW 60
   Of water see Water Microbiology   QW 80
   Veterinary science   QW 70
Bacteriolysis   QW 660
Bacteriophage lambda   QW 161.5.C6
Bacteriophage Typing   QW 25
Bacteriophages   QW 161
Bacteriophages T see T-Phages
Bacteriorhodopsin   QW 52
Bacteriuria   WJ 351
   In urine analysis   QY 185
Bacteroides   QW 133
Bacteroides Infections   WC 200
Bagassosis see Pneumoconiosis
Balance see Equilibrium
Balantidiasis   WC 735
Balantidium   QX 151
Baldness see Alopecia
Balint Psychoanalytic Therapy see Psychoanalytic
   Therapy
Ballistics, Wound see Wounds, Gunshot
Ballistocardiography   WG 141.5.B2
Balloon Angioplasty see Angioplasty, Balloon
Balloon Catheterization see Balloon Dilatation
Balloon Dilatation   WB 365
   In cardiovascular diseases   WG 166.5.B2
   In other diseases, with the disease
Balloon Dilatation, Coronary Artery see
   Angioplasty, Transluminal, Percutaneous
   Coronary
Balloon Tamponade see Balloon Dilatation
Balloon Valvotomy see Balloon Dilatation
Balloon Valvuloplasty see Balloon Dilatation
Balneology   WB 525
Balneotherapy see Balneology
Balsams   QV 241
Banana see Zingiberales
Bancroftian Elephantiasis see Elephantiasis, Filarial
Band 3 Protein   WH 400
Bandages
   First aid   WA 292

   Surgical   WO 167
   See also Occlusive Dressings   WO 167
Bandages, Occlusive see Occlusive Dressings
Bandicoot Rats see Muridae
Bandicota see Muridae
Banding, Chromosome see Chromosome Banding
Bang's Disease see Brucellosis, Bovine
Banks see Blood Banks; Eye Banks; Tissue Banks
   (Form number 23-24 in any NLM schedule where
     applicable)
Bar Codes see Automatic Data Processing
Barany's Test see Caloric Tests
Barbary Ape see Macaca
Barber Surgeons   WO 11
Barbering
   Care of hair   WR 465
   Public health aspects of barber shops   WA 744
   Registration of barbers   WA 32
Barbital   QV 88
Barbitone see Barbital
Barbiturates   QV 88
Barbituric Acid Derivatives see Barbiturates
Barefoot Doctors see Community Health Aides
Barium   QV 618
   As a contrast medium in radiology   WN 160
Barlow's Disease see Scurvy
Barnacles   QX 463
Baroreceptors see Pressoreceptors
Barotrauma
   In high altitude   WD 710
   Underwater   WD 650
   See also Atmospheric Pressure
Barr Bodies see Sex Chromatin
Barrett Esophagus   WI 250
Barriers, Architectural see Architectural
   Accessibility
Bartholin's Glands   WP 200
Bartonella Infections   WC 640
Bartonellaceae Infections   WC 640
Bartonellosis see Bartonella Infections
Bartter's Disease   WK 770
Basal Anesthesia see Preanesthetic Medication
Basal Ganglia   WL 307
Basal Ganglia Diseases   WL 307
   See also names of specific disorders, e.g.,
     Parkinson Disease   WL 359
Basal Metabolism   QU 125
Basal Nuclei see Basal Ganglia
Basal Vein see Cerebral Veins
Base Composition   QU 58
Base Pairs see Base Composition
Base Ratio see Base Composition
Base Sequence   QU 58
Base Sequence Homology see Sequence Homology,
   Nucleic Acid
Baseball   QT 260.5.B2
Basedow's Disease see Goiter, Exophthalmic
Basic Life Support see Cardiopulmonary
   Resuscitation
Basic Pancreatic Trypsin Inhibitor see Aprotinin
Basicranium see Skull Base
Basidiomycetes see Basidiomycota
Basidiomycota   QW 180.5.B2

**ALWAYS CONSULT MAIN SCHEDULES. USE NUMBER ASSIGNED ONLY WHEN
SUBJECT REPRESENTS MAJOR EMPHASIS OF WORK BEING CLASSIFIED**

Basilar Artery   WG 595.B2
Basilar Artery Insufficiency see Vertebrobasilar
   Insufficiency
Basilar Impression see Platybasia
Basilar Membrane   WV 250
Basketball   QT 260.5.B3
Basophilism, Pituitary see Cushing Syndrome
Basophils   WH 200
Basophils, Tissue see Mast Cells
Bathing Beaches   WA 820
Baths
   Hygiene   QT 240
   Mud see Mud Therapy   WB 525
   Public   WA 820
   Sand see Ammotherapy   WB 525
   See also Balneology   WB 525; Thalassotherapy
     WB 750
Baths, Finnish   WB 525
Baths, Sand see Ammotherapy
Bats see Chiroptera
Batten–Spielmeyer–Vogt Disease see Neuronal
   Ceroid–Lipofuscinosis
Battered Child Syndrome   WA 320
Battle Fatigue see Combat Disorders
Baunscheidtism see Acupuncture
Bayer 39 see Inproquone
BCG see Mycobacterium bovis
BCG Vaccine   WF 250
Beaches, Bathing see Bathing Beaches
Beans see Legumes
Beard see Hair
Beauty   BH
   Women   HQ 1219–1220
   Plastic surgery   WO 600
Beauty Culture
   Hygienic aspects   QT 275
   Public health aspects   WA 744
   Registration of beauticians and cosmeticians
     WA 32
Beauty Salons see Beauty Culture
Beavers see Rodentia
Bechterew's Disease see Spondylitis, Ankylosing
Becker Muscular Dystrophy see Muscular
   Dystrophy
Beclomethasone   WK 757
Beclomethasone Dipropionate see Beclomethasone
Bed Capacity, Hospital see Hospital Bed Capacity
Bed Conversion   WX 140
   In special type of facilities, with the facility
Bed Occupancy   WX 16
Bed Size, Hospital see Hospital Bed Capacity
Bedbugs   QX 503
Bedding and Linens   WX 165
   Home care of sick   W 26
Beds
   Home care of sick   W 26
   Hospitals   WX 147
Beds, Swing see Bed Conversion
Bedside Computing see Point–of–Care Systems
Bedside Testing see Point–of–Care Systems
Bedsore see Decubitus Ulcer
Bedsores see Decubitus Ulcer
Bee Venoms   WD 430

Beer
   As a dietary supplement in health or disease
     WB 444
   Chemical technology   TP 577
   Microorganisms of fermentation   QW 85
   See also Alcoholism   WM 274; Alcohol, Ethyl
     QV 84, etc.
Bees   QX 565
Beetles   QX 555
Beggiatoales see Cytophagales   QW 128
Beginning of Life see Biogenesis
Behavior
   Adolescence   WS 462
   Child   WS 105
   Drug effects   WM, QV
   Infant   WS 105
   Psychology (General)   BF 110–149
   Sex see Sex behavior   HQ 12–30.7, etc.
   Special topics, by subject
Behavior, Adaptive see Adaptation, Psychological
Behavior, Addictive   WM 176
Behavior, Adolescent see Adolescent Behavior
Behavior, Animal   QL 750–785.3
Behavior, Compulsive see Compulsive Behavior
Behavior, Dangerous see Dangerous Behavior
Behavior Disorders see Affective Symptoms; Child
   Behavior Disorders; Social Behavior Disorders;
   names of specific disorders
Behavior, Exploratory see Exploratory Behavior
Behavior Modification see Behavior Therapy
Behavior Modifiers see Psychotropic Drugs
Behavior Therapy   WM 425
   Adolescence   WS 463
   Child   WS 350.6
   Infant   WS 350.6
   Nursing texts   WY 160
   See also Counseling   WY 87, etc.;
     Nurse–patient relations   WY 87
Behavior Therapy, Cognitive see Cognitive Therapy
Behavioral Medicine   WB 103
   Special topics, by subject
Behavioral Sciences
   Animals see Ethology   QL 750–785.3
   Educational aspects   LB–LC
   Psychiatric aspects   WM
   Psychological aspects   BF
   Sociological aspects   HM
   Other special topics, by subject, e.g., statistics
    for the behavioral sciences   HA 29
Behaviorism   BF 199
Behcet's Syndrome   WW 240
Bejel see Treponemal Infections
Belching see Eructation
Belgian Hare see Rabbits
Belladonna
   As a medicinal plant   QV 766
   As a sympatholytic   QV 134
   Culture   SB 295.B4
   Poisoning   WD 500
Bell's Palsy see Facial Paralysis
Benactyzine   QV 77.9
Bence Jones Protein   WH 540
Bender–Gestalt Test   WM 145.5.B4

Bends see Decompression Sickness
Beneckea see Vibrio
Benhydramin see Diphenhydramine
Benign Intracranial Hypertension see Pseudotumor
    Cerebri
Benign Monoclonal Gammopathies see Monoclonal
    Gammopathies, Benign
Bensokain see Benzocaine
Benzalacetophenone see Chalcone
Benzalkonium see Benzalkonium Compounds
Benzalkonium Compounds   QV 233
Benzamides   QU 62
    Organic chemistry   QD 341.A7
Benzanthracenes   QZ 202
Benzathine Penicillin see Penicillin G, Benzathine
Benzene
    Organic chemistry   QD 341.H9
    Toxicology   QV 633
Benzene Derivatives
    Organic chemistry   QD 341.H9
    Toxicology   QV 633
Benzene Hexachloride see Lindane
Benzimidazoles
    As anthelmintics   QV 253
    Organic chemistry   QD 401
    Veterinary pharmacology   SF 918.A45
Benzo(a)pyrene   QZ 202
Benzoates   QU 98
    Organic chemistry   QD 341.A2
Benzocaine   QV 115
Benzodiazepine Tranquilizers see Anti-Anxiety
    Agents, Benzodiazepine
Benzoin   QV 241
Benzol see Benzene
Benzophenoneidum
    Toxicology   QV 632
    As a disinfectant   QV 235
Benzopyrans
    Organic chemistry   QD 405
Benzopyrenes
    As carcinogens   QZ 202
Benzothiadiazines
    Organic chemistry   QD 401
Benzoyl Peroxide
    As a dermatological agent   QV 60
Benzoyl Superoxide see Benzoyl Peroxide
Benzylamines
    Biochemistry   QU 61
Benzylideneacetophenone see Chalcone
Benzylpenicillin see Penicillin G
Bereavement   BF 575.G7
    Adolescence   WS 462
    Child   WS 105.5.E5
    Infant   WS 105.5.E5
Bereavement Care see Hospice Care
Berger's Disease see Glomerulonephritis, IGA
Beriberi   WD 122
Berries see Fruit
Berry Aneurysm see Cerebral Aneurysm
Bertielliasis see Cestode Infections
Berylliosis   WF 654
Beryllium   QV 275
Beryllium Disease see Berylliosis

Besnier-Boeck Disease see Sarcoidosis
Besnoitiasis see Protozoan Infections
Bestiality see Paraphilias
beta-Adrenergic Blocking Agents see Adrenergic
    beta-Antagonists
beta-Adrenergic Receptor Agonists see Adrenergic
    beta-Agonists
beta-Adrenergic Receptor Blockaders see
    Adrenergic beta-Antagonists
beta-Adrenergic Receptors see Receptors,
    Adrenergic, beta
beta-Alanine Ketoglutarate Aminotransferase see
    4-Aminobutyrate Transaminase
beta,beta-Dimethylcysteine see Penicillamine
beta-Blockers, Adrenergic see Adrenergic
    beta-Antagonists
Beta Carotene   QU 110
    As a coloring agent   WA 712
    Vitamin A related   QU 167
Beta Cell, Artificial see Insulin Infusion Systems
beta-Cell Tumor see Insulinoma
Beta-Globulins   WH 400
    Clinical analysis   QY 455
beta-Hydroxyphenethylamine see
    2-Hydroxyphenethylamine
beta-Hypophamine see Vasopressins
beta-Lactam Antibiotics see Antibiotics, Lactam
beta-Lactamase I see Penicillinase
beta-Lactamases   QU 136
Beta-naphthol see Naphthols
Beta Particles see Beta Rays
beta-Phenylethanolamine see
    2-Hydroxyphenethylamine
Beta Rays   WN 105
beta 2-Microglobulin   WH 400
    Clinical analysis   QY 455
Betacarotene see Beta Carotene
Betadexamethasone see Betamethasone
Betaine   QV 87
Betamethasone   WK 757
Betatrons see Particle Accelerators
Betel see Areca
Beverages
    As a dietary supplement in health or disease
      WB 433-444
    Chemical technology   TP 500-659
    Microbiology   QW 85
    Public health (General)   WA 695
      Legislation (General)   WA 697
    See also names of specific beverages, e.g.,
      Alcoholic Beverages   WB 444, etc.
Bezoars   WI 300
    Of the intestines   WI 400
    Veterinary   SF 851
Bhang see Cannabis
Bible   BS
    Medicine depicted in   WZ 330
    Special topics, by subject, e.g., medical properties
      of Biblical plants   QV 766
Bibliography
    Of subjects represented in NLM's classification,
      appropriate classification number preceded by
      the letter Z

ALWAYS CONSULT MAIN SCHEDULES. USE NUMBER ASSIGNED ONLY WHEN
SUBJECT REPRESENTS MAJOR EMPHASIS OF WORK BEING CLASSIFIED

Of other subjects, LC's Z schedule
See bibliography section of Introduction for
further instructions
Bibliography, Descriptive   Z 1001
Bibliography, National   Z 1201–4980
Bibliography of Medicine
  General works including monographs and serials
    Issued as monograph   ZWB 100
    Issued as serial   ZW 1
  Of monographs   ZWB 100
    Issued serially   ZW 1
  Of serials   ZW 1
  On specific subject, NLM number for the subject
    preceded by Z
Bibliography, Statistical see Bibliometrics
Bibliometrics   Z 669.8
  Special topics, by subject
Bibliotherapy   WM 450.5.B5
Bicarbonates
  Inorganic chemistry   QD 181.C1
  Pharmacology   QV 138.C1
Bicuculline   QV 103
Bicycle Ergometry Test see Exercise Test
Bicycling   QT 260.5.B5
Bifidobacterium   QW 125.5.A2
Bifocal Lenses see Eyeglasses
Bifunctional Reagents see Cross–Linking Reagents
Biguanides   QU 61
  Organic chemistry   QD 305.A8
Bilayer Fluidity see Membrane Fluidity
Bilayers, Lipid see Lipid Bilayers
Bile   WI 703
Bile Acids and Salts   WI 703
Bile Duct Diseases   WI 750
Bile Duct Neoplasms   WI 765
Bile Duct Obstruction see Cholestasis
Bile Duct Obstruction, Extrahepatic   WI 750
Bile Ducts   WI 750
  See also Common Bile Duct   WI 750; Cystic
    Duct   WI 750; Hepatic Duct   WI 750
Bile Ducts, Intrahepatic   WI 750
Bile Pigments   WI 703
  Clinical pathology   QY 143
Bile Reflux   WI 703
Bile Salts see Bile Acids and Salts
Bilharzia see Schistosoma
Bilharziasis see Schistosomiasis
Biliary Atresia   WI 750
Biliary Calculi see Cholelithiasis
Biliary Calculi, Common Bile Duct see Common Bile
  Duct Calculi
Biliary Fistula   WI 750
Biliary Stasis see Cholestasis
Biliary Stasis, Extrahepatic see Bile Duct
  Obstruction, Extrahepatic
Biliary Surgery see Biliary Tract Surgical
  Procedures
Biliary Tract   WI 700–770
Biliary Tract Diseases   WI 700–770
  General works   WI 700
Biliary Tract Neoplasms   WI 735
Biliary Tract Surgical Procedures   WI 770
Bilingualism see Multilingualism

Bilirubin   WI 703
  Clinical pathology   QY 143
Bilirubin Encephalopathy see Kernicterus
Bilirubinemia see Hyperbilirubinemia
Binding, Competitive
  Bacteriology   QW 570
  Biochemistry (General)   QU 34
  Pharmacology   QV 38
Binding Proteins see Carrier Proteins
Binding Sites
  Antigen–antibody reactions   QW 570
  Biochemistry (General)   QU 34
  Immunochemistry   QW 504.5
  Pharmacology   QV 38
Binding Sites, Antibody   QW 575
  See also Agglutination   QW 640
Binocular Vision see Depth Perception; Eye
  Movements; Accommodation, Ocular; Vision
Bioartificial Liver see Liver, Artificial
Bioassay see Biological assay
Bioavailability see Biological Availability
Biobibliography
  General Z 1010
  Individual   WZ 100
  Of individuals in fields largely unrelated to the
    biological sciences, in the appropriate LC
    number
  Of groups of persons in special fields   WZ
    112–112.5 or in appropriate LC number
Biochemic Medicine see Alternative Medicine
Biochemical Genetics see Genetics, Biochemical
Biochemical Markers see Biological Markers
Biochemical Phenomena
  General   QU 34
Biochemistry   QU
  Biography
    Collective   WZ 112
    Individual   WZ 100
  Cryobiochemistry   QU 25
  Directories   QU 22
  Fetus   WQ 210.5
  Inorganic substances   QU 130
  Nursing texts   QU 4, etc.
  Of respiration   WF 110
  Technique   QU 25
  See also Biochemical Phenomena   QU 34
Biochemists see Biography; Directories   QU 22
  under Biochemistry
Biocompatible Materials   QT 37
  Used for special purposes, by subject, e.g., for
    artificial organs (General)   WO 176
Biocompatible Materials Testing see Materials
Testing
Biodegradation   WA 671
  Waste disposal   WA 778–788
  Special topics, by subject
Bioelectric Energy Sources   QT 34
  Used for special purposes, by subject, e.g. for
    pacemakers   WG 26
Bioenergetics see Energy Metabolism
Bioequivalence see Therapeutic Equivalency
Bioethics   QH 332
  Special topics, by subject

**ALWAYS CONSULT MAIN SCHEDULES.   USE NUMBER ASSIGNED ONLY WHEN
SUBJECT REPRESENTS MAJOR EMPHASIS OF WORK BEING CLASSIFIED**

See also Ethics, Medical   W 50
Biofeedback (Psychology)   WL 103
  Behavior therapy   WM 425.5.B6
Bioflavonoids   QU 220
Biogenesis   QH 325
  Legal establishment of beginning of life   W 789
Biogenic Amines   QU 61
  Special topics, by subject
Biographical Accounts of Disease see Name of diseases, e.g. Mental Retardation
Biographical Clinics see Famous Persons; Psychoanalytic Interpretation; names of particular persons
Biography   CT
  As a form of literature   CT 21
  Of mentally ill   WM 40
  Of other persons with particular diseases, with the disease
  Physicians and specialists of medically related fields
    Collective   WZ 112–150
    Individual   WZ 100
  Scientists and behavioral scientists
    Collective in appropriate LC number
    Individual   WZ 100
  Other professions, in appropriate LC number
  See also names of other groups of persons, e.g., Pharmacists   WZ 112.5.P4
Biohazards Containment see Containment of Biohazards
Bioinformatics see Computational Biology
Biological Assay   QV 771
  Of hormones   QY 330
  Of vitamins   QY 350
Biological Availability   QV 38
  Special topics, by subject
Biological Availability, Nutritional see Nutritive Value
Biological Chemistry see Biochemistry
Biological Clocks   QT 167
  See also special topics under Circadian Rhythm
Biological Dressings   WO 167
Biological Energy Sources see Bioelectric Energy Sources
Biological Markers
  Genetics   QH 438.4.B55
  In the diagnosis of a particular disease, with the disease
Biological Monitoring see Environmental Monitoring
Biological Oscillators see Biological Clocks
Biological Pest Control see Pest Control, Biological
Biological Phenomena
  General   QH 307–307.2
Biological Products   QW 800
  Refrigeration   WA 730
  Tissue extracts   QV 370
  Veterinary   SF 918.B5
  See also Hormones, Synthetic   WK 187
Biological Psychiatry   WM 102
  Special topics, by subject
Biological Pump see Biological Transport, Active
Biological Response Modifiers   QW 800

Biological Therapy
  General works   WB 365
  Of a particular disease, with the disease
  See also names of specific therapies, e.g., Immunotherapy   QW 940–949; Organotherapy   WB 391
Biological Transport   QH 509
  Cytology   QH 601
  Metabolism   QU 120
  See also Osmosis   QH 615, etc.
Biological Transport, Active   QH 509
  Cytology   QH 601
  Metabolism   QU 120
Biological Warfare
  Bacteriological aspects   QW 300
  Military aspects   UG 447.8
Biological Waste Disposal see Medical Waste Disposal
Biologics see Biological Products
Biology   QH 301–705
  General works   QH 307–307.2
  History   QH 305–305.2
  In art   N 72.B5
  Life (Biology)   QH 501
Bioluminescence see Luminescence
Bioluminescent Proteins see Luminescent Proteins
Biomass see Ecology
Biomaterials see Biocompatible Materials
Biomathematics see Mathematics
Biomechanics   WE 103
Biomedical and Dental Materials
  Biomedical and biocompatible materials   QT 37
  Dental materials   WU 190
  Used for special purposes, by subject
Biomedical Engineering   QT 36
  Special topics, by subject
Biomedical Research see Research
Biomedical Technology see Technology, Medical
Biometry   QH 323.5
  Medical   WA 950
Biomodulators see Biological Response Modifiers
Bionator see Activator Appliances
Bionics   Q 317–321
  Used for special purposes, by subject, e.g. in biophysics   QT 34
Bionomics see Ecology
Bioperiodicity see Periodicity
Biopharmaceutics   QV 38
Biophysics   QT 34
  Radiation   WN 110
Biopolymers
  Organic chemistry   QD 380–388
Bioprobes see Biosensing Techniques
Bioprosthesis
  For heart valve   WG 169
  See also Heart Valve Prosthesis
Biopsy
  Clinical diagnosis   WB 379
  Surgical diagnosis   WO 142
  Veterinary   SF 772
  Specific area, by organ; in specific diseases, with the disease
Biopsy, Chorionic Villi see Chorionic Villi Sampling

Biopsy, Needle
   Clinical diagnosis   WB 379
   Surgical diagnosis   WO 142
   Specific area, by organ; in specific diseases, with
     the disease
Biopterin
   As a pteridines   QU 188
   As a growth substance   QU 107
Bioreactors   TP 248.25.B55
   Special biological systems as bioreactors, with
     the system, e.g., Erythrocytes   WH 150;
     Animal cells   TP 248.27.A53
Biorhythms see Biological Clocks; Circadian
   Rhythm; Periodicity
Biosensing Techniques   QT 36
Biosensors see Biosensing Techniques
Biostatistics see Statistics
Biosynthetic Proteins see Recombinant Proteins
Biotechnology   TP 248.13–248.65
   Applied to specific topics, by subject
Biotin   QU 195
Biotransformation
   Metabolism   QU 120
   Pharmacology   QV 38
Biphenyl Compounds
   As carcinogens   QZ 202
   As insecticides   WA 240
   Organic chemistry   QD 341.H9
   Toxicology   QV 633
Bipolar Disorder   WM 207
Bird Diseases   SF 994–995.6
Bird Fancier's Lung   WF 150
Birds
   As laboratory animals   QY 60.B4
   Domestic (Breeding)   SF 460–473
   Wild   QL 671–699
Birds of Prey see Raptors
Birth see Delivery; Biogenesis
Birth Certificates   HA 38–39
Birth Control see Contraception; Family Planning
Birth Defects see Abnormalities
Birth Injuries   WS 405
Birth, Multiple see Pregnancy, Multiple; named
   groups, e.g., Twins
Birth Order
   Psychological aspects in children   WS 105.5.F2
Birth Rate   HB 901–1108
Birth Registration see Birth Certificates
Birth Statistics see Birth Rate; Vital Statistics
Birth Weight
   Newborn   WS 420
   Premature infant   WS 410
   Tables   WS 16
Birthmark see Hemangioma; Nevus; Nevus,
   Pigmented
Bis(Chloromethyl) Ether
   As a carcinogen   QZ 202
Bisexuality
   As a life style   HQ 74
   Psychiatric aspects   WM 611
Bishydroxycoumarin see Dicumarol
Bismuth   QV 290
Bisnorephedrine see 2–Hydroxyphenethylamine

Bite Force   WU 440
Bites and Stings   WD 400–430
   Insects see Insect Bites and Stings   WD 430
   Snake see Snake Bites   WD 410
   Spider and scorpion see Arachnidism   WD 420
   Surgical treatment   WO 700
Bitters see Flavoring Agents; Gastrointestinal Agents
Biundulant Meningo–Encephalitis Virus see
   Encephalitis Viruses, Tick–Borne
Biureas
   Organic chemistry   QD 315
BK Virus see Polyomavirus hominis 1
Black Ape see Macaca
Black Flies see Simuliidae
Black Tongue see Tongue, Hairy
Blacks
   American   E 184.6–185.97
   As physicians
     Collective biography   WZ 150
     History   WZ 80.5.B5
     Individual biography   WZ 100
   In other countries, see name of country in LC
     schedules   D–F
   See also special topics under Ethnic groups
Blackwater Fever   WC 750–770
Bladder   WJ 500–504
Bladder Calculi   WJ 500
Bladder Diseases   WJ 500–504
   General   WJ 500
   See also Vesicovaginal Fistula   WP 180
Bladder Drug Administration see Administration,
   Intravesical
Bladder Exstrophy   WJ 500
Bladder Fistula   WJ 500
Bladder Neck Obstruction   WJ 500
Bladder Neoplasms   WJ 504
Bladder, Neurogenic   WJ 500
Bladder Stones see Bladder Calculi
Bladder Worm see Taenia
Blast Injuries   WO 820
Blast Transformation see Lymphocyte
   Transformation
Blast–2 Antigen, B–Cell see Antigens,
   Differentiation, B–Lymphocyte
Blastocladiella   QW 180.5.P4
Blastocyst Transfer see Embryo Transfer
Blastogenesis see Lymphocyte Transformation
Blastomyces   QW 180.5.A8
Blastomycosis   WC 450
Blastomycosis, North American see Blastomycosis
Blastomycosis, South American see
   Paracoccidioidomycosis
Bleeding see Hemorrhage
Blennorrhea, Inclusion see Conjunctivitis, Inclusion
Bleomycin
   Pharmacology   QV 269
   Therapeutic use   QZ 267
Blepharitis   WW 205
Blepharoplasty   WW 205
Blepharoptosis   WW 205
Blepharospasm   WW 205
Blind see Visually Impaired Persons
Blindness   WW 276

Child   WW 276
Color see Color Blindness   WW 150
Education of blind   HV 1618-2349
Hysterical   WM 173.5
Infant   WW 276
Libraries for the blind   Z 675.B6
Library operations   Z 729-871
Night see Night Blindness   WD 110
Rehabilitation
   Physical & medical   WW 276
   Social   HV 1573-2349
   Veterinary   SF 891
Blister   WR 143
Localized, by site
Block Anesthesia see Anesthesia, Conduction
Blood   WH
Chemistry see Blood chemical analysis   QY
   450-490, etc.
Child   WS 300
Clinical examination   QY 400-490
Corpuscles see Blood Cells   WH 140, etc.;
   Erythocytes   WH 150-180; Leukocytes   WH
   200
Derivatives   WH 450
Fluid elements   WH 400
Flukes see Schistosoma   QX 355
Infant   WS 300
Medicolegal examination   W 750
Physiology see Blood Physiology   WH 100
Substitutes see Plasma Substitutes   WH 450
Typing see Blood Grouping and Crossmatching
   QY 415
Velocity see Blood Flow Velocity   WG 106
See also Anticoagulants   QV 193; Lipids   QU
   85-95; Plasma   WH 400, etc.
Blood, Artificial see Blood Substitutes
Blood Bactericidal Activity   QW 541
Special topics, by subject
Blood Banks   WH 23-24
Procedures   WH 460
Blood-Borne Pathogens   WA 790
Blood-Brain Barrier   WL 200
Blood Cell Count   QY 402
Veterinary   SF 772.67
Blood Cell Count, Red see Erythrocyte Count
Blood Cell Count, White see Leukocyte Count
Blood Cell Number see Blood Cell Count
Blood Cells   WH 140
Clinical examination   QY 402
Drugs affecting   QV 180-185
Blood Cells, Red see Erythrocytes
Blood Cells, White see Leukocytes
Blood Chemical Analysis   QY 450-490
Child   QY 450-490
Infant   QY 450-490
Medicolegal   W 750
Veterinary   SF 772.67
Blood Circulation   WG 103
Child   WG 103
Disorders as a manifestation of disease   QZ 170
Infant   WG 103
Tests   WG 103
See also names of specific types of circulation,

e.g., Pulmonary Circulation   WF 600
Blood Circulation, Collateral see Collateral
   Circulation
Blood Circulation Time   WG 103
Blood Coagulation
Clinical examination   QY 410
Drugs affecting   QV 190-195
Physiology   WH 310
Blood Coagulation Disorders   WH 322
Hemophilia   WH 325
Veterinary   SF 769.5
See also names of specific disorders
Blood Coagulation Factor Inhibitors   WH 310
Clinical examination   QY 410
Pharmacology   QV 193
Blood Coagulation Factors   WH 310
Clinical examination   QY 410
Pharmacology   QV 195
Blood Coagulation Tests   QY 410
Blood Component Removal   WH 460
Blood Component Transfusion   WB 356
Blood Count, Complete see Blood Cell Count
Blood Diseases see Hematologic Diseases
Blood Donors   WH 460
Blood Doping see Doping in Sports
Blood Expanders see Plasma Substitutes
Blood Flow see Rheology
Blood Flow Velocity   WG 106
Blood Gas Analysis   QY 450
Veterinary   SF 774
Blood Gas Monitoring, Transcutaneous   QY 450
Blood Glucose   QU 75
Clinical analysis   QY 470
Blood Glucose Self-Monitoring
In diabetes   WK 850
Blood Group Incompatibility   WH 420
Blood Grouping and Crossmatching   QY 415
Special topics, by subject
Blood Groups   WH 420-425
Medicolegal examination   W 791
Typing see Blood Grouping and Crossmatching
   QY 415
Blood Loss, Postoperative see Postoperative
   Hemorrhage
Blood Loss, Surgical
During surgery for a particular condition, with
   the condition
Blood Physiology   WH 100
Blood Plasma see Plasma
Blood Plasma Volume see Plasma Volume
Blood Platelet Disorders   WH 300
See also Purpura, Thrombopenic   WH 315
Blood Platelet Transfusion see Platelet Transfusion
Blood Plateletpheresis see Plateletpheresis
Blood Platelets   WH 300
Count   QY 402
Blood Poisoning see Septicemia
Blood Preservation   WH 460
Blood Pressure   WG 106
General physical examination   WB 280
High see Hypertension   WG 340
Low see Hypotension   WG 340
Blood Pressure Determination   WG 106

**ALWAYS CONSULT MAIN SCHEDULES. USE NUMBER ASSIGNED ONLY WHEN
SUBJECT REPRESENTS MAJOR EMPHASIS OF WORK BEING CLASSIFIED**

Physical examination   WB 280
Blood Pressure, High see Hypertension
Blood Pressure, Low see Hypotension
Blood Pressure Monitors   WG 26
Blood Pressure, Venous see Venous Pressure
Blood Protein Disorders   WH 400
   Clinical pathology   QY 455
   Specific disorders involving various blood
    elements, with the element
   See other specific disorders under their names
    in the index
Blood Protein Electrophoresis   QY 455
Blood Proteins   WH 400
   Clinical analysis   QY 455
   Coagulation factors   WH 310
    Clinical pathology   QY 410
Blood Sedimentation   QY 408
Blood Serum see Blood
Blood Specimen Collection   QY 26
Blood Substitutes   WH 450
Blood Sugar see Blood Glucose
Blood Sugar Self–Monitoring see Blood Glucose
  Self–Monitoring
Blood Tests see Hematologic Tests
Blood Transfusion   WB 356
   Veterinary   SF 919.5.B55
   See also Blood Banks   WH 23–24, etc.; Blood
    Donors   WH 460
Blood Transfusion, Intrauterine   WQ 210
Blood Typing see Blood Grouping and
  Crossmatching
Blood Vessel Prosthesis   WG 170
Blood Vessel Prosthesis Implantation   WG 170
   Of a particular region or organ, with the region
    or organ
   See also names of specific vessels, e.g., Coronary
    Vessels   WG 300
Blood Vessels
   Peripheral   WG 500–700
   Radiography see Angiography   WG 500
   Surgery see Vascular Surgical Procedures   WG
    170
   Of a particular region or organ, with the region
    or organ
Blood Viscosity   WG 106
   Clinical analysis   QY 408
Blood Volume   WG 106
   Volume index   QY 408
Bloodletting   WB 381
Blotting, Northern   QH 441
Blotting, Southern   QH 441
Blotting, Western   QW 525.5.I32
   Proteins   QU 55
   Peptides   QU 68
Blue–Green Bacteria see Cyanobacteria
Blue Sclera see Abnormalities   WW 230 under
  Sclera
Bluetongue Virus   QW 168.5.R15
BLV Infections see HTLV–BLV Infections
Board, Governing see Governing Board
Boats see Ships
Bodies, Dead see Cadaver
Body Buffer Zone see Personal Space

Body Build see Somatotypes
Body Burden   WN 660
Body Composition   QU 100–110
Body Constitution
   Anthropology   GN 62
   As a cause of disease   QZ 50
Body Fluid Compartments   QU 105
Body Fluids   QU 105
Body Height
   Adult   GN 66
   Child   WS 103
   Infant   WS 103
    Tables   WS 16
Body Image   BF 697.5.B63
   Adolescence   WS 462
   Child   WS 105.5.S3
Body Language see Kinesics
Body Lice see Lice
Body Rocking see Stereotypic Movement Disorder
Body Size see Body Constitution
Body Snatching see Cadaver
Body Surface Area   GN 66
   Veterinary
    Domestic animals   SF 761
    Wild animals   QL 363
Body Temperature   WB 270
   Changes see Body Temperature Changes   QT
    165, etc.
   Child   WS 141
   High see Fever   WB 152
   In antibody production   QW 575
   Infant   WS 141
    Newborn   WS 420
   In ovulation   WP 540
   In physical examination   WB 270
    Veterinary   SF 772.5
   See also Skin Temperature   WR 102
Body Temperature Changes
   Child   WS 141
   In antibody formation   QW 575
   In ovulation   WP 540
   In physical examination   WB 270
   Infant   WS 141
   Physiology   QT 165
   See also Body Temperature   WB 270, etc.; Body
    Temperature Regulation   QT 165, etc.; Fever
     WB 152, etc.; Hypothermia   WD 670, etc.
Body Temperature Regulation   QT 165
   Skin as a factor   WR 102
Body Types see Somatotypes
Body vermin see Lice; Bedbugs
Body Water   QU 105
Body Weight
   Adult   GN 66
   Child   WS 103
   Infant   WS 103
    Tables   WS 16
   Infant, Premature see Birth Weight   WS 410,
    etc.
   Newborn see Birth Weight   WS 420, etc.
   Physiology   QT 104
Body Weight Changes
   Child   WS 103

Infant   WS 103
Signs and symptoms   WB 146
See also Body Weight   GN 66, etc.; Obesity
  WD 210–212; Thinness   GN 66–67.5, etc.;
  Weight Gain   WS 103; Weight Loss   WS 103
Body Weights and Measures
  Adult   GN 66
  Child   WS 103
  Infant   WS 103
    Tables   WS 16
  See also Anthropometry   GN 51–59; Body
    Height   GN 66, etc.; Body Weight   GN 66,
    etc.
Boeck's Sarcoid see Sarcoidosis
Boils see Furunculosis
Bombesin   QU 68
Bombina see Anura
Bond Issues, Construction see Financing,
  Construction
Bonding, Dental see Dental Bonding
Bonding, Human–Pet   WM 460.5.B7
Bonding (Psychology) see Object Attachment
Bonds, Emotional see Object Attachment
Bone Age Measurement see Age Determination by
  Skeleton
Bone and Bones   WE 200–259
  Physiology   WE 200
  Surgery   WE 168–190
  Transplantation   WE 190
  See also Skeleton   WE 100–102
Bone Cements   WE 190
  Used for special purposes, by subject
Bone Conduction   WV 272
Bone Cysts   WE 258
  Localized, by site
Bone Density   WE 200
Bone-Derived Transforming Growth Factor see
  Transforming Growth Factor beta
Bone Development   WE 200
Bone Diseases   WE 225–259
  Child   WS 270
  Infant   WS 270
  Infectious see Bone Diseases, Infectious   WE
    251
  Veterinary   SF 901
Bone Diseases, Developmental   WE 250
Bone Diseases, Endocrine   WE 250
Bone Diseases, Infectious   WE 251
Bone Diseases, Metabolic   WE 250
Bone Dysplasias see Bone Diseases, Developmental
Bone Lengthening   WE 168
  Localized, by site
Bone Loss, Age-Related see Osteoporosis
Bone Loss, Osteoclastic see Bone Resorption
Bone Loss, Perimenopausal see Osteoporosis,
  Postmenopausal
Bone Loss, Periodontal see Alveolar Bone Loss
Bone Loss, Postmenopausal see Osteoporosis,
  Postmenopausal
Bone Marrow   WH 380
Bone Marrow Cells   WH 380
Bone Marrow Diseases   WH 380
  See also Anemia, Aplastic   WH 175; Anemia,

Myelophthisic   WH 175; Leukemoid reaction
  WH 200; Polycythemia vera   WH 180
Bone Marrow Examination   WH 380
Bone Marrow Fibrosis see Myelofibrosis
Bone Marrow Neoplasms   WH 380
Bone Marrow Transplantation   WH 380
Bone Mineral Content see Bone Density
Bone Mineral Density see Bone Density
Bone Mineralization see Calcification, Physiologic
Bone Neoplasms   WE 258
  Veterinary   SF 910.T8
Bone Plates   WE 185
Bone Regeneration   WE 200
Bone Resorption   WE 200
  See also Ainhum   WE 835
Bone Screws   WE 185
Bone Transplantation   WE 190
Bone Tuberculosis see Tuberculosis, Osteoarticular
Bones of Foot see Foot Bones
Bones of Leg see Leg Bones
Bones of Upper Extremity   WE 805
  See also names of specific parts of arm, e.g.,
    Shoulder   WE 810
Bonobo see Pan paniscus
Book Circulation see Library Services
Book Classification   Z 696–697
  Medicine   Z 697.M4
Book Collecting   Z 987–997
  See also Libraries   Z 662–1000; names of specific
    types of libraries
Book Illustration see Books, Illustrated
Book Imprints   Z 242.I3
Book Industry   Z 116.A2–656
Book Ornamentation   Z 276
  See also Medical Illustration   WZ 348
Book Prices   Z 1000
Book Reviews   Z 1035.A1
  Criticism of early works (pre-1801)   WZ 294
  Of books on specific subjects in the bibliography
    number for the subject
  See also Bibliography
Book Selection   Z 689–689.8
Bookbinding   Z 266–276
Booklets see Pamphlets
Bookplates   Z 993–996
  Medical   WZ 340
Books
  History   Z 4–8
  Medicine and related fields
    Americana   WZ 270
    Early imprints   WZ 240–270
      Criticism   WZ 294
      Modern editions   WZ 290
      Modern collections   WZ 292
  See also Incunabula   WZ 230, etc.
Books, Illustrated
  Bibliography   Z 1023
  Techniques   NC
  Special types of books, by subject
  See also Medical Illustration   WZ 348, etc.
Booksellers' Catalogs see Catalogs, Booksellers'
Bookselling   Z 278–549
Boranes   QD 181.B1

ALWAYS CONSULT MAIN SCHEDULES. USE NUMBER ASSIGNED ONLY WHEN
SUBJECT REPRESENTS MAJOR EMPHASIS OF WORK BEING CLASSIFIED

Pharmacology   QV 239
Borates   QD 181.B1
Pharmacology   QV 239
Borderline Personality Disorder   WM 190
Bordetella   QW 131
Bordetella Infections   WC 340
Bordetella pertussis   QW 131
Bordetella Pertussis Toxins see Pertussis Toxins
Boredom
    Adolescence   WS 462
    Child   WS 105.5.E5
    Infant   WS 105.5.E5
    Psychology   BF 575.B67
Boric Acids   QV 239
Bornholm Disease see Pleurodynia, Epidemic
Borohydrides   QD 181.B1
    Pharmacology   QV 239
Boron   QD 181.B1
    Metabolism   QU 130.5
Boron Compounds   QD 181.B1
    As antiseptics   QV 239
    Dental use   WU 190
Borrelia   QW 155
Borrelia Infections   WC 406
    Veterinary   SF 809.B67
Botany   QK
    Economic   SB 107–109
    Medical see Pharmacognosy   QV 752; Plants,
      Medicinal   QV 766, etc.
Botrytis   QW 180.5.D38
    Botany   QK 625.M7
Bottle Feeding   WS 120
Botulism   WC 268
Bouillaud's Disease see Rheumatic Heart Disease
Bourneville's Disease see Tuberous Sclerosis
Bovine Herpesvirus 1 see Herpesvirus 1, Bovine
Bovine Kunitz Pancreatic Trypsin Inhibitor see
    Aprotinin
Bovine Leukemia Virus see Leukemia Virus, Bovine
Bovine Parainfluenza Virus 3 see Paramyxovirus
Bovine Virus Diarrhea–Mucosal Disease   SF
    967.M78
Boxing   QT 260.5.B7
Braces   WE 172
    Catalogs   W 26
Brachial Artery   WG 595.B7
Brachial–Basilar Insufficiency Syndrome see
    Subclavian Steal Syndrome
Brachial Neuralgia see Cervico–Brachial Neuralgia
Brachial Plexus   WL 400
Brachiocephalic Trunk   WG 595.B72
Brachiocephalic Veins   WG 625.B7
Brachytherapy   WN 250.5.B7
Bracyteles see Cebidae
Bradyarrhythmia see Bradycardia
Bradycardia   WG 330
Bradykinin   QU 68
Brain   WL 300–385
    Blood supply   WL 302
      See also Cerebral arteries   WG 595.C37
    Cerebral hemispheres   WL 307
    Cerebrum   WL 307
    Embryology   WL 300

Hemorrhage see Cerebral hemorrhage   WL 355
    Injury   WL 354
    Intracranial complications of ENT diseases   WV
      180
    Radiography   WL 141
    Surgery   WL 368
Brain Abscess   WL 351
Brain Chemistry   WL 300
Brain Concussion   WL 354
Brain Damage, Chronic   WL 354
    Child   WS 340
    Infant   WS 340
Brain Death   W 820
Brain Diseases   WL 348–362
    Child   WS 340
    Infant   WS 340
    Veterinary   SF 895
    See also specific brain diseases
Brain Dysfunction, Minimal see Attention Deficit
    Disorder with Hyperactivity
Brain Edema   WL 348
Brain Electrical Activity Mapping see Brain
    Mapping
Brain Injuries   WL 354
    Child   WS 340
    Infant   WS 340
Brain Mapping   WL 335
Brain Neoplasms   WL 358
    Localized, by site
Brain Revascularization see Cerebral
    Revascularization
Brain Stem   WL 310
Brain Stem Auditory Evoked Potentials see Evoked
    Potentials, Auditory, Brain Stem
Brain Tissue Transplantation   WL 368
Brainwashing see Persuasive Communication
Branched–Chain Ketoaciduria see Maple Syrup
    Urine Disease
Branchial Arches see Branchial Region
Branchial Clefts see Branchial Region
Branchial Cyst see Branchioma
Branchial Region   WE 101
Branchioma   QZ 310
Brassica
    As a dietary supplement in health and disease
      WB 430
    Botany   QK 495.C9
    Culture   SB 317.B65
Brassicaceae see Cruciferae
Bread
    As a dietary supplement in health or disease
      WB 431
    Baking   TX 769
Breakbone Fever see Dengue
Breast   WP 800–910
Breast Cysts see Fibrocystic Disease of Breast
Breast Diseases   WP 840–910
Breast Dysplasia see Fibrocystic Disease of Breast
Breast Feeding   WS 125
    See also Lactation Disorders   WP 825
Breast Implantation   WP 910
Breast Implants   WP 910
Breast Neoplasms   WP 870

**ALWAYS CONSULT MAIN SCHEDULES. USE NUMBER ASSIGNED ONLY WHEN
SUBJECT REPRESENTS MAJOR EMPHASIS OF WORK BEING CLASSIFIED**

Male   WP 870
Breast Prosthesis Implantation see Breast
   Implantation
Breast Xeroradiography see Xeromammography
Breath Tests
   For alcoholic intoxication in traffic accidents
      WA 275
   Forensic medicine   W 780
   In general physical examination   WB 205
   Manifestation of gastroenterological diseases
      WI 143
Breathalyzer Tests see Breath Tests
Breathing see Respiration
Breathing Exercises   WB 541
Breech Presentation   WQ 307
Breeding
   Animal   SF 105-109
   Of laboratory animals   QY 54
   Of plants   SB 123-123.5
   Of individual animals or plants, with animal or
      plant
Brevibacterium   QW 118
Bridged Compounds
   Organic chemistry   QD 341.H9
   Toxicity   QV 633
   Used for special purposes, by subject
Bridges, Dental see Denture, Partial; Tooth,
   Artificial
Brief Psychotherapy see Psychotherapy, Brief
Bright Disease see Glomerulonephritis
Bright's Disease see Nephritis
Brill-Symmers Disease see Lymphoma, Follicular
Brill-Zinsser Disease see Typhus, Epidemic
   Louse-Borne
Brill's Disease see Typhus, Epidemic Louse-Borne
Brine Shrimp see Artemia
Briquet Syndrome see Somatoform Disorders
Bristle-Coated Pits see Coated Pits, Cell-Membrane
BRL 2288 see Ticarcillin
Broad Ligament   WP 275
Broadsides   Z 240.4
Broca Area see Frontal Lobe
Brochures see Pamphlets
Bromchlortrifluorethane see Halothane
Bromhexine   QV 76
Bromides   QV 87
Bromine   QV 231
   Metabolism   QU 130
Bromocriptine   QV 174
Bromocryptin see Bromocriptine
Bromosuccinimide   QV 85
Bromsulphalein see Sulfobromophthalein
Bronchi   WF 500-553
   Blood supply   WF 500
   Calculi   WF 500
   Child   WS 280
   Drugs affecting see names of specific agents
   Infant   WS 280
Bronchial Arteries   WG 595.B76
   See also Blood supply   WF 500 under Bronchi
Bronchial Asthma see Asthma
Bronchial Constriction see Bronchoconstriction
Bronchial Diseases   WF 500-553

Child   WS 280
Infant   WS 280
Veterinary   SF 831
Bronchial Fistula   WF 500
Bronchial Lavage see Bronchoalveolar Lavage
Bronchial Lavage Fluid see Bronchoalveolar Lavage
   Fluid
Bronchial Neoplasms   WF 500
   See also Adenocarcinoma, Bronchiolo-Alveolar
      WF 658; Carcinoma, Bronchogenic   WF
      658
Bronchial Provocation Tests   WF 141.5.B8
Bronchial Spasm   WF 500
Bronchiectasis   WF 544
Bronchiolar Carcinoma see Adenocarcinoma,
   Bronchiolo-Alveolar
Bronchioles see Bronchi
Bronchitis   WF 546
   Veterinary   SF 831
Bronchoalveolar Lavage   WF 600
Bronchoalveolar Lavage Fluid   WF 600
Bronchoconstriction   WF 102
Bronchodilator Agents   QV 120
Bronchography   WF 500
Broncholithiasis see Bronchial Diseases
Bronchopneumonia   WC 202
   Veterinary   SF 831
Bronchopulmonary Dysplasia   WS 410
Bronchoscopy   WF 500
Bronchospasm see Bronchial Spasm
Bronchospasm, Exercise-Induced see Asthma,
   Exercise-Induced
Bronchospirometry   WB 284
Bronze Diabetes see Hemochromatosis
Browning Reaction see Maillard Reaction
Brucella abortus   QW 131
Brucella Vaccine   WC 310
Brucellosis   WC 310
   Veterinary   SF 809.B8
Brucellosis, Bovine   SF 967.B7
Brucine see Strychnine
Brucite see Magnesium Hydroxide
Brugia   QX 301
Bruises see Contusions
Brunhilde Virus see Polioviruses, Human 1-3
Brunner's Gland see Duodenum
Brush Border see Microvilli
Bubo, Climatic or Tropical see Lymphogranuloma
   Venereum
Bubo, Venereal see Sexually Transmitted Diseases
Bubonic Plague see Plague
Bucca see Cheek
Buckthorn see Rhamnus
Buddhism   BQ
   And medical philosophy   W 61
   And psychology   BQ 4570.P76
      See also Religion and Psychology   WM 61,
         etc.
   And psychoanalysis   WM 460.5.R3
   Medicine in religious works   WZ 330
Budding and Appendaged Bacteria   QW 153
Budding Yeast see Saccharomycetales
Budgerigar Fancier's Lung see Bird Fancier's Lung

Budgetary Control see Budgets
Budgets
   Hospitals   WX 157
   General
      Public finance   HJ 2005+
      U.S.   HJ 2050–2053
   For other topics, class by subject if specific; if
     general, in economics number where available
Buerger's Disease see Thromboangiitis Obliterans
Buffaloes   QL 737.U5
   Diseases   SF 997.5.B8
   European bison   QL 737.U53
Buffers   QV 786
   In acid base equilibrium   QU 105
   See also Preservation, Biological   QH 324
Bufo see Bufonidae
Bufonidae   QL 668.E227
   As laboratory animals   QY 60.A6
Bugs see Hemiptera
Buildings, Public Health Aspects see Housing; Public
   Housing; Restaurants; and names of other types
   of buildings; Architecture; Environment,
   Controlled; Sanitation
Bulbar Palsy see Paralysis, Bulbar
Bulbourethral Glands   WJ 600
Bulimia   WM 175
Bulla see Blister
Bullous Skin Diseases see Skin Diseases,
   Vesiculobullous
Bumetanide   QV 160
Bundle–Branch Block   WG 330
Bundle of His   WG 201–202
Bundle of Kent see Heart Conduction System
Bunion see Hallux Valgus
Bunostomiasis see Hookworm Infections
Bunostomum see Ancylostomatoidea
Bunyaviridae   QW 168.5.B9
Bunyaviridae Infections   WC 501
Bunyavirus Infections see Bunyaviridae Infections
Buphthalmos see Hydrophthalmos
Bupivacaine   QV 115
Bupranolol   QV 132
Buprenorphine   QV 92
Burial   WA 846
Burial Grounds see Mortuary Practice
Burkitt Herpesvirus see Herpesvirus 4, Human
Burkitt Lymphoma   WH 525
   Localized by site
   Veterinary in the appropriate LC SF number,
     by site
Burkitt Tumor see Burkitt Lymphoma
Burkitt's Lymphoma Virus see Herpesvirus 4,
   Human
Burning Mouth Syndrome   WU 140
Burnout, Professional   WM 172
Burns   WO 704
   Death from (medicolegal aspects)   W 843
   Localized, by site
   Nursing   WY 161
   See also Sunburn   WR 150
Burns, Chemical   WO 704
Burns, Electric   WO 704
Burns, Inhalation   WO 704

Bursa–Dependent Lymphocytes see B–Lymphocytes
Bursa, Synovial   WE 400
Bursine see Choline
Bursitis   WE 400
Burst–Promoting Factor, Erythrocyte see
   Interleukin–3
Buserelin   WK 515
   Used for treatment of particular disorders, with
    the disorder
Buses see Automobiles
Bush Babies see Galago
Business see Commerce
Business Administration see Hospital Administration;
   Organization and Administration; Practice
   Management, Dental; Practice Management,
   Medical
Business Coalitions (Health Care) see Health Care
   Coalitions
Buspirone   QV 77.9
Busulfan   QV 269
   Cancer chemotherapy   QZ 267
Busulphan see Busulfan
Butacaine   QV 115
Butanoic Acids see Butyric Acids
Butesin Picrate see Butylamines
Butorphanol   QV 92
Butter
   As a dietary supplement in health or disease
    WB 425
   Biochemistry   QU 86
   Manufacture   SF 263
   Public health aspects   WA 715
Butter Yellow see p–Dimethylaminoazobenzene
Butterflies   QX 560
Buttermilk see Milk
Buttocks   WE 750
Butylamines   QU 61
   As local anesthetics   QV 115
Butylated Hydroxyanisole
   Toxicology   QV 632
   As a food preservative   WA 712
Butylated Hydroxytoluene
   As a food preservative   WA 712
Butylcarbamide see Carbutamide
Butylhydroxyanisole see Butylated Hydroxyanisole
Butylhydroxytoluene see Butylated Hydroxytoluene
Butyn see Butacaine
Butyribacterium see Eubacterium
Butyric Acids   QU 90
Butyrophenone Antipsychotic Agents see
   Antipsychotic Agents, Butyrophenone
Butyrophenone Tranquilizers see Antipsychotic
   Agents, Butyrophenone
Butyrophenones   QV 77.9
By–Products, Industrial see Industrial Waste; names
   of specific products
Bylaws see Constitution and Bylaws
Bypass, Coronary Artery see Coronary Artery
   Bypass
Byssinosis   WF 654
B16 Melanoma see Melanoma, Experimental

**ALWAYS CONSULT MAIN SCHEDULES. USE NUMBER ASSIGNED ONLY WHEN
SUBJECT REPRESENTS MAJOR EMPHASIS OF WORK BEING CLASSIFIED**

I–38

C

C Fibers see Nerve Fibers
c–Ha–ras Genes see Genes, ras
c–Ki–ras Genes see Genes, ras
c–N–ras Genes see Genes, ras
C–Peptide   WK 820
CA Antigens see Antigens, Tumor–Associated, Carbohydrate
CA–125 Antigen see Antigens, Tumor–Associated, Carbohydrate
CA–15–3 Antigen see Antigens, Tumor–Associated, Carbohydrate
CA–19–9 Antigen see Antigens, Tumor–Associated, Carbohydrate
Ca(2+) Mg(2+)-ATPase   QU 136
Ca(2+)-Transporting ATPase   QU 136
CA–50 Antigen see Antigens, Tumor–Associated, Carbohydrate
Cabbage see Brassica
Cacajao see Cebidae
Cacao
    As a dietary supplement in health or disease   WB 438
    Chemical technology   TP 640
    Cultivation   SB 267
    Diseases of   SB 608.C17
    Pharmacology   QV 107
    See also Beverages   WB 438, etc.; Candy   WU 113.7, etc.
Cachectin see Tumor Necrosis Factor
Cachexia   WB 146
    Associated with malnutrition   WD 100
    Pituitary see Hypopituitarism   WK 550
Cacodylic Acid   QU 143
    As amebicides   QV 255
    As antisyphilitic agents   QV 262
Cadaver   WA 840–847
    Body snatching   WZ 320
    Destruction of human body   W 822
    Identification   W 800
    Resurrectionists   WZ 320
    See also Autopsy   QZ 35, etc.; Coroners and Medical Examiners   W 800; Death Certificates   WA 54; Dissection   QS 130, etc.; Embalming   WA 844; Mortuary Practice   WA 840–847
Cadmium   QV 290
Caduceus see Emblems and Insignia
Caenorhabditis   QX 203
Caerulein Receptors see Receptors, Cholecystokinin
Caeruloplasmin see Ceruloplasmin
Caesarean Section see Cesarean Section
Cafeterias see Restaurants
Caffea see Coffee
Caffeine   QV 107
Caffeine Receptors see Receptors, Purinergic
Caimans see Alligators and Crocodiles
Caisson Disease see Decompression Sickness
Calcaneus   WE 880
Calciferols see Ergocalciferols
Calcification, Pathologic see Calcinosis
Calcification, Physiologic   WE 200

    See also Ossification, Physiologic   WE 200
Calcinosis   WD 200.5.C2
    Intervertebralis   WE 740
    See also Ossification, Pathologic   QZ 180
Calciphylaxis   WD 200.5.C2
Calcitonin   WK 202
Calcium   QV 276
    Inorganic chemistry   QD 181.C2
Calcium–Activated Neutral Protease see Calpain
Calcium Adenosinetriphosphatase see Ca(2+)-Transporting ATPase
Calcium Antagonists, Exogenous see Calcium Channel Blockers
Calcium ATPase see Ca(2+)-Transporting ATPase
Calcium–Binding Proteins
Calcium Blockaders, Exogenous see Calcium Channel Blockers
Calcium Carbimide see Cyanamide
Calcium Channel Blockers   QV 150
Calcium Channels   QH 603.I54
Calcium Cyanamide see Cyanamide
Calcium–Dependent Activator Protein see Calmodulin
Calcium–Dependent Neutral Proteinase see Calpain
Calcium–Dependent Regulator see Calmodulin
Calcium, Dietary   QU 130
    As a supplement in health or disease   WB 428
Calcium Diphosphate see Calcium Pyrophosphate
Calcium Hydroxide
    Dentistry   WU 190
    Inorganic chemistry   QD 181.C2
    Pharmacology   QV 276
Calcium Inhibitors, Exogenous see Calcium Channel Blockers
Calcium Isotopes
    Inorganic chemistry   QD 181.C2
    Pharmacology   QV 276
Calcium Leucovorin see Leucovorin
Calcium Magnesium Adenosinetriphosphatase see Ca(2+) Mg(2+)-ATPase
Calcium Magnesium ATPase see Ca(2+) Mg(2+)-ATPase
Calcium Metabolism Disorders   WD 200.5.C2
    Decalcification, Pathologic   WE 250
Calcium Oscillations see Calcium Signaling
Calcium Oxalate
    Biochemistry   QU 98
Calcium Phosphates
    Inorganic chemistry   QD 181.C2
    Of bone in general   WE 200
    Of teeth   WU 101
Calcium Pyrophosphate   QV 285
Calcium Signaling
    Cytology   QH 601
    Special topics, by subject
    See also Calcium   QV 276, etc.; Calcium–Binding Proteins   QU 55; Calcium Channels   QH 603.I54; Calmodulin   QU 55
Calcium Sulfate
    In density   WU 190
    In casting models   QY 35
    In surgical casts   WO 170
Calcium Transport Proteins see Calcium–Binding Proteins

Calcium Waves see Calcium Signaling
Calculators, Programmable see Computers
Calculi   QZ 180
   Biliary see Cholelithiasis   WI 755
   Bladder see Bladder Calculi   WJ 500
   Common bile duct see Common Bile Duct Calculi
     WI 755
   Kidney see Kidney Calculi   WJ 356
   Salivary duct see Salivary Duct Calculi   WI
     230
   Ureteral see Ureteral Calculi   WJ 400
   Urinary see Urinary Calculi   WJ 140
   See also Lithiasis   QZ 180, etc.
Calculosis see Lithiasis
Caldesmon see Calmodulin–Binding Proteins
Calibration
   Special topics, by subject
California Encephalitis Virus see California Group
   Viruses
California Group Viruses   QW 168.5.B9
Californium   WN 420
   Nuclear physics   QC 796.C45
   For other specific aspects use numbers listed in
     this index under Radioisotopes
Calisthenics see Gymnastics
Callicebinae see Cebidae
Callithricidae see Callitrichinae
Callitrichinae   QL 737.P92
   As laboratory animals   QY 60.P7
   Diseases   SF 997.5.P7
Callosities   WR 500
   Foot   WE 880
   Toes   WE 835
   Other locations, by site
Callotasis see Osteogenesis, Distraction
Calmette–Guerin Bacillus see Mycobacterium bovis
Calmette–Guerin Immunization see BCG Vaccine
Calmodulin   QU 55
Calmodulin–Binding Proteins   QU 55
Caloric Intake see Energy Intake
Caloric Tests   WV 255
Caloric Value of Foods see Nutrition
Calorie Deficiency see Deficiency Diseases;
   Protein–Energy Malnutrition
Calorimetry   QU 125
Calpain   QU 136
Calspectin see Calmodulin–Binding Proteins
Camelids, New World   QL 737.U54
   Diseases   SF 997.5.C3
Camellia see Tea
Camels   QL 737.U54
   Diseases   SF 997.5.C3
Camphor   QV 65
Campimetry see Perimetry
Camping   QT 250
   Special topics, by subject, e.g., discussion of camp
     safety act   WA 33
Campylobacter fetus   QW 154
Campylobacter pylori see Helicobacter pylori
Cancer see Neoplasms
Cancer–Associated Carbohydrate Antigens see
   Antigens, Tumor–Associated, Carbohydrate

Cancer Care Facilities   QZ 23–24
Cancer Chemotherapy see Drug therapy   QZ 267
   under Neoplasms or names of specific types of
   neoplasm
Cancer Genes see Oncogenes
Cancer Research see Neoplasms, Experimental   QZ
   206 or names of specific types of neoplasm
Cancer Staging see Neoplasm Staging
Cancer Vaccines   QZ 266
   For particular neoplasms, with the neoplasm
Candida   QW 180.5.D38
Candidiasis   WC 470
Candidiasis, Cutaneous   WR 300
Candidiasis, Oral   WC 470
Candy
   As a dietary supplement in health or disease
     WB 400
   In dental health   WU 113.7
Canine Tooth see Cuspid
Canis lupus see Wolves
Canker Sore see Stomatitis, Aphthous
Cannabidiol
   As an anticonvulsant   QV 85
   As a hallucinogen   QV 77.7
Cannabinoids   QV 77.7
Cannabis
   Abuse see Marijuana Abuse   WM 276
   Associated with hallucinogens   QV 77.7
Cannabis Abuse see Marijuana Abuse
Cannabis Smoking see Marijuana Smoking
Canned Foods see Food Preservation;
   Food–Processing Industry
Canned Milk see Milk
Cannulation see Catheterization
Cantharides see Cantharidin
Cantharidin   QV 65
Caoutchouc see Rubber
CAPD see Peritoneal Dialysis, Continuous
   Ambulatory
Capgras Syndrome   WM 202
Capillaries   WG 700
Capillaries, Lymphatic see Lymphatic System
Capillarity   QC 183
Capillary Electrophoresis see Electrophoresis,
   Capillary
Capillary Endothelium see Endothelium, Vascular
Capillary Fragility   WG 700
Capillary Leak Syndrome   WG 700
Capillary Permeability   WG 700
Capillary Resistance   WG 106
Capillary Resistance, Hematologic see Capillary
   Fragility
Capital Expenditures
   Medicine   W 74
   Other fields, by subject, in the number for
     economics when available
Capital Financing
   Hospitals   WX 157
   For other specific subject, class in economics
     number where applicalble
Capitalism see Political Systems
Capitation Fee
   Dental   WU 77

**ALWAYS CONSULT MAIN SCHEDULES. USE NUMBER ASSIGNED ONLY WHEN
SUBJECT REPRESENTS MAJOR EMPHASIS OF WORK BEING CLASSIFIED**

Hospital   WX 157
Medical   W 74
Nursing   WY 77
With other specialties, class in economics number
  where applicable
Capnography   WF 141.5.C2
  Used for general anesthesia monitoring   WO 275
Caprines see Goats
Caproates   QU 90
Caprolactam
  As an industrial poison   WA 465
  Special topics, by subject
Capsaicin   QU 90
Capsules   QV 785
Captopril
  As an antihypertensive agent   QV 150
  As an enzyme inhibitor   QU 143
Carassius auratus see Goldfish
Carassius carassius see Carp
Carbachol   QV 122
Carbamates   QU 98
  As insecticides   WA 240
  Organic chemistry
    Aliphatic compounds   QD 305.A2
Carbamazepine   QV 85
Carbamylcholine see Carbachol
Carbarsone see Arsenicals
Carbenicillin   QV 354
Carbenicillin Phenyl Sodium see Carfecillin
Carbenoxalone see Carbenoxolone
Carbenoxolone   QV 66
Carbocaine see Mepivacaine
Carbocysteine
  Biochemistry   QU 60
  Pharmacology   QV 76
Carbofuran
  Agriculture   SB 952.C3
  Public health   WA 240
Carbohydrate Antigens, Tumor-Associated see
  Antigens, Tumor-Associated, Carbohydrate
Carbohydrate Conformation   QU 75
Carbohydrate Linkage see Carbohydrate
  Conformation
Carbohydrate Metabolism, Inborn Errors   WD
  205.5.C2
Carbohydrates   QU 75
  Clinical analysis   QY 470
  See also Dietary Carbohydrates   WB 427, etc.
Carbolic Acid see Phenols
Carbolines
  As tranquilizing agents   QV 77.9
  Organic chemistry   QD 401
Carbon   QD 181.C1
  Pharmacology   QV 138.C1
Carbon Compounds, Inorganic   QD 181.C1
  Pharmacology   QV 138.C1
Carbon Dioxide   QV 314
Carbon Dioxide Partial Pressure Determination,
  Transcutaneous see Blood Gas Monitoring,
  Transcutaneous
Carbon Disulfide   QD 181.C1
  Toxicological effects   QV 633

Carbon Isotopes
  Inorganic chemistry   QD 181.C1
  Pharmacology   QV 138.C1
Carbon Monoxide   QV 662
Carbon Monoxide Poisoning   QV 662
Carbon Tetrachloride
  As an anthelmintic   QV 253
  Organic chemistry   QD 305.H5
Carbon Tetrachloride Poisoning   QV 633
Carbonate Dehydratase   QU 139
Carbonate Dehydratase Inhibitors see Carbonic
  Anhydrase Inhibitors
Carbonate Dehydratase Isoenzymes see Carbonate
  Dehydratase
Carbonates
  Inorganic chemistry   QD 181.C1
  Organic chemistry   QD 305.A2
  Pharmacology   QV 138.C1
Carbonic Acid   QV 138.C1
Carbonic Anhydrase see Carbonate Dehydratase
Carbonic Anhydrase Inhibitors   QV 160
  Enzymology   QU 143
Carbonic Anhydrase Isoenzymes see Carbonate
  Dehydratase
Carbonic Anhydride see Carbon Dioxide
Carbonization see Drug Compounding
Carbonyl Chloride see Phosgene
Carboxy-Lyases   QU 139
Carboxybenzyl Penicillin see Carbenicillin
Carboxyl (Acid) Proteinases see Aspartic Proteinases
Carboxylic Acids   QU 98
  Organic chemistry
    Aliphatic compounds   QD 305.A2
    Aromatic compounds   QD 341.A2
Carboxymethylcysteine see Carbocysteine
Carbuncle   WR 235
Carbutamide   WK 825
Carcinoembryonic Antigen   QW 570
  Neoplasm immunology   QZ 310
Carcinogen Markers see Tumor Markers, Biological
Carcinogenesis see Neoplasms
Carcinogenicity Tests   QZ 202
Carcinogens   QZ 202
Carcinogens, Environmental   QZ 202
Carcinoid Heart Disease   WG 210
Carcinoid Tumor   WI 435
  Localized, by site
Carcinoma   QZ 365
  Localized, by site
Carcinoma, Adenoid Cystic   QZ 365
  Localized, by site
Carcinoma, Alveolar see Adenocarcinoma,
  Bronchiolo-Alveolar
Carcinoma, Bronchial see Carcinoma, Bronchogenic
Carcinoma, Bronchiolo-Alveolar see
  Adenocarcinoma, Bronchiolo-Alveolar
Carcinoma, Bronchogenic   WF 658
Carcinoma, Hepatocellular   WI 735
Carcinoma, Hypernephroid see Carcinoma, Renal
  Cell
Carcinoma, Renal Cell   WJ 358
Carcinosarcoma   QZ 310
Cardamom see Zingiberales

Cardia   WI 300
  Neoplasms   WI 320
Cardiac Arrest see Heart Arrest
Cardiac Complexes, Premature   WG 330
Cardiac Depressants see Anti-Arrhythmia Agents
Cardiac Electroversion see Electric Countershock
Cardiac Emergencies   WG 205
Cardiac Failure see Heart Failure, Congestive
Cardiac Glycosides   QV 153
Cardiac Hypertrophy see Heart Hypertrophy
Cardiac Neurosis see Neurocirculatory Asthenia
Cardiac Output   WG 106
Cardiac Output, Low   WG 210
Cardiac Pacemaker, Artificial see Pacemaker,
  Artificial
Cardiac Pacing, Artificial   WG 168
  See also Pacemaker, Artificial   WG 26
Cardiac Remodeling, Ventricular see Ventricular
  Remodeling
Cardiac Rupture, Traumatic see Heart Injuries
Cardiac Stimulants see Cardiotonic Agents
Cardiac Surgical Procedures   WG 169
  Child   WS 290
  Infant   WS 290
Cardiac Transplantation see Heart Transplantation
Cardiac Volume   WG 106
Cardiography, Impedance   WG 141.5.C15
  Special topics, by subject, e.g., in the diagnosis
  of Tachycardia   WG 330
Cardiologists, Directories see Directories   WG 22
  under Cardiology
Cardiology   WG
  General works WG 100
  Directories   WG 22
  Child   WS 290
  Experimental studies   WG 110
  Infant   WS 290
  Nursing   WY 152.5
Cardiomyopathies see Myocardial Diseases
Cardiomyopathy, Alcoholic   WG 280
Cardiomyopathy, Chagas see Chagas
  Cardiomyopathy
Cardiomyopathy, Congestive   WG 280
Cardiomyopathy, Dilated see Cardiomyopathy,
  Congestive
Cardiomyopathy, Restrictive   WG 280
Cardiomyoplasty   WG 169
Cardiopulmonary Arrest see Heart Arrest
Cardiopulmonary Resuscitation
  First Aid   WA 292
Cardiospasm see Esophageal Achalasia
Cardiotocography   WQ 209
Cardiotonic Agents   QV 150
Cardiotonic Steroids see Cardiac Glycosides
Cardiovascular Abnormalities   WG 220
Cardiovascular Agents   QV 150-156
Cardiovascular Disease (Specialty) see Cardiology
Cardiovascular Diseases   WG
  General works   WG 120
  Child   WS 290
  In pregnancy see Pregnancy Complications,
    Cardiovascular   WQ 244
  Infant   WS 290

  Neoplasms (General)   WG 120
    See also Neoplasms, Vascular Tissue   QZ 340
  Nursing   WY 152.5
  Veterinary   SF 811
Cardiovascular Physiology   WG 102
Cardiovascular Surgical Procedures   WG
  168-169.5
Cardiovascular System   WG
  Abnormalities see Cardiovascular Abnormalities
    WG 220
  Child   WS 290
  Drugs affecting   QV 150-156
  Experimental studies   WG 110
  Infant   WS 290
  Physiology see Cardiovascular Physiology   WG
    102
  Radiography (General)   WG 141.5.R2
  Radionuclide imaging   WG 141.5.R3
  Surgery see Cardiovascular Surgical Procedures
    WG 168-169.5
  Tomography   WG 141.5.T6
Cardioversion see Electric Countershock
Carditis, Bacterial see Endocarditis, Bacterial
Care, Surgical see Postoperative Care; Preoperative
  Care; Perioperative Nursing
Career Choice
  Dentistry   WU 21
  Nursing   WY 16
  Ophthalmology   WW 21
  Pharmacy   QV 21
  Physicians   W 21
  Psychiatry   WM 21
  Surgery   WO 21
  In other fields, by subject
Career Counseling see Vocational Guidance
Career Ladders see Career Mobility
Career Mobility
  Social conditions   HN
  Vocational guidance   HF 5381-5382.5
  Specific careers, by subject, e.g. Nursing   WY
    16
Caregivers
  In particular fields, by subjects
  See also names of specific caregivers
Carfecillin   QV 354
Caricatures   NC 1300-1763
  Medical   WZ 336
  See also Medical Illustration   WZ 348
Caries see Dental Caries
Caries, Dental see Dental Caries
Cariogenic Agents   WU 270
  See also Diet, Cariogenic   WU 113.7
Carnitine   QU 187
Carnitine O-Palmitoyltransferase   QU 141
Carnitine Palmitoyltransferase see Carnitine
  O-Palmitoyltransferase
Carnivora   QL 737.C2-737.C28
  Diseases   SF 600-1100
  Specific carnivora or groups, by animal or group
Carnosine   QU 68
Carotene   QU 110
  Animal biochemistry wild   QP 671.C3
  Plants   QK 898.C35

Vitamin A related   QU 167
Carotenoids   QU 110
  Animal biochemistry wild   QP 671.C35
  Plants   QK 898.C35
  Vitamin A related   QU 167
Carotid Arteries   WG 595.C2
Carotid Artery Diseases   WL 355
Carotid Artery, External   WG 595.5.C2
Carotid Artery, Internal   WG 595.5.C2
Carotid Artery Thrombosis   WL 355
Carotid Body   WL 102.9
Carotid Body Tumor   WL 102.9
Carotid Sinus   WG 595.5.C2
  Carotid sinus syndrome   WG 560
Carp   QL 638.C94
  Diseases   SH 179.C3
  As laboratory animals   QY 60.F4
Carpal Bones   WE 830
Carpal Tunnel Syndrome   WL 500
Carphenazine see Phenothiazine Tranquilizers
Carpus see Wrist
Carrageenan   QU 83
Carrier Ampholytes see Ampholyte Mixtures
Carrier Proteins   QU 55
  In immunochemistry   QW 504.5
  Special topics, by subject
  See also names of specific proteins, e.g.,
    Ferrodoxins   QW 52, etc.
Carrier State   QW 700
  Veterinary   SF 757.2
Carriers, Genetic see Heterozygote
Carriers, Genetic, Detection see Heterozygote
  Detection
Carriers of Infection see Carrier State; Disease
  Vectors; Insect Vectors
Carriers, Public see Railroads   WA 810, etc. and
  names of other forms of transportation
Carrion's Disease see Bartonella Infections
Carsickness see Motion Sickness
Cartilage   WE 300
Cartilage, Articular   WE 300
Cartilage Diseases   WE 300
  Child   WS 270
  Infant   WS 270
Cartilage, Epiphyseal see Growth Plate
Cartoons   WZ 336
Caryophanales see Bacteria
Casanthranol see Cascara
Cascara   QV 75
Case-Base Studies see Case-Control Studies
Case-Comparison Studies see Case-Control Studies
Case-Control Studies
  In epidemiology   WA 105
  Of particular disorders, with the disorder
Case Management   W 84.7
  In nursing   WY 100
Case Management, Insurance see Managed Care
  Programs
Case Mix see Diagnosis-Related Groups
Case-Mix Adjustment see Risk Adjustment
Case-Referent Studies see Case-Control Studies
Case reports see Case studies

Case studies
  Medicine   WB 293
  Psychiatry   WM 40-49
  Surgery   WO 16
  Special topics, by subject
Case Taking see Medical History Taking
Caseins   WA 716
  Dairy science   SF 253
  Food and milk microbiology   QW 85
Cassava
  As a dietary supplement in health or disease
    WB 431
  Cultivation   SB 211.C3
  Poisoning   WD 500
Caste see Social Class
Castor see Rodentia
Castor Bean Lectin see Ricin
Castor Oil   QV 75
Castration
  Female   WP 660
  Male   WJ 868
  Veterinary   SF 889
Castration, Male see Orchiectomy
Casts see Models, Structural; Dental Casting
  Investment
Casts, Surgical   WO 170
Cat Diseases   SF 985-986
CAT Scan, Radionuclide see Tomography,
  Emission-Computed
CAT Scan, X-Ray see Tomography, X-Ray
  Computed
CAT Scanners, X-Ray see Tomography Scanners,
  X-Ray Computed
Cat-Scratch Disease   WC 593
Catabolism see Metabolism
Catalase   QU 140
Catalepsy   WM 197
  Catatonic   WM 203
  Hysterical neurosis   WM 173
  Neurologic manifestation   WL 390
Cataloging   Z 693-695.83
Catalogs see Types of catalogs or product being
  announced, e.g., Catalogs, Drug   QV 772
Catalogs, Booksellers'   Z 998-1000.5
  General catalogs of modern books   Z 1036
  On particular subjects, in bibliography number
  for the subject
Catalogs, Commercial   HF 5861-5862
  Embryology   QS 626
  Medical supplies   W 26
  Non-book materials (Form number 18.2 in any
    NLM schedule where applicable)
    Embryology   QS 618.2
    Histology   QS 518.2
  Specialty catalogs   W 26
  See also names of specific types of catalogs
Catalogs, Drug   QV 772
Catalogs, Library   Z 881-980
  Private libraries   Z 997-997.2
  Other particular classes of libraries (not LC
    practice)   Z 675.A-Z
Catalogs, Publishers'   Z 1217-4980
  Booksellers   Z 998-1000.5

General catalogs of modern books   Z 1036
On particular subjects, in bibliography number
  for the subject
Catalogs, Union
  Books or general   Z 695.83
  Serials   Z 6945
  On particular subjects, in bibliography number
    for the subject
Catalysis
  Enzymatic   QU 135
  Organic chemistry   QD 281.C3
  Pharmaceutical chemistry   QV 25
  Physical chemistry   QD 505
  Therapeutics see Alternative Medicine   WB 890
  Applications in other areas, by subject
Cataphoresis see Electrophoresis
Cataplexy   WM 197
  Associated with narcolepsy   WM 188
Cataract   WW 260
Cataract Extraction   WW 260
Catarrhina see Cercopithecidae
Catastrophic Health Insurance see Insurance, Major
  Medical
Catastrophic Illness
  Special topics, by subject
  See also Disease
Catatonia   WM 197
  Associated with schizophrenia   WM 203
Catatonic Schizophrenia see Schizophrenia,
  Catatonic
Catchment Area (Health)   WA 541
  Geriatrics   WT 30
Catechin
  In dyeing and tanning   TP 925.C38
  Special topics by subject
Catechinic Acid see Catechin
Catechol Estrogens see Estrogens, Catechol
Catecholamines   WK 725
Catechols
  Organic chemistry   QD 341.P5
Catechu see Catechin
Catechuic Acid see Catechin
Caterpillars see Lepidoptera
Catharsis   WM 420.5.A2
Cathartics   QV 75
Cathepsins   QU 136
Catheterization
  General   WB 365
  Heart see Heart Catheterization   WG 141.5.C2
  Surgical technique   WO 500
  Urinary see Urinary Catheterization   WJ 500
Catheterization, Balloon see Balloon Dilatation
Catheterization, Bronchial see Catheterization,
  Peripheral
Catheterization, Cardiac see Heart Catheterization
Catheterization, Heart see Heart Catheterization
Catheterization, Peripheral
  General   WB 365
Catheterization, Peripheral Arterial see
  Catheterization, Peripheral
Catheterization, Peripheral Venous see
  Catheterization, Peripheral
Catheterization, Ureteral see Urinary Catheterization

Catheterization, Urethral see Urinary Catheterization
Catheterization, Urinary see Urinary Catheterization
Catheters, Indwelling
  (Form number 26 in any NLM schedule where
    applicable)
  See also names of various types of catheterization
Cathode see Electrodes
Cathode Ray Tube Display see Data Display
Cathode Rays see Beta Rays
Catholicism   BX 800–4795
  And birth control   HQ 766.3
  And psychiatry   WM 61
  Medical ethics   W 50
  Other special topics, by subject, e.g., nursing
    ethics according to Catholic standards   WY
    85
  See also Religion and Medicine   WB 885, etc.;
    other headings beginning with Religion
Cations   QV 275–278
Cations, Divalent   QV 275
Cations, Monovalent   QV 275
Catnip see Lamiaceae
Cats
  As laboratory animals   QY 60.C2
    Anatomy   QL 813.C38
  Culture   SF 441–450
  Diseases see Cat Diseases   SF 985–986
  Wild   QL 737.C23
Cattell Personality Factor Questionnaire   WM
  145.5.C3
  In psychology   BF 698.8.S5
Cattle
  Anatomy   SF 767.C3
  Culture   SF 191–219
  Physiology   SF 768.2.C3
Cattle Diseases   SF 961–967
Cattle Leukemia Virus see Leukemia Virus, Bovine
Cattle Plague see Rinderpest
Caucasoid Race
  Anthropology   GN 537
  See also special topics under Ethnic Groups
Caudal Anesthesia see Anesthesia, Epidural
Caudata see Urodela
Caudate Nucleus   WL 307
Causalgia   WL 544
Cause of Death   WA 900
  Special topics, by subject
Causes of Disease see Pathogenesis   QZ 40–109
  under Disease
Caustics   QV 612
Cautery   WO 198
Cavernous Sinus   WG 625.C7
CAVH see Hemofiltration
Cavia see Guinea Pigs
Caviidae see Guinea Pigs
Cavities, Dental see Dental Cavity Preparation
Cavus Deformity see Foot Deformities
Cazenave's Lupus see Lupus Erythematosus, Discoid
CD-ROM
  Catalogs and works about (Form number 18.2
    in any NLM schedules where applicable)
  Special topics, by subject
CDP Choline see Cytidine Diphosphate Choline

CD25 Antigens see Receptors, Interleukin–2
CD4 Antigens see Antigens, CD4
CD4 Molecule see Antigens, CD4
CD4 Receptors see Antigens, CD4
Cebidae   QL 737.P925
   Diseases   SF 997.5.P7
   As laboratory animals   QY 60.P7
Cebuella see Callitrichinae
Cebus   QL 737.P925
   Diseases   SF 997.5.P7
   As laboratory animals   QY 60.P7
Cecal Diseases   WI 530
Cecal Neoplasms   WI 530
Cecum   WI 530
Cefacler see Cephalexin
Cefaclor   QV 350.5.C3
Cefalotin see Cephalothin
Cefamandole   QV 350.5.C3
Cefotaxime   QV 350.5.C3
Cefoxitin   QV 350.5.C3
Ceftazidime   QV 350.5.C3
Ceftriaxone   QV 350.5.C3
Cefuroxime   QV 350.5.C3
Celebes Ape see Macaca
Celiac Artery   WG 595.C3
Celiac Disease   WD 175
Celiac Ganglia see Ganglia, Sympathetic
Celioscopy see Laparoscopy
Cell Adhesion Molecules
   Biochemistry   QU 55
Cell Aggregation   QH 604.2
Cell Aging
   General   QH 608
      Human   WT 104
      Plants   QK 725
Cell Anoxia see Cell Hypoxia
Cell Communication   QH 604.2
   Nerve cells   WL 102.8
Cell Compartmentation   QH 604.3
Cell Count   QH 585.5
   Of neoplasms   QZ 202
   Of particular organs, with the organ
Cell Culture   QH 585.2–585.45
   In histology   QS 530
      Techniques   QS 525
Cell Cycle   QH 605–605.3
Cell Death   QH 671
Cell Degranulation   QH 631
Cell Density see Cell Count
Cell Differentiation
   Animals
      Domestic   SF 767.5
      Wild   QL 963.5
   General and human   QH 607
Cell Division   QH 605–605.3
   Plants   QK 725
Cell Fractionation   QH 585.5.C43
   Special topics, by subject
Cell–Free System   QH 581–581.2
Cell Fusion   QH 451
Cell Growth see Cell Division
Cell Growth Inhibitors see Growth Inhibitors
Cell Hypoxia   QH 633

Cell Isolation see Cell Separation
Cell Line   QH 585.4–585.45
Cell Line, Tumor see Tumor Cells, Cultured
Cell–Mediated Immunity see Immunity, Cellular
Cell–Mediated Lympholytic Cells see
   T–Lymphocytes, Cytotoxic
Cell Membrane   QH 601–601.2
   Bacterial   QW 51–52
   See also Nuclear Membrane   QH 601.2
Cell–Membrane Coated Pits see Coated Pits,
   Cell–Membrane
Cell Membrane Lipids see Membrane Lipids
Cell Membrane Permeability
   Cytology   QH 611
   Metabolism   QU 120
Cell Membrane Proteins see Membrane Proteins
Cell Movement   QH 647
Cell Nucleolus   QH 596
Cell Nucleus   QH 595
Cell Number see Cell Count
Cell Organelles see Organelles
Cell Physiology   QH 631
Cell Protection see Cytoprotection
Cell Respiration   QH 633
Cell Segregation see Cell Separation
Cell Separation   QH 585.5.C44
Cell Surface Antigens see Antigens, Surface
Cell Surface Glycoproteins see Membrane
   Glycoproteins
Cell Surface Proteins see Membrane Proteins
Cell Surface Receptors see Receptors, Cell Surface
Cell Survival
   Effect of physical and chemical agents   QH
      650–659
   Metabolism   QH 634.5
   Special topics, by subject
   See also Cell Aging   QH 608, etc.; Cell Death
      QH 671; Cell Physiology   QH 631
Cell Therapy see Tissue Therapy
Cell Transformation, Neoplastic   QZ 202
Cell Transformation, Viral   QH 604
   Of neoplasms   QZ 202
Cell Transplants see Transplants
Cell Viability see Cell Survival
Cell Wall
   Bacterial   QW 51–52
   Plant   QK 725
Cellophane
   Plastics manufacture   TP 1180.C4
   Used for special purposes, by subject, e.g.; in
      hemodialysis   WJ 378
Cells   QH 573–659
   Eukaryotic see Eukaryotic Cells   QH 581–581.2
   Histology   QS 504–532
   Pathology
      Animal   QH 671
      Human   QZ 4, etc.
   Radiation effects   WN 620
   Of a specific tissue, with the tissue, e.g., Muscle
      cells   WE 500
   See also more specific terms, e.g., Cell Aging
      QH 608, etc.; Cell Physiology   QH 631;
      Chromosome Abnormalities   QS 677

Cells, Cultured   QH 585.2–585.45
   In histology   QS 530
      Techniques   QS 525
Cells, Immobilized
   Cytology   QH 585.5.I45
   Biotechnology   TP 248.25.I55
   Special topics, by subject
Cellular Immunity see Immunity, Cellular
Cellular Inclusions see Inclusion Bodies
Cellular Neurobiology see Neurobiology
Cellular Respiration see Cell Respiration
Cellulitis   WR 220
   Phlegmon   WD 375
Cellulitis, Pelvic see Parametritis
Cellulose
   Biochemistry   QU 83
   Deficiency   WD 105
   Organic chemistry   QD 323
   Plastics manufacture   TP 1180.C6
   Therapeutic use by diet   WB 427
   Used for special purposes, by subject, e.g., in the
      treatment of kidney calculi   WJ 356
CELSS see Ecological Systems, Closed
Cement, Dental see Dental Cementum
Cement Fillings see Dental Cements; Silicate Cement
Cementation   WU 300
   Crowns   WU 515
   Inlays   WU 360
   See also Dental Cements   WU 190
Cementoblasts see Dental Cementum
Cementoma   WU 280
Cementoperiostitis see Periodontitis
Cementum see Dental Cementum
Cemeteries see Mortuary Practice
Censuses   HA 154–4737
   See also Demography   HB 848–3697
Centenarian see Aged, 80 and over
Centers for Health Planning see Health Planning
   Organizations
Centipedes see Arthropods
Central Nervous System   WL 300–405
   Drugs affecting   QV 76.5–115
Central Nervous System Agents   QV 76.5
   Psychotropic drugs   QV 77.2–77.9
   See also Central Nervous System Stimulants
      QV 100–107
Central Nervous System Depressants   QV 80–98
   Local anesthetics   QV 110–115
   See also specific depressants and specific types
      of depressants
Central Nervous System Diseases   WL 300–405
   General works   WL 300
   Associated eye diseases   WW 460
   Child   WS 340–342
   Diagnosis   WL 141
   Infant   WS 340–342
   Nursing   WY 160.5
   Veterinary   SF 895
Central Nervous System Infections
   General works   WL 300
   Child   WS 340
   Diagnosis   WL 141
   Infant   WS 340
   Nursing   WY 160.5

Central Nervous System Neoplasms   WL 358
Central Nervous System Stimulants   QV 100–107
Central Retinal Artery see Retinal Artery
Central Retinal Vein see Retinal Vein
Central Supply, Hospital   WX 165
Central Venous Pressure   WG 106
Centralized Hospital Services   WX 150
Centrally Acting Muscle Relaxants see Muscle
   Relaxants, Central
Centrifugation
   Biological research   QH 324.9.C4
   Chemical engineering   TP 159.C4
   Chemical techniques   QD 54.C4
   Clinical chemistry   QY 90
   See also Ultracentrifugation   QD 54.C4, etc.
Centrifugation, Density Gradient
   Clinical chemistry   QY 90
   Histochemistry   QS 531
   Other special topics, by subject
Centrioles   QH 597
Centrophenoxine see Meclofenoxate
Cenuriasis see Cestode Infections
Cephalalgia see Headache
Cephalexin   QV 350.5.C3
Cephalins see Phosphatidylethanolamines
Cephalometry
   Anthropology (medieval and modern)   GN
      71–131
   General dental diagnosis   WU 141.5.C3
   Used for diagnosis of particular disorders, with
      the disorder
Cephalopelvic Disproportion see Labor
   Complications
Cephalopelvic Proportion see Pelvimetry
Cephalopelvimetry see Pelvimetry
Cephalosporins   QV 350.5.C3
Cephalothin   QV 350.5.C3
Cephamycins   QV 350.5.C3
Cephradine   QV 350.5.C3
Ceramics
   Chemical technology   TP 785–842
   Dentistry   WU 190
   Medicine   QT 37.5.C4
   Used for special purposes, by subject
Ceratodon see Mosses
Ceratopogonidae   QX 505
Cercopithecidae   QL 737.P93
   Diseases   SF 997.5.P7
   As laboratory animals   QY 60.P7
Cercopithecus aethiops   QL 737.P93
   Diseases   SF 997.5.P7
   As laboratory animals   QY 60.P7
Cercopithecus pygerythrus see Cercopithecus
   aethiops
Cercopithecus sabeus see Cercopithecus aethiops
Cercopithecus tantalus see Cercopithecus aethiops
Cereals
   As a dietary supplement in health or disease
      WB 431
   Cultivation   SB 188–192
   Processing   TS 2120–2159
Cerebellar Ataxia   WL 320

**ALWAYS CONSULT MAIN SCHEDULES. USE NUMBER ASSIGNED ONLY WHEN
SUBJECT REPRESENTS MAJOR EMPHASIS OF WORK BEING CLASSIFIED**

Cerebellar Cortex   WL 320
Cerebellar Diseases   WL 320
Cerebellar Neoplasms   WL 320
Cerebellar Nuclei   WL 320
Cerebellopontile Angle see Cerebellopontine Angle
Cerebellopontine Angle   WL 320
Cerebellum   WL 320
Cerebral Aneurysm   WL 355
   Traumatic   WL 354
Cerebral Angiography   WL 141
Cerebral Anoxia   WL 355
Cerebral Arteries   WG 595.C37
   See also Blood supply   WL 302 under Brain
Cerebral Arteriosclerosis   WL 355
Cerebral Arteriovenous Malformations   WL 355
Cerebral Artery Diseases   WL 355
Cerebral Cortex   WL 307
Cerebral Decortication   WL 307
Cerebral Dominance see Dominance, Cerebral
Cerebral Edema see Brain Edema
Cerebral Embolism and Thrombosis   WL 355
Cerebral Hemispheres see Brain
Cerebral Hemorrhage   WL 355
   Localized, by site
Cerebral Infarction   WL 355
Cerebral Ischemia   WL 355
Cerebral Ischemia, Transient   WL 355
Cerebral Meningitis see Meningitis
Cerebral Palsy   WS 342
   Adult   WL 354
Cerebral Peduncle see Mesencephalon
Cerebral Revascularization   WL 355
Cerebral Sclerosis, Diffuse   WL 348
Cerebral Thrombosis see Cerebral Embolism and
   Thrombosis
Cerebral Vasospasm see Cerebral Ischemia,
   Transient
Cerebral Veins   WG 625.C3
Cerebral Ventricle Neoplasms   WL 358
Cerebral Ventricles   WL 307
Cerebral Ventriculography   WL 141
   Child   WS 340
   Infant   WS 340
Cerebrospinal Fluid   WL 203
   Clinical analysis   QY 220
   General diagnosis   WB 377
Cerebrospinal Fluid Pressure   WL 203
Cerebrospinal Fluid Proteins   WL 203
   Clinical examination   QY 220
Cerebrospinal Meningitis, Epidemic see Meningitis,
   Meningococcal
Cerebrovascular Circulation   WL 302
   Disorders   WL 355
Cerebrovascular Disorders   WL 355
Cerebrum see Brain
Ceremonial Behavior
   Coming of age (Primitive customs)   GN 483.3
   Religious (Primitive customs)   GN 473–473.6
   Royalty and nobility   GT 5010–5090
Cerium
   Inorganic chemistry   QD 181.C4
   Pharmacology   QV 290

Cerium Isotopes
   Inorganic chemistry   QD 181.C4
   Pharmacology   QV 290
Ceroid–Lipofuscinosis, Neuronal see Neuronal
   Ceroid–Lipofuscinosis
Certificate of Need
   Relating to health facilities   WX 157
   Relating to regional health planning   WA 541
   For other special purposes, by subject
Certification
   (Form number 21 in any NLM schedule where
   applicable)
   Of paraprofessionals, with the general number
   for the type
Certification of the Dead see Death Certificates
Ceruloplasmin   WH 400
   Clinical examination   QY 455
Cerumen   WV 222
   Impacted   WV 222
Cervical Manipulation see Manipulation, Spinal
Cervical Rib Syndrome   WL 500
Cervical Smears see Vaginal Smears
Cervical Vertebrae   WE 725
Cervicitis   WP 475
Cervico–Brachial Neuralgia   WL 400
Cervix Diseases   WP 470
   Veterinary   SF 871
Cervix Dysplasia   WP 480
Cervix Erosion   WP 470
Cervix Mucus   WP 470
Cervix Neoplasms   WP 480
Cervix Uteri   WP 470–480
   Dilatation (in labor)
     Obstetrical surgery   WQ 400
     Physiology   WQ 305
Cesarean Section   WQ 430
   Veterinary   SF 887
Cesium
   Inorganic chemistry   QD 181.C8
   Pharmacology   QV 275
Cesium Isotopes
   Inorganic chemistry   QD 181.C8
   Pharmacology   QV 275
Cesium Radioisotopes   WN 420
   Nuclear physics   QC 796.C8
   See also special topics under Radioisotopes
Cestoda   QX 400
Cestode Infections   WC 830–840
   Veterinary   SF 810.C5
Cetacea   QL 737.C4
   Paleozoology   QE 882.C5
Chagas Cardiomyopathy   WC 705
Chagas' Disease see Trypanosomiasis, South
   American
Chagas Disease   WC 705
Chalazion see Eyelid Diseases   WW 205
Chalcone
   Pharmacology   QV 150
Chalicosis see Pneumoconiosis
Chalones see Growth Inhibitors
CHAMPUS see Health Benefit Plans, Employee
Chancroid   WC 155
Channel Blockers, Calcium see Calcium Channel
   Blockers

**ALWAYS CONSULT MAIN SCHEDULES. USE NUMBER ASSIGNED ONLY WHEN
SUBJECT REPRESENTS MAJOR EMPHASIS OF WORK BEING CLASSIFIED**

I–47

Chaplaincy Service, Hospital WX 187
Character BF 818–839
 Disorders see Antisocial Personality WM 190;
  Personality Disorders WM 190
Charbon see Anthrax
Charcoal QV 601
Charcot-Marie Disease WE 550
Charcot-Marie-Tooth Disease see Charcot-Marie
 Disease
Charcot's Joint see Arthropathy, Neurogenic
Charge Nurses see Nursing, Supervisory
Charges see Fees and Charges
Charlatanry see Quackery
Charting, Clinical see Medical Records
Charts
 Statistical (Form number 16 in any NLM schedule
  where applicable)
Chaulmoogra Oil QV 259
Chediak-Higashi Syndrome WD 308
Cheek WE 705
Cheese
 As a dietary supplement in health or disease
  WB 428
 Dairying SF 270–274
 Home economics TX 382
 Sanitary processing WA 715
Cheilitis WI 200
Cheilosis see Riboflavin Deficiency
Chelating Agents QV 290
Chelidonium see Plants, Medicinal
Chemexfoliation WO 600
Chemical Analysis see Chemistry, Analytical
Chemical Elements see Elements; Isotopes;
 Radioisotopes
Chemical Engineering TP 155–156
Chemical Face Peeling see Chemexfoliation
Chemical Genetics see Genetics, Biochemical
Chemical Industry HD 9650–9663
 Occupational medicine WA 400, etc.
 Industrial waste WA 788
Chemical Models see Models, Chemical
Chemical Technology see Technology
Chemical Toxicology see Toxicology
Chemical Vaccines see Vaccines, Synthetic
Chemical Warfare Agents QV 663–667
Chemical Water Pollution see Water Pollution,
 Chemical
Chemicals see Chemistry; Drugs; and names of
 particular chemicals and groups of chemicals, e.g.,
 Inorganic Chemicals; Organic Chemicals; Poisons
Chemistry QD
 Bacterial QW 52
 Biological see Biochemistry QU
 Chemicals as a cause of disease QZ 59
 Dental WU 170
 Forensic W 750
 Industrial TP
 Industrial protection WA 465
 Milk, Public health aspects WA 716
 Physiological QU
 Water analysis WA 686
 See also Blood Chemical Analysis QY 450–490;

 Histocytochemistry QS 531
Chemistry, Agricultural S 583–587.7
Chemistry, Analytical
 Inorganic QD 71–142
 Methods in clinical pathology QY 90
 Of air WA 750
 Of food see Food Analysis QU 50, etc.
 Of milk WA 716
 Of water WA 686
Chemistry, Clinical QY 90
 Animal SF 772.66
Chemistry, Inorganic QD 146–197
Chemistry, Organic QD 241–441
 Aliphatic compounds QD 300–315
 Aromatic compounds QD 330–341
 Physical QD 476
Chemistry, Pharmaceutical QV 744
Chemistry, Physical QD 450–731
Chemistry Tests, Clinical see Clinical Chemistry
 Tests
Chemodectoma see Paraganglioma, Extra-Adrenal
Chemolysis, Intervertebral Disk see Intervertebral
 Disk Chemolysis
Chemonucleolysis see Intervertebral Disk
 Chemolysis
Chemoprevention
 General WB 330
 Neoplasms QZ 267
Chemoprophylaxis see Chemoprevention
Chemoreceptors WL 102.9
Chemosterilants WA 240
Chemotactic Factor, Macrophage-Derived see
 Interleukin-8
Chemotactic Factor, Neutrophil, Monocyte-Derived
see Interleukin-8
Chemotactic Factors
 In immune reaction QW 700
 In phagocytosis QW 690
Chemotaxins see Chemotactic Factors
Chemotaxis
 Cells (General) QH 647
 In phagocytosis QW 690
 Special topics, by subject
Chemotaxis, Leukocyte
 In phagocytosis QW 690
Chemotherapy see Drug Therapy
Chenic Acid see Chenodeoxycholic Acid
Chenodeoxycholate see Chenodeoxycholic Acid
Chenodeoxycholic Acid WI 703
Chenodiol see Chenodeoxycholic Acid
Chenopodium QV 766
 As an anthelmintic QV 253
Chest see Thorax
Chest Injuries see Thoracic Injuries
Chest Pain WF 970
Chest X-Ray see Mass Chest X-Ray; Radiography,
 Thoracic
Chewing see Mastication
Chewing Tobacco see Tobacco, Smokeless
Ch'i
 Philosophy B 127.C49
 Special topics, by subject

Chick Embryo
    General works   QL 959
Chicken Sarcoma Virus B77 see Sarcoma Viruses, Avian
Chicken Tumor 1 Virus see Sarcoma Viruses, Avian
Chickenpox   WC 572
Chickenpox Vaccine   WC 572
Chickenpox Virus see Herpesvirus 3, Human
Chickens
    Anatomy   SF 767.P6
    Culture   SF 481–503.52
    Diseases   SF 995–995.6
    Physiology   SF 768.2.P6
Chief Cells, Gastric
    Cytology   WI 301
    Physiology   WI 302
Chiggers see Mites
Chilblains   WG 530
Child   WS
    Abnormal see Child, Exceptional   WS 105.5.C3, etc.
    Adopted see Adoption   WS 105.5.F2, etc.
    Anesthesia   WO 440
    Care and training see Child Care   WS 113
    Dentistry see Pedodontics   WU 480
    Labor   HD 6228–6250.5
    Nursing see Pediatric Nursing   WY 159
    Radiography   WN 240
    School child see School Health Services   WA 350–352
    Surgery   WO 925
    Tuberculosis see Tuberculosis in Childhood   WF 415
Child Abuse   WA 320
Child Abuse, Sexual   WA 320
    Abuser's psychological aspect   WM 610
Child Advocacy   WA 320
    Special topics, by subject
Child Behavior   WS 105
Child Behavior Disorders   WS 350.6
Child Care   WS 113
Child Custody
    Special topics, by subject
Child Day Care Centers
    Public health   WA 310–320
    Sociology   HV 851–861
Child Development   WS 105
    Educational measurement   LB 3051–3060.87
    Evaluation (General)   WS 105.5.E8
    External influences   WS 105.5.E9
    Intelligence tests   BF 432.C48
    Of the mentally retarded child   WS 107.5.D3
    Physical see Growth   WS 103, etc.
Child Development Deviations see Developmental Disabilities
Child Development Disorders see Developmental Disabilities
Child Development Disorders, Pervasive   WS 350
Child Development Disorders, Specific see Developmental Disabilities
Child, Disabled see Disabled Children
Child, Exceptional
    Education   LC 3951–4000

    Rearing (General)   WS 105.5.C3
    See also Child Gifted   LC 3991–4000, etc.;
       Education of Mentally Retarded   LC 4601–4640.4; Mental Retardation   WS 107–107.5, etc.
Child, Gifted
    Care   WS 113
    Education   LC 3991–4000
    Guidance   WS 350
    Mental development   WS 105
Child Guidance   WS 350–350.8
Child Guidance Clinics   WS 27–28
    Directories   WS 22
Child Health see Child Welfare
Child Health Services   WA 320
    Mother and child   WA 310
    In school   WA 350
       See also School Health   WA 350
Child, Hospitalized   WS 105.5.H7
Child, Institutionalized
    Public health aspects   WA 310–320
    Retarded child   WS 107.5.I4
    Sociological aspects   HV 959–1420.5
    See also Child, Hospitalized   WS 105.5.H7
Child Language   WS 105.5.C8
Child Molestation, Sexual see Child Abuse, Sexual
Child Neglect see Child Abuse
Child Nutrition
    Feeding   WS 130
    Requirements   WS 115
Child Nutrition Disorders   WS 115
Child of Impaired Parents   WS 105.5.F2
    Special topics, by subject
Child, Preschool
    General works   WS 440
    Other topics, by subject within the WS or other schedules
Child Psychiatry   WS 350–350.8
    As a career   WS 350
    Case studies in mental retardation   WS 107.5.C2
Child Psychology   WS 105
Child Reactive Disorders   WS 350.6
Child Rearing   WS 105.5.C3
    Physiological needs see Child Care   WS 113
Child, Unwanted   HV 873
    Effect on pregnancy   WQ 240
    Parent–child relations   WS 105.5.F2
    See also Child Welfare   WA 310, etc.
Child Welfare
    Public health aspects   WA 310–320
    Sociology   HV 701–1420.5
Childbirth see Labor; Popular works   WQ 150 under Pregnancy; Natural Childbirth
Childbirth at Home see Home Childbirth
Childbirth Injuries see Birth Injuries; Labor Complications
Childhood Schizophrenia see Schizophrenia, Childhood
Children, Disabled see Disabled Children
Children of Impaired Parents see Child of Impaired Parents
Children with Disabilities see Disabled Children
Chills see Shivering; Hypothermia; Freezing; Frostbite

Chimera   QH 445.7
Chimeric Toxins see Immunotoxins
Chimpanzee see Pan troglodytes
Chimpanzee Coryza Agent see Respiratory Syncytial
    Viruses
Chimpanzee, Pygmy see Pan paniscus
Chin   WE 705
    See also Mandible   WU 101, etc.
Chinacrin see Quinacrine
Chinchilla   QL 737.R636
    Culture   SF 405.C45
    Diseases   SF 997.5.C5
Chinese see Mongoloid Race
Chinese Americans see Asian Americans
Chinese Herbal Drugs see Drugs, Chinese Herbal
Chinese Liver Fluke see Opisthorchis
Chinese Medicine, Traditional see Medicine, Chinese
    Traditional
Chiniofon see Hydroxyquinolines
Chipmunks see Sciuridae
Chironex Venoms see Coelenterate Venoms
Chironomidae   QX 505
Chironomus see Chironomidae
Chiropody see Podiatry
Chiropotes see Cebidae
Chiropractic   WB 905–905.9
Chiropractic Adjustment see Manipulation, Spinal
Chiroptera   QL 737.C5
    Diseases   SF 997.5.B38
Chitin   QU 83
Chitinase   QU 136
Chlamydia   QW 152
Chlamydia Infections   WC 600
    Veterinary   SF 809.C45
    Specific infection, by type
Chlamydiales   QW 152
Chloral Hydrate   QV 85
Chlorambucil   QV 269
Chloramiphene see Clomiphene
Chloramphenicol   QV 350.5.C5
Chlorbutol see Chlorobutanol
Chlordecone
    Agriculture   SB 952.C44
    Public health   WA 240
Chlordiazepoxide   QV 77.9
Chlorella   QK 569.C49
Chlorethazine see Mechlorethamine
Chlorhexidine   QV 220
Chloride Channels   QH 603.I54
Chlorides
    Inorganic chemistry   QD 181.C5
    Pharmacology   QV 280
    Water purification   WA 690
Chlorimipramine see Clomipramine
Chlorinated Hydrocarbons see Hydrocarbons,
    Chlorinated
Chlorine   QV 231
    Toxicology   QV 663
Chlorine Compounds
    Inorganic chemistry   QD 181.C5
    Pharmacology   QV 231
    Water purification   WA 690

Chlormequat
    As a plant growth regulator   QK 745
    Organic chemistry   QD 305.A8
Chlormerodrin   QV 160
Chlormeroprin see Chlormerodrin
Chlormethine see Mechlorethamine
Chlorobutanol   QV 115
Chlorodinitrobenzene see Dinitrochlorobenzene
Chloroethylene see Vinyl Chloride
Chloroethylene Polymer see Polyvinyl Chloride
Chloroform   QV 81
Chloroiodoquine see Clioquinol
Chloromethyl Ether see Bis(Chloromethyl) Ether
Chlorophenols   QV 223
Chlorophenyl GABA see Baclofen
Chlorophyll   QK 898.C5
Chloropicrin   QV 664
Chloroplast Coupling Factor see H(+)–Transporting
    ATP Synthase
Chloroplasts   QK 898.C5
Chloroprene
    As a carcinogen   QZ 202
    Toxicology   QV 633
Chloroquine   QV 256
Chlorosis see Anemia, Hypochromic
Chlorosis, Egyptian see Hookworm Infections
Chlorphenamine see Chlorpheniramine
Chlorpheniramine   QV 157
Chlorpromazine   QV 77.9
Chlorprophenpyridamine see Chlorpheniramine
Chlorprothixene   QV 77.9
Chlortetracycline   QV 360
Chocolate see Cacao
Choice Behavior   BF 608–618
    Special topics, by subject
Choked Disk see Papilledema
Choking see Airway Obstruction
Cholagogues and Choleretics   QV 66
Cholalic Acids see Cholic Acids
Cholangiography   WI 750
Cholangiopancreatography, Endoscopic Retrograde
    WI 750
Cholecalciferol   QU 173
Cholecystectomy   WI 750
Cholecystitis   WI 755
Cholecystography   WI 750
Cholecystokinin   WK 170
Cholecystokinin Octapeptide Receptors see
    Receptors, Cholecystokinin
Cholecystokinin–Pancreozymin Receptors see
    Receptors, Cholecystokinin
Cholecystokinin Receptors see Receptors,
    Cholecystokinin
Cholecystostomy   WI 750
Choledocholithiasis see Common Bile Duct Calculi
Choledochus see Common Bile Duct
Cholelithiasis   WI 755
Cholelithiasis, Common Bile Duct see Common Bile
    Duct Calculi
Cholera   WC 262–264
Cholera Toxin   WC 262
Cholera Vaccine   WC 262
Choleragen see Cholera Toxin

Choleragenoid see Cholera Toxin
Choleretics see Cholagogues and Choleretics
Cholestasis   WI 703
Cholestasis, Extrahepatic see Bile Duct Obstruction,
     Extrahepatic
Cholesteatoma   QZ 365
     Localized, by site
Cholesterol   QU 95
Cholesterol, Dietary   QU 95
     Control in sickness or health   WB 425
     Cookbooks   WB 425
Cholesterol HDL see Lipoproteins, HDL
     Cholesterol
Cholesterol Inhibitors see Anticholesteremic Agents
Cholesterol LDL see Lipoproteins, LDL Cholesterol
Cholesterol 7 alpha-Monooxygenase   QU 140
Cholesterol-7-Hydroxylase see Cholesterol 7
     alpha-Monooxygenase
Cholic Acids   WI 703
Choline   QU 87
     Esters   QV 122
Choline Acetylase see Choline O-Acetyltransferase
Choline Acetyltransferase see Choline
     O-Acetyltransferase
Choline Deficiency   WD 120
Choline O-Acetyltransferase   QU 141
Choline Phosphoglycerides see Phosphatidylcholines
Cholinergic Agents   QV 122
Cholinergic Antagonists   QV 124
Cholinergic-Blocking Agents see Cholinergic
     Antagonists
Cholinergic Receptors see Receptors, Cholinergic
Cholinesterase Inhibitors   QV 124
Cholinesterase Reactivators   QV 124
Cholinesterases   QU 136
Cholinoceptive Sites see Receptors, Cholinergic
Cholinoceptors see Receptors, Cholinergic
Cholinolytics see Cholinergic Antagonists
Cholinomimetics see Cholinergic Agents
Chondroblastoma   QZ 340
Chondrocytes   WE 300
Chondrodysplasia, Hereditary Deforming see
     Exostoses, Multiple Hereditary
Chondrodysplasia Punctata   WE 250
Chondrodystrophia Calcificans Congenita see
     Chondrodysplasia Punctata
Chondrodystrophia Fetalis see Achondroplasia
Chondrogenesis   WE 300
Chondroitin   QU 83
Chondroma   QZ 340
Chorda Tympani Nerve   WL 330
Chordata   QL 605-739.8
     See also special aspects, e.g., Embryology   QL
     958, etc.
Chordoma   QZ 310
     Localized, by site
Chorea   WL 390
     Associated with rheumatic fever   WC 220
Chorea, Hereditary see Huntington Chorea
Chorioadenoma see Hydatidiform Mole, Invasive
Choriocarcinoma   WP 465
     Pathology   QZ 310
Chorioepithelioma see Choriocarcinoma

Chorion   WQ 210
     Animal   QL 977
     Embryology   QS 645
Chorionic Somatomammotropin, Human see
     Placental Lactogen
Chorionic Villi   WQ 210
     Animal   QL 977
     Embryology   QS 645
Chorionic Villi Sampling   WQ 209
Chorioretinitis   WW 270
Choroid   WW 245
     Edema   WW 245
Choroid Diseases   WW 245
Choroid Neoplasms   WW 245
Choroid Plexus   WL 307
Choroidal Neovascularization   WW 245
Choroiditis   WW 245
Christ-Siemens-Touraine Syndrome see Ectodermal
     Dysplasia
Christian Science   BX 6903-6997
     Healing   WB 885
     See also Mental Healing   WB 885, etc.
Christianity   BR
     And medicine   W 61
          See also Religion and Medicine   BL 65.M4,
          etc.
     And psychiatry   WM 61
          See also Religion and Psychology   BL 53,
          etc
     And psychoanalysis   WM 460.5.R3
     General works   BR 120-126
     Medical ethics   W 50
     Other special topics, by subject
Christmas Disease see Hemophilia B
Chromaffin System
     Endocrinology   WK 102
     Of particular glands or other organs, by gland
     or organ
Chromatin   QU 56
     Cytology   QH 599
Chromatin, Sex see Sex Chromatin
Chromatium   QW 145
Chromatography
     Analytical chemistry (General)   QD 79.C4
     Organic analysis (General)   QD 272.C4
     Qualitative analysis   QD 98.C4
     Quantitative analysis   QD 117.C5
     Used for special purposes, by subject, e.g., in
     Assay of Hormones   QY 330
Chromatography, Affinity
     Biochemistry   QU 25
Chromatography, Gas
     Analytical chemistry   QD 79.C45
     Organic analysis   QD 272.C44
Chromatography, Gas-Liquid see Chromatography,
     Gas
Chromatography, High Performance Liquid see
     Chromatography, High Pressure Liquid
Chromatography, High Pressure Liquid
     Analytical chemistry   QD 79.C454
Chromatography, High Speed Liquid see
     Chromatography, High Pressure Liquid

Chromatography, Paper
    Analytical chemistry   QD 79.C46
Chromatography, Thin Layer
    Analytical chemistry   QD 79.C8
    Organic analysis   QD 272.C45
Chromatophores   QS 532.5.E7
Chromium   QV 290
    Metabolism   QU 130.5
Chromium Isotopes
    Inorganic chemistry   QD 181.C7
    Pharmacology   QV 290
Chromogenic Compounds
    Analytical chemistry   QD 77
    Pharmaceutical chemistry   QV 744
    Used for special purposes, by subject
Chromogenic Substrates see Chromogenic
    Compounds
Chromomycins   QV 269
Chromophobe Adenoma see Adenoma,
    Chromophobe
Chromosomal Probes see DNA Probes
Chromosomal Translocation see Translocation
    (Genetics)
Chromosome Aberrations   QH 462.A1
    See also Chromosome Deletion   QH 462.D4;
        Inversion (Genetics)   QH 462.I5;
        Translocation (Genetics)   QH 462.T7
Chromosome Abnormalities   QS 677
    See also Trisomy   QH 461, etc.
Chromosome Banding   QH 600
Chromosome Breakage   QH 462.B7
Chromosome Deletion   QH 462.D4
Chromosome Fragile Sites see Chromosome
    Fragility
Chromosome Fragility   QH 461.A1
Chromosome Mapping   QH 445.2
Chromosome Markers see Genetic Markers
Chromosome 21 see Chromosomes, Human, Pair 21
Chromosomes   QH 600
    See also Sex Chromosomes   QH 600.5
Chromosomes A see Chromosomes, Human, 1-3
Chromosomes, Bacterial   QW 51-52
Chromosomes D see Chromosomes, Human, 13-15
Chromosomes, Human   QH 600
Chromosomes, Human, Pair 21   QH 600
Chromosomes, Human, 1-3   QH 600
Chromosomes, Human, 13-15   QH 600
Chronic Disease   WT 500
    Child   WS 200
    Infant   WS 200
    Nursing   WY 152
    Social problems   WT 30
Chronic Fatigue Syndrome see Fatigue Syndrome,
    Chronic
Chronic Hepatitis C see Hepatitis C, Chronic
Chronic Illness see Chronic Disease
Chronic Limitation of Activity see Activities of
    Daily Living
Chronic Motor or Vocal Tic Disorder see Tic
    Disorders
Chronic Obstructive Pulmonary Disease see Lung
    Diseases, Obstructive
Chronobiology   QT 167

Chronologies, Medicine see Chronologies   WZ 30
    under Medicine; Chronology
Chronology   CE
    Historical   D-F
    Medical   WZ 30
Chronotherapy   WB 340
    For particular diseases, with the disease
Chronotropism, Cardiac see Heart Rate
Chrysanthemum see Pyrethrum
Chrysenes   QV 138.C1
    Organic chemistry   QD 395
Chrysotherapeutic Agents see Antirheumatic
    Agents, Gold
Church see Catholicism; Religion
Churg-Strauss Syndrome   WG 515
Chyle   WI 402
Chylomicrons   QU 85
Chylothorax   WF 700
Chymopapain   QU 136
Chymosin   QU 136
    In milk analysis   WA 716
CI-581 see Ketamine
Cicatrix   WR 143
    Wound healing   WO 185
    Localized, by site
Ciguatera see Ciguatoxin
Ciguatoxin   QW 630
Cilastatin   QU 90
    As a protease inhibitor   QU 136
Cilia   QS 532.5.E7
    In animals   QP 310.C5
    Specific to an organ, with the organ
Ciliary Body   WW 240
Ciliary Dyskinesia see Ciliary Motility Disorders
Ciliary Motility Disorders   WF 140
    Cilia of specific organs, with the organ
Ciliata see Ciliophora
Ciliate Infections see Balantidiasis   WC 735 or
    names of other parasitic diseases caused by Ciliata
Ciliophora   QX 151
Cimetidine   QV 157
    As an anti-ulcer agent   QV 69
Cimex see Bedbugs
Cincain see Dibucaine
Cinchocain see Dibucaine
Cinchona   QV 257
Cinchophen   QV 95
Cine-CT see Tomography, X-Ray Computed
Cineangiography   WG 500
Cinefluorography see Cineradiography
Cineradiography   WN 220
    Heart   WG 141.5.R2
    Diagnosis of specific disease with the disease or
    organ
Ciprofloxacin   QV 250
Circadian Rhythm   QT 167
    Animals   QP 84.6
    Biology (General)   QH 527
Circular Dichroism   QD 473
Circulation see Blood Circulation; Cerebrovascular
    Circulation; Collateral Circulation; Coronary
    Circulation; Liver Circulation; Microcirculation;
    Pulmonary Circulation

**ALWAYS CONSULT MAIN SCHEDULES. USE NUMBER ASSIGNED ONLY WHEN
SUBJECT REPRESENTS MAJOR EMPHASIS OF WORK BEING CLASSIFIED**

Circulation of Books see Circulation   Z 712-714
under Library Services
Circulatory Disorders see Blood Circulation;
Cerebrovascular Circulation; Disorders   WI 720
under Liver Circulation
Circulatory Function Tests see Blood Circulation
Circulatory System see Cardiovascular System
Circumcision
    Anthropology   GN 484
    Judaism   BM 705
    Medical procedure   WJ 790
Circumcision, Female
    Anthropology   GN 484
    Medical procedure   WP 200
Cirrhosis see Liver Cirrhosis; Pulmonary Fibrosis
Cirrhosis, Liver see Liver Cirrhosis
cis-Diammincdichloroplatinum(II) see Cisplatin
cis-Dichlorodiammineplatinum(II) see Cisplatin
Cisapride
    As a gastrointestinal agent   QV 66
    Biochemistry   QU 62
    Used in the treatment of particular diseases, with
    the disease
Cisplatin   QV 269
    Therapeutic use for neoplasms   QZ 267
Cisterna Chyli see Thoracic Duct
Cisterna Magna   WL 200
Cisternal Puncture see Punctures
Cisternography, Myelographic see Myelography
Cisternography, Pneumoencephalographic see
Pneumoencephalography
Citellus see Sciuridae
Citicoline see Cytidine Diphosphate Choline
Citizen Participation see Consumer Participation
Citrate see Citric Acid
Citrated Calcium Cyanamide see Cyanamide
Citrates   QU 98
    Organic chemistry
        Aliphatic compounds   QD 305.A2
Citric Acid   QU 98
Citric Acid Cycle   QU 98
Citrin see Bioflavonoids
Citrovorum Factor see Leucovorin
Citrus
    As a dietary supplement in health or disease
    WB 430
    Sanitary control   WA 703
City Planning   HT 165.5-169.9
    Architecture and engineering   NA 9000-9428
    Public health aspects in   WA
    See also Urban Renewal   HT 170-178, etc.
Civil Defense   UA 926-929
    Psychological aspects   UA 926.5
Civil Rights   JC 571-628
    Constitutional law (U.S.)   KF 4741-4785
        Control of individual rights   KF 4791-4856
    Mentally disabled   WM 30-32
    Political rights   JF 800-1191
    Other special topics, by subject, e.g., Medical
    records and privacy rights   WX 173, etc.
Civilian Protection see Civil Defense
Civilization   CB
    General works   CB 23-161

Sociological aspects   HM
Other special topics, by subject, e.g. civilization
and disease   WA 30
Claims Review see Insurance Claim Review
Clairvoyance see Parapsychology
Clams   QX 675
    Food poisoning   WC 268
    Food sanitation   WA 703; WA 710
Clarification, Pharmaceutical see Drug
Compounding
Class I Genes see Genes, MHC Class I
Class II Antigens see Histocompatibility Antigens
Class II
Class II Genes see Genes, MHC Class II
Class II Human Antigens see HLA-D Antigens
Classical Complement Pathway see Complement
Pathway, Classical
Classification
    (Form number 15 in any NLM schedule where
    applicable)
    See also Book Classification   Z 696-697 and
    subjects or objects being classified
Clastogens see Mutagens
Claustrophobia see Phobic Disorders
Claustrum see Basal Ganglia
Clavicle   WE 810
Clavulanate see Clavulanic Acid
Clavulanic Acid   QV 350
Clavulanic Acids   QV 350
Claw see Hoof and Claw
Cleanliness, Personal see Cleanliness   QT 240 under
Hygiene
Cleansing Agents see Detergents
Cleavage, Cell see Cell Division
Cleft Lip   WV 440
Cleft Palate   WV 440
Cleft Palate Prosthesis see Palatal Obturators
Clemastine   QV 157
Clerambault Syndrome see Delirium, Dementia,
Amnestic, Cognitive Disorders
Clergy   BV 659-683
    See also Psychology, Pastoral   WM 61
Clerical Medicine see Pastoral Care
Clethrionomys see Microtinae
Client-Centered Therapy see Nondirective Therapy
Climacteric
    Female   WP 580
        See also Menopause   WP 580
    Male   WJ 702
    Postmenopausal see Menopause   WP 580
Climate
    Climatology (Physics)   QC 980-999
    Prescribed for health   WB 750
    Prescribed for tuberculosis   WF 330
    Relation to disease   WB 700-710
    See also Acclimatization   QT 145, etc.; Cold
    Climate   QT 160, etc.; Desert Climate   QT
    150, etc.; Environment   QT 230, etc.;
    Meteorological Factors   WA 30, etc.; Tropical
    Climate   QT 150, etc.; Weather   WB
    700-710, etc.
Climatology, Medical see Climate; Weather
Climatotherapy see Climate; Health Resorts;
Thalassotherapy

Clinical Capillary Leak Syndrome see Capillary
Leak Syndrome
Clinical Charting see Medical Records
Clinical Chemistry see Chemistry, Clinical
Clinical Chemistry Tests   QY 90
Clinical Competence   W 21
    As an educational measurement
        Works about (Form number 18 in any NLM
        schedule where applicable)
        Actual tests (Form number 18.2 in any NLM
        schedule where applicable)
Clinical Decision Support Systems see Decision
Support Systems, Clinical
Clinical Departments see Hospital Departments
Clinical Engineering see Biomedical Engineering
Clinical Equivalency see Therapeutic Equivalency
Clinical Ethics see Ethics, Medical
Clinical Informatics see Medical Informatics
Clinical Investigators see Research Personnel
Clinical Laboratory Information Systems   QY 26.5
Clinical Ladders see Career Mobility
Clinical Markers see Biological Markers
Clinical Medicine   WB 102
    Case studies   WB 293
Clinical Nurse Specialists see Nurse Clinicians
Clinical Nursing Research   WY 20.5
Clinical Pathology see Pathology, Clinical
Clinical Pathways see Critical Pathways
Clinical Pharmacology see Pharmacology, Clinical
Clinical Pharmacy Service see Pharmacy Service,
Hospital
Clinical Practice Nursing Research see Clinical
Nursing Research
Clinical Practice Patterns see Physician's Practice
Patterns
Clinical Practice Variations see Physician's Practice
Patterns
Clinical Protocols
    Used for special purposes, by subject
Clinical Psychology see Psychology, Clinical
Clinical Refraction see Refraction, Ocular
Clinical Skills see Clinical Competence
Clinical Trials
    Drugs   QV 771
    Vision research   WW 20
    For other purposes, by subject or specific drug
    or procedure
Clinical Trials, Controlled see Controlled Clinical
Trials
Clinical Trials, Randomized see Randomized
Controlled Trials
Clinics, Dental see Dental Clinics
Clinics, Free–Standing see Ambulatory Care
Facilities
Clinics, Outpatient see Outpatient Clinics, Hospital
Clioquinol   QV 255
Clitoridectomy see Circumcision, Female
Clitoris   WP 200
Cloaca   WJ 101
Clofibric Acid
    As an anticholesteremic agent   QU 95
Clofibrinic Acid see Clofibric Acid

Clomifene see Clomiphene
Clomiphene   QV 170
Clomipramine   QV 77.5
Clone Cells   QH 585
    Nuclear cloning   QH 442.2
Cloning, Embryo see Cloning, Organism
Cloning, Human see Cloning, Organism
Cloning, Molecular   QH 442.2
Cloning, Organism   QH 442.2
Cloning Vectors see Genetic Vectors
Clonogenic Cell Assay see Colony–Forming Units
Assay
Clonogenic Cell Assay, Tumor see Tumor Stem Cell
Assay
Clonorchis sinensis   QX 353
Cloranfenicol see Chloramphenicol
Closed–Circuit Anesthesia see Anesthesia,
Closed–Circuit
Closed Cohort Studies see Cohort Studies
Closed Ecologic Life Support Systems see
Ecological Systems, Closed
Clostridiopeptidase A see Microbial Collagenase
Clostridium   QW 127.5.C5
Clostridium botulinum   QW 127.5.C5
Clostridium histolyticum Collagenase see Microbial
Collagenase
Clostridium Infections   WC 368–375
    See also Botulism   WC 268; Hemoglobinuria,
    Bacillary   WJ 344; Wound Infection   WC
    255
Clostridium perfringens   QW 127.5.C5
Clostridium welchii see Clostridium perfringens
Closure of Wounds see Wounds and Injuries
Clothing   QT 245
    See also Protective Clothing   WA 260, etc.
Clouston's Syndrome see Ectodermal Dysplasia
Clove see Rosales
Clubfoot   WE 883
    Veterinary   SF 901
Clumping see Agglutination
Clumping, Erythrocytic see Hemagglutination
Cluster Headache   WL 344
Clysis see Enema
Clyster see Enema
CMHC see Community Mental Health Centers
Cnidaria   QX 195
CoA see Coenzyme A
Coagulants   QV 195
Coagulase   WH 310
    Special topics, by subject
Coagulation see Blood Coagulation; Laser
Coagulation; Light Coagulation
Coagulation Factors see Blood Coagulation Factors
Coal   TP 325–326
    Poisoning   QV 633
    See also Pneumoconiosis   WF 654 and related
    disorders
Coal Mining
    Occupational accidents   WA 485
    Occupational medicine   WA 400–495
    Industrial waste   WA 788
Coal Tar   QV 60
    Anti–infective dyes derived from   QV 235

**ALWAYS CONSULT MAIN SCHEDULES. USE NUMBER ASSIGNED ONLY WHEN
SUBJECT REPRESENTS MAJOR EMPHASIS OF WORK BEING CLASSIFIED**

I–54

Toxicology   QV 633
    See also Cresols   QV 223, etc.; Phenols   QV 223, etc.
Coated Pits, Cell–Membrane   QH 603.C63
Cobalamin see Vitamin B 12
Cobalt
    Inorganic chemistry   QD 181.C6
    Metabolism   QU 130.5
    Pharmacology   QV 290
Cobalt Isotopes
    Inorganic chemistry   QD 181.C6
    Pharmacology   QV 290
Cobalt Radioisotopes   WN 420
    Nuclear physics   QC 796.C6
    See also special topics under Radioisotopes
Coca   QV 113
Cocaine   QV 113
    Dependence   WM 280
Cocaine–Related Disorders   WM 280
Cocarboxylase see Thiamine Pyrophosphate
Cocarcinogenesis   QZ 202
Cocci, Gram–Positive see Gram–Positive Cocci
Coccidia   QX 123
Coccidioides   QW 180.5.P4
Coccidioidomycosis   WC 460
Coccidiosis   WC 730
    Veterinary   SF 792
        Avian diseases   SF 995.6.C6
Coccygeal Region see Sacrococcygeal Region
Coccyx   WE 725
Cochlea   WV 250
Cochlear Aqueduct   WV 250
Cochlear Diseases   WV 250
Cochlear Implantation   WV 274
Cochlear Implants   WV 274
Cochlear Microphonic Potentials   WV 270
Cochlear Nerve   WL 330
    Physiology of hearing   WV 272
Cochlear Prosthesis see Cochlear Implants
Cochlear Prosthesis Implantation see Cochlear Implantation
Cochliobolus see Ascomycota
Cockroaches   QX 570
Cocoa see Cacao
Coconut
    Diets for control of fats   WB 425
    Diets for control of proteins   WB 426
    Plant culture   SB 401.C6
Cocos see Coconut
Cod Liver Oil   QU 86
Codeine   QV 92
    Dependence   WM 286
Codes of Ethics see Bioethics; Ethics; Ethics, Medical; ethics in other specialties
Codes, Sanitary see Legislation   WA 32–33 under Sanitation
Codon   QU 58.7
Coelenterata see Cnidaria
Coelenterate Venoms   WD 405
Coendou see Rodentia
Coenuriasis see Cestode Infections
Coenzyme A   QU 135
Coenzyme I see NAD

Coenzyme II see NADP
Coenzyme M see Mesna
Coenzyme Q see Ubiquinone
Coenzymes   QU 135
Coercion
    Special topics, by subject
Coffea see Coffee
Coffee
    As a dietary supplement in health or disease   WB 438
    Cultivation   SB 269
    See also Caffeine   QV 107
Coformycin
    As an antineoplastic agent   QV 269
    As an immunosuppressant   QW 920
Cognition   BF 311–499
    Adolescence   WS 462
    Aged   WT 145
    Child   WS 105.5.C7
    Cognition & age (adulthood)   BF 724.55.C63
    Infant   WS 105.5.C7
Cognition Disorders
    General and psychotic   WM 204
    Aged   WT 150
    Other special topics by subject, e.g., Amnesia   WM 173.7
Cognitive Dissonance   BF 337.C63
Cognitive Symptoms   WM 204
    Aged   WT 150
Cognitive Therapy   WM 425.5.C6
    Child   WS 350.6
Cohort Analysis see Cohort Studies
Cohort Studies
    In epidemiology   WA 105
    Special topics, by subject
Coin Lesion, Pulmonary   WF 658
Coins see Numismatics
Coinsurance see Deductibles and Coinsurance
Coitus
    Animal (General) see Copulation   QL 761
    Human   HQ 19–30.7
    Psychophysiologic problems   WM 611
        Female   WP 610
        Male   WJ 709
Cola see Beverages
Colchicine   QV 98
Colchicum   QV 98
Cold
    Adverse effects   QZ 57
    In anesthesia see Anesthesia, Refrigeration   WO 350
    Therapeutic use   WB 473
Cold Agglutinin Disease see Anemia, Hemolytic, Autoimmune
Cold Climate
    Physiological effects   QT 160
    Winter temperatures (meteorology)   QC 905
Cold, Common see Common Cold
Cold–Insoluble Globulins see Fibronectins
Cold Therapy see Cryotherapy
Colectomy   WI 520
Coleonol see Forskolin
Coleoptera   QX 555

Colic
  Abdominal WI 147
  Other specific region or organ, with the region
    or organ
Colicines see Colicins
Colicins QV 350
Coliform Bacilli see Enterobacteriaceae
Coliphage lambda see Bacteriophage lambda
Coliphages QW 161.5.C6
Coliphages T see T-Phages
Colistin QV 350
Colitis WI 522
  Amebic see Dysentery, Amebic WC 285
Colitis, Amebic see Dysentery, Amebic
Colitis, Granulomatous see Crohn Disease
Colitis, Mucous see Colonic Diseases, Functional
Colitis, Ulcerative WI 522
Collagen QU 55
Collagen Diseases WD 375
  See also names of specific diseases
Collagen Type I see Collagen
Collagen Type II see Collagen
Collagen Type III see Collagen
Collagen Type IV see Collagen
Collagen Type IX see Collagen
Collagen Type V see Collagen
Collagen Type VI see Collagen
Collagen Type VII see Collagen
Collagen Type VIII see Collagen
Collagen Type X see Collagen
Collagen Type XI see Collagen
Collagen Type XII see Collagen
Collagen Type XIII see Collagen
Collagenase, Microbial see Microbial Collagenase
Collapse Therapy WF 350
Collateral Circulation WG 103
Collected Correspondence
  Physicians and specialists of medically related
    fields
    Collective WZ 112-150
    Individual WZ 100
  Special topics, by subject
Collected works
  By several authors (Form number 5 in any NLM
    schedule where applicable)
  By individual authors (Form number 7 in any
    NLM schedule where applicable)
Collection of Fees see Fees and Charges; Fees,
  Dental; Fees, Medical; Fees, Pharmaceutical
Collections see Form numbers 5-7 in any NLM
  schedule where applicable
Collective Bargaining HD 6971.5-6971.6
  Hospitals and hospital personnel WX 159.8
  Industry and health services WA 412
    Mental health services WA 495
  Industry and health insurance W 125-270
  Nurses WY 30
    With hospital staff WX 159.8
  Special topics, by subject
College Admission Test LB 2353-2353.8
  Works about (Form number 18 in any NLM
    schedule where applicable)
  Actual tests (Form number 18.2 in any NLM

    schedule where applicable)
  See also Educational Measurement LB
    3051-3059, etc.
College Students, Health see Student Health Services
Colleges, Medical see Schools, Medical
Collodion
  Pharmaceutic aids QV 800
  Photographic processing TR 390
Colloids
  As dosage form QV 785
  Biochemistry QU 133
Colobus QL 737.P93
  Diseases SF 997.5.P7
  As laboratory animals QY 60.P7
Colocynth QV 75
Colon WI 520-529
  Surgery WI 520
Colon, Irritable see Colonic Diseases, Functional
Colonialism see Political Systems
Colonic Diseases WI 520-529
Colonic Diseases, Functional WI 520
Colonic Neoplasms WI 529
Colonic Polyps WI 529
Colonoscopes see Endoscopes
Colonoscopy WI 520
Colony-Forming Units see Stem Cells
Colony-Forming Units Assay QH 585
Colony-Forming Units Assay, Tumor see Tumor
  Stem Cell Assay
Colony-Forming Units, Hematopoietic see
  Hematopoietic Stem Cells
Colony-Forming Units, Neoplastic see Tumor Stem
  Cells
Colony-Stimulating Factor, Mast-Cell see
  Interleukin-3
Colony-Stimulating Factor, Multipotential see
  Interleukin-3
Colony-Stimulating Factor 2 Alpha see
  Interleukin-3
Colony-Stimulating Factors
  In hematopoiesis WH 140
Color QC 494-496.9
  Psychology BF 789.C7
  Therapeutic use see Color Therapy WB 890
  See also Eye Color WW 101; Food Additives
    WA 712; Hair Color WR 450;
    Pigmentation WR 102, etc.
Color Blindness see Color Vision Defects
Color Perception WW 150
Color Therapy WB 890
  For particular diseases, with the disease
Color Vision see Color Perception
Color Vision Defects WW 150
Colorectal Neoplasms WI 529
Colorectal Neoplasms, Hereditary Nonpolyposis
  WI 529
Colorectal Surgery WI 650
  See also Surgery WI 520 under Colon; Surgery
    WI 650 under Rectum
Colorimetry QD 113
  Clinical pathology QY 90
Coloring Agents see Dyes
Coloring Agents, Food see Food Coloring Agents

**ALWAYS CONSULT MAIN SCHEDULES. USE NUMBER ASSIGNED ONLY WHEN
SUBJECT REPRESENTS MAJOR EMPHASIS OF WORK BEING CLASSIFIED**

Coloring Agents, Hair see Hair Dyes
Colostomy   WI 520
Colostrum   WP 825
Colpohysterectomy see Hysterectomy, Vaginal
Colposcopy   WP 250
Coma   WB 182
    Diabetic see Diabetic Coma   WK 830
    Hepatic see Hepatic Encephalopathy   WI 700
Coma, Hyperglycemic Hyperosmolar Nonketotic see
    Hyperglycemic Hyperosmolar Nonketotic Coma
Combat Disorders   WM 184
Combat Psychiatry see Military Psychiatry
Combination Chemotherapy see Drug Therapy,
    Combination
Combined Modality Therapy
    General   WB 300
    For neoplasms   QZ 266
Combining Site see Binding Sites
Comfort Stations see Toilet Facilities
Commerce   HF
    General works   HF 1003–1008
Commercial Oils see Industrial Oils
Commercial Preparations see Drugs,
    Non-prescription
Comminution, Pharmaceutical see Drug
    Compounding
Commitment of Mentally Ill   WM 32–33
Common Bile Duct   WI 750
Common Bile Duct Calculi   WI 755
Common Bile Duct Diseases   WI 750
Common Bile Duct Neoplasms   WI 765
Common Cold   WC 510
Common Cold Virus see Rhinovirus
Common Hepatic Duct see Hepatic Duct, Common
Common Porpoises see Porpoises
Communicable Disease Contact Tracing see Contact
    Tracing
Communicable Disease Control   WA 110–240
    Disinfestation   WA 240
    Notifiable disease registration   WA 55
    See also Quarantine   WA 230, etc.; names of
    various types of control, e.g., Pest control
    WA 240
Communicable Diseases   WC
    General works   WC 100
    Child   WC
    Drugs used in   QV 250–268.5
    In pregnancy see Pregnancy, Complications,
    Infectious   WQ 256
    Infant   WC
    Nursing   WY 153
    Prevention see Communicable Disease Control
    WA 110, etc.; Insect Control   QX 600;
    Quarantine   WA 230, etc.
    Transmission
        Epidemiological aspects   WA 110
        Insect vectors   QX 650
        Mechanisms   QW 700
        Veterinary   SF 781–809
Communication
    Adolescence   WS 462
    Child   WS 105.5.C8
    In mentally retarded   WM 307.C6

    Child   WS 107.5.C6
    Infant   WS 107.5.C6
    In psychoanalysis   WM 460.5.C5
    Infant   WS 105.5.C8
    Information systems   Z 699, etc.
    Manual   HV 2474–2480
    Medical writing and publishing   WZ 345
    Nonverbal see Nonverbal communication
    BF 637.N66
    Philology and linguistics   P 87–96
    Physician's interpersonal relations   W 62
    Psychology   BF 637.C45
    Social psychology   HM 258
    Telecommunication (General)   TK 5101–5105.9
Communication Aids for Disabled
    For communicative disorders   WL 340.2
    See also specific types of aids
Communication Aids for Handicapped see
    Communication Aids for Disabled
Communication, Animal see Animal Communication
Communication Barriers
    Adolescence   WS 462
    Child   WS 105.5.C8
    In mentally retarded   WM 307.C6
    Infant   WS 105.5.C8
    Physician's interpersonal relations   W 62
    Psychological aspects   BF 637.C45
    Social psychology aspects   HM
Communication Boards see Communication Aids for
    Disabled
Communication Disorders
    General   WL 340.2
    Psychogenic   WM 475
    Neurologic   WL 340.2
Communication Methods, Total   HV 2497
Communications Media   P 87–96
    See also Mass Media; specific types of media,
    e.g., Computer Communication Networks,
    Newspapers, Periodicals, Radio,
    Telecommunications, Television, etc.
    Special topics, by subject
Communicative Disorders see Communication
    Disorders
Communism   HX 72–73, 626–780.7
    As practiced in special countries in JN or in the
    history number for the country
    Special topics, by subject, e.g., State medicine
    in a Communist country   W 225
Community Action see Consumer Participation
Community Care Networks see Community
    Networks
Community Dentistry   WU 113
Community Health Aides   W 21.5
Community Health Care see Community Health
    Services
Community Health Education see Health Education
Community Health Networks see Community
    Networks
Community Health Nursing   WY 106
Community Health Services   WA 546
Community–Institutional Relations
    Hospital   WX 160
    Other types of institutions, by subject

ALWAYS CONSULT MAIN SCHEDULES. USE NUMBER ASSIGNED ONLY WHEN
SUBJECT REPRESENTS MAJOR EMPHASIS OF WORK BEING CLASSIFIED

Community Medicine   W 84.5
Community Mental Health Centers   WM 29
Community Mental Health Services   WM 30
  For infants or children and other age groups
    WM 30
    Special population groups   WA 305
    See also Hospitals, Psychiatric   WM 27–28, etc.;
     Social Work, Psychiatric   WM 30.5
Community Networks
    In community health services   WA 546
    As information systems   W 26.55.I4
Community Pharmacies see Pharmacies
Community Pharmacy Services   QV 737
Community Psychiatry   WM 30.6–31.5
    Etiological factors in mental disorders   WM 31
    Preventive measures   WM 31.5
    Social psychiatry   WM 30.6–31.5
Comorbidity
    Of particular disorders, with the disorder
Compact Disk Read–Only Memory see CD–ROM
Comparative Anatomy see Anatomy, Comparative
Comparative Pathology see Pathology
Comparative Physiology see Physiology,
    Comparative
Comparative Psychology see Psychology,
    Comparative
Compartment Syndromes   WE 550
Compensation, Disability see Veterans Disability
    Claims; Disability Evaluation; Workers'
    Compensation
Competence, Clinical see Clinical Competence
Competence, Immunologic see Immunocompetence
Competence, Professional see Professional
    Competence
Competency–Based Education
    General works   LC 1031–1034.5
    In a particular field (Form number 18 in any NLM
     schedule where applicable)
Competition, Economic see Economic Competition
Competition, Managed see Managed Competition
Competitive Behavior   HM
Competitive Bidding
    Medical work   W 74
    Other fields, in economics number by subject
Competitive Binding see Binding, Competitive
Complement   QW 680
Complement Activating Enzymes   QW 680
    Biochemistry   QU 135
Complement Activation   QW 680
Complement Fixation Tests   QY 265
Complement Pathway, Classical   QW 680
Complement Proteins see Complement
Complement Receptors see Receptors, Complement
Complement 1   QW 680
Complement 1 Esterase Inhibitors see Complement
    1 Inactivators
Complement 1 Inactivators   QW 680
    Biochemistry   QU 136
Complement 1 Inhibitors see Complement 1
    Inactivators
Complement 3   QW 680
Complement 3 Convertase   QW 680
Complement 5 Convertase see Complement 3

Convertase
Complexons see Chelating Agents
Compliant Behavior see Cooperative Behavior
Composite Resins   WU 190
Compound Fractures see Fractures, Open
Compound Q see Trichosanthin
Comprehensive Dental Care   WU 29
Comprehensive Health Care   W 84.5
Comprehensive Health Insurance see Insurance,
    Major Medical
Comprehensive Health Planning see Regional Health
    Planning
Comprehensive Health Planning Agencies see Health
    Systems Agencies
Comprehensive Health Plans, Local see Health
    Systems Plans
Comprehensive Health Plans, State see State Health
    Plans
Compressed Air Disease see Decompression Sickness
Compression of the Brain see Brain Injuries
Compression of the Spinal Cord see Spinal Cord
    Compression
Compulsive Behavior   WM 176
    See also Obsessive–Compulsive Disorder   WM
     176
Compulsive Personality see Compulsive Personality
    Disorder
Compulsive Personality Disorder   WM 190
Compulsory Health Insurance see Insurance, Health
Computational Biology   QH 506
Computed Tomography Scanners, X–Ray see
    Tomography Scanners, X–Ray Computed
Computer Architecture see Computer Systems
Computer–Assisted Decision Making see Decision
    Making, Computer–Assisted
Computer–Assisted Diagnosis see Diagnosis,
    Computer–Assisted
Computer–Assisted Image Processing see Image
    Processing, Computer–Assisted
Computer–Assisted Instruction
    (Form number 18.2 in any NLM schedule where
     applicable)
    Embryology   QS 618.2
    General works   LB 1028.5
    Histology   QS 518.2
Computer–Assisted Radiotherapy see Radiotherapy,
    Computer–Assisted
Computer–Assisted Radiotherapy Planning see
    Radiotherapy Planning, Computer–Assisted
Computer–Assisted Therapy see Therapy,
    Computer–Assisted
Computer Communication Networks   TK
    5105.5–5105.9
    In medicine (General)   W 26.5
    In other special fields (Form number 26.5 in any
     NLM schedule where applicable)
    Used for special purposes, by subject
    See also Internet   TK 5105.875.I57, etc.
Computer Data Processing see Automatic Data
    Processing
Computer Graphics   T 385
Computer Hardware see Computers
Computer Literacy   QA 76.9.C64

Computer Models see Computer Simulation
Computer Network Management see Computer
 Communication Networks
Computer Programs see Software
Computer Reasoning see Artificial Intelligence
Computer Simulation   QA 76.9.C65
  Used for special purposes, by subject
Computer Software see Software
Computer Systems
  As equipment in special fields (Form number 26.5
   in any NLM schedule where applicable)
  Used for particular fields, by subject
Computer Systems Development see Computer
 Systems
Computer Systems Evaluation see Computer
 Systems
Computer Systems Organization see Computer
 Systems
Computer Terminals   TK 7887.8.T4
Computer User Training   QA 76.27
  In form number 26.5 in any NLM schedule where
   applicable
Computer Vision Systems see Artificial Intelligence
Computerized Emission Tomography see
 Tomography, Emission–Computed
Computerized Tomography, X–Ray see
 Tomography, X–Ray Computed
Computers   QA 75–76.95
  As equipment in special fields
   In medicine (General)   W 26.55.C7
   (Form number 26.5 in any other NLM schedule
    where applicable)
  Computer engineering   TK 7885–7895
  Digital   QA 76.5–76.73
  Machine theory   QA 267–268.5
  Space medicine   WD 751.6
  See also Automatic Data Processing   W
   26.55.A9, etc.; Information Systems   Z 699,
   etc.
Computers, Analog   QA 76.4
  As equipment in special fields
   In medicine (General)   W 26.55.C7
   (Form number 26.5 in any other NLM schedule
    where applicable)
  Computer engineering   TK 7885–7985
  See also Automatic Data Processing   W
   26.55.A9, etc.; Information Systems   Z 699,
   etc.
Computers, Digital see Computers
Computers, Personal see Microcomputers
Computing Methodologies
  In medicine (General)   W 26.5
  In other special fields (Form number 26.5 in any
   NLM schedule where applicable)
  Used for special purposes, by subject
Concanavalin A
  As antibodies   QW 575
  Diagnostic use, with disease being diagnosed, e.g.,
   in nephritis   WJ 353
  Other special topics, by subject
Concentration see Attention
Concentration Camps   HV 8963–8964
Concept Formation   BF 443

Child   WS 105.5.D2
Infant   WS 105.5.D2
Conception see Fertilization
Conchae Nasales see Turbinates
Concurrent Review   WX 153
Concurrent Studies see Cohort Studies
Concussion see Brain Concussion   WL 354 and
 other localized injuries, e.g. of the spinal cord
Condiments
  As a dietary supplement in health or disease
   WB 447
  Cookery   TX 819
Conditioned Reflexes see Conditioning, Classical
Conditioning, Classical   BF 319
Conditioning, Operant   BF 319.5.O6
Conditioning (Psychology)   BF 319
Conditioning Therapy see Behavior Therapy
Conditioning, Transplantation see Transplantation
 Conditioning
Condoms   WJ 710
Condoms, Female   WP 640
Conduct Disorder
  Adolescence   WS 463
  Adult   WM 190
  Child   WS 350.6
Conduct Disorders, Child see Child Behavior
 Disorders
Conduction Anesthesia see Anesthesia, Conduction
Conduction Blocking Anesthetics see Anesthetics,
 Local
Conduction of Nerve Impulses see Neural
 Conduction
Conductometry   QD 116.C65
  Clinical chemistry   QY 90
Condurango see Gastrointestinal Agents
Conferences see Congresses
Confidentiality
  Dentistry, Forensic   W 705
  United States   KF 8958–8959.5
  Medicolegal (General)   W 700
  Psychiatry, Forensic   W 740
Confined Spaces
  Related to occupational health   WA 400–495
  Special topics, by subject
  See also Air Pollutants, Occupational   WA 450;
   Ecological Systems, Closed   WD 756;
   Ventilation   WA 770, etc.
Conflict of Interest   W 50
  Economic aspects   W 58
Conflict (Psychology)
  Child   WS 105.5.M5
  Infant   WS 105.5.M5
  Interpersonal   BF 637.I48
  Psychoanalysis   WM 460.5.M6
  Social psychology   HM
Conformal Radiotherapy see Radiotherapy,
 Conformal
Conformity, Social see Social Conformity
Confusion
  Aged   WT 150
  Related to psychoses   WM 204
Congenital Anomalies see Abnormalities
Congenital Defects see Abnormalities

**ALWAYS CONSULT MAIN SCHEDULES. USE NUMBER ASSIGNED ONLY WHEN
SUBJECT REPRESENTS MAJOR EMPHASIS OF WORK BEING CLASSIFIED**

Congestive Cardiomyopathy see Cardiomyopathy,
   Congestive
Congestive Heart Failure see Heart Failure,
   Congestive
Congo Red   QV 240
Congo Virus Infection see Hemorrhagic Fever,
   Crimean
Congresses   W3
   Directories   W 3.5
   See also NLM Classification Practices, preceding
      the Schedules
Conjoined Twins see Twins, Conjoined
Conjugation, Genetic   QW 51
Conjugative Pili see Pili, Sex
Conjunctiva   WW 212-215
Conjunctival Diseases   WW 212
Conjunctivitis   WW 212
   Contagious granular see Trachoma   WW 215
Conjunctivitis, Acute Hemorrhagic   WW 212
Conjunctivitis, Allergic   WW 212
Conjunctivitis, Atopic see Conjunctivitis, Allergic
Conjunctivitis, Giant Papillary see Conjunctivitis,
   Allergic
Conjunctivitis, Inclusion   WW 212
Conjunctivitis, Vernal see Conjunctivitis, Allergic
Connecting Peptide see C-Peptide
Connective Tissue   QS 532.5.C7
   Aging   WT 104
Connective Tissue Cells   QS 532.5.C7
Connective Tissue Disease, Mixed see Mixed
   Connective Tissue Disease
Connective Tissue Diseases   WD 375
   See also names of specific diseases, e.g., Cellulitis
      WR 220
Conn's Disease see Hyperaldosteronism
Conradi-Hunermann Syndrome see
   Chondrodysplasia Punctata
Consanguinity
   Forensic medicine   W 791
   Marriage   HQ 1026
   Primitive customs   GN 480
   See also Inbreeding   SF 105, etc.
Conscience   BJ 1471
   Psychoanalysis   WM 460.5.R3
Conscious Sedation
   General works   WO 200
   Child   WO 460
   In dentistry   WO 460
   Infant   WO 440
Consciousness
   Child   WS 105.5.C7
   General diagnosis   WB 182
   Infant   WS 105.5.C7
   Neurologic manifestation of disease   WL 341
   Physiological aspects   WL 705
   Psychology   BF 309-499
   See also Unconsciousness   WB 182 etc.
Consciousness Disorders   WL 341
Consensus Development Conferences
   On specific topics, by subject
Consensus Development Conferences, NIH
   On specific topics, by subject
Consensus Sequence   QU 58

Consensus Workshops see Consensus Development
   Conferences
Conservation of Energy Resources   TJ 163.3-163.5
   In hospitals   WX 140
   Other special topics, by subject
Conservation of Natural Resources   S 900-954
   Forestry   SD 411-428
   Game and bird conservation and protection   SK
      351-579
   Nature   QH 75-77
   Wildlife   QL 81.5-84.77
   See also Ecology   QH 540-549, etc.
Constipation   WI 409
   Pregnancy   WQ 240
Constitution and Bylaws
   Special topics, by subject, e.g. in Hospital
      Administration   WX 150
Constitution, Body see Body Constitution
Constitutional Psychopathic Personality see
   Antisocial Personality Disorder
Constriction, Pathologic
   Of blood vessels   WG 560
   Of duodenum   WI 505
   Special topics, by subject
Constrictive Pericarditis see Pericarditis,
   Constrictive
Construction Loans see Financing, Construction
Construction Materials   TA 401-492
   Industrial wastes   WA 788
Consultants
   Medical   W 64
   Nursing   WY 90
   Psychiatric   WM 64
   Surgical   WO 64
   In other specific specialties in the number for
      interpersonal relationships or lacking that, in
      the general works number
Consultation see Referral and Consultation
Consumer Advocacy   WA 288
   Environmental control   WA 670-847
   General   HC 79.C63
   In special areas, by subject
Consumer Involvement see Consumer Participation
Consumer Organizations   HC 79.C6-79.C63
   By country   HC 94-1085 (with topical
      breakdown as given in HC 79, etc.)
   Consumer protection   HC 79.C63
      By country (as above)
   For community health planning   WA 546
   For special purposes, by subject
Consumer Participation
   In mental health planning   WM 30
   In special areas, in the administrative number for
      the area or lacking that, in the general number,
      e.g., in community health organizations   WA
      546
   See also Patient Participation   WX 158.5
Consumer Preference see Consumer Satisfaction
Consumer Price Index see Economics
Consumer Product Safety   WA 288
   Special topics, by subject
Consumer Protection see Accident Prevention;
   Consumer Organizations

**ALWAYS CONSULT MAIN SCHEDULES.   USE NUMBER ASSIGNED ONLY WHEN
SUBJECT REPRESENTS MAJOR EMPHASIS OF WORK BEING CLASSIFIED**

Consumer Satisfaction
    General works HF 5415.3–5415.5
    With hospitals WX 158.5
    With health services, medical treatment, etc.
      W 85
    With mental hospitals WM 29.5
    With other services or products, by subject
Consumption Coagulopathy see Disseminated
    Intravascular Coagulation
Contact Dermatitis see Dermatitis, Contact
Contact Lens Solutions WW 355
Contact Lenses WW 355
Contact Lenses, Extended–Wear WW 355
Contact Lenses, Hydrophilic WW 355
Contact Prevention in Illness see Communicable
    Disease Control; Patient Isolation; Quarantine
Contact Tracing
    Of particular disorders, with the disorder
Contactants as Allergens see Allergens
Contagious Diseases see Communicable Diseases
Contagious Pustular Dermatitis see Ecthyma,
    Contagious
Containment of Biohazards
    In the environment WA 671
    In genetic engineering QH 442
    In other areas, by subject
Contingent Negative Variation WL 102
Continued Stay Review see Concurrent Review
Continuing Care Retirement Centers see Housing for
    the Elderly
Continuity of Patient Care W 84.6
Continuum of Care see Continuity of Patient Care
Contour Perception see Form Perception
Contraception WP 630
    By prevention of ovulation WP 630
    Male WJ 710
    Religious aspects HQ 766.2
      Catholicism HQ 766.3
      Protestantism HQ 766.35
      Islam HQ 766.374
      Other HQ 766.4, A–Z
    Sociological aspects HQ 763–766
    See also Abortion WQ 225, etc.
Contraception Behavior
    General works HQ 766
Contraception, Immunologic WP 630
Contraceptive Agents QV 177
    See also specific topics under Contraception
Contraceptive Agents, Female QV 177
Contraceptive Agents, Male QV 177
Contraceptive Devices WP 640
Contraceptive Devices, Female WP 640
    See also Intrauterine Devices WP 640
Contraceptive Devices, Intrauterine see Intrauterine
    Devices
Contraceptive Devices, Male WJ 710
Contraceptives, Oral QV 177
Contraceptives, Oral, Combined QV 177
Contraceptives, Oral, Hormonal QV 177
Contraceptives, Oral, Sequential QV 177
Contraceptives, Oral, Synthetic QV 177
Contraceptives, Postcoital QV 177

Contract Services
    In medicine (General) W 74
    Other topics, class by subject if specific; if general,
      in economics number where available
    See also Outsourced Services W 74, etc.
Contracture
    Fingers, wrist see Volkmann's Contracture WE
    835
    Hand see Dupuytren's Contracture WE 830
    Hip see Hip Contracture WE 855
    Joint WE 300
    Muscle (General) WE 545
Contrast Media
    In radiology
      Supplies WN 150
      Technique of use WN 160
    Used for special purposes, by subject
Contrast Sensitivity WW 105
    As a measure of visual acuity WW 145
Controlled Clinical Trials
    Drugs QV 771
    For other purposes, by subject or specific drug
      or procedure
Controlled Clinical Trials, Randomized see
    Randomized Controlled Trials
Controlled Hypotension see Hypotension,
    Controlled
Controlled Vocabulary see Vocabulary, Controlled
Contusions WO 192
    First aid WA 292
    Localized, by site
Convalescence WB 545
    After surgery WO 183
    Convalescence from particular disorder, by the
      disorder
    Particular forms of convalescence, by subject
Convallaria QV 153
Convergence, Ocular WW 410
Convergent Strabismus see Esotropia
Conversion Disorder WM 173.5
Convulsants QV 103
Convulsions WL 340
    Child WL 340
    Drugs checking see Anticonvulsants QV 85
    In epilepsy WL 385
    In pregnancy see Eclampsia WQ 215
    Infant WL 340
    Veterinary SF 895
Convulsions, Febrile WL 340
Convulsive Disorders see Chorea; Epilepsy
Convulsive Therapy WM 410–412
    With pentylenetetrazole WM 410
Convulsive Therapy, Electric see Electroconvulsive
    Therapy
Cookery
    Army UC 720–735, UH 487
    Diabetic diet WK 819
    For hospitals WX 168
    Institutional (General) TX 820
    Navy VC 370–375
    Obesity diet see Diet, Reducing WD 210, etc.
    Therapeutic diet (General) WB 405
    See also names of specific diets and diseases for

which diet is being administered
Cooley's Anemia see Thalassemia
Coombs' Test   QY 265
    Diagnosis of erythroblastosis fetalis   WH 425
    Used for other special purposes, by subject
Coon's Technique see Fluorescent Antibody
    Technique
Cooperative Behavior   HM
COPD see Lung Diseases, Obstructive
Coping Behavior see Adaptation, Psychological
Copper   QV 65
    Metabolism   QU 130.5
Copulation   QL 761
    Human see Coitus
    Particular animals, in QL or SF number for the
        animal
Copying Processes   Z 265–265.5
Copyright   Z 551–656
Cor Pulmonale see Pulmonary Heart Disease
Coramine see 1 Nikethamide
Cord, Umbilical see Umbilical Cord
Cordials see Alcoholic Beverages
Corethamid see Nikethamide
Corium see Dermis
Corn
    As a dietary supplement in health or disease
        WB 430
    Cultivation   SB 191.M2, 351.C7
Cornea   WW 220
    Eye bank procedures   WW 170
    Transplantation   WW 220
Corneal Arcus see Arcus Senilis
Corneal Diseases   WW 220
Corneal Endothelium see Endothelium, Corneal
Corneal Epithelium see Epithelium, Corneal
Corneal Epithelium, Anterior see Epithelium,
    Corneal
Corneal Opacity   WW 220
Corneal Topography   WW 220
Corneal Transplantation   WW 220
Corneal Ulcer   WW 220
Corns see Callosities
Coronary Angioplasty, Transluminal Balloon see
    Angioplasty, Transluminal, Percutaneous
    Coronary
Coronary Arteries see Coronary Vessels
Coronary Arteriosclerosis   WG 300
Coronary Arteritis see Coronary   WG 300 under
    Arteritis
Coronary Artery Bypass   WG 169
Coronary Artery Disease see Coronary Disease
Coronary Artery Vasospasm see Coronary
    Vasospasm
Coronary Atherosclerosis see Coronary
    Arteriosclerosis
Coronary Care Units   WG 27–28
Coronary Circulation   WG 300
Coronary Disease   WG 300
    Popular works   WG 113
Coronary Embolism see Embolism
Coronary Heart Disease see Coronary Disease
Coronary Infarction see Myocardial Infarction
Coronary-Prone Personality see Type A Personality

Coronary Reperfusion see Myocardial Reperfusion
Coronary Thrombosis   WG 300
Coronary Vasospasm   WG 300
Coronary Vessel Anomalies   WG 220
Coronary Vessels   WG 300
Coronaviridae   QW 168.5.C8
Coroners and Medical Examiners   W 800
Coronoid Fossa see Humerus
Corpora Bigemina see Optic Lobe
Corpora Quadrigemina   WL 310
Corporate Practice see Professional Corporations
Corpses see Cadaver
Corpulence see Obesity
Corpus Callosum   WL 307
Corpus Cardiacum see Neurosecretory Systems
Corpus Luteum   WP 320
    Endocrine functions   WP 530
        See also Corpus Luteum Hormones   WP 530
Corpus Luteum Cyst see Ovarian Cysts
Corpus Luteum Hormones   WP 530
Corpus Pineale see Pineal Body
Corpus Striatum   WL 307
Corpuscles, Blood see Blood Cells; Erythrocytes;
    Leukocytes
Correspondence
    Physicians and specialists of medically related
        fields
        Collective   WZ 112–150
        Individual   WZ 100
    Special topics, by subject
Correspondence Courses see Education, Distance
Corridor Disease see Theileriasis
Corrosion   TA 462
    In dentistry   WU 180
    In orthopedics   WE 26
    In other areas, by subject
Corrosion Casting   QS 525
Corrosive Poisons see Poisons
Corset see Braces; Clothing
Cortex see Adrenal Cortex; Auditory Cortex;
    Cerebellar Cortex; Cerebral Cortex; Kidney
    Cortex; Motor Cortex; Somatosensory Cortex;
    Visual Cortex
Cortexone see Desoxycorticosterone
Cortical Depression, Spreading see Spreading
    Cortical Depression
Cortical Hormones see Adrenal Cortex Hormones
Corticoids see Adrenal Cortex Hormones
Corticospinal Tracts see Pyramidal Tracts
Corticosteroid Receptors see Receptors,
    Glucocorticoid
Corticosteroids see Adrenal Cortex Hormones
Corticosterone   WK 755
Corticotropin   WK 515
Corticotropin–Releasing Factor see
    Corticotropin–Releasing Hormone
Corticotropin–Releasing Hormone   WK 515
Corticotropin–Releasing Hormone–41 see
    Corticotropin–Releasing Hormone
Corti's Organ see Organ of Corti
Cortisol see Hydrocortisone
Cortisone   WK 755
Corynebacteriaceae see Actinomycetales

**ALWAYS CONSULT MAIN SCHEDULES. USE NUMBER ASSIGNED ONLY WHEN
SUBJECT REPRESENTS MAJOR EMPHASIS OF WORK BEING CLASSIFIED**

Corynebacterium   QW 118
Corynebacterium diphtheriae   QW 118
Corynebacterium Diphtheriae Toxin see Diphtheria
  Toxin
Corynebacterium Infections   WC 318–320
Coryneform Group   QW 118
Coryza, Acute see Common Cold
Coryza Viruses see Rhinovirus
Cosmetic Surgery see Surgery, Plastic
Cosmetic Techniques
  Surgical (General)   WO 600
    Skin   WR 650
    Specific location, by site
  Used for special purposes, by subject
  See also Reconstructive Surgical Procedures;
    Surgery, Plastic; names of specific procedures,
    e.g., Blepharoplasty   WW 205; Mammaplasty
      WP 910; Rhinoplasty   WV 312
Cosmetics
  Chemical technology   TP 983
  Public health aspects   WA 744
  See also Beauty Culture   QT 275, etc.
Cosmetics, Hair see Hair Preparations
Cosmetology see Beauty Culture
Cosmic Radiation   WN 415
  Adverse effects   WN 610–650
  Biophysics   QT 34
  Cosmic physics   QC 809.R3
  Medical safety measures   WN 650
  Radiation physics   QC 484.8–485.9
Cosmids   QW 51
  As genetic vectors   QH 442.2
Cost Allocation
  Medicine   W 74
  Other topics, class by subject if specific; if general,
    in economics number where available
Cost Apportionment see Cost Allocation
Cost–Benefit Analysis   HD 47.4
  Of particular procedures, by subject if specific,
    e.g., value of a diagnostic test   WB 141; if
    general, in economics number for the specialty,
    e.g., economics of medical practice   W 74;
    lacking an economics number, in the general
    number
Cost–Benefit Data see Cost–Benefit Analysis
Cost Containment see Cost Control
Cost Control
  General   HD 47.3
  Dentistry   WU 77
  Hospitals   WX 157
  Medicine   W 74
  Nursing   WY 77
  Pharmacy   QV 736
Cost Effectiveness see Cost–Benefit Analysis
Cost Shifting see Cost Allocation
Costen's Syndrome see Temporomandibular Joint
  Dysfunction Syndrome
Costs and Cost Analysis
  Dentistry   WU 77
  Hospitals   WX 157
  Medicine   W 74
  Nursing   WY 77
  Pharmacy   QV 736

Costs, Direct Service see Direct Service Costs
Cot Death see Sudden Infant Death
Cotton
  Agriculture   SB 245–251.5
  Diseases from dust   WF 654
  Industrial wastes   WA 788
    Control in work atmosphere   WA 450
  Used for special purposes, by subject
Cottonseed see Cottonseed Oil
Cottonseed Oil   WB 431
  As dietary protein
    In animal feed   SF 99.C6
    In human nutrition   WB 426
  Biochemistry   QU 86
Cough   WF 143
Coumaphos
  Agriculture   SB 952.P5
  Public health   WA 240
Coumarins   QV 193
Counseling   WM 55
  Adolescence   WS 462
  By nurses   WY 87
  Child   WS 105.5.C3
  Divorce   WM 55
  Genetic see Genetic Counseling   WZ 50, etc.;
  Infant   WS 105.5.C3
  Marriage   WM 55
  Pastoral care   WM 61
  Sex   WM 55
  Special population groups   WA 305, etc.
  Students   LB 1027.5–1027.9
    Extension. Adult education   LC 5225.C68
    Secondary education   LB 1620.4–1620.53
    Higher education   LB 2343
    (Form number 18 or other appropriate
    education number in any NLM schedule
    where applicable)
    See also Mental Health Services   WA
    352–353, etc.
  Vocational   HF 5381–5382.5
  Workers   HD 5549.5.C8
  Mental health   WA 495
Counseling, Sex see Sex Counseling
Counterimmunoelectrophoresis   QY 250–275
  Used for diagnostic monitoring, or evaluation
    tests in special fields, with the field
Counterirritants see Irritants
Counterirritation see Therapeutic Use under Irritants
Countertransference (Psychology)   WM 62
Couples Therapy   WM 430.5.M3
Coupling Factor 1 see H(+)-Transporting ATP
  Synthase
Court Plaster see Bandages
Courtship   HQ 801–801.5
  Animal   QL 761
Cowper's Glands see Bulbourethral Glands
Coxa see Hip
Coxa Plana see Legg–Perthes Disease
Coxarthrosis see Osteoarthritis, Hip
Coxiella   QW 150
Coxsackievirus Infections   WC 500
Coxsackieviruses   QW 168.5.P4
CPR see Cardiopulmonary Resuscitation

Crabs, Horseshoe see Horseshoe Crabs
Crackles see Respiratory Sounds
Cramp see Muscle Cramp
Cranial Base see Skull Base
Cranial Fossa, Posterior   WE 705
Cranial Nerve Diseases   WL 330
Cranial Nerve Neoplasms   WL 330
Cranial Nerves   WL 330
   See individual nerves under name of nerve
Cranial Sinus Thrombosis see Sinus Thrombosis
Cranial Sinuses   WG 625.C7
Cranial Sutures   WE 705
Craniofacial Abnormalities   WE 705
Craniofacial Dysostosis   WE 705
Craniology   GN 71-131
Craniomandibular Disorders   WU 140.5
Craniometry   GN 71-131
Craniopharyngioma   QZ 310
Craniosynostoses   WE 705
Craniotomy   WL 368
Cranium see Skull
Crataegus see Rosales
Crayfish   QX 463
CRD-401 see Diltiazem
Creatine   QU 61
Creatine Kinase   QU 141
Creatine Kinase Isoenzymes   QU 141
   Used for special purposes, by subject
Creatine Kinase Isozymes see Creatine Kinase
   Isoenzymes
Creatine Phosphate see Phosphocreatine
Creatine Phosphokinase see Creatine Kinase
Creatinine   QU 65
Creativeness   BF 408-426
   Adolescence   WS 462
   Child   WS 105.5.C7
   Infant   WS 105.5.C7
   In psychoanalysis   WM 460.5.C7
Credentialing
   (Form number 21 in any NLM schedule where
    applicable)
   Nursing   WY 16
   See also specific methods, e.g., Licensure,
    Medical   W 40
Credit and Collection, Patient see Patient Credit and
   Collection
Cremation see Mortuary Practice
Crenothrix see Bacteria
Creosote
   As an anti-infective agent   QV 223
   Toxicology   QV 627
Cresols
   As an anti-infective agent   QV 223
   Organic chemisty   QD 341.P5
Cresylic Acid see Cresols
Cretinism   WK 252
CRF-41 see Corticotropin-Releasing Hormone
Crib Death see Sudden Infant Death
Cribriform Plate see Ethmoid Bone
Cricetidae see Microtinae
Cricetinae see Hamsters
Cricetulus   QL 737.R666
   As laboratory animals   QY 60.R6

   As pets   SF 459.H3
Cricetus see Hamsters
Crigler-Najjar Syndrome   WD 205.5.H9
Crime   HV 6251-7220.5
   Compensation to victims   W 910
   Therapy for victims   WM 401
   Specific types, by subject
Crime Victims   HV 6250-6250.4
   Crisis intervention   WM 401
   Psychological aspects (General)   WM 165
Criminal Justice see Criminal Law
Criminal Law
   Psychiatric aspects   W 740
Criminal Psychology   HV 6080-6113
Criminal Violence Victims see Crime Victims
Criminology   HV 6001-9960
Crippled see Disabled
Crisis Intervention
   Community programs   WM 30
   General   WM 401
   Adolescence   WS 463
   Child   WS 350.2
   In preventing suicide   HV 6545
   See also Emergency Services, Psychiatric   WM
   401
Critical Care   WX 218
   Child   WS 366
    Administration of hospital unit   WS 27-28
   In emergencies (not in hospital)   WB 105
   Infant   WS 366
    Administration of hospital unit   WS 27-28
   Nursing   WY 154
    Pediatric   WY 159
   Of a particular disease or in a particular field
    General, with the disease or field
    Nursing, with the nursing specialty
Critical Illness
   General   WX 218
   Emergencies (not in hospital)   WB 105
    Pediatric   WS 205
   Nursing   WY 154
    Pediatric   WY 159
   A particular disease, with the disease
    Nursing, with the nursing specialty
Critical Pathways   W 84.7
   In nursing   WY 100
Criticism see Book Reviews
Crocodiles see Alligators and Crocodiles
Crohn Disease   WI 512
   Affecting the colon only   WI 522
Cromolyn Sodium   QV 120
Cronkhite-Canada Syndrome see Churg-Strauss
   Syndrome
Cross-Cultural Comparison
   Comparative civilization   CB 151
   Ethnology   GN 378
   Ethnopsychology   GN 270-279
   Mental development   WS 105
   Special topics by subject, e.g., Cross-National
    MMPI Research   WM 145
Cross-Eye see Strabismus
Cross Infection   WC 195
   Prevention and control in hospitals   WX 167

ALWAYS CONSULT MAIN SCHEDULES. USE NUMBER ASSIGNED ONLY WHEN
SUBJECT REPRESENTS MAJOR EMPHASIS OF WORK BEING CLASSIFIED

Cross–Linking Reagents
    Analytical chemistry QD 77
    Pharmaceutical chemistry QV 744
    Used for special purposes, by subject
Cross–Sectional Studies
    In epidemiology WA 105
    Special topics, by subject
Crossing Over (Genetics) QH 445
Crossmatching, Blood see Blood Grouping and Crossmatching
Crossmatching, Tissue see Histocompatibility Testing
Crotalid Venoms WD 410
Croton Oil QV 75
Croup WV 510
Crouzon's Disease see Craniofacial Dysostosis
Crowding
    Animal population QL 752
    Housing WA 795
    Human population HB 871
Crown Compounds see Ethers, Cyclic
Crowns WU 515
Cruciferae
    As dietary supplements in health and disease WB 430
    As medicinal plants QV 766
    Botany QK 495.C9
Crude Oil see Petroleum
Cruor see Postmortem Changes
Crush Injuries see Wounds and Injuries
Crush Syndrome
    Kidney failure WJ 342
    Wounds and injuries WO 700–820
Crustacea QX 463
Crutches WE 26
Crying
    Child WS 105.5.E5
    Emotions BF 575.C88
    Grief BF 575.G7
    Infant WS 105.5.E5
    Neuroses WM 170–184, etc.
Cryoablation see Cryosurgery
Cryoanesthesia see Hypothermia, Induced
Cryobiochemistry see Biochemistry; Freezing
Cryobiology see Freezing
Cryofixation see Cryopreservation
Cryogenic Surgery see Cryosurgery
Cryoglobulinemia WH 400
Cryopreservation QH 324.9.C7
Cryoprotective Agents
    In blood preservation WH 460
    In microbiology QW 25–26
    See also Freezing
Cryosurgery WO 510
    Used for special purposes, by subject
    See also Cryotherapy WB 473; Freezing WO 665, etc.
Cryotherapy WB 473
    Used for special purposes, by subject
    See also Cryosurgery WO 510
Cryptococcosis WC 475
Cryptococcus QW 180.5.D38
Cryptorchidism WJ 840

    Veterinary SF 871
Cryptorchism see Cryptorchidism
Cryptosporidiosis WC 730
    Veterinary SF 792
Cryptosporidium QX 123
Crystal Violet see Gentian Violet
Crystalline Lens see Lens, Crystalline
Crystallins WW 101
Crystallization
    Crystal structure and growth QD 921
    Pharmaceutical chemistry QV 744
    Physical and theoretical chemistry QD 548
    Other special topics, by subject
Crystallography QD 901–999
CTG, Antepartum see Cardiotocography
Cu–Zn Superoxide Dismutase see Superoxide Dismutase
Cuban Americans see Hispanic Americans
Cubital Fossa see Elbow; Humerus
Cues
    Conditioned response BF 319
    Prediction (Logic) BC 181
Culdoscopy WP 141
Culex QX 530
Culicidae QX 510–530
    See also Aedes QX 525; Anopheles QX 515; Culex QX 530
Culicoides see Ceratopogonidae
Cults, Medical see Alternative Medicine
Cultural Characteristics
    Special topics, by subject
Cultural Deprivation
    Adolescents WS 462
    Child WS 105.5.D3
    Education LC 4051–4100.4
    Infant WS 105.5.D3
Cultural Disadvantagement see Cultural Deprivation
Cultural Diversity
    Personnel management HF 5549.5.M5
    As social factor in public health WA 30
    Special topics, by subject
Cultural Evolution HM 106+
    Special topics, by subject
Culture CB
    Anthropology GN 301–499
    General works CB 23–113
    Sociology HM
Culture Media QW 25–26
Cultured Cells see Cells, Cultured
Cultured Tumor Cells see Tumor Cells, Cultured
Cumulative Survival Rate see Survival Rate
Cumulative Trauma Disorders WE 175
Cupping see Alternative Medicine
Curare QV 140
Curare–Like Agents see Neuromuscular Nondepolarizing Agents
Curariform Drugs see Neuromuscular Nondepolarizing Agents
Cures, Special see Alternative Medicine
Curettage WO 500
    Localized, by site
    See also Dilatation and Curettage WP 470, etc.
Curietherapy see Brachytherapy

Curiosities, Medical see Folklore; Superstitions
Curiosity see Exploratory Behavior
Curium   WN 420
   Nuclear physics   QC 796.C55
   See also special topics under Radioisotopes
Curriculum
   (Form number 18 in any NLM schedule where
    applicable)
   Education extension   LC 5219
   Elementary schools   LB 1570–1571
   Secondary schools   LB 1628–1629.8
   Universities and colleges   LB 2361–2365
   University extension   LC 6223
Curvatures, Spinal see Spinal Curvatures
Cushing Syndrome   WK 770
Cushion Liners see Denture Liners
Cuspid   WU 101
Custody, Child see Child Custody
Customized Drugs see Designer Drugs
Customs see Culture
Cutaneous Drug Administration see Administration,
   Cutaneous
Cutaneous Leishmaniasis see Leishmaniasis
Cutaneous Oximetry see Blood Gas Monitoring,
   Transcutaneous
Cutis Elastica see Ehlers–Danlos Syndrome
Cutting Wounds see Wounds, Penetrating
Cyanamide   QV 610
Cyanates   QV 280
Cyanidanol–3 see Catechin
Cyanides   QV 610
Cyanobacteria   QW 131
Cyanocobalamin see Vitamin B 12
Cyanophyceae see Cyanobacteria
Cyanosis   WG 142
Cybernetics   Q 300–390
   Used for special purposes, by subject
   See also Information Theory   Q 350–390
Cyclamates   WA 712
Cyclandelate   QV 243
Cyclic AMP   QU 57
   Pharmacology   QV 185
Cyclic GMP   QU 58
   Pharmacology   QV 185
Cyclic N–Oxides
   Organic chemistry   QD 401
Cyclicity see Periodicity
Cyclitis, Heterochromic see Iridocyclitis
Cycloamylose see Cyclodextrins
Cyclodextrins   QU 83
Cycloheptaamylose see Cyclodextrins
Cyclohexanes
   Organic chemistry   QD 305.H9
Cyclohexanones
   As carcinogens   QZ 202
   Toxicology   QV 633
Cycloheximide   QV 252
Cyclopentanes
   Organic chemistry   QD 305.H9
Cyclophosphamide   QV 269
   Cancer chemotherapy   QZ 267
   Immunosuppression   QW 920
Cycloplegics see Mydriatics

Cyclopropanes   QV 81
Cycloserine   QV 268
Cyclosporins   QW 920
Cyclostomes   QL 638.12–638.25
Cyclothymic Disorder   WM 171
Cyclothymic Personality see Cyclothymic Disorder
Cyclothymic Psychosis see Bipolar Disorder
Cylindroma see Carcinoma, Adenoid Cystic
Cyprinidae   SH 167.C3
   Anatomy and physiology   QL 638.C94
   Diseases   SH 179.C3
Cyprinus see Carp
Cyproheptadine   QV 157
Cyproterone   WJ 875
Cyprus Fever see Brucellosis
Cystadenocarcinoma   QZ 365
   Localized, by site
Cystadenoma   QZ 365
   Localized, by site
Cystadenoma Lymphomatosum, Papillary see
   Adenolymphoma
Cysteamine   QU 61
   As a radiation–protective agent   WN 650
   Organic chemistry   QD 305.A8
Cysteinamine see Cysteamine
Cysteine   QU 60
Cysteinyldopa   WK 725
   As a disease marker, class with the specific disease
Cystic Disease of Breast see Fibrocystic Disease of
   Breast
Cystic Duct   WI 750
Cystic Fibrosis   WI 820
Cysticercosis   WC 838
   Localized, by site
   Veterinary   SF 810.C5
Cysticercus   QX 400
Cystine   QU 60
Cystinosis   WJ 301
Cystitis   WJ 500
Cystocele see Bladder Diseases
Cystopyelitis see Pyelitis
Cystosarcoma Phyllodes see Phyllodes Tumor
Cystoscopes see Endoscopes
Cystoscopy   WJ 500
Cysts   QZ 200
   Bone see Bone Cyst   WE 258
   Breast   WP 840
   Dermoid see Dermoid Cyst   QZ 310
   Kidney see Kidney, Cystic   WJ 358
   Mediastinum see Mediastinal Cyst   WF 900
   Mesentery see Mesenteric Cyst   WI 500
   Nonodontogenic see Nonodontogenic Cysts
    WU 280
   Odontogenic see Odontogenic Cysts   WU 280
   Ovary see Ovarian Cysts   WP 322
   Pancreatic see Pancreatic Cyst   WI 810
   Periodontal see Periodontal Cyst   WU 240
   Pilonidal see Pilonidal Sinus   WE 750
   Radicular see Radicular Cyst   WU 240
   Sebaceous see Epidermal Cyst   WR 420
   Thyroglossal see Thyroglossal Cyst   WK 270
   Vaginal   WP 250
   Vulval   WP 200

Other localities, by site
Cysts, Hydatid see Echinococcosis
Cytarabine   QV 269
Cytidine Diphosphate Choline   QU 87
Cytidine Phosphates see Cytosine Nucleotides
Cytochemistry see Histocytochemistry
Cytochrome aa3 see Cytochrome–c Oxidase
Cytochrome–c Oxidase   QU 140
Cytochrome Oxidase see Cytochrome–c Oxidase
Cytochrome P–450(arom) see Aromatase
Cytochromes   WH 190
    Clinical examination   QY 455
Cytodiagnosis   QY 95
    Neoplasms   QZ 241
    Gynecology   WP 141
    Used for diagnosis of particular disorders, with
      the disorder or system
Cytofluorometry, Flow see Flow Cytometry
Cytogenetics   QH 441.5
    General   QH 441.5
    Human   QH 431
      Blood analysis   QY 402
      Predisposition to disease see Genetic
        Predisposition to Disease   QZ 50
Cytokeratin see Keratin
Cytokines   QW 568
Cytokinesis see Cell Division
Cytokinetics see Cell Cycle
Cytological Techniques   QH 585
    Clinical pathology   QY 95
Cytology   QH 573–671
    Cell pathology, with specific subject in NLM
      schedules
    See also Cells   QH 573–659, etc. and related
      headings
Cytolysins see Cytotoxins
Cytomegalic Inclusion Disease see Cytomegalovirus
    Infections
Cytomegalovirus   QW 165.5.H3
Cytomegalovirus Infections   WC 500
Cytometry, Flow see Flow Cytometry
Cytopathic Effect, Viral see Cytopathogenic Effect,
    Viral
Cytopathogenic Effect, Viral   QW 160
Cytophagales   QW 128
Cytophotometry   QH 585.5.C984
    Clinical pathology   QY 95
Cytoplasm   QH 591
Cytoplasmic Filaments see Cytoskeleton
Cytoplasmic Granules   QH 603.M35
Cytoplasmic Inclusions see Inclusion Bodies
Cytoprotection
    Pharmacology (General)   QV 38
    Special topics, by subject
Cytosine
    In nucleic acids   QU 58
Cytosine Arabinoside see Cytarabine
Cytosine Nucleotides   QU 57
Cytoskeletal Filaments see Cytoskeleton
Cytoskeletal Proteins   QU 55
Cytoskeleton   QH 603.C96
Cytosol Aminopeptidase see Leucyl Aminopeptidase
Cytostatic Agents see Antineoplastic Agents

Cytotaxinogens see Chemotactic Factors
Cytotaxins see Chemotactic Factors
Cytotoxic Antibiotics see Antibiotics, Antineoplastic
Cytotoxic Drugs see Antineoplastic Agents
Cytotoxic T–Lymphocytes see T–Lymphocytes,
    Cytotoxic
Cytotoxicity, Antibody–Dependent Cell see
    Antibody–Dependent Cell Cytotoxicity
Cytotoxicity, Immunologic   QW 568
Cytotoxicity Tests, Immunologic   QW 568
    Used for special purposes, by subject
Cytotoxin–Antibody Conjugates see Immunotoxins
Cytotoxins   QW 630.5.C9
    See also Antibiotics, Antineoplastic   QV 269;
      names of toxins specific to particular cells, e.g.,
      Enterotoxins   QW 630.5.E6
C1 Esterase Inhibitors see Complement 1
    Inactivators
C1 Inactivators see Complement 1 Inactivators
C3 Activator see Complement 3 Convertase
C3 Convertase see Complement 3 Convertase
C5 Cleaving Enzyme see Complement 3 Convertase

D

D–Amino–Acid Oxidase   QU 140
D–Glucuronolactone Dehydrogenase see Aldehyde
    Dehydrogenase
D 600 see Gallopamil
DAB see p–Dimethylaminoazobenzene
Dacryocystitis   WW 208
Dacryocystorhinostomy   WW 208
Dacryocystostomy see Dacryocystorhinostomy
Dactinomycin   QV 269
Dactylolysis Spontanea see Ainhum
Dairy Products   SF 250.5–275
    As dietary supplement in health or disease   WB
      428
    Bacteriology   QW 85
    Home economics   TX 759–759.5
    Sanitation   WA 715
Dairying   SF 221–250
    Public health aspects   WA 715–719
    Pasteurization   WA 719
Dall Porpoises see Porpoises
Danazol   WP 522
Dance Therapy   WM 450.5.D2
Dancing
    Injuries   WA 487.5.D4
    Physiological aspects   QT 255
Dandruff see Scalp Dermatoses
Dandy–Walker Syndrome   WL 350
Dane Particle see Hepatitis B Virus
Dangerous Behavior
    As a social behavior disorder   WM 600
    Adolescence   WS 463
    Child   WS 350.8.A4
    Infant   WS 350.8.A4
Dantrolene   QV 140
Dapsone   QV 259
Dark Adaptation   WW 109
Darkness
    Physiological effects   QT 162.L5

**ALWAYS CONSULT MAIN SCHEDULES. USE NUMBER ASSIGNED ONLY WHEN
SUBJECT REPRESENTS MAJOR EMPHASIS OF WORK BEING CLASSIFIED**

See also Nyctalopia   WD 110; Visual Perception
  WW 105
Data Analysis, Statistical see Data Interpretation,
  Statistical
Data Collection   WA 950
  For particular purposes, by subject
Data Display   TK 7882.I6
  (Form number 26.5 in any NLM schedule where
    applicable)
  Special topics, by subject
Data Interpretation, Statistical
  Special topics, by subject
Data Processing, Automatic see Automatic Data
  Processing
Data Systems see Information Systems
Database Management Systems   W 26.5
  Used for special purposes, by subject
Databases   Z 699–699.5
  By subject   Z 699.5.A–Z
  In medicine (General)   W 26.55.I4
  In other special fields (Form number 26.5 in any
    NLM schedule where applicable)
  See also Databases, Bibliographic   Z 699–699.5,
    etc.
Databases, Bibliographic   Z 699–699.5
  By subject   Z 699.5.A–Z
  In medicine (General)   W 26.55.I4
  In other special fields (Form number 26.5 in any
    NLM schedule where applicable)
Databases, Distributed see Computer
  Communication Networks
Datura see Stramonium
Day Blindness see Vision Disorders
Day Care
  Aged   WT 29
  Of the mentally ill   WM 29
  Of the physically ill and disabled   WX 29
  See also Child Day Care Centers   WA 310–320,
    etc.
Day Dreams see Fantasy
DDAVP see Desmopressin
DDD   WA 240
DDE   WA 240
DDT   WA 240
DDX see DDE
De Lange's Syndrome   QS 675
Dead Bodies see Cadaver
Deadly Nightshade see Belladonna
DEAE-Dextran   QU 83
Deaf see Hearing Impaired Persons
Deaf-Mutism see Deafness; Mutism
Deafness   WV 270–280
  Child   WV 271
  Infant   WV 271
  Rehabilitation
    Physical and medical aspects   WV 270–280
    Social aspects   HV 2353–2990.5
    See also Rehabilitation of Hearing Impaired
      WV 270–280, etc.
  Therapy   WV 276
Deafness, Conductive see Hearing Loss, Conductive
Deafness, Partial see Hearing Loss, Partial
Deafness, Sensorineural see Deafness

Deafness, Sudden   WV 270
Deamination   QD 281.A6
  Biochemistry   QU 25
Deamino Arginine Vasopressin see Desmopressin
Death
  Attitude see Attitude to Death   BF 789.D4
  Aged   WT 116
  Child   WS 200
  Infant   WS 200
  Legal establishment of   W 820
    See also Death certificates   WA 54
  Medicolegal aspects   W 800–867
  Registration   WA 54
  Speculative philosophy   BD 443.8–445
  Statistics see Mortality   HB 1321–1528, etc.
  See also Brain death   W 820; Fetal death   WQ
    225
Death Certificates   WA 54
Death Rate see Mortality
Death, Sudden   W 820
  Special topics, by subject, e.g., when associated
    with coronary disease   WG 300
  See also Death, Sudden, Cardiac   WG 205;
    Sudden Infant Death   WS 430
Death, Sudden, Cardiac   WG 205
Death with Dignity see Right to Die
Debridement   WO 700–820
  Localized, by site
Decalcification, Pathologic   WE 250
Decalcification Technique   QS 525
Decamethonium Compounds   QV 140
Decarboxylases see Carboxy-Lyases
Decay, Dental see Dental Caries
Decayed, Missing, and Filled Teeth see DMF Index
Deceleration   WD 720
Deception   BJ 1420–1428
  Applied psychology   BF 637.D42
  Adolescence   WS 463
  Child   WS 350.8.D2
  Infant   WS 350.8.D2
Decerebrate State   WL 340
Decidua   WQ 210
  Embryology   QS 645
Decidual Cell Reaction see Ovum Implantation
Decision Analysis see Decision Support Techniques
Decision Making   BF 448
  Adolescence   WS 462
  Child   WS 105.5.D2
  Infant   WS 105.5.D2
  Special topics, by subject, e.g., in local health
    administration   WA 546
Decision Making, Computer-Assisted
  In medicine (General)   W 26.55.D2
  In other special fields (Form number 26.5 in any
    NLM schedule where applicable)
  Used for special purpose, by subject
Decision Making, Organizational
  Management   HD 30.23
  Psychology   BF 448
  Special topics, by subject
Decision Modeling see Decision Support Techniques
Decision Support Systems, Clinical
  In medicine (General)   W 26.55.D2

In other special fields (Form number 26.5 in any
  NLM schedule where applicable)
  Used for special purpose, by subject
Decision Support Systems, Management   W 26.5
  In other areas, by subject
Decision Support Techniques
  Special topics, by subject, e.g., Diagnosis   WB
  141
Decision Theory
  In mathematical statistics   QA 279.4–279.7
  In special topics, by subject
Decision Trees
  In mathematical statistics   QA 279.4
  In special topics, by subject
Decoctions see Solutions
Decoloration, Drug see Drug Compounding
Decompression
  Aerospace medicine   WD 710
  Submarine medicine   WD 650
  Other special topics, by subject
Decompression, Explosive
  Aerospace medicine   WD 710
  Submarine medicine   WD 650
  Other special topics, by subject
Decompression Sickness
  Altitude effects   WD 712
  Aviation medicine   WD 712
  Diving problem   WD 650
  Submarine medicine   WD 650
Decompression, Surgical   WO 500
  Localized, by site
  For special purposes, by subject
Decongestants see Nasal Decongestants
Decontamination
  Chemical warfare agents   QV 663
  Radiation   WN 650
Decortication, Cerebral Cortex see Cerebral
  Decortication
Decubitus Ulcer   WR 598
Decussation, Pyramidal see Pyramidal Tracts
Dedications see Anniversaries and Special Events
Deductibles and Coinsurance
  Medical insurance   W 100–275
  See also specific types of insurance, e.g.
  Insurance, Health   W 100–275
Deer Fly Fever see Tularemia
Defecation   WI 600
  See also Encopresis   WI 600; Fecal incontinence
  WI 600
Defectives, Mental see Mental Retardation
Defects, Equipment see Equipment Failure
Defense Mechanisms   WM 193–193.5
  Child   WS 350.8.D3
  Infant   WS 350.8.D3
Defensive Medicine   W 44
  Dentistry   WU 44
  Nursing   WY 44
  (Form number 33 in any other NLM schedule
  where applicable)
Defensive Practice see Defensive Medicine
Deferoxamine   QV 183
Defibrillation, Electric see Electric Countershock
Defibrillators, Implantable   WG 330

Deficiency Diseases   WD 105–155
  Veterinary   SF 854–855
Defoliants, Chemical
  Plant culture   SB 951.4
  Public health aspects   WA 240
Deformities see Abnormalities
Degeneration see Atrophy; Hepatolenticular
  Degeneration; Lipoidosis; Nerve Degeneration;
  Retinal Degeneration
Degeneration, Social see Skid Row Alcoholics;
  Social Alienation; Social Behavior Disorders
Degenerative Processes in Disease see Disease
Deglutition   WI 102
Deglutition Disorders   WI 250
Degus see Rodentia
Dehydration
  Diagnostic significance   WB 158
  In water–electrolyte imbalance   WD 220
Dehydrocholesterol see Cholecalciferol
Dehydrocortisone see Prednisone
Dehydrogenases see Oxidoreductases
Dehydromethyltestosterone see Methandrostenolone
Deinstitutionalization   W 84.7
  See also Home Care Services   WY 115, etc.
Deja Vu   WM 173.7
Delayed–Action Preparations   QV 785
Delayed Effects, Prenatal Exposure see Prenatal
  Exposure Delayed Effects
Deletion (Genetics) see Chromosome Deletion
Delhi Sore see Leishmaniasis
Delirium
  Neurologic manifestations   WL 340
  Psychotic   WM 204
  Specific disease associations, with the disease
Delirium, Dementia, Amnestic, Cognitive Disorders
  Organic mental disorders   WM 140
  Organic mental disorders, psychotic   WM 220
  See also names of specific disorders, e.g., Amnesia
  WM 173.7; Cognition Disorders   WM 204,
  etc.,; Delirium   WL 340, etc.; Dementia
  WM 220, etc.
Delirium Tremens see Alcohol Withdrawal Delirium
Delivery   WQ 415
  Drugs affecting see Oxytocics   QV 173
  Methods   WQ 415–430
    Forceps   WQ 425
    See also Cesarean section   WQ 430
  Version   WQ 415
  Veterinary   SF 887
  See also Natural Childbirth   WQ 152; Home
  Childbirth   WQ 155
Delivery, Abdominal see Cesarean Section
Delivery, Home see Home Childbirth
Delivery of Dental Care see Delivery of Health Care
Delivery of Health Care   W 84
  In developing countries   WA 395
  In rural areas   WA 390
Delivery of Health Care, Integrated   W 84
Delphi Technique
  Research (Form number 20 or 20.5 in any NLM
  schedule where applicable)
  Used for particular purposes, by subject
Delta Agent see Hepatitis Delta Virus

Delta Hepatitis see Hepatitis D
Delta Infection see Hepatitis D
Delta Sleep–Inducing Peptide   WL 104
   Biochemistry   QU 68
Delta Superinfection see Hepatitis D
Delta Virus see Hepatitis Delta Virus
delta(9)–THC see Tetrahydrocannabinol
Deltavirus see Hepatitis Delta Virus
Delusions   WM 204
Dementia   WM 220
   Senile   WT 155
Dementia, Multi–Infarct   WM 220
Dementia Paralytica see Paresis
Dementia Praecox see Schizophrenia
Dementia, Presenile see Dementia
Dementia, Primary Degenerative, Senile see
   Dementia
Dementia, Senile see Dementia
Dementia, Vascular   WM 220
Demethyl Epipodophyllotoxin Ethylidine Glucoside
see Etoposide
Demography   HB 848–3697
Demulcents see Dermatologic Agents
Demyelinating Diseases
   General works   WL 140
   Manifestation of disease, with the disease
Demyelination see Demyelinating Diseases
Dendrites   WL 102.5
Dendritic Cells   QW 568
Dendritic Cells, Follicular see Dendritic Cells
Denervation   WL 368
Denervation, Autonomic see Autonomic
   Denervation
Denervation, Sympathetic see Sympathectomy
Dengue   WC 528
Dengue Fever see Dengue
Dengue Hemorrhagic Fever   WC 528
Dengue Shock Syndrome see Dengue Hemorrhagic
   Fever
Denial (Psychology)   WM 193.5.D3
   Adolescence   WS 463
   Child   WS 350.8.D3
   Infant   WS 350.8.D3
Densitometry
   Photometry (Optics)   QC 391
   Radiography   WN 160
     Technique in radiography of special systems
     with the radiography number for the system
     or disease being diagnosed
Dental Abrasion see Tooth Abrasion
Dental Acid Etching see Acid Etching, Dental
Dental Alloys   WU 180
Dental Amalgam   WU 180
Dental Anesthesia see Anesthesia, Dental
Dental Arch   WU 101
Dental Articulators   WU 26
Dental Assistants   WU 90
Dental Attrition see Tooth Attrition
Dental Attrition see Tooth Attrition
Dental Audit   WU 29
   Of a hospital dental service   WU 27
Dental Auxiliaries   WU 90
Dental Bonding   WU 190

Dental Bridgework see Denture, Partial
Dental Calculus   WU 250
Dental Care   WU 29
   Aged see Dental Care for Aged   WU 490
   For infants and children see Pediatric Dentistry
     WU 480
   School clinics see School Dentistry   WA
     350–351, etc.
Dental Care for Aged   WU 490
Dental Care for Children   WU 480
Dental Care for Chronically Ill   WU 460
Dental Care for Disabled   WU 470
Dental Care for Handicapped see Dental Care for
   Disabled
Dental Care Plans see Insurance, Dental
Dental Caries   WU 270
Dental Casting Investment   WU 180
Dental Casting Technique   WU 25
Dental Cavity Preparation   WU 350
Dental Cements   WU 190
   See also Silicate Cement   WU 190
Dental Cementum   WU 230
Dental Chemistry see Chemistry
Dental Clinics   WU 27–28
   School Dental Clinics   WA 350–351
Dental Crowns see Crowns
Dental Decay see Dental Caries
Dental Deposits   WU 250
Dental Digital Radiography see Radiography,
   Dental, Digital
Dental Economics see Economics, Dental
Dental Education see Education, Dental
Dental Education, Continuing see Education, Dental,
   Continuing
Dental Education, Graduate see Education, Dental,
   Graduate
Dental Enamel   WU 220
   See also Fluorosis, Dental   WU 220
Dental Enamel Solubility   WU 220
Dental Equipment   WU 26
Dental Facilities   WU 27–28
Dental Fillings, Permanent see Dental Restoration,
   Permanent
Dental Fillings, Temporary see Dental Restoration,
   Temporary
Dental Focal Infection see Focal Infection, Dental
Dental Granuloma see Periapical Granuloma
Dental Health Education see Health Education,
   Dental
Dental Health Services   WU 29
Dental Health Surveys   WU 30
Dental High–Speed Equipment   WU 26
Dental High–Speed Technique   WU 25
Dental Hygiene see Oral Hygiene
Dental Hygienists   WU 90
Dental Implantation   WU 640
Dental Implants   WU 640
Dental Implants, Single–Tooth   WU 640
Dental Impression Materials   WU 190
Dental Impression Technique   WU 25
Dental Infection Control see Infection Control,
   Dental
Dental Inlays see Inlays

ALWAYS CONSULT MAIN SCHEDULES. USE NUMBER ASSIGNED ONLY WHEN
SUBJECT REPRESENTS MAJOR EMPHASIS OF WORK BEING CLASSIFIED

Biography
  Collective   WZ 112.5.D3
  Individual   WZ 100
  Directories   WU 22
  Interprofessional and public relations   WU 61
  Licensure see Licensure, Dental   WU 40
  Supply & distribution   WU 77
Dentist's Practice Patterns   WU 29
Dentists, Women   WU 21
  See also special topics under Dentistry where
    applicable
Dentition   WU 210
Dentition, Adult see Dentition, Permanent
Dentition, Permanent   WU 210
Dentition, Secondary see Dentition, Permanent
Dentoalveolar Abscess, Apical see Periapical
  Abscess
Dentoalveolar Cyst see Periodontal Cyst
Denture Bases   WU 500
Denture, Complete   WU 530
Denture, Complete, Immediate   WU 530
Denture, Implant–Supported see Dental Prosthesis,
  Implant–Supported
Denture Liners   WU 500
Denture, Overlay   WU 515
Denture, Partial   WU 515
Denture, Partial, Fixed   WU 515
Denture, Partial, Immediate   WU 515
Denture, Partial, Removable   WU 515
Denture Precision Attachment   WU 515
Denture Retention   WU 500
Denture Stability see Denture Retention
Denture Wear see Dental Restoration Wear
Dentures see Dental Prosthesis   WU 500–530; types
  of dentures
Denturists   WU 150
Deodorants   WA 744
Deontological Ethics see Ethics
Deoxycorticosterone see Desoxycorticosterone
Deoxyephedrine see Methamphetamine
Deoxyglucose   QU 75
Deoxyribonucleases   QU 136
Deoxyribonucleic Acid see DNA
Deoxythymidine Kinase see Thymidine Kinase
Deoxyursocholic Acid see Ursodeoxycholic Acid
Dependency (Psychology)   BF 575.D34
Dependent Personality Disorder   WM 190
Depersonalization   WM 171
Depersonalization Disorder see Depersonalization
Depilation see Hair Removal
Depolarizing Muscle Relaxants see Neuromuscular
  Depolarizing Agents
Depot Preparations see Delayed–Action
  Preparations
Depreciation
  Hospital administration   WX 157
  Other topics, class by subject if specific; if general,
    in economics number where available
Deprenalin see Selegiline
Deprenil see Selegiline
Deprenyl see Selegiline
Depressants see Alcohols; Analgesics; Anesthetics;
  Anticonvulsants; Hypnotics and Sedatives; names

of specific depressants
Depression   WM 171
  Bipolar see Bipolar Disorder   WM 207
  Neurotic see Depressive Disorder   WM 171
Depression, Bipolar see Bipolar Disorder
Depression, Chemical   QV 38
Depression, Endogenous see Depressive Disorder
Depression, Involutional   WM 207
Depression, Neurotic see Depressive Disorder
Depression, Postpartum   WQ 500
Depression, Reactive see Adjustment Disorders
Depression, Unipolar see Depressive Disorder
Depressive Disorder   WM 171
  Psychotic   WM 207
Depressive Symptoms see Depression
Depressive Syndrome see Depressive Disorder
Deprivation see Names of types of deprivation, e.g.,
  Maternal Deprivation, Psychosocial Deprivation,
  Sleep Deprivation, etc.
Deprivation Diseases see Deficiency Diseases
Depth Intoxication see Inert Gas Narcosis
Depth Perception   WW 105
Dercum's disease see Adiposis Dolorosa
Derealization see Depersonalization
Dermabrasion   WO 600
Dermal Drug Administration see Administration,
  Cutaneous
Dermal Sinus see Spina Bifida Occulta
Dermatalgia see Skin Diseases
Dermatitis   WR 160–190
  General works   WR 160
  Occupational see Occupational Dermatitis   WR
  600
Dermatitis, Adverse Drug Reaction see Drug
  Eruptions
Dermatitis, Atopic   WR 160
  Veterinary   SF 901
Dermatitis, Contact   WR 175
Dermatitis, Contagious Pustular see Ecthyma,
  Contagious
Dermatitis, Eczematous see Eczema
Dermatitis, Exfoliative   WR 180
Dermatitis Herpetiformis   WR 200
Dermatitis Medicamentosa see Drug Eruptions
Dermatitis, Occupational   WR 600
Dermatitis, Radiation–Induced see Radiodermatitis
Dermatitis, Seborrheic   WR 415
Dermatitis Seborrheica see Dermatitis, Seborrheic
Dermatitis, Toxicodendron   WR 175
Dermatitis Venenata see Dermatitis, Contact
Dermato–neuroses see Neurodermatitis
Dermatoglyphics
  Anatomical structure   WR 101
  Criminal anthropometry   HV 6074–6078
  Physiological anthropology   GN 191–192
  Used for diagnosis of particular disorders, with
    the disorder, or system, e.g., of chromosome
    abnormalities   QS 677
Dermatologic Agents   QV 60–65
  Adsorbents   QV 63
  Demulcents   QV 63
  Emollients   QV 63
  Protectives   QV 63

**ALWAYS CONSULT MAIN SCHEDULES. USE NUMBER ASSIGNED ONLY WHEN
SUBJECT REPRESENTS MAJOR EMPHASIS OF WORK BEING CLASSIFIED**

See also Astringents   QV 65; Irritants   QV 65, etc.; Anti-Infective Agents, Local   QV 220–239
Dermatologists, Directories see Directories   WR 22 under Dermatology
Dermatology   WR
  Child   WS 260
  Directories   WR 22
  Infant   WS 260
  Nursing texts   WY 154.5
Dermatomycoses   WR 300–340
  General works   WR 300
  Veterinary   SF 901
Dermatomyositis   WE 544
Dermatophytes   QW 180.5.D3
Dermatophytoses see Dermatomycoses
Dermatoplasty see Skin Transplantation
Dermatosclerosis see Scleroderma, Circumscribed
Dermatoses see Skin Diseases
Dermatotoxins see Dermotoxins
Dermatotropic Virus Infections see Skin Diseases, Infectious
Dermis   WR 101
Dermoid see Dermoid Cyst
Dermoid Cyst   QZ 310
Dermotoxins   QW 630
Desensitization, Immunologic   QW 900
  For particular diseases of hypersensitivity, with the disease
Desensitization, Psychologic   WM 425.5.D4
  Adolescence   WS 463
  Child   WS 350.6
Desert Climate   QC 993.7
  Diseases of geographic areas   WB 710
  Physiological effects   QT 150
Desferrioxamine see Deferoxamine
Desiccated Stomach see Tissue Extracts
Desickling Agents see Antisickling Agents
Design and Construction, Hospital see Hospital Design and Construction
Design, Equipment see Equipment Design
Designer Drugs
  Abuse   WM 270
  General works   QV 55
  Pharmacology   QV 38
Desipramine   QV 77.5
Desmethylimipramine see Desipramine
Desmoid see Fibromatosis, Aggressive
Desmolases see Lyases
Desmopressin   WK 520
Desoxycorticosterone   WK 755
Desoxycortone see Desoxycorticosterone
Desoxyribonucleases see Deoxyribonucleases
Desoxyribonucleic Acid see DNA
Detachment, Choroid see Choroid
Detachment, Retinal see Retinal Detachment
Detergents   QV 233
Determination of Health Care Needs see Needs Assessment
Detoxication, Drug, Metabolic see Metabolic Detoxication, Drug
Deuterium   QV 275
  Inorganic chemistry   QD 181.H1

Deuteromycetes   QW 180.5.D38
Deuterons see Deuterium
Developing Countries
  Economics   HC 59.69–59.72
  Public health   WA 395
  Other special topics, by subject
Development see Bone Development; Child Development; Growth; Language Development; Maxillofacial Development; Personality Development; Psychosexual Development
Development, Urban see Urban Renewal
Developmental Biology   QH 491
  Genetics   QH 453
Developmental Bone Diseases see Bone Diseases, Developmental
Developmental Conditions as a Cause of Disease see Pathogenesis   QZ 45 under Growth Disorders
Developmental Coordination Disorder see Motor Skills Disorders
Developmental Delay Disorders see Developmental Disabilities
Developmental Disabilities   WS 350.6
  Adult (General)   WM 140
    Sociological aspects   HV 1570–1570.5
    See also Mentally Disabled Persons   LC 4815, etc.; Mental Retardation   WM 300–308, etc.
  Special topics, by subject
Deviant Behavior, Social see Social Behavior Disorders
Deviants, Sexual see Paraphilias
Device Design see Equipment Design
Device Failure see Equipment Failure
Device Safety see Equipment Safety
Devices see Equipment and Supplies
Dexamethasone   QV 60
Dexpropranolol see Propranolol
Dextranase   QU 136
Dextrans   WH 450
Dextrins   QU 83
dextro-Amino Acid Oxidase see D-Amino-Acid Oxidase
Dextrose see Glucose
Dextrosulfenidol see Thiamphenicol
DFP see Isoflurophate
Diabetes, Autoimmune see Diabetes Mellitus, Insulin-Dependent
Diabetes, Bronze see Hemochromatosis
Diabetes Insipidus   WK 550
Diabetes Mellitus   WK 810–850
  See also Obesity in Diabetes   WK 835; Pregnancy in Diabetes   WQ 248; Prediabetic State   WK 810
Diabetes Mellitus, Adult-Onset see Diabetes Mellitus, Non-Insulin-Dependent
Diabetes Mellitus, Brittle see Diabetes Mellitus, Insulin-Dependent
Diabetes Mellitus, Experimental   WK 810
Diabetes Mellitus, Insulin-Dependent   WK 810
Diabetes Mellitus, Juvenile-Onset see Diabetes Mellitus, Insulin-Dependent
Diabetes Mellitus, Ketosis-Prone see Diabetes Mellitus, Insulin-Dependent
Diabetes Mellitus, Ketosis-Resistant see Diabetes Mellitus, Non-Insulin-Dependent

Diabetes Mellitus, Non-Insulin-Dependent WK 810

Diabetes Mellitus, Stable see Diabetes Mellitus, Non-Insulin-Dependent

Diabetes Mellitus, Type 1 see Diabetes Mellitus, Insulin-Dependent

Diabetes Mellitus, Type 2 see Diabetes Mellitus, Non-Insulin-Dependent

Diabetic Acidosis see Acidosis, Diabetic

Diabetic Angiopathies WK 835

Diabetic Coma WK 830

Diabetic Diet WK 818–819

Diabetic Foot WK 835

Diabetic Ketoacidosis WK 830

Diabetic Ketosis see Diabetic Ketoacidosis

Diabetic Nephropathies WK 835

Diabetic Neuropathies WK 835

Diabetic Retinopathy WK 835

Diacetylmorphine see Heroin

Diagnosis WB 141–293
    Aged WT 141
    Breast diseases WP 815
    Cardiovascular diseases WG 141
    Child WS 141
    Ear diseases WV 210
    Endocrine diseases WK 140
    Eye diseases WW 141–145
    Gastrointestinal diseases WI 141
    Gynecologic diseases WP 141
    Infant WS 141
    Mental disorders WM 141
    Musculoskeletal system WE 141
    Neoplasms QZ 241
    Nervous system diseases WL 141
    Otorhinolaryngologic diseases WV 150
    Physical WB 200–288
      See also Physical Examination WB 205, etc.
    Pregnancy WQ 202
      See also Pregnancy Complications WQ 240; Pregnancy Tests QY 335; Sex Determination (Analysis) WQ 206
    Prenatal see Prenatal Diagnosis WQ 209
    Radioisotope WN 445
    Radioscopic see Fluoroscopy WN 220
    Respiratory tract diseases WF 141
    Signs and symptoms WB 143
    Skin diseases WR 141
    Thoracic diseases WF 975
    Tooth diseases WU 141
    Tuberculosis WF 220–225
    Urologic WJ 141
    For diagnosis of other diseases see specific headings below or general works number for disease, organ or system

Diagnosis, Computer-Assisted
    General WB 141
    Used for diagnosis of particular disorders, with the disorder or system

Diagnosis, Differential WB 141.5
    Child WS 141
    Infant WS 141

Diagnosis, Immunological see Immunologic Tests

Diagnosis, Laboratory see Laboratory Techniques and Procedures

Diagnosis, Nursing see Nursing Diagnosis

Diagnosis, Oral WU 141

Diagnosis, Prenatal see Prenatal Diagnosis

Diagnosis–Related Groups WX 157.8

Diagnosis, Surgical see Diagnostic Techniques, Surgical

Diagnostic Equipment
    (Form number 26 in any NLM schedule where applicable)
    General WB 26
    See also indentions under Equipment and Supplies; Equipment and Supplies, Hospital

Diagnostic Errors WB 141
    In special fields, in the diagnosis number for the field

Diagnostic Imaging WN 180
    Child WN 240
    Dental WN 230
    Infant WN 240
    Instrumentation WN 150

Diagnostic Reagent Kits see Reagent Kits, Diagnostic

Diagnostic Services WA 243

Diagnostic Skin Tests see Skin Tests

Diagnostic Techniques and Procedures
    General works WB 141
    Aged WT 141
    Child WS 141
    Infant WS 141
    See also Laboratory Techniques and Procedures QY, etc.; names of specific diagnostic techniques; and diagnostic techniques for specific organ systems, e.g., Diagnostic Techniques, Cardiovascular WG 141

Diagnostic Techniques, Cardiovascular WG 141
    See also specific diagnostic procedures, e.g., Angiocardiography WG 141.5.A3; Echocardiography WG 141.5.E2

Diagnostic Techniques, Digestive System WI 141

Diagnostic Techniques, Endocrine WK 140

Diagnostic Techniques, Neurological WL 141

Diagnostic Techniques, Obstetrical and Gynecological
    For gynecological conditions (General) WP 141
    For obstetrical conditions (General) WQ 202
      See also Pregnancy Complications WQ 240, etc.; Pregnancy Tests QY 335; Prenatal Diagnosis WQ 209

Diagnostic Techniques, Ophthalmological WW 141–145

Diagnostic Techniques, Otological WV 210

Diagnostic Techniques, Respiratory System WF 141

Diagnostic Techniques, Surgical WO 141

Diagnostic Techniques, Urological WJ 141

Diagnostic Tests, Routine WB 200
    Used for specific purposes, by subject

Diagnosticians, Directories see Directories W 22 under Medicine

Dialysis
    Biochemical technique QU 25

Organic chemistry (General)   QD 281.D47
 See also Hemodialysis   WJ 378, etc.
Dialysis, Extracorporeal see Hemodialysis
Diamine Oxidase see Amine Oxidase
 (Copper-Containing)
Diaminodiphenylsulfone see Dapsone
Diammonium Chloroplatinum Compounds
 Inorganic chemistry   QD 181.P8
 Pharmacology   QV 290
Diamond-Blackfan Anemia see Fanconi's Anemia
Diamorphine see Heroin
Diaper Pins see Infant Care
Diaper Rash   WS 420-430
Diapers, Infant see Infant Care
Diaphanography see Transillumination
Diaphanoscopy see Transillumination
Diaphorase see Lipoamide Dehydrogenase
Diaphoretics see Drugs for   QV 122 under
 Hypohidrosis
Diaphragm   WF 800-810
Diaphragmatic Eventration   WF 800
Diaphragmatic Hernia see Hernia, Diaphragmatic
Diaphragmatic Hernia, Traumatic see Hernia,
 Diaphragmatic, Traumatic
Diaphragmatic Paralysis see Respiratory Paralysis
Diaphyseal Aclasis see Exostoses, Multiple
 Hereditary
Diarrhea   WI 407
 Child   WS 312
 Infant   WS 312
 Veterinary   SF 851
Diarrhea, Infantile   WS 312
Diarsenol see Arsphenamine
Diastase see Amylase
Diastematomyelia see Spina Bifida Occulta
Diastole   WG 280
Diathermy   WB 510
 Surgical see Electrocoagulation   WO 198
Diathermy, Surgical see Electrocoagulation
Diathesis see Disease Susceptibility
Diathetic Disease see Disease Susceptibility
Diatrizoate
 As contrast medium   WN 160
 Organic chemistry   QD 341.A2
Diazepam   QV 77.9
Diazinon
 Public health   WA 240
Diazonium Compounds   QU 54
 Organic chemistry
  Aliphatic compounds   QD 305.A9
  Aromatic compounds   QD 341.A9
Diazoxide   QV 150
Dibekacin   QV 268
Dibenzazepines
 As antidepressive agents   QV 77.5
 Organic chemistry   QD 401
Dibothriocephalus see Diphyllobothrium
Dibucaine   QV 115
Dichlorodiethyl Sulfide see Mustard Gas   QV 666
 under Mustard Compounds
Dichlorodiphenyldichloroethane see DDD
Dichloroethanes see Ethylene Dichlorides

Dichloroethylenes
 Toxicology   QV 633
Dichloromethane see Methylene Chloride
Dichloromethyl Ether see Bis(Chloromethyl) Ether
Dichotic Listening Tests   WV 272
Diclofenac
 As an analgesic   QV 95
 Biochemistry   QU 98
Diclophenac see Diclofenac
Dicoumarin see Dicumarol
Dicrostonyx see Microtinae
Dictionaries
 (Form number 13 in any NLM schedule where
 applicable)
 Others, in appropriate LC number
Dictionaries, Chemical   QD 5
Dictionaries, Classical   DE 5
Dictionaries, Dental   WU 13
Dictionaries, Medical   W 13
Dictionaries, Pharmaceutic   QV 13
Dictionaries, Polyglot   P 361
 Of a specific subject, with the subject
Dictyocaulus   QX 248
Dictyoptera see Orthoptera
Dictyostelium   QW 180.5.M9
Dictyostelium discoideum see Dictyostelium
Dicumarol   QV 193
Didelphis see Opossums
Dideoxykanamycin B see Dibekacin
Dieldrin   WA 240
Diemal see Barbital
Diencephalon   WL 312
Diet   QT 235
 And oral health   WU 113.7
 Child   WS 115-130
 Diabetic see Diabetic Diet   WK 818-819
 In disease see Diet Therapy   WB 400-449
 Infant   WS 115-130
 Low sodium see Diet, Salt-Free   WB 424
 Raw food   WB 432
 See also Nutrition   QU 145; Vegetarianism
  WB 430; names of particular foods used in
  special diets; particular diseases for which diet
  is prescribed
Diet, Atherogenic   WG 550
Diet, Cariogenic   WU 113.7
Diet, Chemically Defined see Food, Formulated
Diet, Diabetic see Diabetic Diet
Diet, Elemental see Food, Formulated
Diet Fads   WB 449
Diet, Formula see Food, Formulated
Diet, Low-Salt see Diet, Sodium-Restricted
Diet, Macrobiotic   WB 422
Diet, Reducing   WD 210-212
 Popular works   WD 212
Diet, Salt-Free see Diet, Sodium-Restricted
Diet, Sodium-Restricted   WB 424
 Cookery   WB 424
Diet Surveys   QU 146
Diet, Synthetic see Food, Formulated
Diet Therapy   WB 400-449
 Child   WS 366
 Infant   WS 366

Dietary Calcium see Calcium, Dietary
Dietary Carbohydrates   QU 75
   As a supplement in health or disease   WB 427
   Cookery for carbohydrate control   WB 427
     See also Diet, Reducing   WD 210–212
Dietary Cholesterol see Cholesterol, Dietary
Dietary Fats   QU 86
   As a supplement in health or disease   WB 425
   Cookery for fat control   WB 425
   See also Butter   QU 86, etc.; Cholesterol,
     Dietary   QU 95, etc.; Diet, Reducing   WD
     210–212; Margarine   QU 86, etc.
Dietary Fats, Unsaturated   QU 86
   As a supplement in health or disease   WB 425
   Cookery for fat control   WB 425
Dietary Fiber   QU 83
   As a supplement in health or disease   WB 427
Dietary Formulations see Food, Formulated
Dietary Habits see Food Habits
Dietary Iron see Iron, Dietary
Dietary Modification see Food Habits
Dietary Oils see Dietary Fats, Unsaturated
Dietary Proteins   QU 55
   As a supplement in health or disease   WB 426
   Cookery for protein control   WB 426
Dietary Services
   Hospitals   WX 168
     See also Food Service, Hospital   WX 168
   Public health aspects   WA 695–722
   See also Dietetics   WB 400; Food Services
     WA 350, etc.
Dietary Sodium see Sodium, Dietary
Dietary Sucrose   QU 83
   As a sweetening agent   WA 712
Dietary Sugars see Dietary Sucrose
Dietary Supplementation see Dietary Supplements
Dietary Supplements   QU 145.5
   See also names of specific supplements, e.g.,
     Vitamins   QU 160–220, etc.
Dietetic Departments in Hospitals see Dietary
   Services; Food Service, Hospital
Dietetics   WB 400
   Child   WS 115
   Infant   WS 115
Diethyl Ether see Ether, Ethyl
Diethyldithiocarbamate see Ditiocarb
Diethylmalonylurea see Barbital
Diethylnicotinamid see Nikethamide
Diethylnitrosamine
   As a carcinogen   QZ 202
Diethylstilbestrol   WP 522
   Animal Feed   SF 98.H67
   Organic chemistry   QD 341.H9
Dietotherapy see Diet Therapy
Differential Diagnosis see Diagnosis, Differential
Differential Leukocyte Count see Leukocyte Count
Differential Thermal Analysis   QD 79.T38
   Of a particular substance, with the substance
Differentiation Antigens see Antigens,
   Differentiation
Differentiation Antigens, B–Cell see Antigens,
   Differentiation, B–Lymphocyte
Differentiation Antigens, B–Lymphocyte see

Antigens, Differentiation, B–Lymphocyte
Differentiation Antigens, Hairy Cell Leukemia see
   Antigens, Differentiation
Differentiation Antigens, Leukocyte, Human see
   Antigens, CD
Differentiation Markers see Antigens, Differentiation
Difficult Labor see Dystocia
Diffuse Lewy Body Disease see Parkinson Disease
Diffusion
   Biochemistry   QU 34
   Biophysics   QT 34
   Solution chemistry   QD 543
Diffusion of Innovation
   Special topics, by subject
Diflucortolone
   As a dermatologic agent   QV 60
Diflunisal   QV 95
   As a dermatological agent   QV 60
Digenic Acid see Kainic Acid
Digestants see Gastrointestinal Agents
Digestion   WI 102
   Liver function in   WJ 704
Digestive Physiology   WI 102
Digestive System   WI
   Animal   SF 851
   Child   WS 310
   Infant   WS 310
Digestive System Abnormalities   WI 101
   Child   WS 310
   Infant   WS 310
Digestive System Diseases   WI 140
   Child   310
   Diagnosis   WI 141
   Infant
   Signs and symptoms see Signs and Symptoms,
     Digestive   WI 143
   Surgery   WI 900
Digestive System Fistula   WI 140
Digestive System Neoplasms   WI 149
Digestive System Surgical Procedures   WI 900
Digital Radiography see Radiographic Image
   Enhancement
Digital Radiography, Dental see Radiography,
   Dental, Digital
Digital Signal Processing see Signal Processing,
   Computer–Assisted
Digitalis   QV 153
Dihydrodiethylstilbestrol see Hexestrol
Dihydrofolate Dehydrogenase see Tetrahydrofolate
   Dehydrogenase
Dihydrofolate Reductase see Tetrahydrofolate
   Dehydrogenase
Dihydrolipoamide Dehydrogenase see Lipoamide
   Dehydrogenase
Dihydrotachysterol   QU 95
Dihydroxycholecalciferols   QU 173
Dihydroxyphenylalanine see Dopa
Dihydroxyvitamins D see Dihydroxycholecalciferols
Diiodohydroxyquin see Iodoquinol
Diiodotyrosine Receptors see Receptors, Thyroid
   Hormone
Diisocyanatotoluene see Toluene 2,4–Diisocyanate
Diisopropylfluorophosphate see Isoflurophate

Dilatation
   Of the cervix
      Obstetrical surgery   WQ 400
      Physiology   WQ 305
   Of the pupil   WW 240
Dilatation and Curettage   WP 470
   Used for special purposes, by subject
Dilatation, Balloon see Balloon Dilatation
Dilatation, Pathologic
   Of the blood vessels   WG 578
   Of the colon see Megacolon   WI 528
   Of the heart see Heart Hypertrophy   WG 210
   Of the pupil   WW 240
   Of the stomach see Stomach Dilatation   WI 300
   Of other specific parts, with the part
Dilatation, Transluminal Arterial see Angioplasty,
   Balloon
Dilated Cardiomyopathy see Cardiomyopathy,
   Congestive
Diltiazem   QV 150
Dilution Techniques see Indicator Dilution
   Techniques
Dimenhydrinate   QV 73
Dimethoxystrychnine see Brucine
Dimethyl Sulfoxide   QV 60
Dimethylaminoazobenzene see
   p–Dimethylaminoazobenzene
Dimethylaminophenazone see Aminopyrine
Dimethylcysteine see Penicillamine
Dimethylguanylguanidine see Metformin
Dimexide see Dimethyl Sulfoxide
Dinitrochlorobenzene
   Toxicology   QV 633
Dinitrophenols
   As fungicides   WA 240, etc.
   Pharmaceutical indicators or reagents   QV 744
   Toxicology   QV 632
Dinoflagellida   QX 70
Dinoprost   QU 90
   As an abortifacient agent   QV 175
Diodone see Iodopyracet
Diodoquin see Diiodohydroxyquin
Diodoxyquinoline see Iodoquinol
Diosgenin
   Biochemistry   QU 85
Diothane Hydrochloride see Anesthetics, Local
Dioxanes   WA 240
   As a carcinogen   QZ 202
Dioxins
   Organic chemistry   QD 405
Dioxoles
   As pesticides   WA 240
   Organic chemistry   QD 405
Dipeptidyl Aminopeptidases see Dipeptidyl
   Peptidases
Dipeptidyl Peptidases   QU 136
Diphasic Milk Fever Virus see Encephalitis Viruses,
   Tick-Borne
Diphenhydramine   QV 157
Diphenhydramine Theoclate see Dimenhydrinate
Diphenyl Oxides see Phenyl Ethers
Diphenylamine
   Toxicology   QV 632

Diphenylbutazone see Phenylbutazone
Diphenylhydantoin see Phenytoin
Diphenylhydramin see Diphenhydramine
Diphosgene see Phosgene
Diphosphates   QV 285
Diphosphopyridine Nucleotide see NAD
Diphtheria   WC 320
Diphtheria Antitoxin   WC 320
Diphtheria Toxin   WC 320
Diphtheria Toxoid   WC 320
Diphtheria Vaccine see Diphtheria Toxoid
Diphyllobothrium   QX 400
Diploidy   QH 461
Diplopia   WW 410
Dipropyl Acetate see Valproic Acid
Diptera   QX 505
Dipylidiasis see Cestode Infections
Dipyridamole   QV 150
Dipyrine see Aminopyrine
Dipyrone   QV 95
Direct Service Costs
   By subject, in economics number where
      applicable
Directories
   (Form number 22 in any NLM schedule where
      applicable)
   Embryology   QS 622
   Forensic medicine   W 622
   Optometry   WW 722
   Pharmacies   QV 722
   Toxicology   QV 605
Dirofilaria immitis   QX 301
Dirofilariasis   WC 880
Disability Compensation see Veterans Disability
   Claims; Workers' Compensation
Disability Evaluation
   Medicolegal aspects of insurance   W 900
   Medicolegal aspects of occupational disease and
      injury   W 925
   Other special topics, by subject, e.g., in epilepsy
      WL 385; in ophthalmology   WW 32; in
      otolaryngology   WV 32
Disability Insurance see Medicare
Disabled Children
   Education   LC 4001–4806.5
   Psychological problems   WS 105.5.H2
   Readers for disabled children   PE 1126.D4
   Rehabilitation
      Mentally retarded   WS 107.5.R3
      Physically disabled   WS 368
Disabled Persons
   Consumer rights   HD 7255–7256
   Education
      Adults   LC 4812–4824
         Mentally disabled   LC 4815
         Socially disabled   LC 4822–4824
      Children see Education   LC 4001–4806.5
         under Disabled Children
   Psychological problems
      Group psychotherapy   WM 430.5.H2
      Adults
         Counseling   WM 55
         Special problems, by subject, e.g., Neurotic

ALWAYS CONSULT MAIN SCHEDULES. USE NUMBER ASSIGNED ONLY WHEN
SUBJECT REPRESENTS MAJOR EMPHASIS OF WORK BEING CLASSIFIED

Disorders   WM 170–184
Children see Psychological problems   WS
105.5.H2 under Disabled Children
Rehabilitation   WB 320
Adults   WB 320
Children see Rehabilitation   WS 368 under
Disabled Children
Sociological aspects only   HD 7255–7256
See also other entries under Rehabilitation;
names of disabilities
Sociological aspects   HV 1551–3024
Transportation
Mentally disabled   HV 3005.5
Physically disabled   HV 3022
Vocational guidance
Mentally disabled   HV 3005
Physically disabled   HV 3018–3019
See also Disabled Children; Mentally Disabled
Persons; Hearing Impaired Persons; Visually
Impaired Persons; names of specific disabilities
Disaccharides   QU 83
Disaster Planning   WX 185
See also special topics under Disasters
Disasters   HC 79.D45
First aid   WA 292
Hospital emergency service   WX 215
Hospital programs see Disaster Planning   WX
185
Medical emergencies   WB 105
Relief (General)   HV 553–555
Nursing   WY 154
Specific types of disaster, by subject
See also Civil Defense   UA 926–929, etc.
Discharge Planning see Patient Discharge
Disclosure, Truth see Truth Disclosure
Discolysis see Intervertebral Disk Chemolysis
Discrete Subaortic Stenosis see Aortic Valve
Stenosis
Discretionary Adjustment Factor see Prospective
Payment System
Discriminant Analysis   QA 278.65
Special topics, by subject
Discrimination Learning
Animal   QL 785
Educational psychology   LB 1059
General psychology   BF 318
Discrimination (Psychology)   BF 697
Racial see Prejudice   BF 575.P9
Sex see Women's Rights   HQ 1154, etc.
See also Race Relations   HT 1503–1595, etc.
Disease
General manifestations   QZ 140–190
Degenerative processes   QZ 180
Pathogenesis   QZ 40–109
Bacterial   QZ 65
Special topics, by subject, e.g., endocrine aspects
of disease processes   WK 140
Disease Frequency Surveys see Cross–Sectional
Studies
Disease Management   W 84.7
Disease Models, Animal   QY 58
Disease Outbreaks   WA 105
Cholera   WC 264

History   WA 11
Plague   WC 350–355
Smallpox   WC 590
Statistics and surveys   WA 900
Typhus   WC 610
Veterinary   SF 781
Yellow fever   WC 532
Disease Reservoirs   WA 106
Endemic to a particular locality   WB 710
Pathogenesis   QZ 40
Veterinary   SF 780.9
See also names of particular diseases
Disease Resistance see Immunity, Natural
Disease Susceptibility   QZ 50
Disease Vectors
Bacteriology   QW 700
Parasitology
Arthropod Vectors   QX 460, etc.
Insect Vectors   QX 650
Public health aspects   WA 110
See also Insect Control   QX 600
Diseases in Twins   QZ 50
Particular deseases, with the disease
Disgerminoma see Dysgerminoma
Disinfectants   QV 220–239
Disinfection
In hospitals   WX 165
In preventive medicine   WA 240
In surgery   WO 113
Disinfection, Hand see Handwashing
Disinfestation see Communicable Disease Control;
Ectoparasitic Infestations; Mite Infestations; Tick
Infestations
Disk, Herniated see Intervertebral Disk
Displacement
Disk, Intervertebral see Intervertebral Disk
Disk, Temporomandibular Joint see
Temporomandibular Joint Disk
Dislocation, Tooth see Tooth Avulsion
Dislocations   WE 175
Hip see Hip Dislocation   WE 860
Jaw   WU 610
Shoulder see Shoulder Dislocation   WE 810
Tooth see Tooth Avulsion   WU 158
Of other specific bones or joints, with the bone
or joint
Disodium Cromoglycate see Cromolyn Sodium
Disopyramide   QV 150
Dispensaries, Outpatient see Outpatient Clinics,
Hospital
Dispensatories   QV 740
Dispensing Fees see Prescription Fees
Dispensing, Pharmaceutical see Drug Compounding;
Pharmacy Service, Hospital; Pharmaceutical
Services
Displacement (Psychology)   WM 193.5.D5
Adolescence   WS 463
Child   WS 350.8.D3
Infant   WS 350.8.D3
Disposable Equipment   W 26
Disposal of the Dead see Cadaver; Mortuary
Practice
Disruptive Behavior Disorder see Attention Deficit

and Disruptive Behavior Disorders
Dissection   QS 130–132
   Veterinary   SF 762
Disseminated Intravascular Coagulation   WH 322
Dissertations, Academic
   General   Z 5053
   Presented to medical, dental, pharmacy, nursing,
   public health and veterinary schools or
   departments.
      American schools   W 4A
      Foreign schools   W4
Dissociation see Dissociative Disorders
Dissociative Disorders   WM 173.6
Dissociative Identity Disorder see Multiple
   Personality Disorder
Distance Education see Education, Distance
Distance Learning see Education, Distance
Distance Perception   WW 105
Distemper Virus, Canine   QW 168.5.P2
Distraction Osteogenesis see Osteogenesis,
   Distraction
Distributed Systems see Computer Communication
   Networks
Disulfides   QV 280
Disulfiram
   Organic chemistry   QD 305.S3
   Used in treatment of alcoholism   WM 274
   Used for other particular purposes, by subject.
Dithranol see Anthralin
Ditiocarb
   As a chelating agent   QV 290
Diuresis   WJ 303
Diuretics   QV 160
Diuretics, Mercurial   QV 160
Diuretics, Osmotic   QV 160
Diuretics, Sulfamyl   QV 160
Diurnal Rhythm see Circadian Rhythm
Divalproex see Valproic Acid
Divers' Paralysis see Decompression Sickness
Diverticulitis   WI 425
Diverticulitis, Colonic   WI 425
Diverticulosis see Diverticulum
Diverticulosis, Colonic   WI 425
Diverticulosis, Esophageal see Esophageal
   Diverticulum
Diverticulum   WI 425
Diving   QT 260.5.D6
   Accidents   QT 260.5.D6
   Anoxia associated with   WD 650
   Industrial accidents   WA 485
   Submarine and deep-water   VM 975–989
Divorce   HQ 811–960.7
   Counseling   WM 55
   Effect on adolescents   WS 462
   Effect on children   WS 105.5.F2
     See also Maternal Deprivation   WS 105.5.D3;
     Paternal Deprivation   WS 105.5.D3
Dixamon Bromide see Methantheline
Dizziness   WL 340
DMF Index   WU 30
DMSO see Dimethyl Sulfoxide
DNA   QU 58.5
DNA, Antisense   QU 58.5

DNA, Bacterial   QW 52
DNA-Binding Proteins   QU 58.5
DNA Cytosine-5-Methylase see DNA
   (Cytosine-5-)-Methyltransferase
DNA (Cytosine-5-)-Methyltransferase   QU 141
DNA Damage   QH 465
   By specific agent, A–Z, e.g., Chemicals   QH
   465.C5
DNA-Dependent RNA Polymerases see
   DNA-Directed RNA Polymerase
DNA-Directed DNA Polymerase   QU 141
DNA-Directed RNA Polymerase   QU 141
DNA, Double-Stranded see DNA
DNA Fingerprinting
   As a genetic technique   QH 441
   In forensic medicine   W 700–791
DNA Footprinting
   As a genetic technique   QH 441
DNA-Gyrase see DNA Topoisomerase
   (ATP-Hydrolysing)
DNA Helix Destabilizing Proteins see
   DNA-Binding Proteins
DNA Injury see DNA Damage
DNA Insertion Elements see DNA Transposable
   Elements
DNA Joinases see DNA Ligases
DNA Ligases   QU 138
DNA Markers see Genetic Markers
DNA Methylation   QU 58.5
DNA Mutational Analysis   QU 58.5
DNA, Neoplasm   QZ 200
DNA Nicking-Closing Protein see DNA
   Topoisomerase
DNA Nucleotidylexotransferase   QU 141
DNA Probes   QU 58.5
DNA Rearrangement see Gene Rearrangement
DNA, Recombinant   QU 58.5
   Genetic and ethical emphasis   QH 438.7
DNA Recombinant Proteins see Recombinant
   Proteins
DNA Relaxing Enzyme see DNA Topoisomerase
DNA Repair   QH 467
   Biochemistry   QU 58.5
DNA Repair Enzymes see DNA Ligases
DNA Replication   QH 462.D8
   Biochemistry   QU 58.5
DNA Restriction Enzymes   QU 136
DNA, Satellite   QU 58.5
DNA Sequence see Base Sequence
DNA Sequence Analysis see Sequence Analysis,
   DNA
DNA, Single-Stranded   QU 58.5
   Phages   QW 161
DNA Synthesis Inhibitors see Nucleic Acid
   Synthesis Inhibitors
DNA Topoisomerase   QU 58.5
DNA Topoisomerase (ATP-Hydrolysing)   QU 137
DNA Topoisomerase I see DNA Topoisomerase
DNA Topoisomerase II see DNA Topoisomerase
   (ATP-Hydrolysing)
DNA Transposable Elements   QH 462.I48
DNA Transposons see DNA Transposable Elements
DNA Tumor Viruses   QW 166
   Directory of research   QW 22

**ALWAYS CONSULT MAIN SCHEDULES. USE NUMBER ASSIGNED ONLY WHEN
SUBJECT REPRESENTS MAJOR EMPHASIS OF WORK BEING CLASSIFIED**

DNA Untwisting Enzyme see DNA Topoisomerase
DNA Untwisting Protein see DNA Topoisomerase
DNA Vaccines see Vaccines, DNA
DNA, Viral   QW 165
DNA Viruses
   General works   QW 165
   Specific viruses   QW 165.5A–Z
DNAase see Deoxyribonucleases
DNase see Deoxyribonucleases
DNCB see Dinitrochlorobenzene
Do–Not–Resuscitate Orders see Resuscitation
   Orders
Dobutamine
DOCA see Desoxycorticosterone
Docimasia, Pulmonary see Autopsy; Biogenesis
Docosenoic Acids see Erucic Acids
Doctor–Patient Relations see Physician–Patient
   Relations
Doctors see Physicians
Documentation   Z 1001
Documents, Serial see Periodicals
Dog Diseases   SF 991–992
Dog Heartworm see Dirofilaria immitis
Dogfish   QL 638.95.S84
Dogs
   As laboratory animals   QY 60.D6
   Domestic   SF 421–440.2
   Anatomy   SF 767.D6
   Wild   QL 737.C22
Dolphins   QL 737.C432
Domestic Medicine see Popular works   WB 120
   under Medicine; Self Medication
Domestic Violence
   Crime against the person   HV 6626–6626.23
   Forensic medicine   W 860
Domiciliary Care see Home Care Services
Dominance, Cerebral   WL 335
Dominance, Social see Social Dominance
Dominance–Subordination
   In animals   QL 775
   Sociology   HM
Donors, Living see Living Donors
Donovanosis see Granuloma Inguinale
Dopa   WK 725
Dopa Decarboxylase   QU 139
Dopamine   WK 725
Dopamine Agents   QV 76.5
Dopamine Agonists   QV 76.5
Dopamine Antagonists   QV 76.5
Dopamine Receptor Agonists see Dopamine
   Agonists
Dopamine Receptor Antagonists see Dopamine
   Antagonists
Dopamine Receptors see Receptors, Dopamine
Dopaminergic Agonists see Dopamine Agonists
Dopaminergic Antagonists see Dopamine
   Antagonists
Doping in Sports   QT 261
Doppler Echocardiography see Echocardiography,
   Doppler
Doppler Effect
   Biophysics   QT 34

   Health physics   WN 110
   Special topics, by subject
Doppler Shift see Doppler Effect
Doppler Ultrasound see Ultrasonics
Dormice see Rodentia
Dosage see Drug Administration Schedule; Drug
   Therapy; Prescriptions, Drug; Radiation Dosage;
   Radiotherapy Dosage
Dosage Forms   QV 785
   See also names of specific forms
Dose Fractionation
   Radioisotopes   WN 450
   Radium   WN 340
   X–rays   WN 250.5.X7
   See also Radiation Dosage   WN 665
Dose–Response Relationship, Drug   QV 38
Dose–Response Relationship, Radiation
   Non–ionizing radiation   WB 460
   Radioisotopes   WN 450
   Radium   WN 340
   X–rays   WN 250.5.X7
   Ultraviolet rays   WB 480
   Other specific types of radiation, by type
   Specific disease treated, with the disease
Dosimetric System of Therapeutics see Alternative
   Medicine
Dosimetry Calculations, Computer–Assisted see
   Radiotherapy Planning, Computer–Assisted
Dot Immunoblotting see Immunoblotting
Double Bind Theory
   In parent–child communication   WS 105.5.F2
   In psychotherapy   WM 420
   Other applications, by subject
Double–Stranded RNA see RNA, Double–Stranded
Double Vision see Diplopia
Down Syndrome   WS 107
   Adult   WM 300
Downsizing, Staff see Personnel Downsizing
Doxorubicin   QV 269
Doxylamine   QV 157
   As enzyme inhibitors   QU 143
   Organic chemistry   QD 401
   As sedatives   QV 85
DPN see NAD
Dracunculus   QX 203
Dracunculus medinensis see Dracunculus
Dragon Worm see Dracunculus
Drainage   WO 188
   Localized, by site
Drainage, Sanitary   WA 670
Drainage, Suction see Suction
Drama
   Related to medicine   WZ 330
   Related to psychiatry   WM 49
Drama Therapy in Psychiatry see Psychodrama
Drawings
   (Form number 17 in any NLM schedule where
    applicable)
Dreams
   Child   WS 105.5.D8
   Infant   WS 105.5.D8
   Parapsychology   BF 1074–1099
   Psychoanalysis   WM 460.5.D8

Sleep, Normal   WL 108
Dress see Clothing; Protective Clothing
Dressings see Bandages
Dressings, Biological see Biological Dressings
Dressings, Occlusive see Occlusive Dressings
Dressings, Surgical see Bandages; Occlusive
   Dressings
DRG see Diagnosis–Related Groups
Dried Milk see Dairy Products; Milk
Drill see Papio
Drinking   WI 102
   See also Alcohol Drinking   WM 274, etc.; Water
      Supply   WA 675–690
Drinking, Alcohol see Alcohol Drinking
Drinking Behavior
   Customs   GT 2850–2930
Drinks see Beverages
Drip Infusions see Infusions, Intravenous
Drive   BF 501–505
   Adolescence   WS 462
   Child   WS 105.5.M5
   Infant   WS 105.5.M5
   Psychoanalysis   WM 460.5.M6
Dromedary see Camels
Dropsy see Edema
Drosophila   QX 505
Drought see Natural Disasters
Drowning
   Resuscitation   WA 292
   Statistics   HB 1323.D7
   Swimming, accidents   QT 260.5.S9
Drowsiness see Sleep Stages
Drug Abuse see Substance–Related Disorders
Drug Abuse, Intravenous see Substance Abuse,
   Intravenous
Drug Abuse, Parenteral see Substance Abuse,
   Intravenous
Drug Abuse, Sports see Doping in Sports
Drug Abuse Testing see Substance Abuse Detection
Drug Action see Pharmacology; Drug Interactions;
   Dose–Response Relationship, Drug   QV 38 and
   other specific actions
Drug Addiction see Substance–Related Disorders
Drug Administration, Bladder see Administration,
   Intravesical
Drug Administration, Dermal see Administration,
   Cutaneous
Drug Administration, Inhalation see Administration,
   Inhalation
Drug Administration, Intranasal see Administration,
   Intranasal
Drug Administration, Oral see Administration, Oral
Drug Administration, Rectal see Administration,
   Rectal
Drug Administration, Respiratory see
   Administration, Inhalation
Drug Administration Routes   WB 340–356
Drug Administration Schedule   WB 340
Drug Administration, Topical see Administration,
   Topical
Drug Adulteration see Drug Contamination
Drug Aerosol Therapy see Administration,
   Inhalation

Drug and Narcotic Control
   Laws (sales)   QV 32–33
   Laws (use)   WM 32–33
   Sociological aspects   HV 5800–5840
   Special topics, by subject
Drug Antagonism   QV 38
Drug Approval   QV 771
Drug Benefit Plans see Insurance, Pharmaceutical
   Services
Drug Carriers   QV 785
Drug Catalogs see Catalogs, Drug
Drug Combinations   QV 785
   See also Drug Therapy, Combination   WB 330
      and names of specific drugs, or diseases for
      which the drug combinations are prescribed
Drug Combinations, Antineoplastic see
   Antineoplastic Agents, Combined
Drug Compounding   QV 778
Drug Containers and Closures see Drug Packaging
Drug Contamination
   Fraud   QV 773
   Legislation and jurisprudence   QV 32–33
   Public health aspects   WA 730
Drug Counterfeiting see Drug Contamination
Drug Delivery Systems, Implantable see Infusion
   Pumps, Implantable
Drug Dependence see Substance–Related Disorders
Drug Design   QV 744
Drug Detoxication, Metabolic see Metabolic
   Detoxication, Drug
Drug Eruptions   WR 165
Drug Evaluation   QV 771
   See also Drug Screening   QV 771
Drug Evaluation, Preclinical see Drug Screening
Drug Exanthems see Drug Eruptions
Drug Habituation see Substance–Related Disorders
Drug Hypersensitivity   WD 320
Drug Incompatibility   QV 746
Drug Industry   QV 736
   Fraud   QV 773
      See also Ethics, Pharmacy   QV 21
   Occupational medicine   WA 400–495
   Industrial waste   WA 788
Drug Information Services
   Computerized   QV 26.5
   Services in particular fields, by subject
Drug Infusion Systems see Infusion Pumps
Drug Insurance see Insurance, Pharmaceutical
   Services
Drug Interactions   QV 38
Drug Kinetics see Pharmacokinetics
Drug Labeling   QV 835
Drug Laws see Legislation, Drug
Drug Modeling see Drug Design
Drug Monitoring
   Of drugs administered therapeutically   WB 330
Drug Packaging   QV 825
Drug Potentiation see Drug Synergism
Drug Precursors see Prodrugs
Drug Recall see Drug and Narcotic Control
Drug Receptors see Receptors, Drug
Drug Regulations see Drug and Narcotic Control

ALWAYS CONSULT MAIN SCHEDULES.   USE NUMBER ASSIGNED ONLY WHEN
SUBJECT REPRESENTS MAJOR EMPHASIS OF WORK BEING CLASSIFIED

Drug Residues
    Food contamination   WA 701
    Public health   WA 730
Drug Resistance   WB 330
    In particular diseases, with the disease
Drug Resistance, Antineoplastic see Drug
    Resistance, Neoplasm
Drug Resistance, Microbial   QW 52
    In drug therapy   WB 330
    Of particular organisms, with the organism
    To particular drugs, with the drug
Drug Resistance, Neoplasm
    In drug therapy (General)   QZ 267
    In particular neoplasms, with the neoplasm
    See also Antineoplastic Agents   QV 269, etc.
Drug Screening   QV 771
    See also Drug Evaluation   QV 771
Drug Screening Assays, Antitumor
    Used in testing antineoplastic agents   QV 269
Drug Screening Tests, Tumor-Specific see Drug
    Screening Assays, Antitumor
Drug Sensitivity Assay, Microbial see Microbial
    Sensitivity Tests
Drug Stability   QV 754
Drug Storage   QV 754
    Public health aspects   WA 730
Drug Stores see Pharmacies
Drug Surveillance, Postmarketing see Product
    Surveillance, Postmarketing
Drug Synergism   QV 38
Drug Therapy   WB 330
    Adverse effects   QZ 42
    Aged   WT166
    Child   WS 366
    Infant   WS 366
    Mental Disorders   WM 402
        Child   WS 350.2
        Infant   WS 350.2
    Neoplasms   QZ 267
    Pregnancy   WQ 200
    Veterinary   SF 915–919.5
    For particular diseases, with the disease
Drug Therapy, Combination   WB 330
    Anti-neoplastic   QZ 267
    For other particular diseases, with the disease
    See also Drug Combinations   QV 785
Drug Tolerance   QV 38
Drug Toxicity   QZ 42
    Special topics, by subject
Drug Use Disorders see Substance-Related
    Disorders
Drug Utilization   WB 330
Drug Withdrawal Symptoms see Substance
    Withdrawal Syndrome
Drugs see Pharmaceutical Preparations
Drugs, Chinese Herbal   QV 767
    See also Medicine, Herbal   WB 925
Drugs, Essential
    General works   QV 704
    Economic aspects   QV 736
Drugs, Investigational   QV 771
Drugs, Non-Prescription   QV 772
Drugs of Abuse see Street Drugs

Drugs, Veterinary see Veterinary Drugs
Dry Eye Syndromes   WW 208
DSIP see Delta Sleep-Inducing Peptide
Dual Personality see Multiple Personality Disorder
Dubin–Johnson Syndrome see Jaundice, Chronic
    Idiopathic
Duchenne Muscular Dystrophy see Muscular
    Dystrophy
Ducks
    Anatomy   SF 767.P6
    Culture   SF 504.7–505.63
    Diseases
        Domestic and wild   SF 995.2
        Wild   SF 510.D8
Ductless Glands see Endocrine Glands
Ductus Arteriosus   WQ 210.5
Ductus Arteriosus, Patent   WG 220
Ductus Deferens see Vas Deferens
Due Process see Jurisprudence
Duffy Blood-Group System   WH 420
Duhring's Disease see Dermatitis Herpetiformis
Dumbness, Hysteric see Mutism
Dumping Syndrome   WI 380
Duncan's Syndrome see Lymphoproliferative
    Disorders
Duodenal Contents see Analysis   QY 130 under
    Duodenum
Duodenal Diseases   WI 505
Duodenal Neoplasms   WI 505
Duodenal Obstruction   WI 505
Duodenal Papilla, Major see Vater's Ampulla
Duodenal Papilla, Minor see Pancreatic Ducts
Duodenal Ulcer   WI 370
Duodenitis   WI 505
Duodenogastric Reflux   WI 302
Duodenoscopy   WI 505
Duodenum   WI 505
    Analysis   QY 130
    Feeding by see Tube Feeding   WB 410
Duplicating Processes see Copying Processes
Dupuytren's Contracture   WE 830
Dura Mater   WL 200
Durable Power of Attorney see Living Wills
Dwarfism   WE 250
    See also Cretinism   WK 252
Dwarfism, Pituitary   WK 550
Dwellings see Housing
Dye Dilution Technique   WG 141
    In hemodynamics   WG 106
Dye Exclusion Assays, Antitumor see Drug
    Screening Assays, Antitumor
Dyes
    As anti-infective agents   QV 235
    As reagents, indicators, etc.   QV 240
    Used in particular procedures, with the procedure
    See also Staining   QW 25, etc.
Dyes, Hair see Hair Dyes
Dynorphins   QU 68
Dysarthria   WL 340.2
    Psychogenic   WM 475
Dysautonomia see Autonomic Nervous System
    Diseases
Dysautonomia, Familial   WL 600

Dyschondroplasias see Osteochondrodysplasias
Dysembryoma see Teratoma
Dysentery   WC 280–285
    Veterinary   SF 809.D87
Dysentery, Amebic   WC 285
Dysentery, Bacillary   WC 282
Dysgammaglobulinemia   WD 308
Dysgerminoma   QZ 310
    Localized, by site
Dyskinesia see Movement Disorders
Dyskinesia, Drug–Induced   WL 390
Dyskinesia, Tardive see Dyskinesia, Drug–Induced
Dyslexia
    Neurologic   WL 340.6
    Psychogenic   WM 475.6
    Remedial teaching   LB 1050.5
Dyslexia, Acquired
    Neurologic   WL 340.6
    Psychogenic   WM 475.6
    Remedial teaching   LB 1050.5
Dyslexia, Congenital see Dyslexia
Dyslexia, Developmental see Dyslexia
Dysmenorrhea   WP 560
Dysmyelopoietic Syndromes see Myelodysplastic
    Syndromes
Dysostosis, Craniofacial see Craniofacial Dysostosis
Dyspareunia   WP 610
Dyspepsia   WI 145
Dysphagia see Deglutition Disorders
Dysphasia see Aphasia
Dysphonia see Voice Disorders
Dyspituitarism see Hyperpituitarism;
    Hypopituitarism
Dysplasia Epiphysialis Punctata see
    Chondrodysplasia Punctata
Dysplastic Nevus Syndrome   WR 500
    Pathology   QZ 310
Dyspnea   WF 143
Dyspnea, Paroxysmal   WG 370
Dyssocial Behavior see Antisocial Personality
    Disorder
Dysthymic Disorder   WM 171
    Psychotic   WM 207
Dystocia   WQ 310
Dystonia   WL 390
Dystonia Musculorum Deformans   WE 550
Dystrophic Skin Disorders see Skin Diseases   WR
    140, etc. or name of specific disorders, e.g.,
    Scleroderma, Circumscribed
Dystrophy, Progressive Muscular see Muscular
    Dystrophy

E

E Antigens see Hepatitis B e Antigens
E–B Virus see Herpesvirus 4, Human
E. coli Infections see Escherichia coli Infections
E–Mail see Computer Communication Networks
EAC142 see Complement 3 Convertase
Ear   WV 200–290
    Surgery   WV 200
Ear Canal   WV 222
Ear Deformities, Acquired   WV 220

Deformities of other than the external ear, by
    part
Ear Diseases   WV 200–290
    General works   WV 200
    Child   WV 200–290
    Infant   WV 200–290
    Nursing   WY 158.5
Ear Drum see Tympanic Membrane
Ear, External   WV 220–222
Ear, Inner see Labyrinth
Ear, Internal see Labyrinth
Ear, Middle   WV 230–233
Ear Molds see Hearing Aids
Ear Neoplasms   WV 290
    Localized, by site
Ear Ossicles   WV 230
Ear Protective Devices   WV 26
Ear Trumpets see Hearing Aids
Ear Wax see Cerumen
Early Gene Transcription see Transcription, Genetic
Earthquakes see Natural Disasters
Earthworms see Oligochaeta
East Coast Fever see Theileriasis
Eating Behavior see Feeding Behavior
Eating Disorders
    Child   WS 130
    Infant   WS 120
    Manifestation of disease   WI 143
    Psychophysiological   WM 175
Ebola Hemorrhagic Fever see Hemorrhagic Fever,
    Ebola
Ebola Virus Disease see Hemorrhagic Fever, Ebola
Ebstein's Anomaly   WG 220
EBV see Herpesvirus 4, Human
EBV Infections see Epstein–Barr Virus Infections
EC Cells see Tumor Stem Cells
EC–IC Arterial Bypass see Cerebral
    Revascularization
Eccentro–Osteochondrodysplasia see
    Mucopolysaccharidosis IV
Eccrine Glands   WR 400
Ecdysone   SF 768.3
    Zoology   QL 868
ECG see Electrocardiography
Echinococcosis   WC 840
    Veterinary   SF 810.H8
Echinococcosis, Hepatic   WI 700
Echinococcosis, Hepatic Alveolar see
    Echinococcosis, Hepatic
Echinococcosis, Pulmonary   WF 600
Echinococcus   QX 442
Echinopanax see Ginseng
Echo–Endoscopy see Endosonography
Echo Viruses see Echoviruses
Echocardiography   WG 141.5.E2
Echocardiography, Continuous Doppler see
    Echocardiography, Doppler
Echocardiography, Contrast see Echocardiography
Echocardiography, Cross–Sectional see
    Echocardiography
Echocardiography, Doppler   WG 141.5.E2
Echocardiography, Doppler, Color   WG 141.5.E2
Echocardiography, Doppler, Pulsed   WG 141.5.E2

Echocardiography, Four–Dimensional   WG 141.5.E2

Echocardiography, M–Mode see Echocardiography

Echocardiography, Three–Dimensional   WG 141.5.E2

Echocardiography, Transesophageal   WG 141.5.E2

Echocardiography, Two–Dimensional see Echocardiography

Echocardiography, Two–Dimensional Doppler see Echocardiography, Doppler

Echoencephalography   WL 154

Echography see Ultrasonography

Echolalia   WM 475

Echolocation   QL 782.5

Echothiophate Iodide   QV 124

Echoviruses   QW 168.5.P4

Eck Fistula see Portacaval Shunt, Surgical

Eclampsia   WQ 215

Eclecticism   WB 920

Eco DNA Topoisomerase II see DNA Topoisomerase (ATP–Hydrolysing)

Ecological Monitoring see Environmental Monitoring

Ecological Systems, Closed   WD 756

Ecology
 General and animal   QH 540–549.5
 Human   GF
  General works   GF 31–48
 Plant   QK 901–938

Economic Competition
 By subject, in economics number where applicable

Economic Factors see Socioeconomic Factors

Economic Inflation see Inflation, Economic

Economics
 Land, agriculture, industry   HD
  General works   HD 31–37
 National production   HC
  General works   HC 21
 Pharmacy   QV 736
 Theory   HB
  General works   HB 151–181

Economics, Dental   WU 77–79

Economics, Hospital   WX 157

Economics, Medical   W 74–80

Economics, Nursing   WY 77

Economics, Pharmaceutical   QV 736

Ecosystem see Ecology

Ecothiopate Iodide see Echothiophate Iodide

ECT (Psychotherapy) see Electroconvulsive Therapy

Ectasia, Alveolar see Pulmonary Emphysema

Ecthyma   WR 225

Ecthyma, Contagious   WC 584

Ectodermal Defect, Congenital see Ectodermal Dysplasia

Ectodermal Dysplasia   WR 218

Ectogenesis   WQ 205

Ectohormones see Pheromones

Ectoparasitic Infestations   WC 900
 Disinfestation   WC 900
 Veterinary   SF 810

Ectopia Cordis see Heart Defects, Congenital

Ectopic Hormone Syndromes see Neoplastic Endocrine–Like Syndromes

Ectopic Pregnancy see Pregnancy, Ectopic

Ectropion   WW 205

Eczema   WR 190
 Veterinary   SF 901

Eczema, Atopic see Dermatitis, Atopic

Eczema, Contact see Dermatitis, Contact

Eczema, Dyshidrotic   WR 200

Eczema, Infantile see Dermatitis, Atopic

Eczema, Vesicular Palmoplantar see Eczema, Dyshidrotic

Edathamil see Edetic Acid

Edema
 Angioneurotic see Angioneurotic Edema   WR 170
 Brain see Brain Edema   WL 348
 Bronchial   WF 500
 Diagnostic significance   WB 158
 Drugs affecting   QV 160
 Laryngeal see Laryngeal Edema   WV 500
 Lymph see Lymphedema   WH 700, etc.
 Manifestation of Disease   QZ 170
 Optic papilla see Papilledema   WW 280
 Pulmonary see Pulmonary Edema   WF 600
 See also names of body parts with which the edema is associated

Edema, Cardiac   WG 370

Edema–Proteinuria–Hypertension Gestosis see Gestosis, EPH

Edentata see Xenarthra

Edetates see Edetic Acid

Edetic Acid   QV 276

EDTA see Edetic Acid

Education
 (Form number 18 in any NLM schedule where applicable)
 Elementary   LB 1555–1602
 Health see Health Education   WA 590, etc.; Health Education, Dental   WU 113
 Higher   LB 2300–2430
 Physical see Physical Education and Training   QT 255
 Safety   WA 250
 Secondary   LB 1603–1696.6
 Sex see Sex Education   QT 225, etc.
 Vocational see Vocational Education   LC 1041–1048
 See also subheading Education under names of disabilities, specialties, etc.

Education, Competency–Based see Competency–Based Education

Education, Continuing   LC 5201–6660.4
 See also specific continuing education terms, e.g., Education, Dental, Continuing; Education, Medical, Continuing; Education, Pharmacy, Continuing; etc.

Education, Dental   WU 18

Education, Dental, Continuing   WU 20

Education, Dental, Graduate   WU 20

Education, Dental Health see Health Education, Dental

Education, Distance
(Form number 18 in any NLM schedule where applicable)
In particular subjects, by subject
Education, Graduate   LB 2371-2372
Education, Health see Health Education
Education, Medical   W 18
Education, Medical, Continuing   W 20
In psychiatry   WM 19.5
Education, Medical, Graduate   W 20
In psychiatry   WM 19.5
Education, Medical, Undergraduate   W 18
Education, Nursing   WY 18
See also Education   WY 18.8 under Nursing, Practical
Education, Nursing, Associate   WY 18
Education, Nursing, Baccalaureate   WY 18
Education, Nursing, Continuing   WY 18.5
Education, Nursing, Diploma Programs   WY 18
Education, Nursing, Graduate   WY 18.5
Education of Mentally Defective see Education of Mentally Retarded
Education of Mentally Retarded   LC 4601-4640.4
Sex education   HQ 54.3
Health education   LC 4613
Education of Patients see Patient Education
Education, Pharmacy   QV 18
Education, Pharmacy, Continuing   QV 20
Education, Pharmacy, Graduate   QV 20
Education, Predental   WU 18
Education, Premedical   W 18
Education Research, Nursing see Nursing Education Research
Education, Sex see Sex Education
Education, Special
Blind children   HV 1618-2349
Children with behavior disorders   LC 4801-4803
Deaf children   HV 2417-2990.5
Disabled adults   LC 4812-4824
Disabled children   LC 4001-4043
Mentally ill children   LC 4165-4184
Mentally retarded children see Education of Mentally Retarded   LC 4601-4640.4
Other ill children   LC 4580-4599
Physically disabled children   LC 4201-4243
Slow learning or under achieving children   LC 4661-4700.4
Socially disabled children   LC 4051-4100.4
See also subheading Education under names of disabilities, specialties, etc.
Education, Veterinary   SF 756.3-756.37
Educational Achievement see Educational Status
Educational Measurement   LB 3051-3060.87
In a particular field
Works about (Form number 18 in any NLM schedule where applicable)
Actual tests (Form number 18.2 in any NLM schedule where applicable)
Other special topics, by subject
Educational Needs Assessment see Needs Assessment

Educational Status
General official reports, by country   L 111-791
School surveys   LB 2823
Relation to special topics, by subject
Special classes of people   LC 1390-5160.3
Educational Technology   LB 1028.3
Special topics, by subject
Educational Therapy in Psychiatry see Occupational Therapy; Education of Mentally Retarded
EEG see Electroencephalography
Eel, Congo see Urodela
Efficiency
Industrial   T 58.8
Use of time   BF 637.T5
Effort see Exertion
Effort Syndrome see Neurocirculatory Asthenia
EGF-URO Receptors see Receptors, Epidermal Growth Factor-Urogastrone
Egg see Ovum
Egg Proteins   QU 55
In diet therapy   WB 426
Egg Shell Proteins see Egg Proteins
Egg White Proteins see Egg Proteins
Egg Yolk Proteins see Egg Proteins
Eggs
As a dietary supplement in health and disease
Cholesterol content   WB 425
Protein content   WB 426
See also Egg Proteins   QU 55
Sanitary handling   WA 703
Ego
Child psychology   WS 105.5.S3
Psychoanalysis   WM 460.5.E3
See also Self Concept   BF 697, etc.
Ehlers-Danlos Syndrome   WR 218
Ehrlichia   QW 150
Eicosanoids   QU 90
Eidetic Imagery   WL 705
Eigenmannia see Electric Fish
Ejaculation
Physiology   WJ 750
Psychological disorders   WM 611
Ejaculatory Ducts   WJ 750
Ejection Seats   WD 740
EKG see Electrocardiography
Elaeophoriasis see Filariasis
Elastic Stockings see Bandages
Elastic Tissue   QS 532.5.E5
Elastica see Rubber
Elasticity   QC 191
Of arteries, bones, etc. in general   QT 34
Of specific organs or parts, by subject
Of a particular material, with material
Elastin   QU 55
Elastomers see Rubber
Elastomers, Silicone see Silicone Elastomers
Elbow   WE 820
Elbow Joint   WE 820
Elder Abuse   HV 6626.3
For the aged being abused   WT 30
For the abusers' aggressive behavior   WM 600
Elderly see Aged
Elderly, Frail see Frail Elderly

ALWAYS CONSULT MAIN SCHEDULES. USE NUMBER ASSIGNED ONLY WHEN SUBJECT REPRESENTS MAJOR EMPHASIS OF WORK BEING CLASSIFIED

Electric Anesthesia see Electronarcosis
Electric Burns see Burns, Electric
Electric Conductance, Skin see Galvanic Skin
   Response
Electric Conductivity
   Human   QT 34
   Physics   QC 610.3–612
Electric Countershock   WG 330
Electric Fish   QL 639.1
   As laboratory animals   QY 60.F4
Electric Injuries   WD 602
   Industrial   WA 485
   See also Burns, Electric   WO 704
Electric Organ
   In fishes   QL 639.1
Electric Power Plants see Power Plants
Electric Shock see Electric Injuries;
   Electroconvulsive Therapy; Electroshock
Electric Stimulation
   Neurophysiology   WL 102
   Therapeutic use see Electric Stimulation Therapy
     WB 495
   Diagnostic use see Electrodiagnosis   WB 141
Electric Stimulation Therapy   WB 495
   See also Electroconvulsive Therapy   WM 412
Electric Stimulation, Transcutaneous see
   Transcutaneous Electric Nerve Stimulation
Electricity
   Adverse effects   WD 602
     See also Electric Injuries   WD 602
   Atmospheric   QC 960.5–969
     See also Lightning   WD 602, etc.
   Death by (Medicolegal aspects)   W 843
   Physics   QC 501–718.8
     Electric currents   QC 601–625
Electroacoustic Impedance Tests see Acoustic
   Impedance Tests
Electroacupuncture   WB 369
Electroanalgesia see Transcutaneous Electric Nerve
   Stimulation
Electroanesthesia see Electronarcosis
Electrocardiography   WG 140
   Child   WS 290
   Infant   WS 290
   Veterinary   SF 811
Electrocardiography, Ambulatory   WG 140
Electrocardiography, Dynamic see
   Electrocardiography, Ambulatory
Electrocardiography, Holter see
   Electrocardiography, Ambulatory
Electrocautery see Electrocoagulation
Electrochemistry   QD 551–575
   Electrochemical analysis   QD 115
   Industrial   TP 250–261
   Organic compounds   QD 273
Electrocoagulation   WO 198
Electrocochleography see Audiometry, Evoked
   Response
Electroconvulsive Therapy   WM 412
   See also Electroshock   WM 25
Electrocution, Accidental see Electric Injuries
Electrodeposition see Electroplating
Electrodermal Response see Galvanic Skin Response

Electrodes   QD 571
   Biomedical engineering   QT 36
   In electric stimulation therapy   WB 495
   Used for special purposes, by subject, e.g., in
     Urinalysis   QY 185
   See also Microelectrodes   QT 36, etc.
Electrodes, Enzyme see Biosensing Techniques
Electrodes, Miniaturized see Microelectrodes
Electrodiagnosis   WB 141
   Used for diagnosis of particular disorders, with
     the disorder or system
Electroencephalography   WL 150
Electroencephalography, Alpha Rhythm see Alpha
   Rhythm
Electrofocusing see Isoelectric Focusing
Electrogalvanism, Intraoral   WU 180
Electrohydraulic Shockwave Lithotripsy see
   Lithotripsy
Electroimmunoblotting see Immunoblotting
Electroimmunodiffusion Test see Immunodiffusion
Electrokymography   WN 100
   Cardiovascular   WG 141.5.K9
   Used for diagnosis of particular disorders, with
     the disorder or system
Electrolysis   QD 551–575
   In electrotherapy   WB 495
   In hair removal   WR 450
   Special topics, by subject
Electrolytes   QV 270
   Analytical chemistry   QD 139.E4
   Bacteriology   QW 52
   Electrochemistry   QD 565
   Physiological effects (General)   QT 162.E4
   See also Water–Electrolyte Balance   QU 105;
     Water–Electrolyte Imbalance   WD 220
Electrolytic Depilation see Hair Removal
Electromagnetic Energy see Radiation
Electromagnetic Fields
   Biophysics   QT 34
   Physics   QC 665.E4
Electromagnetic Radiation see Radiation
Electromagnetic Radiation, Ionizing see Radiation,
   Ionizing
Electromagnetic Radiation, Nonionizing see
   Radiation, Nonionizing
Electromagnetic Waves see Radiation
Electromagnetics
   Biophysics   QT 34
   Electromyography   WE 500
Electromyography   WE 500
   Special topics, by subject
Electron Microscope see Microscopy, Electron
Electron Microscopy see Microscopy, Electron
Electron Microscopy, Transmission see Microscopy,
   Electron
Electron Nuclear Double Resonance see Electron
   Spin Resonance Spectroscopy
Electron Paramagnetic Resonance see Electron Spin
   Resonance Spectroscopy
Electron Probe Microanalysis
   Qualitative analysis   QD 98.E4
   Quantitative analysis   QD 117.E42
   Special topics, by subject

Electron Spin Resonance Spectroscopy
    Biological research
        General   QH 324.9.E36
        Medically oriented   QT 34
    Chemistry   QD 455.2
    Used for special purposes, by subject
Electron Theory, Roentgenographic see Health
    Physics
Electron Transport   QU 125
Electronarcosis
    Anesthesiology   WO 275
    Psychiatry   WM 412
Electronic Data Processing see Automatic Data
    Processing
Electronic Mail see Computer Communication
    Networks
Electronics   TK 7800-8360
Electronics, Medical   QT 34
    See also Biomedical Engineering   QT 36
Electrons   WN 415-450
    In general nuclear physics   QC
    793.5.E62-793.5.E629
    In health physics   WN 110
Electronystagmography   WW 410
Electrooculography   WW 143
Electrophoresis
    Analytical chemistry (General)   QD 79.E44
    Biology   QH 324.9.E4
        Medically oriented   QU 25
    Microbiology   QW 25
    Organic chemistry (General)   QD 272.E43
    Quantitative analysis   QD 117.E45
    Used for other special purposes, by subject
    See also Blood Protein Electrophoresis   QY 455;
        Isoelectric focusing   QW 25, etc.
Electrophoresis, Agar Gel   QU 25
    Special topics, by subject
Electrophoresis, Agarose Gel see Electrophoresis,
    Agar Gel
Electrophoresis, Capillary   QU 25
    Analytical chemistry (General)   QD 79.E44
    Biotechnology   TP 248.25.C37
    Used for special purposes, by subject
Electrophoresis, Gel, Two-Dimensional   QU 25
    Special topics, by subject
Electrophysiology   QT 34
    Animals (General)   QP 341
        Domestic   SF 768
        Wild   QP 341
    Biology (General)   QH 517
    Nervous system   WL 102
    Plants   QK 845
    Other systems involved, in physiology number
    for the system or part
Electroplating   TS 670-693
Electroretinography   WW 270
Electroshock   WM 25
    See also Electric injuries   WD 602;
        Electroconvulsive therapy   WM 412
Electroshock Therapy see Electroconvulsive
    Therapy
Electrosleep see Electronarcosis
Electrosurgery   WO 198

    Dental   WU 600
Electrosyneresis see Counterimmunoelectrophoresis
Electrotherapy see Electric Stimulation Therapy
Electroversion, Cardiac see Electric Countershock
Elements
    Biochemistry   QU 130
    Inorganic chemistry   QD 181
    Non-metallic (pharmacology)   QV 138
    Physical chemistry   QD 466-469
    See also Isotopes   QD 181, etc.; Radioisotopes
        WN 420, etc. and specific chemical elements
Elements, Radioactive
    General works   WN 420
    See also specific radioactive elements, e.g.,
        Radium   WN 300-340
Elephantiasis   WH 700
Elephantiasis, Bancroftian see Elephantiasis, Filarial
Elephantiasis, Filarial   WC 880
Elephants   QL 737.P98
    Diseases   SF 997.5.E4
Eligibility Determination
    For Medicaid   W 250
    For Medicare   WT 31
    Medicolegal aspects
        Of insurance   W 900
        Of occupational disease & injury   W 925
    Eligibility for other benefits and services, by
        subject
    See also Disability Evaluation, W 900, etc.
ELISA see Enzyme-Linked Immunosorbent Assay
Elixirs, Pharmacy see Pharmaceutic Aids
Emaciation   WB 146
    Malnutrition   WD 100, etc.
    Metabolic diseases   WD 200
Emasculation see Castration
Embalming   WA 844
Emblems and Insignia
    In medicine and related fields   WZ 334
    Seals   CD 5005-6471
Embolic Tumor Cells see Neoplasm Circulating
    Cells
Embolism   QZ 170
    Arterial   WG 540
    Cerebral see Cerebral Embolism and Thrombosis
        WL 355
    Coronary   WG 300
    Pulmonary see Pulmonary Embolism   WG 420
    Venous   WG 610
Embolism, Air   QZ 170
    As an effect of high altitude   WD 710
    In decompression sickness   WD 712
    In other disorders, with the disorder
Embolism, Amniotic Fluid   WQ 244
Embolism, Fat   QZ 170
Embolism, Gas see Embolism, Air
Embolism, Paradoxical   WG 540
Embolism, Tumor see Neoplasm Circulating Cells
Embolization, Therapeutic
    General works   WH 310
    Performed in interventional radiology   WN 200
    Used for the control of operative hemorrhage
        WO 500
    Used for particular diseases, with the disease

**ALWAYS CONSULT MAIN SCHEDULES. USE NUMBER ASSIGNED ONLY WHEN
SUBJECT REPRESENTS MAJOR EMPHASIS OF WORK BEING CLASSIFIED**

See also Hemostasis, Surgical   WO 500, etc.;
   Hemostatic Techniques   WH 310
Embolus see Embolism
Embryo   QS 604
   Animals
      Domestic   SF 767.5
      Wild animals   QL 971
      Specific animals, with the animal
Embryo, Chick see Chick Embryo
Embryo Cloning see Cloning, Organism
Embryo Development see Fetal Development
Embryo Transfer
   Human   WQ 208
Embryologists, Directories see Directories   QS 622
   under Embryology
Embryology   QS 604–681
   Directories   QS 622
   Domestic animals   SF 767.5
   Experimental   QS 604
   Gynecology   WP 150
   Twinning   QS 642
      See also Twins   WQ 235, etc.; Pregnancy,
        Multiple   WQ 235
   Zoology   QL 951–991
   See also special topics under Anatomy
   Localized, by site
Embryonal Carcinoma Cells see Tumor Stem Cells
Embryonic Induction   QH 607
Embryonic Structures   QS 604
Embryopathies see Fetal Diseases
Embryos, Plant see Seeds
Embryotomy   WQ 435
Embryotoxins see Teratogens
Emergencies
   General   WB 105
   Cardiac   WG 205
   Child   WS 205
   Dental (General)   WU 105
   First aid   WA 292
   Infant   WS 205
   Medical see Emergency Medicine   WB 105
   Surgical   WO 700–820
   Veterinary (General)   SF 778
   Veterinary surgery   SF 914.3–914.4
   See also Crisis Intervention   WM 401, etc.
Emergency Care see Emergency Medical Services
Emergency Care Information Systems see
   Information Systems
Emergency Health Services see Emergency Medical
   Services
Emergency Medical Service Communication
   Systems see Emergency Medical Services   WX
   215, etc.
Emergency Medical Services   WX 215
   Occupational   WA 412
   See also Emergency Services, Psychiatric   WM
      401; Emergency Service, Hospital   WX 215;
      names of particular types of service, e.g., Mobile
      Health Units   WX 190
Emergency Medical Tags   W 26
Emergency Medical Technicians   W 21.5
   Services provided   WX 215
Emergency Medicine   WB 105

Child   WS 205
Infant   WS 205
Emergency Mobile Units see Ambulances
Emergency Nursing   WY 154
Emergency Outpatient Unit see Emergency Service,
   Hospital
Emergency Service, Hospital   WX 215
Emergency Services, Psychiatric   WM 401
Emergency Surgery see Surgery
Emergency Treatment
   General   WB 105
   Cardiac   WG 205
   Child   WS 205
   Dental (General)   WU 105
   First aid   WA 292
   Infant   WS 205
   Surgical   WO 700–820
   Veterinary (General)   SF 778
   Veterinary surgery   SF 914.3–914.4
   For specific emergencies, with the emergency,
      injury, disease, or organ system involved
   See also Crisis Intervention   WM 401, etc.;
      Emergencies   WG 205, etc.; Emergency
      Medical Services   WX 215, etc.
Emergicenters see Emergency Medical Services
Emerogenes see Genes, Suppressor, Tumor
Emetics   QV 73
Emetine   QV 255
Emigration and Immigration   JV 6008–6348
   Emigration   JV 6061–6149
   General works   JV 6008–6049
   Immigration   JV 6201–6348
   Of health manpower   W 76
   See also Transients and Migrants   WA 300, etc.
Emmenagogues see Menstruation–Inducing Agents
Emollients   QV 63
Emotional Bonds see Object Attachment
Emotional Disturbances see Affective Symptoms
Emotional Maladjustment see Affective Symptoms
Emotional Stress see Stress, Psychological
Emotions   BF 531–593
   Adolescence   WS 462
   Child   WS 105.5.E5
   Disorders see Affective Symptoms   WS 350.6,
      etc.
   Infant   WS 105.5.E5
   Physiology   WL 103
Empathy   BF 575.E55
   Adolescence   WS 462
   Child   WS 105.5.E5
   Infant   WS 105.5.E5
Emphysema   QZ 140
   Mediastinal see Mediastinal Emphysema   WF
      900
   Pulmonary see Pulmonary Emphysema   WF 648
Emphysema, Mediastinal see Mediastinal
   Emphysema
Emphysema, Pulmonary see Pulmonary Emphysema
Empiricism
   Medical philosophy
      History (Ancient)   WZ 51
Employee Assistance Programs (Health Care) see
   Occupational Health Services

ALWAYS CONSULT MAIN SCHEDULES. USE NUMBER ASSIGNED ONLY WHEN
SUBJECT REPRESENTS MAJOR EMPHASIS OF WORK BEING CLASSIFIED

Employee Discipline
    Hospital   WX 159
    Nursing   WY 30
    Psychiatry   WM 30
    In other areas, by subject
Employee Grievances
    Hospital   WX 159
    Nursing   WY 30
    Psychiatry   WM 30
    In other areas, by subject
Employee Health see Occupational Health
Employee Health Benefit Plans see Health Benefit
    Plans, Employee
Employee Health Services see Occupational Health
    Services
Employee Orientation Programs see Inservice
    Training
Employee Performance Appraisal
    Hospital Personnel   WX 159
    Nursing   WY 30
    Psychiatry   WM 30
Employee Strikes see Strikes, Employee
Employee Turnover see Personnel Turnover
Employment
    Child   HD 6228–6250.5
    Employment agencies   HD 5860–6000.7
    Health problems see Occupational Medicine
       WA 400–495
    Labor market   HD 5701–5856
    Migrants see Transients and Migrants   WA 300,
       etc.
    Nurses   WY 29
    Women   HD 6050–6223
       See also Physicians, Women   W 21, etc.
    Other special topics, by subject
    See also Rehabilitation, Vocational   HD
       7255–7256; Unemployment   HD 5707.5–5851;
       Vocational Guidance   HF 5381, etc.
Employment Application see Job Application
Employment Termination see Employment
Emporiatrics see Travel
Empyema   WF 745
Empyema, Gallbladder see Cholecystitis
Empyema, Tuberculous   WF 745
EMS Communication Systems see Emergency
    Medical Service Communication Systems
Emulsifying Agents see Excipients
Emulsions   QV 785
EN–1639A see Naltrexone
Enalapril   QV 150
Enalapril Maleate see Enalapril
Enallynymalum see Methohexital
Enamel see Dental Enamel
Enamel Microabrasion   WU 220
Encephalitis   WL 351
    Equine see Encephalomyelitis, Equine   SF
       959.E5, etc.
    Meningeal see Meningoencephalitis   WL 351,
       etc.
Encephalitis, Central European see Encephalitis,
    Tick-Borne
Encephalitis, Epidemic   WC 542
Encephalitis, Equine see Encephalomyelitis, Equine

Encephalitis, Japanese   WC 542
    Veterinary   SF 809.E62
Encephalitis, Japanese B see Encephalitis, Japanese
Encephalitis, Post-Vaccinal see Encephalomyelitis,
    Acute Disseminated
Encephalitis, St. Louis   WC 542
Encephalitis, Tick-Borne   WC 542
    Veterinary   SF 809.E62
Encephalitis Virus, California see California Group
    Viruses
Encephalitis Virus, Central European see
    Encephalitis Viruses, Tick-Borne
Encephalitis Virus, St. Louis   QW 168.5.A7
Encephalitis Virus, Venezuelan Equine   QW
    168.5.A7
Encephalitis Viruses   QW 168.5.A7
Encephalitis Viruses, Tick-Borne   QW 168.5.A7
Encephalocele
    Congenital   WL 350
    Traumatic   WL 354
Encephalography see Cerebral Angiography;
    Electroencephalography; Radiography   WL 141
    under Brain; Cerebral Ventriculography
Encephalomalacia   WL 348
    Associated with cerebral infarction   WL 355
Encephalomyelitis   WL 351
    Equine see Encephalomyelitis, Equine   SF
       959.E5
       As a communicable disease   SF 809.E7
Encephalomyelitis, Acute Disseminated   WL 351
Encephalomyelitis, Allergic   WL 351
Encephalomyelitis, Equine   SF 959.E5
    In humans   WC 542
Encephalomyelitis, Experimental Allergic see
    Encephalomyelitis, Allergic
Encephalomyelitis, Myalgic see Fatigue Syndrome,
    Chronic
Encephalomyelitis Virus, Venezuelan Equine see
    Encephalitis Virus, Venezuelan Equine
Enchondroma see Chondroma
Enclomifene see Clomiphene
Encopresis   WI 600
    Toilet training   WS 113
    See also Defecation   WI 600; Fecal Incontinence
       WI 600
Encounter Groups
    In psychotherapy   WM 430.5.S3
    In sociology   HM
Encyclopedias   AE
    (Form number 13 in any NLM schedule where
      applicable)
    Science   Q 121
    On other topics, by subject
End-Stage Renal Disease see Kidney Failure,
    Chronic
Endamoeba see Entamoeba
Endarterectomy   WG 170
Endarteritis   WG 515
Endbrain see Telencephalon
Endemic Diseases   WA 105
    Statistics and surveys   WA 900
    Specific diseases, with the disease
Endemic Typhus see Typhus, Endemic Flea-Borne

Endocardial Cushion Defects WG 220
Endocarditis WG 285
Endocarditis, Bacterial WG 285
Endocarditis Lenta see Endocarditis, Subacute
  Bacterial
Endocarditis, Subacute Bacterial WG 285
Endocardium WG 285
Endocavitary Fulguration see Electrocoagulation
Endocrine Cells, Gastrointestinal see Endocrine
  Cells of Gut
Endocrine Cells of Gut WI 101
  See also Gastrointestinal Hormones WK 170
Endocrine Diseases WK
  General works WK 140
  Child WS 330
  Infant WS 330
  Nursing WY 155
Endocrine Drugs see Hormones; Hormones,
  Synthetic; Hypoglycemic Agents
Endocrine Glands WK
  Of children WS 330
  Of domestic animals SF 768.3
  Of wild animals QP 187
  See also Corpus Luteum WP 530, etc.; Ovary
    WP 520–530, etc.; Testis WJ 875, etc.;
    names of other specific glands
Endocrine Surgical Procedures WK 148
Endocrine System WK
  General works WK 100
  Of children WS 330
  Physiology WK 102
Endocrinologists, Directories see Directories WK
  22 under Endocrinology
Endocrinology WK
  Child WS 330
  Directories WK 22
  Infant WS 330
Endocrinology and Metabolism (Specialty) see
  Endocrinology
Endoderm WQ 205
Endodermal Sinus Tumor
  In the ovary WP 322
Endodontics WU 230
Endolymph WV 250
Endolymphatic Duct WV 255
Endolymphatic Sac WV 255
Endometrial Cycle see Menstrual Cycle
Endometriosis WP 390
Endometritis WP 451
Endometrium WP 400
Endomycetales see Saccharomycetales
Endomycopsis see Saccharomycetales
Endophthalmitis WW 212
Endoplasmic Reticulum QH 603.E6
ENDOR see Electron Spin Resonance Spectroscopy
Endorphins QU 68
  Neurochemistry WL 104
  Other special topics, by subject
Endoscopes
  (Form number 26 in any NLM schedule where
    applicable)
Endoscopic Retrograde Cholangiopancreatography
  see Cholangiopancreatography, Endoscopic

Retrograde
Endoscopic Surgical Procedures see Surgical
  Procedures, Endoscopic
Endoscopic Ultasonography see Endosonography
Endoscopy WB 141
  Used for diagnosis of particular disorders, with
    the disorder or system
  See also specific types of endoscopy
Endoscopy, Digestive System WI 141
Endoscopy, Echo see Endosonography
Endoscopy, Gastrointestinal WI 141
Endoscopy, Ultrasonic see Endosonography
Endoscopy, Uterine see Hysteroscopy
Endosomes QH 591
Endosonography WN 208
  Used for special purposes, by subject
Endospore–Forming Bacteria
  General works QW 50
  See also Bacteria QW, etc.
Endothelin–1 see Endothelins
Endothelin–2 see Endothelins
Endothelin–3 see Endothelins
Endothelins
  As vasoconstrictors QV 150
  Biochemistry QU 68
Endothelium
  Histology QS 532.5.E7
  See also organ–specific terms, e.g., Endothelium,
    Corneal WW 220
Endothelium, Anterior Chamber see Endothelium,
  Corneal
Endothelium, Corneal WW 220
  Anterior chamber epithelium WW 210
  Eyebank procedures WW 170
Endothelium–Derived Relaxing Factor QV 150
Endothelium–Derived Vasoconstrictor Factors see
  Endothelins
Endothelium, Vascular WG 500–700
  Histology QS 532.5.E7
Endotoxemia WC 240
Endotoxins QW 630.5.E5
Endotracheal Anesthesia see Anesthesia,
  Intratracheal
Endowments see Financial Management
Enema WB 344
Energy Expenditure see Energy Metabolism
Energy–Generating Resources
  Special topics, by subject, e.g. Environmental
    Health WA 30
Energy Intake
  In normal diet QT 235
  Nutritional requirements QU 145
Energy Metabolism QU 125
Energy Resources Conservation see Conservation of
  Energy Resources
Energy Transfer QU 34
Enflurane QV 81
Engineering TA
  Biomedical see Biomedical Engineering QT 36
  General works TA 144–145
  Hospital maintenance WX 165
  Sanitary see Sanitary Engineering WA 671, etc.
Engineering, Hospital see Maintenance and

Engineering, Hospital
Engineering Psychology see Human Engineering
English Literature see Literature   P, etc. and
    related headings
Enhancer Elements (Genetics)   QH 450.2
Enkephalins   QU 68
    Neurochemistry   WL 104
    Other special topics, by subject
Enoxacin   QV 250
    As an urinary anti-infective agent   QV 243
Enoxaparin   QV 193
Enoxolone see Glycyrrhetinic Acid
Enriched Food see Food, Fortified
Entamoeba   QX 55
Entamoebiasis   WC 285
Entamoebiasis, Hepatic see Liver Abscess, Amebic
Entamoebiasis, Intestinal see Dysentery, Amebic
Enteral Feeding see Enteral Nutrition
Enteral Nutrition   WB 410
Enteric Fever see Typhoid
Enteric Hormones see Gastrointestinal Hormones
Enteric Infections see Enterobacteriaceae Infections;
    Enterovirus Infections; Intestinal Diseases,
    Parasitic; names of specific infections
Enterically-Transmitted Non-A, Non-B Hepatitis
    see Hepatitis E
Enteritis   WI 420
Enteritis, Granulomatous see Crohn Disease
Enteritis, Regional see Crohn Disease
Enterobacter   QW 138.5.E5
Enterobacteriaceae   QW 138
Enterobacteriaceae Infections   WC 260-290
    Veterinary   SF 809.E63
Enterobiasis see Oxyuriasis
Enterocele see Hernia
Enterochromaffin Cells   WI 400
    Physiology   WI 402
Enteroclysis see Enema
Enterocolitis   WI 420
Enterocolitis, Necrotizing   WI 420
Enterocolitis, Pseudomembranous   WI 420
Enteroendocrine Cells see Endocrine Cells of Gut
Enteropathy, Exudative see Protein-Losing
    Enteropathies
Enteropathy, HIV see HIV Enteropathy
Enterostomy   WI 480
Enterotoxins   QW 630.5.E6
Enterovirus   QW 168.5.P4
Enterovirus Infections   WC 500
    Veterinary   SF 809.E64
    See also names of specific infections, e.g.,
    Poliomyelitis   WC 555-556
Enterovirus 70 see Enterovirus
Entomology   QL 461-599.82
    Medical   QX 500-650
    See also Insects   QX 500-650, etc.
Entrapment Neuropathy see Nerve Compression
    Syndromes
Entropion   WW 205
Entropy
    Biochemistry   QU 34
    Physics   QC 318.E57
Enuresis   WJ 146

Child   WS 322
Environment
    Living space   QT 230
    Physical
        Adaptation to   QT 140-165
        As a cause of disease (Pathology)   QZ 57
        See also Climate   WB 750, etc. and related
            headings
    Relation to general public health see
        Environmental Health   WA 30, etc.
    Relation to mental health   WM 31
    Social see Social Environment   HM
    See also Ecology   QH 540-549.5
Environment, Controlled   WA 670-847
    General works   WA 671
    In hospitals
        General   WX 165
        Intensive care   WX 218
    In industry   WA 440-491
    Of laboratory animals   QY 56
    See also Extraterrestrial Environment   WD 758;
        Germ-Free Life   QY 56, etc.; Incubators
        QS 530, etc.; Ecological Systems, Closed   WD
        756, etc.; names of specific types of control, e.g.,
        Ventilation   WA 770, etc.
Environment Design   TA 170
    Government policy
        General   HC 79.E5
        By country   HC 94-1085
    See also City Planning   HT 165.5-169.9, etc.;
        Environment, Controlled   WA 670-847, etc.
Environmental Air Pollutants see Air Pollutants,
    Environmental
Environmental Exposure   QT 140-162
    In workplace   WA 400-495
    To air pollution (General)   WA 754
    To radiation   WN 415-650
    To other specific conditions, by subject
Environmental Factors see Environmental Exposure;
    Meteorological Factors; Socioeconomic Factors;
    names of physical agents, e.g., Heat
Environmental Health   WA 30
    Diseases of geographic areas   WB 710
    Psychiatric aspects   WM 31
    See also Environment, Controlled   WA 671, etc.
Environmental Hypersensitivity see Environmental
    Illness
Environmental Illness
    General   WA 30.5
    Due to specific etiology, by subject, e.g., Food
        Hypersensitivity   WD 310; Air Pollution,
        Indoor   WA 754
Environmental Medicine   WA 30.5
Environmental Microbiology   QW 55
Environmental Monitoring   QH 541.15.M64
    In occupational health   WA 400-495
    Of environmental pollutants   WA 671
    Of air pollutants   WA 754
    Of water pollutants   WA 689
    Of radioactive pollutants   WN 615
    Of other specific conditions, by subject
Environmental Pollutants   WA 671
Environmental Pollution   WA 670

See also specific types of pollution; e.g., Water
Pollution   WA 689
Environmental Pollution, Tobacco Smoke see
Tobacco Smoke Pollution
Enzymatic Zonulolysis see Cataract Extraction
Enzyme Activation   QU 135
Enzyme Immunoassay see Immunoenzyme
Techniques
Enzyme Induction   QU 135
Enzyme Inhibitors   QU 143
Enzyme–Labeled Antibody Technique see
Immunoenzyme Techniques
Enzyme–Linked Immunosorbent Assay   QW
525.5.E6
   Used for diagnostic, monitoring, or evaluation
   tests in special fields, with the field
Enzyme Precursors   QU 142
Enzyme Reactivators   QU 144
Enzyme Repression   QU 135
Enzyme Tests   QY 490
Enzymes   QU 135–141
   Blood chemistry   QY 490
Enzymes, Immobilized   QU 135–141
Enzymologic Gene Expression Regulation see Gene
Expression Regulation, Enzymologic
Enzymology see Enzymes
EOG see Electrooculography
Eosinophilia   WH 200
Eosinophilic Granuloma   WH 650
   Localized, by site
Eosinophils   WH 200
Ependyma   WL 307
EPH Gestosis see Gestosis, EPH
Ephedrine   QV 129
Ephemeral Fever   SF 967.T47
Epidemic Non–A, Non–B Hepatitis see Hepatitis E
Epidemics see Disease Outbreaks
Epidemiologic Determinants see Epidemiologic
Factors
Epidemiologic Factors
   In a particular subject, with the subject
Epidemiologic Methods   WA 950
Epidemiologic Research Design
   General works   WA 105
   Statistics   WA 900
      Theory or methods   WA 950
Epidemiologic Studies   WA 105
   Specific topics, by subject
Epidemiological Monitoring see Environmental
Monitoring
Epidemiology   WA 105–106
   Statistics   WA 900
      As a form subdivision (Form number 16 in
      any NLM schedule where applicable)
      See also Epidemiologic Methods   WA 950
   Of particular disorders, with the disorder
Epidermal Cyst   WR 420
Epidermal Growth Factor see Epidermal Growth
Factor–Urogastrone
Epidermal Growth Factor Receptors see Receptors,
Epidermal Growth Factor–Urogastrone
Epidermal Growth Factor–Urogastrone   WK 170
   As a growth substance   QU 107

As an antacid   QV 69
Epidermal Necrolysis, Toxic   WR 165
Epidermis   WR 101
Epidermoid Cyst see Epidermal Cyst
Epidermolysis Bullosa   WR 200
Epidermophytosis see Tinea
Epidermotoxins see Dermotoxins
Epididymis   WJ 800
Epidural Analgesia see Analgesia, Epidural
Epidural Anesthesia see Anesthesia, Epidural
Epidural Space   WE 725
Epiglottis   WV 500
Epilation see Hair Removal
Epilepsy   WL 385
   Experimental see Convulsions   WL 385, etc.
Epilepsy, Abdominal see Epilepsy, Temporal Lobe
Epilepsy, Absence   WL 385
Epilepsy, Cryptogenic see Epilepsy
Epilepsy, Focal see Epilepsy, Partial
Epilepsy, Generalized Secondary see Epilepsy,
Partial
Epilepsy, Grand Mal see Epilepsy, Tonic–Clonic
Epilepsy, Localization–Related see Epilepsy, Partial
Epilepsy, Myoclonic   WL 385
Epilepsy, Myoclonus see Epilepsy, Myoclonic
Epilepsy, Partial   WL 385
Epilepsy, Petit Mal see Epilepsy, Absence
Epilepsy, Post–Traumatic   WL 385
Epilepsy, Simple Partial see Epilepsy, Partial
Epilepsy, Temporal Lobe   WL 385
Epilepsy, Tonic–Clonic   WL 385
Epilepsy, Traumatic see Epilepsy, Post–Traumatic
Epilepsy, Uncinate see Epilepsy, Temporal Lobe
Epinephrine   WK 725
Epiphyseal Cartilage see Growth Plate
Epiphyseal Plate see Growth Plate
Epiphyses   WE 200
Epiphyses, Slipped   WE 175
Epiphyses, Stippled see Chondrodysplasia Punctata
Epiphysiolysis see Epiphyses, Slipped
Epiphysis Cerebri see Pineal Body
Episiotomy   WQ 415
Episomes see Plasmids
Epispadias   WJ 600
Epistaxis   WV 320
Epistropheus see Axis
Epithalamus   WL 312
Epithelial Attachment   WU 240
Epithelial Cells   QS 532.5.E7
Epithelioma see Carcinoma
Epithelium
   Dermatology   WR 101
   Histology   QS 532.5.E7
   Neoplasms   QZ 365
Epithelium, Anterior Chamber see Endothelium,
Corneal
Epithelium, Anterior Corneal see Epithelium,
Corneal
Epithelium, Corneal   WW 220
Epithelium, Retinal Pigment see Pigment Epithelium
of Eye
Epitopes   QW 573
   Special topics, by subject

Eponyms
 Disease (General) WB 15
 In specialties (Form number 15 in NLM schedule
  or in appropriate LC number)
Epoprostenol QV 180
 Biochemistry QU 90
Epoxides see Epoxy Compounds
Epoxy Compounds
 Organic chemistry QD 305.E7
Epoxy Resins
 Chemical technology TP 1180.E6
 Dentistry WU 190
 Used for special purposes, by subject
Epoxytrichothecenes see Trichothecenes
Epsom Salts see Magnesium Sulphate
Epstein-Barr Virus see Herpesvirus 4, Human
Epstein-Barr Virus Infections WC 571
Epstein-Barr Virus Syndrome, Chronic see Fatigue
 Syndrome, Chronic
Epulis, Giant Cell see Granuloma, Giant Cell
Equilibrium WV 255
 See also Acid-Base Equilibrium QU 105;
  Water-Electrolyte Balance QU 105
Equine Infectious Anemia SF 959.A6
Equipment Alarm Systems see Equipment Failure
Equipment and Supplies
 (Form number 26 in any NLM schedule where
  applicable)
 Anesthetic WO 240
 Catalogs (medical and surgical) W 26
 Dental see Dental Equipment WU 26; Dental
  High Speed Equipment WU 26; Dental
  Instruments WU 26
 Disposable see Disposable Equipment W 26
 Immunology QW 526
 Orthopedic see Orthopedic Equipment WE 26
 Pharmaceutical QV 26; QV 785-835
  Military UH 420-425
 Radiological WN 150
 Surgical see Surgical Equipment WO 162, etc.
 See also particular types of equipment or supplies
Equipment and Supplies, Hospital WX 147
 See also particular items, e.g., Beds WX 147,
 etc.
Equipment Contamination
 Of particular equipment, with the equipment
 See also Equipment and Supplies
Equipment Design
 Of a specific equipment, with the equipment
Equipment Failure
 of a specific equipment, with the equipment
Equipment Safety
 Of a specific equipment, with the equipment
Equivalency, Therapeutic see Therapeutic
 Equivalency
ERCP see Cholangiopancreatography, Endoscopic
 Retrograde
Eremothecium see Saccharomycetales
Ergastoplasm see Endoplasmic Reticulum
Ergobasin see Ergonovine
Ergocalciferols QU 173
Ergolines
 Pharmacology QV 174

Ergometrin see Ergonovine
Ergometrine see Ergonovine
Ergonomics see Human Engineering
Ergonovine QV 173
Ergot Alkaloids QV 174
Ergot Poisoning see Ergotism
Ergotamine QV 174
Ergotamine Derivatives QV 174
Ergotamine Tartrate see Ergotamine
Ergotism WD 505
Ergotoxine QV 174
Erosion, Cervix see Cervix Erosion
Erotica HQ 450-472
Erucic Acids QU 90
Eructation WI 143
Eruption, Skin see Exanthema; Exanthema Subitum
Erysipelas WC 234
Erysipeloid WC 234
Erysipelothrix Infections
 Swine SF 977.E7
Erythema WR 150
 Migrans see Glossitis, Benign Migratory WI
 210
Erythema Multiforme WR 150
Erythema Nodosum WR 150
Erythermalgia see Erythromelalgia
Erythremia see Polycythemia Vera
Erythrina QV 140
Erythroblastic Anemia see Thalassemia
Erythroblastosis, Fetal WH 425
Erythroblasts WH 150
Erythrocebus patas QL 737.P93
 Diseases SF 997.5.P7
 As laboratory animals QY 60.P7
Erythrocyte Aggregation, Intravascular WH 150
Erythrocyte Aging WH 150
Erythrocyte Anion Transport Protein see Band 3
 Protein
Erythrocyte Aplasia see Red-Cell Aplasia, Pure
Erythrocyte Burst-Promoting Factor see
 Interleukin-3
Erythrocyte Count QY 402
Erythrocyte Ghost see Erythrocyte Membrane
Erythrocyte Membrane WH 150
Erythrocyte Membrane Band 3 Protein see Band 3
 Protein
Erythrocyte Number see Erythrocyte Count
Erythrocyte Sedimentation see Blood Sedimentation
Erythrocyte Sialoglycoprotein see Glycophorin
Erythrocyte Substitutes see Blood Substitutes
Erythrocyte Survival see Erythrocyte Aging
Erythrocyte Transfusion WB 356
Erythrocyte Volume WG 106
Erythrocyte Volume, Packed see Hematocrit
Erythrocytes WH 150-180
 Clinical examination QY 402
Erythrocytes, Abnormal WH 150
Erythrocythemia see Polycythemia; Polycythemia
 Vera
Erythrocytosis see Polycythemia
Erythroderma see Dermatitis, Exfoliative
Erythroderma, Maculopapular see Parapsoriasis
Erythromelalgia WG 578

Erythromycin   QV 350.5.E7
Erythropoiesis   WH 150
Erythropoietin   WH 150
    Special topics, by subject
Erythroxylon see Coca
Escape Reaction   BF 319.5.A9
Escharotics see Caustics
Escherichia coli   QW 138.5.E8
Escherichia coli Infections   WC 290
    Veterinary   SF 809.E82
        In swine   SF 977.E83
Escherichia coli Phages see Coliphages
Eserine see Physostigmine
Eskimos   E99.E7
    See also special topics under Ethnic Groups
Esophageal Achalasia   WI 250
Esophageal and Gastric Varices   WI 720
Esophageal Atresia   WI 250
Esophageal Diseases   WI 250
Esophageal Diverticulum   WI 250
Esophageal Dysmotility see Esophageal Motility
    Disorders
Esophageal Fistula   WI 250
Esophageal Motility Disorders   WI 250
Esophageal Neoplasms   WI 250
Esophageal Reflux see Gastroesophageal Reflux
Esophageal Stenosis   WI 250
Esophageal Stricture see Esophageal Stenosis
Esophageal Varices see Esophageal and Gastric
    Varices
Esophagitis   WI 250
Esophagogastroduodenoscopy see Endoscopy,
    Digestive System
Esophagoplasty   WI 250
Esophagotracheal Fistula see Tracheoesophageal
    Fistula
Esophagus   WI 250
Esophagus, Barrett see Barrett Esophagus
Esotropia   WW 415
Esox see Salmonidae
ESRD see Kidney Failure, Chronic
Essays see Form number 9 in any NLM schedule
    where applicable
Essences see Solutions
Essential Amino Acids see Amino Acids, Essential
Essential Oils see Oils, Volatile
Essential Polyarteritis see Polyarteritis Nodosa
Esterases   QU 136
Esthetic Surgery see Surgery, Plastic
Esthetics   BH
    Plastic surgery   WO 600
    Transplantation   WO 660
    Women   HQ 1219-1220
Esthetics, Dental   WU 100
    Special methods, by subject, e.g. Orthodontics
        WU 400-440
Estradiol   WP 522
Estradiol-17 beta see Estradiol
Estramustine   QV 269
Estramustinphosphate see Estramustine
Estriol   WP 522
Estrogen Analogs see Estrogens, Synthetic
Estrogen Antagonists   WP 522

Estrogen Receptors see Receptors, Estrogen
Estrogen Replacement Therapy   WP 522
Estrogenic Substances, Conjugated see Estrogens,
    Conjugated
Estrogens   WP 522
Estrogens, Catechol   WP 522
Estrogens, Conjugated   WP 522
Estrogens, Synthetic   WP 522
    Used for special purposes, by subject
Estrone   WP 522
Estrous Cycle see Estrus
Estrus   SF 105
ESWL (Extracorporeal Shockwave Lithotripsy) see
    Lithotripsy
ET-1 see Endothelin-1
ET-2 see Endothelin-2
ET-3 see Endothelin-3
Etching, Dental see Acid Etching, Dental
Ethambutol   QV 268
Ethanol
    Organic chemistry   QD 305.A4
    Pharmacology   QV 84
Ethanolamine Phosphoglycerides see
    Phosphatidylethanolamines
Ethanolamines   QV 84
    Organic chemistry   QD 305.A4
Ether, Ethyl   QV 81
Ethers
    As anesthetics   QV 81
    Organic chemistry
        Aliphatic compounds   QD 305.E7
        Aromatic compounds   QD 341.E7
    Spectra   QC 463.E7
    Used for special purposes, by subject
Ethers, Cyclic
    Organic chemistry   QD 305.E7
    Used for special purposes, by subject
Ethics   BJ
    General works   BJ 991-1185
    Special applications, by subject
Ethics, Dental   WU 50
Ethics in Publishing see Scientific Misconduct
Ethics, Institutional
    Special topics, by subject, e.g., in hospitals   WX
    150
Ethics, Medical   W 50
    In psychiatry   WM 62
    For other specialties (Form number 21 in any
        NLM schedule where applicable)
Ethics, Nursing   WY 85
Ethics, Pharmacy   QV 21
Ethics, Professional   BJ 1725
    Of special groups, by name of group
Ethinyl Estradiol   WP 522
    As a contraceptive   QV 177
Ethinyl Estradiol 3-Methyl Ether see Mestranol
Ethinyl Trichloride see Trichloroethylene
Ethinylestrenol see Lynestrenol
Ethinylnortestosterone see Norethindrone
Ethiofos see Amifostine
Ethionamide   QV 268
Ethioniamide see Ethionamide
Ethmoid Bone   WE 705

**ALWAYS CONSULT MAIN SCHEDULES. USE NUMBER ASSIGNED ONLY WHEN
SUBJECT REPRESENTS MAJOR EMPHASIS OF WORK BEING CLASSIFIED**

I-94

Ethmoid Sinus   WV 355
Ethnic Groups
    Anthropology   GN 301–673
    Diseases   WB 720
    Education   LC 3701–3747
    General works   DA 125, E 184–185, F 1035, etc.
    Health surveys   WA 300
    Medical biography   WZ 150
    Medical history   WZ 80
    Mental ability assessment   BF 432
    Nutrition surveys   QU 146
    Psychology   GN 270–279
    Public health (including mental health)   WA 300–305
    Other special topics, by subject
    See also names of specific groups
Ethnobotany   GN 476.73
    In medicine
        Plants, Medicinal   QV 766–770
        Medicine, Traditional   WB 50
           History   WZ 309
Ethnography see Anthropology, Cultural
Ethnology   GN 307–673
    See also Anthropology, Cultural   GN 307–673
Ethnomedicine see Medicine, Traditional
Ethnopsychology   GN 270–279
Ethoform see Benzocaine
Ethology   QL 750–785.3
    Veterinary sciences   SF 756.7
Ethoxy Compounds see Ethyl Ethers
Ethyl Aminobenzoate see Benzocaine
Ethyl Carbamate see Urethane
Ethyl Chloride   QV 81
Ethyl Ether see Ether, Ethyl
Ethyl Ethers   QV 81
    Organic chemistry   QD 305.E7
Ethyl Methanesulfonate
    As an antineoplastic agent   QV 269
Ethylamines   QU 61
    Organic chemistry   QD 305.A8
Ethylbarbital see Barbital
Ethyldithiourame see Disulfiram
Ethylene Chlorohydrin   QV 82
Ethylene Dibromide   QV 633
    Public health aspects   WA 240
Ethylene Dichlorides
    Toxicology   QV 633
Ethylene Oxide
    As a fungicide   SB 951.3
    Organic chemistry   QD 305.E7
Ethylene Polymers see Polyethylenes
Ethylenediaminetetraacetic Acid see Edetic Acid
Ethyleneimines see Aziridines
Ethylenes   QV 81
    Organic chemistry   QD 305.H7
Ethylenethiourea
    As a carcinogen   QZ 202
    Biochemistry   QU 65
Ethylestrenolone see Norethandrolone
Ethylnortestosterone see Norethandrolone
Ethynyl Estradiol see Ethinyl Estradiol
Etiology see Pathogenesis   QZ 40–109 under

Disease; names of particular diseases
Etoposide   QV 269
Etretinate   QU 167
    Used in treating a particular skin disease, with the disease
Etryptamine see Indoles
Etymology see Dictionaries; Nomenclature
Eubacterium   QW 120
Eugenics   HQ 750–755.5
Euglena   QX 50
Euglobulins see Serum Globulins
Eukaryotic Cells   QH 581–581.2
Eunuchism   WJ 840
Euoticus see Galago
Euphausia see Crustacea
Euphoria   BF 575.E5
    Adolescence   WS 462
    Child   WS 105.5.E5
Europium
    Inorganic chemistry   QD 181.E8
    Pharmacology   QV 290
Eustachian Tube   WV 230
Eutamias see Sciuridae
Eutelegenesis see Insemination, Artificial
Euthanasia   W 50
Euthanasia, Passive   W 50
Evaluation, Program see Program Evaluation
Evaluation Research, Nursing see Nursing Evaluation Research
Evaluation Studies
    Health services   W 84
    Other special topics, by subject being evaluated
Evaluation Studies, Drug see Drug Evaluation
Evaluation Studies, Drug, Pre–Clinical see Drug Screening
Evaluation Studies, Postmarketing see Product Surveillance, Postmarketing
Evidence–Based Medicine   WB 102
Evidential Material see Forensic Medicine
Evoked Potentials   WL 102
Evoked Potentials, Auditory   WV 270
Evoked Potentials, Auditory, Brain Stem   WV 270
Evoked Potentials, Somatosensory   WL 102
Evoked Potentials, Visual   WW 103
Evoked Response Audiometry see Audiometry, Evoked Response
Evoked Responses, Auditory, Brain Stem see Evoked Potentials, Auditory, Brain Stem
Evolution   QH 359–425
    Darwin's works   QH 365
    General works   QH 366–366.2
    Periodicals, numbered congresses, serial collections, yearbooks, in appropriate NLM numbers
    Single organs with the organ
    See also Ontogeny   QH 359–425, etc.; Phylogeny   QH 367.5
Evolution, Molecular
    In biogenesis   QH 325
    See also Evolution   QH 359–425, etc.; Genetics QH 426–470, etc.; Molecular Biology   QH 506
Ewing's Tumor see Sarcoma, Ewing's

Examination see Diagnosis; names of specific types of examination, e.g., Neurologic Examination

Examination questions
(Form number 18.2 in any NLM schedule where applicable)

Exanthema   WR 220
Veterinary   SF 901

Exanthema Subitum   WC 570

Exchange Transfusion, Whole Blood   WB 356
RH factor   WH 425

Excipients   QV 800

Excitotoxins see Neurotoxins

Excretion of Drugs see Metabolism   QV 38 under Drugs

Exercise
Movement   WE 103
Physical education   QT 255
Sports   QT 260

Exercise, Aerobic see Exercise

Exercise-Induced Asthma see Asthma, Exercise-Induced

Exercise-Induced Bronchospasm see Asthma, Exercise-Induced

Exercise, Isometric see Exercise

Exercise, Physical see Exercise

Exercise Test   WG 141.5.F9

Exercise Therapy   WB 541
In water see Hydrotherapy   WB 520

Exertion
Movement   WE 103
Physical education   QT 255
Sports   QT 260

Exfoliative dermatitis see Dermatitis Exfoliativa

Exhaustion see Fatigue; Heat exhaustion; Neurasthenia

Exhibitionism   WM 610

Exhibitions
(Form numbers 27-28 in any NLM schedule where applicable)

Exhibits   T 391-999
(Form numbers 27-28 in any NLM schedule where applicable)

Existential Psychology see Existentialism

Existentialism
Philosophy
General   B 105.E8
Modern   B 819
Psychoanalysis   WM 460.5.E8
Psychology   BF 204.5

Exocrine Glands   QT 172
Skin glands   WR 101
Specific glands, with system where located, e.g.
Sebaceous glands   WR 410

Exodontia see Tooth Extraction

Exodontics see Tooth Extraction

Exomphalos see Hernia, Umbilical

Exophthalmic Goiter see Graves' Disease

Exophthalmos   WW 210
See also Graves' Disease   WK 265

Exostoses   WE 250
Localized, by site

Exostoses, Familial see Exostoses, Multiple Hereditary

Exostoses, Hereditary Multiple see Exostoses, Multiple Hereditary

Exostoses, Multiple see Exostoses, Multiple Hereditary

Exostoses, Multiple Cartilaginous see Exostoses, Multiple Hereditary

Exostoses, Multiple Hereditary   WE 250

Exotoxins   QW 630

Expectation (Psychology)   BF 323.E8

Expectorants   QV 76

Expeditions
Medical   W 10
Scientific expeditions   Q 115-116

Expenditures, Health see Health Expenditures

Experimental Design see Research Design

Experimental Psychology see Psychology, Experimental

Experimental works in specialties other than psychology see Under the specialty

Expert Systems   QA 76.76.E95
In medicine (General)   W 26.55.A7
In other special fields (Form number 26.5 in any NLM schedule where applicable)

Expert Testimony
Chemistry   W 750
Dentistry   W 705
Medicine   W 725
Psychiatry   W 740
Special topics, by subject

Expiratory Forced Flow Rates see Forced Expiratory Flow Rates

Expiratory Peak Flow Rate see Peak Expiratory Flow Rate

Exploratory Behavior   BF 323.C8
Child   WS 105.5.M5
Infant   WS 105.5.M5

Exploratory Surgery see Diagnostic Techniques, Surgical

Explosions
Hospital emergency service   WX 215
In industry   WA 485
Mining   WA 485
Nuclear explosions   WN 610
Nursing in emergency situations   WY 154
Prevention & control   WA 288
In industry   WA 485
Thermochemistry   QD 516

Explosive Decompression see Decompression, Explosive

Exposure (Radiology) see Environmental Exposure; conditions under which exposure takes place, e.g., Radiotherapy

Expressed Emotion   BF 531-593
Specific emotions, with the emotion
Towards patients with specific disorders, with the disorder

Expression, Pharmacy see Drug Compounding

Extended Care Facilities see Skilled Nursing Facilities

External Degree Programs, Nursing see Education, Nursing, Baccalaureate

External Ear see Ear, External

External Influences on Child see Child Development;

Television; related topics
Extinction (Psychology)   BF 319.5.E9
Extracellular Fluid see Extracellular Space
Extracellular Matrix   QH 603.E93
   Body fluids   QU 105
Extracellular Matrix Proteins   QU 55
Extracellular Space   QU 105
Extrachromosomal Inheritance   QW 51
Extracorporeal Circulation   WG 168
Extracorporeal Dialysis see Hemodialysis
Extracorporeal Shockwave Lithotripsy see
   Lithotripsy
Extracranial–Intracranial Arterial Bypass see
   Cerebral Revascularization
Extraction, Obstetrical   WQ 415
Extraction of Teeth see Tooth Extraction
Extracts see Dosage Forms, Liver Extracts;
   Pancreatic Extracts; Placental Extracts; Thymus
   Extracts; Tissue Extracts
Extramarital Relations   HQ 806
Extraordinary Treatment see Life Support Care
Extrapyramidal Disorders see Basal Ganglia Diseases
Extrapyramidal Tracts   WL 400
Extrasensory Perception see Parapsychology
Extrasystole see Cardiac Complexes, Premature
Extraterrestrial Environment   WD 758
Extraversion (Psychology)
   Personality   BF 698.35.E98
   Psychoanalysis   WM 460.5.E9
Extremities   WE 800–890
   Blood supply   WG 500–700
      Specific extremities, with the part, e.g. Blood
       supply to the leg   WE 850
   Lower extremities   WE 850–890
   Upper extremities   WE 805–835
Extremities, Artificial see Artificial Limbs
Extremity, Lower see Leg
Extremity, Upper see Arm
Exudates and Transudates   QU 105
   Clinical examination   QY 210
Eye   WW
   Blood supply   WW 101–103
      See also names of particular arteries and veins,
       e.g., Ophthalmic Artery   WG 595.O7
   Conservation   WW 113
   Innervation   WW 101–103
      See also Optic Nerves   WW 280, etc.
   Pathology due to diseases of central nervous
     system   WW 460
   Pathological eye conditions in other diseases
     WW 475
   Physiology see Ocular Physiology   WW 103
   Posterior chamber   WW 210
   Surgery see Ophthalmologic Surgical Procedures
     WW 168
Eye Abnormalities   WW 101
Eye, Artificial   WW 358
Eye Banks   WW 23–24
   Procedures   WW 170
Eye Burns   WW 100
Eye Color   WW 101
Eye Conservation see Eye
Eye Diseases   WW

General works   WW 140
Aged   WW 620
Child   WW 600
Disability evaluation   WW 32
Infant   WW 600
Neurologic manifestation   WW 460
Nursing   WY 158
Surgery   WW 168
Therapy   WW 166
Veterinary   SF 891
Eye Diseases, Hereditary   WW 140
Eye Enucleation   WW 168
Eye Foreign Bodies   WW 525
Eye Hemorrhage   WW 140
Eye Infections, Parasitic   WW 160
Eye Injuries   WW 525
   Disability evaluation   WW 32
Eye Injuries, Penetrating   WW 525
Eye Manifestations   WW 475
   Ocular disorders due to neurological disorders
     WW 460
   Of particular diseases, with the disease
Eye Motility Disorders see Ocular Motility
   Disorders
Eye Movements   WW 400–460
   General works   WW 400
Eye Neoplasms   WW 149
   Of parts of the eye, with the part
Eye Protective Devices   WW 113
Eye Proteins   WW 101
Eyeball see Eye
Eyebrows   WW 205
Eyedrops see Ophthalmic Solutions
Eyeglasses   WW 350–354
Eyelashes   WW 205
Eyelid Diseases   WW 205
Eyelids   WW 205

F

F Factor   QW 51
F-2 Toxin see Zearalenone
Face   WE 705–707
Facial Bones   WE 705
   Maxillofacial injuries   WU 610
   Physiological works for the dentist   WU 102
Facial Dermatoses   WR 140
Facial Expression   BF 592.F33
   Child   WS 105.5.C8
   Infant   WS 105.5.C8
   Physical examination   WB 275
   Physiology   WE 705
   See also Nonverbal Communication   HM
     etc.; Physiognomy   BF 840–861
Facial Injuries   WE 706
Facial Muscles   WE 705
Facial Neoplasms   WE 707
Facial Nerve   WL 330
Facial Nerve Diseases   WL 330
Facial Neuralgia   WL 544
Facial Pain   WE 705
   In dentistry   WU 140
Facial Paralysis   WL 330

Facies
    General physiology WE 705
    Characteristic of a disease, with the disease
Facility Access see Architectural Accessibility
Facility Construction see Facility Design and
    Construction
Facility Design and Construction
    Health facilities WX 140
      For the specialties (Form number 27–29 in any
        NLM schedule where applicable)
    Hospital departments WX 200–225
    Public health aspects of houses and public
      buildings WA 795–799
    See also Design and Construction, Hospital WX
      140, etc.
Facility Regulation and Control WX 153
    See also names of particular types of facility, e.g.,
      Rehabilitation Centers WM 29, etc.
Facteur Thymique Serique see Thymic Factor,
    Circulating
Factor Analysis, Statistical QA 278.5
    In psychology BF 39.2.F32
    Used in diagnosis, in the diagnosis number for
      the disease or specialty or lacking that in the
      general works number
    Used in other studies, by subject
Factor Construct Rating Scales (FCRS) see
    Psychiatric Status Rating Scales
Factor I see Fibrinogen
Factor II see Prothrombin
Factor III see Thromboplastin
Factor IV see Calcium
Factor IX Deficiency see Hemophilia B
Factor, RH see RH–HR Blood Group System
Factor VII WH 310
    Clinical examination QY 410
Factor VIII Deficiency see Hemophilia A
Factor VIII-Related Antigen see von Willebrand
    Factor
Factor XIII, Activated see Protein–Glutamine
    gamma–Glutamyltransferase
Factor XIII Transamidase see Protein–Glutamine
    gamma–Glutamyltransferase
Factor XIIIa see Protein–Glutamine
    gamma–Glutamyltransferase
Faculty
    (Form number 19 in any NLM schedule where
      applicable)
    Superintendents and principals LB
      2831.7–2831.99
    Teaching personnel LB 2832–2844.47
Faculty, Medical
    General W 19
    Graduate W 20
    Undergraduate W 19
Faculty, Nursing
    General WY 19
    Graduate WY 18.5
    Undergraduate WY 19
Faculty, Pharmacy see Faculty
FAD QU 135
Fads, Food see Diet Fads
Fagine see Choline

Failure, Equipment see Equipment Failure
Failure to Thrive WS 104
Fainting see Syncope
Faith Cures see Mental Healing
Faith Healing see Mental Healing
Fallopian Tube Diseases WP 300
Fallopian Tube Neoplasms WP 300
Fallopian Tubes WP 300
    Neoplasms WP 300
    In pregnancy see Pregnancy, Tubal WQ 220
    Sterilization see Sterilization, Tubal WP 660
Fallot's Tetralogy see Tetralogy of Fallot
Falls, Accidental see Accidental Falls
False Allegations see Deception
Familial Atypical Multiple Mole–Melanoma see
    Dysplastic Nevus Syndrome
Familial Erythroblastic Anemia see Thalassemia
Familial Jaundice see Spherocytosis, Hereditary
Familial Mediterranean Fever see Periodic Disease
Family
    Adjustment to mentally retarded child WS
      107.5.R5
    Ethnology GN 480–480.65
    Health see Family Health WA 308
    Relations see Family Relations WS 105.5.F2,
      etc.
      See also specific relationship terms, e.g.,
        Father–Child Relations WS 105.5.F2;
        Mother–Child Relations WS 105.5.F2;
        Parent–Child Relations WS 105.5.F2;
        Sibling Relations WS 105.5.F2
    Sociology HQ 503–1064
Family Caregivers see Caregivers
Family Characteristics HQ 503–743
Family Health WA 308
Family Leave
    General works HD 6065–6065.5
Family Life Cycles see Family
Family–Patient Lodging see Housing
Family Physicians see Physicians, Family
Family Planning HQ 763.5–767.7
Family Practice
    As a profession W 89
    Texts and treatises WB 110
Family Relations
    Child WS 105.5.F2
    Ethnology GN 480–480.65
    Infant WS 105.5.F2
    Relations to health see Family Health WA 308
    Relations with the mentally retarded child WS
      107.5.R5
    Sociology HQ 503–1064
    See also specific relationship terms, e.g.,
      Father–Child Relations WS 105.5.F2;
      Mother–Child Relations WS 105.5.F2;
      Parent–Child Relations WS 105.5.F2; Sibling
      Relations WS 105.5.F2
Family Relationship see Family Relations
Family, Single–Parent see Single Parent
Family Size see Family Characteristics
Family Therapy WM 430.5.F2
Famotidine
    As an anti-ulcer agent QV 69

Famous Persons
   Biography
      Collective
         In the field of medicine and related sciences
           WZ 112–150
         In other fields, by subject in LC schedules
         Individual   WZ 100
   Illnesses   WZ 313
Fanconi's Anemia   WH 175
Fangotherapy see Mud Therapy
Fantasy   BF 408–411
   Adolescence   WS 462
   Child   WS 105.5.C7
   Infant   WS 105.5.C7
   Psychiatry   WM 193.5.S8
Far Eastern Russian Encephalitis see Encephalitis,
   Tick–Borne
Faradic Currents see Electric Conductivity; Electric
   Stimulation Therapy; Electricity
Farcy see Glanders
Farm Animals see Animals, Domestic
Farmer's Lung   WF 652
   Veterinary   SF 831
Farsightedness see Hyperopia
Fascia   WE 500
   Localized, by site
Fascicular Block see Bundle–Branch Block
Fasciola   QX 365
Fascioliasis   WC 805
   Veterinary   SF 810.F3
Fasciolopsiasis see Trematode Infections
Fast Electrons see Electrons
Fast Neutrons
   Nuclear physics   QC 793.5.F32–793.5.F329
   In health physics   WN 110
Fasting   WB 420
Fat Emulsions, Intravenous   QU 86
   In parenteral feeding   WB 410
Fat Substitutes   QU 86
Father–Child Relations   WS 105.5.F2
Fathers
   Popular works   HQ 756–756.7
   Special topics, by subject
Fatigue
   Aviation   WD 735
   Occupational
      General   WA 475
      Mental   WA 495
      Physical   WA 475
   Nervous see Fatigue, Mental   WM 174, etc.
   Physical (General)   WB 146
Fatigue Fractures see Fractures, Stress
Fatigue, Mental see Mental Fatigue
Fatigue Syndrome, Chronic
   As a virus disease   WC 500
   Etiology unknown   WB 146
Fatigue Syndrome, Postviral see Fatigue Syndrome,
   Chronic
Fats   QU 86
   Public health aspects   WA 722
   See also Dietary Fats   WB 425, etc.
Fats, Unsaturated   QU 86
Fatty Acids   QU 90

Fatty Acids, Essential   QU 90
Fatty Acids, Free see Fatty Acids, Nonesterified
Fatty Acids, Monounsaturated   QU 90
Fatty Acids, Nonesterified   QU 90
Fatty Acids, Omega–3   QU 90
   As a supplement in health or disease   WB 425
Fatty Acids, Polyunsaturated see Fatty Acids,
   Unsaturated
Fatty Acids, Unsaturated   QU 90
Fatty Acids, Volatile   QU 90
Fatty Liver   WI 700
   In chickens   SF 995.6.F3
Fatty Liver, Alcoholic   WI 700
Fatty Streak, Arterial see Atherosclerosis
Fatty Tissue see Adipose Tissue
Fatty Tumor see Lipoma
Favism   WD 515
Favus see Tinea Favosa
Fc Receptors see Receptors, Fc
Fear   WM 178
   Adolescence   WS 462
   Child   WS 105.5.E5
   Infant   WS 105.5.E5
   In aviation & space flight   WD 730; WD 754
   See also Phobic Disorders   WM 178
Febrifuges see Anti–Inflammatory Agents,
   Non–Steroidal
Fecal Incontinence   WI 600
   See also Defecation   WI 600; Encopresis   WI
   600
Feces   QY 160
   Analysis   QY 160
      Veterinary diagnosis   SF 772.7
Feces, Impacted   WI 460
Fecundity see Fertility
Federal Aid see Financial Support
Federal Health Insurance Plans, United States see
   National Health Insurance, United States
Federal Regulations see Names of Legislation; in
   products or specialties being regulated, e.g., Drug
   and Narcotic Control
Fee, Capitation see Capitation Fee
Fee for Service, Medical see Fees, Medical
Fee Schedules
   Dental   WU 77
   Hospital   WX 157
   Medical   W 74
   Nursing   WY 77
   Pharmaceutical   QV 736
   For other services, by subject
Fee–Splitting
   Dental   WU 58
   Medical   W 58
   See also Fees, Dental   WU 77; Fees, Medical
   W 80; Fees and Charges   W 74, etc.
Feeble–Mindedness see Mental Retardation
Feedback
   Electronics   TK 7871.58.F4
   Mechanical engineering   TJ 216
   Psychophysiology   WL 103
   See also Biofeedback (Psychology)   WL 103,
   etc.
Feedback, Psychophysiologic see Biofeedback
   (Psychology)

**ALWAYS CONSULT MAIN SCHEDULES. USE NUMBER ASSIGNED ONLY WHEN
SUBJECT REPRESENTS MAJOR EMPHASIS OF WORK BEING CLASSIFIED**

Feeding see Child Nutrition; Food Supply; Infant
  Nutrition
Feeding Behavior
  Customs   GT 2850–2960
  Disorders (Neurosis)   WM 175
Feeding Methods
  General   WB 410
  Child   WS 115–130
  Infant   WS 115–130
  See also names of specfic feeding methods, e.g.,
    Bottle Feeding   WS 120; Breast Feeding   WS
    125; Enteral Nutrition   WB 410; Parenteral
    Nutrition   WB 410
Feeding Patterns see Feeding Behavior
Feelings see Emotions
Fees and Charges   W 74
  Fee-splitting
    Dental   WU 58
    Medical   W 58
  Hospitals   WX 157
  Nursing   WY 77
  See also Economics, Medical   W 74 and
    economics in other specialties
Fees, Dental   WU 77
  Fee-splitting   WU 58
Fees, Medical   W 80
  Fee-splitting   W 58
Fees, Pharmaceutical   QV 736
Fees, Prescription see Prescription Fees
Feigned Diseases see Malingering
Feldshers see Physician Assistants
Feline Fibrosarcoma Virus see Sarcoma Virus,
  Feline
Feline Sarcoma Virus see Sarcoma Virus, Feline
Fellowships and Scholarships
  Dental   WU 20
  Medical   W 20
  Nursing   WY 18.5
  Pharmacy   QV 20
Female Circumcision see Circumcision, Female
Female Condoms see Condoms, Female
Female Genitalia see Genitalia, Female
Feminism   HQ 1101–1870.9
Feminist Ethics see Feminism
Femoral Artery   WG 595.F3
Femoral Fractures   WE 865
Femoral Head Prosthesis see Hip Prosthesis
Femoral Hernia see Hernia, Femoral
Femoral Neck Fractures   WE 865
Femoral Nerve   WL 400
Femoral Vein   WG 625.F3
Femur   WE 865
Femur Head   WE 865
Femur Neck   WE 865
Fenazoxine see Nefopam
Fendiline   QV 150
Fenestration, Labyrinth   WV 265
  See also Otosclerosis   WV 265
Fenfluramine   QV 129
Fenformin see Phenformin
Fenilbutazon see Phenylbutazone
Fenitoin see Phenytoin

Fenoterol
Fentanyl   QV 89
Fermentation   QU 34
  Industrial   QW 75
  Of beverages   QW 85
Ferments see Enzymes
Ferredoxins
  In bacteriological chemistry   QW 52
  In photosynthesis   QK 882
  Other special topics, by subject
Ferrets   QL 737.C25
  As laboratory animals   QY 60.M2
  As pets   SF 459.F47
  Diseases   SF 997.3
Ferrihemoglobin see Methemoglobin
Ferriprotoporphyrin see Hemin
Ferritin   QV 183
Ferrocyanides
  Inorganic chemistry   QD 181.F4
  Pharmacology   QV 183
Ferroprotoporphyrin see Heme
Ferrous Compounds   QV 183
Ferroxidase see Ceruloplasmin
Fertility   WP 565
  Animals
    Domestic   SF 871
    Wild   QP 273
  Drugs affecting   QV 170
  Drug effects   WP 565
  Male   WJ 702
  Radiation effects   WN 620
Fertility Agents   QV 170
Fertility Factor see F Factor
Fertilization   WQ 205
  Animals
    Domestic   SF 871
    Wild   QP 273
  Biology (General)   QH 485
  Plants   QK 828
Fertilization, Delayed see Fertilization
Fertilization in Vitro   WQ 208
Fertilization, Polyspermic see Fertilization
Fertilized Ovum see Zygote
Fertilizers   S 631–667
Festivals see Holidays
Fetal Alcohol Syndrome   WQ 211
Fetal Anoxia   WQ 211
Fetal Circulation, Persistent see Persistent Fetal
  Circulation Syndrome
Fetal Death   WQ 225
  Veterinary   SF 887
Fetal Development   WQ 210.5
Fetal Diseases   WQ 211
Fetal Distress   WQ 211
Fetal Growth Retardation   WQ 211
Fetal Heart   WQ 210.5
Fetal Heart Rate see Heart Rate, Fetal
Fetal Hemoglobin   WQ 210.5
Fetal Maturity, Chronologic see Gestational Age
Fetal Maturity, Functional see Fetal Organ Maturity
Fetal Membranes
  Embryology   QS 645
  Neoplasms   QZ 310

Obstetrics WQ 210
   See also Chorion WQ 210 etc.
Fetal Monitoring WQ 209
Fetal Organ Maturity WQ 210.5
Fetal Presentation see Labor Presentation
Fetal Presentation, Breech see Breech Presentation
Fetal Structures see Embryonic Structures
Fetal Transfusion see Blood Transfusion, Intrauterine
Fetal Ultrasonography see Ultrasonography,
  Prenatal
Fetal Viability WQ 210.5
Fetishism (Psychiatric) WM 610
Fetoplacental Function Tests see Placental Function
  Tests
Fetoscopy WQ 209
Fetotoxins see Teratogens
Fetuins see alpha Fetoproteins
Fetus WQ 210–211
   Disproportion WQ 310
   Effect of labor on WS 405
   Embryology QS 645
   Experimentation W 20.5
   Manipulation WQ 415
   Monitoring WQ 209
   Presentation see Labor Presentation WQ 307,
    etc.
   Version see Delivery WQ 415, etc.
Fever WB 152
   Drugs relieving see Analgesics,
    Anti–Inflammatory QV 95
   Therapeutic use see Hyperthermia, Induced
    WB 469, etc.
Fever Blister Virus see Simplexvirus
Fever Therapy see Hyperthermia, Induced
Fiber Optics QC 447.9–448.2
   In endoscopy WB 141
   See also use in specific types of endoscopy
Fiberglass Casts see Casts, Surgical
Fibrillation see Atrial Fibrillation; Ventricular
  Fibrillation
Fibrin WH 310
   Clinical examination QY 410
Fibrinogen WH 310
   Clinical examination QY 410
Fibrinogen Deficiency see Afibrinogenemia
Fibrinokinase see Streptodornase and Streptokinase
Fibrinoligase see Protein–Glutamine
  gamma–Glutamyltransferase
Fibrinolysis WH 310
Fibrinolytic Agents QV 190
Fibrinolytic Therapy see Thrombolytic Therapy
Fibroblast Growth Factor QU 107
Fibrocystic Disease of Breast WP 840
Fibrocystic Disease of Pancreas see Cystic Fibrosis
Fibrocystic Mastopathy see Fibrocystic Disease of
  Breast
Fibroid see Fibroma; Leiomyoma
Fibroid Tumor see Leiomyoma
Fibroids, Uterine see Uterine Neoplasms
Fibroma QZ 340
Fibroma, Shope see Tumor Virus Infections
Fibromatosis, Aggressive QZ 340
   Localized, by site

Fibromyalgia WE 544
Fibronectins QU 55
Fibrosarcoma Virus, Feline see Sarcoma Virus,
  Feline
Fibrosis QZ 150
   Localized, by site
Fibrosis, Bone Marrow see Myelofibrosis
Fibrosis, Liver see Liver Cirrhosis
Fibrositis see Fibromyalgia
Fibrous Dysplasia of Bone WE 250
Fibula WE 870
Fiedler's Disease see Weil's Disease
Field–Block Anesthesia see Anesthesia, Conduction
Field Dependence–Independence BF 323.F45
Figural Aftereffect WW 105
Filaria see Filarioidea
Filarial Elephantiasis see Elephantiasis, Filarial
Filariasis WC 880
Filariasis, Lymphatic see Elephantiasis, Filarial
Filarioidea QX 301
Filarioidea Infections see Filariasis
Fillings, Dental see Inlays; Dental Materials; specific
  types of material used
Film, Radiographic see X–Ray Film
Film–Screen Systems, X–Ray see X–Ray
  Intensifying Screens
Film, X–Ray see X–Ray Film
Films see Motion Pictures
Filth, Epidemic Factor see Communicable Disease
  Control; Environmental Health
Filtration QD 63.F5
Finances see Economics; headings beginning with
  Fee or Fees, etc.
Financial Audit
   Dental administration WU 77
   Hospital administration WX 157
   Medical administration W 80
   Nursing administration WY 77
   Pharmacy administration QV 736
   In other specific fields, by subject
Financial Management
   Dentistry WU 77
   Medicine W 80
   Nursing WY 77
   Pharmacy QV 736
Financial Management, Hospital WX 157
Financial Risk Sharing see Risk Sharing, Financial
Financial Support
   For health planning WA 525–546
   For research (Form number 20–20.5 in any NLM
    schedule where applicable)
   For training (Form number 18 in any NLM
    schedule where applicable)
   See also Health Planning Support; Research
    Support; Training Support.
Financing, Capital see Capital Financing
Financing, Construction WX 157
Financing, Government HJ
   Education (Form number 18 in any NLM
    schedule where applicable)
   Health insurance W 275, etc.
   Hospitals WX 157
   Public health organizations WA 540
   Other special topics, by subject

Floods see Natural Disasters
Floor of Mouth see Mouth Floor
Floppy Mitral Valve see Mitral Valve Prolapse
Florafur see Tegafur
Flour
    As a dietary supplement in health or disease
    WB 431
    Sanitary control   WA 695-701
Flow Cytometry   QH 585.5.F56
    Clinical pathology   QY 95
Flow Microfluorimetry see Flow Cytometry
Flow, Pulsating see Pulsatile Flow
Flowmeters
    Measuring blood flow velocity   WG 106
    Measuring fluids   TJ 935
    Measuring gases   TJ 1025
    Measuring water   TC 177
Flowmetry see Rheology
Floxuridine   QV 268.5
Flubenisolone see Betamethasone
Flufenazin see Fluphenazine
Fluid Balance see Water-Electrolyte Balance
Fluid Therapy   WD 220
Flukes see Trematoda
Flumazenil   QV 77.9
Flumazepil see Flumazenil
Flunarizine   QV 150
Fluocortolone
    As dermatologic agent   QV 60
Fluocortolone Caproate see Fluocortolone
Fluocortolone Pivalate see Fluocortolone
Fluoren-2-ylacetamide see 2-Acetylaminofluorene
Fluorenes   QZ 202
Fluorescein Angiography   WG 500
    Ocular diagnosis   WW 141
Fluoresceins   QV 240
Fluorescence
    Physics   QC 477-477.4
    Qualitative and quantitative analysis
    (Fluorimetry)   QD 79.F4
        Quantitative analysis   QD 117.F5
    Special topics, by subject, e.g., in urinalysis   QY
    185
Fluorescence-Activated Cell Sorting see Flow
    Cytometry
Fluorescence Angiography see Fluorescein
    Angiography
Fluorescence Microscopy see Microscopy,
    Fluorescence
Fluorescent Antibody Technique   QW 525.5.F6
    In clinical pathology   QY 250
    Used for special purposes, by subject
Fluorescent Antinuclear Antibodies see Antibodies,
    Antinuclear
Fluorescent Antinuclear Antibody Test see
    Fluorescent Antibody Technique
Fluorescent Dyes   QV 240
Fluorescent Probes see Fluorescent Dyes
Fluorescent Protein Tracing see Fluorescent
    Antibody Technique
Fluoridation   WU 270
Fluoride Poisoning   QV 282
    Dentistry   WU 270

    Veterinary   SF 757.5
Fluoride Varnishes see Fluorides, Topical
Fluorides   QV 282
Fluorides, Topical   QV 282
    Dental pharmacology   QV 50
Fluorimetry see Fluorometry
Fluorinated Hydrocarbons see Hydrocarbons,
    Fluorinated
Fluorine   QV 282
    Metabolism   QU 130.5
    Toxicity in animals   SF 757.5
Fluormethyldehydrocorticosterone see
    Fluocortolone
Fluorochromes see Fluorescent Dyes
Fluorodeoxyuridine see Floxuridine
Fluorotur see Tegafur
Fluoroimmunoassay   QW 525.5.F6
    In clinical pathology   QY 250
    Used for special purposes, by subject
Fluorometry
    Analytical chemistry (General)   QD 79.F4
    Laboratory diagnosis   QY 25
    Quantitative analysis   QD 117.F5
    Used for particular purposes, by subject
Fluorophotometry   WW 143
Fluoroscopy   WN 220
    Used for diagnosis of particular disorders, with
    the disorder or system
Fluorosis, Dental   WU 220
Fluorouracil   QV 269
Fluostigmine see Isoflurophate
Fluoxetine
    As a serotonin uptake inhibitor   QV 126
    As an antidepressive agent   QV 77.5
    Biochemistry   QU 61
Fluphenazine   QV 77.9
Flurazepam   QV 77.9
Flurbiprofen   QV 95
    Biochemistry   QU 98
Flutter, Auricular see Auricular Flutter
FMN   QU 135
Focal Epilepsy see Epilepsy, Focal
Focal Infection   WC 230
Focal Infection, Dental   WU 290
Fogarty Balloon Catheterization see Balloon
    Dilatation
Folate Polyglutamates see Pteroylpolyglutamic
    Acids
Foley Balloon Catheterization see Balloon Dilatation
Folic Acid   QU 188
Folic Acid Deficiency   WD 120
Folic Acid Reductase see Tetrahydrofolate
    Dehydrogenase
Folie a Deux see Shared Paranoid Disorder
Folinic Acid see Leucovorin
Folk Medicine see Medicine, Traditional
Folklore   GR
    Curiosities   WZ 308
    Medical   WZ 309
    General works   GR 60-71
Follicle-Stimulating Hormone see FSH
Follicular Lymphoma see Lymphoma, Follicular
Folliculostatin see Inhibin

Follow–Up Studies
  (Form number 20 in any NLM schedule where
    applicable)
  In a particular area, with the subject of the
    original study, e.g., Heart Diseases WG 210
Food
  Adulteration see Food Contamination WA 701
  Allergy see Food Hypersensitivity WD 310
  Assimilation QU 120
  Chemical technology see Food Technology TP
    368–456, etc.
  Chemistry QU 50
  Deficiency diseases WD 105–155
  Digestion WI 102
  Fads see Diet Fads WB 449
  For children WS 115–130
  For infants see Infant Food WS 115–125
  Fresh WA 703
  Hospital service see Food Service, Hospital
    WX 168
  Laws see Legislation, Food WA 697;
    subheading legislation under heading beginning
    with Food
  Nutritive value QU 145.5
  Public health aspects WA 695–722
  Therapeutic use see Diet Therapy WB 400–449;
    names of specific foods
Food Additives WA 712
Food Adulteration see Food Contamination
Food Allergy see Food Hypersensitivity
Food Analysis
  Bacteriology QW 85
  Biochemistry QU 50
  Home Economics TX 501–597
  Nutrition QU 145.5
  Sanitation WA 695–722
  Analysis for specific nutritive agents QU 50–98,
    etc.
Food, Artificial see Food, Formulated
Food–Borne Diseases see Communicable Diseases;
  Food Contamination; Food Poisoning
Food Browning see Maillard Reaction
Food, Canned see Food Preservation
Food Coloring Agents WA 712
Food Contamination WA 701
  Poisoning from see Food Poisoning WC 268,
    etc.
Food Contamination, Radioactive WN 612
Food Deprivation
  Experimental biochemistry QU 34
  Experimental pharmacology QV 34
  See also Hunger QU 146, etc.
    Deficiency Diseases WD 105–155, etc.
Food, Dried see Food Preservation
Food, Drug and Cosmetic Act see Legislation, Drug
Food Fads see Diet Fads
Food, Formulated WB 447
  Special types or for special purposes, by subject
Food, Fortified QU 145.5
  Food processing (General) TP 370
Food, Frozen see Frozen Foods
Food Habits GT 2850–2960

Food Handling
  Restaurant sanitation WA 799
  Sanitation WA 695–722
  Technology TP 368–684
Food, Health see Health Food
Food Hypersensitivity WD 310
Food Industry
  Economics HD 9000–9495
  Occupational medicine aspects WA 400–495
  Public health aspects WA 695–722
  Technology TP 368–684
  See also Food Handling WA 799, etc.; Food
    Packaging TP 374, etc.; Food–Processing
    Industry TP 368–684, etc.; Food Technology
      TP 368–456, etc.; Meat–Packing Industry
    TS 1970–1973, etc.; names of specific industries
    and food processing activities
Food, Infant see Infant Food
Food Inspection WA 695
Food Intake Regulation see Appetite Regulation
Food, Irradiated see Food Irradiation
Food Irradiation WA 710
Food Laws see Legislation, Food
Food Microbiology QW 85
Food, Organic see Health Food
Food Packaging
  Chemical technology TP 374
  Public health aspects WA 695–722
Food Parasitology WA 701
Food Plants see Plants, Edible
Food Poisoning WC 268
  Veterinary SF 757.5
    See also Mushroom Poisoning WD 520; Plant
      Poisoning WD 500–530, etc.; Salmonella
      Food Poisoning WC 268; Staphylococcal
      Food Poisoning WC 268 and specific types
      of poisoning or poisoning agents
Food Preferences
  Health aspects QT 235
  Institutional cooking TX 820
Food Preservation WA 710
Food Preservatives WA 712
Food, Preserved see Food Preservation
Food Processing see Food Handling
Food–Processing Industry
  Chemical technology TP 368–684
  Economic aspects HD 9000–9495
  Occupational medicine WA 400–495
  Industrial waste WA 788
Food Selection see Food Preferences
Food Service, Hospital WX 168
Food Services
  Public health aspects WA 695–722
  Schools
    Elementary and Secondary WA 350
    University and College WA 351
  See also Dietary Services WX 168, etc.;
    Restaurants WA 799
Food, Supplemented see Dietary Supplements
Food Supplements see Dietary Supplements
Food Supply
  Home economics TX 351–354.5
  Public health aspects WA 695–722

Food Technology
  Chemical technology   TP 368–456
  Public health aspects   WA 695–722
  See also Meat   WA 707, etc.; names of other specific foods
Food Values see Nutritive value
Foot   WE 880–886
Foot-and-Mouth Disease   SF 793
Foot-and-Mouth Disease Virus see Aphthovirus
Foot Bones   WE 880
  Deformities see Foot Deformities   WE 883
Foot Deformities   WE 883
Foot Deformities, Acquired   WE 883
Foot Deformities, Congenital   WE 883
Foot Dermatoses   WR 140
  See also Tinea pedis   WR 310
Foot Diseases   WE 880
  Veterinary (General)   SF 906
Foot Joint see Tarsal Joint
Foot Ulcer, Diabetic see Diabetic Foot
Football   QT 260.5.F6
Footprints, DNA see DNA Footprinting
Foramen of Monro see Cerebral Ventricles
Foramen Ovale, Patent see Heart Septal Defects, Atrial
Forced Expiratory Flow Rates   WF 102
  As a diagnostic test   WF 141
  General physical examination   WB 284
Forced Expiratory Flow 0.2–1.2 see Maximal Expiratory Flow Rate
Forced Expiratory Flow 200–1200 see Maximal Expiratory Flow Rate
Forceps Delivery see Methods   WQ 425 under Delivery; Obstetrical Forceps
Forearm   WE 820
Forearm Injuries   WE 820
Forebrain see Embryology   WL 300 under Brain
Forecasting   CB 158
  Agriculture   HD 1401–2210
  Business   HB 3730
  Civilization   CB 428–430
  Environment   HC 79.E5
  Health manpower   W 76
  Hospitals   WX 140
  Natural resources
    Conservation   S 900–954
    Economics   HC 55
    Land   HD 1635 1741; S 950–954
  Urban areas   HT 165.5–178
  Other special topics, by subject
Forefoot, Human   WE 880
Foreign Aid see International Cooperation
Foreign Bodies
  As a cause of disease   QZ 55
  In the ear   WV 222
  Localization by radiography   WN 210
  Removal   WO 700
  Localized, by site
  See also Bezoars   WI 300, etc.; Eye Foreign Bodies   WW 525
Foreign Medical Graduates
  Education   W 18–20
  Supply & distribution   W 76

Foreign Professional Personnel
  Health sciences (General)   W 76
  Science   Q 147–149
  See also Foreign Medical Graduates   W 76, etc.
Forelimb   QL 950.7
Forensic Chemistry see Chemistry
Forensic Dentistry   W 601–925
  General works   W 705
Forensic Examination of Blood see Blood Chemical Analysis
Forensic Medicine   W 601–925
  Directories   W 622
  Examination of evidential material   W 750
    Postmortem   W 825
  Medical evidence for establishing responsibility   W 725
  Medicolegal examination   W 775–867
  Nineteenth century works   W 600
  See also Jurisprudence   W 32.5–32.6
Forensic Psychiatry   W 740
  As a career   W 740
Foreskin see Penis
Forestier–Certonciny Syndrome see Polymyalgia Rheumatica
Forests see Trees
Form Perception   WW 105
Formaldehyde
  Organic chemistry   QD 305.A6
  Pharmacology   QV 225
Formalin see Formaldehyde
Formalin Test see Pain Measurement
Formates   QU 98
  Organic chemistry
    Aliphatic compounds   QD 305.A2
Formicoidea Venoms see Ant Venoms
Forms and Records Control   W 80
  Special field, by subject
Formularies   QV 740
Formularies, Dental   QV 50
Formularies, Homeopathic   WB 930
Formularies, Hospital   QV 740
Forskolin
  Biochemistry   QU 85
  Toxicology   QV 633
Fosfomycin   QV 350
Fossils   QE 701–996.5
  Special topics, by subject
Foster Home Care   HV 875
  Public health aspects   WA 310–320
  Of persons with various disabilities, with the disability, e.g., of mental patients   WM 29; of the mentally retarded child   WS 107.5.F6
Fourier Analysis   QA 403.5–404.5
  Biomedical mathematics   QT 35
Fowl Paralysis see Marek's Disease
Fowl Pest see Fowl Plague
Fowl Plague   SF 995.6.F59
Fowl Plague Virus see Influenza A Virus, Avian
Fowls, Domestic see Poultry
Foxes   QL 737.C22
Foxglove see Digitalis
Fractionation
  Of a particular substance, with the substance, e.g.,

Blood protein fractionation   QY 455
See also Cell Fractionation   QH 585.5.C43
Fracture Fixation   WE 185
Veterinary   SF 914.4
Fracture Fixation, Internal   WE 185
Fracture Fixation, Intramedullary   WE 185
Fractures   WE 175–185
Child   WE 175–180
Infant   WE 175–180
See also types of fracture by site, e.g., Skull
Fractures   WL 354
Fractures, Compound see Fractures, Open
Fractures, Fatigue see Fractures, Stress
Fractures, March see Fractures, Stress
Fractures, Open   WE 182
Fractures, Pathological see Fractures, Spontaneous
Fractures, Spontaneous   WE 180
Fractures, Stress   WE 180
Fractures, Ununited   WE 180
Fragile Sites, Chromosome see Chromosome
Fragility
Fragile X Syndrome   QS 677
Fragilitas Ossium see Osteogenesis Imperfecta
Frail Elderly   WT
See special topics under Aged
Frail Older Adults see Frail Elderly
Frambesia see Yaws
Frames (Spectacles) see Eyeglasses
Frangula see Rhamnus
Fraternities see Societies; names of specialties
Fraud   HV 6691–6699
Special topics, by subject
Fraud, Drug Manufacture and Sales see Drug
Industry
Fraud, Scientific see Scientific Misconduct
Fraudulent Data see Scientific Misconduct
Freckles see Lentigo
Free Association   WM 460.5.F8
Free Fatty Acids see Fatty Acids, Nonesterified
Free Radicals   QD 471
Freedom
Political theory   JC 585–599
Sociology   HM
Special topics, by subject
Freeze Drying
Blood   WH 460
Food   WA 710
Research techniques   QH 324.9.C7
Tissue   QS 525
See also Tissue Preservation   WO 665, etc.
Freeze Fracturing   QH 236.2
Freezing
Anesthesia see Hypothermia, Induced   WO 350
Biochemical technique   QU 25
Blood   WH 460
Food   WA 710
Normal effects on cells   QH 653
Research techniques   QH 324.9.C7
Special aspects, by subject
Tissue   WO 665
Frei's Disease see Lymphogranuloma Venereum
Frenum, Labial see Labial Frenum
Fresh Foods see Food

Fresh Frozen Plasma see Plasma
Fresh Water   WA 675–690
Freudian Theory   WM 460
Friedlaender's Pneumonia see Pneumonia
Friedreich's Ataxia   WL 390
Friedreich's Disease see Myoclonus
Frigidity see Sexual Dysfunctions, Psychological
Fringe Benefits see Salaries and Fringe Benefits
Froehlich's Syndrome   WK 550
Frog Venoms see Amphibian Venoms
Frogs and Toads see Anura
Frontal Bone   WE 705
Frontal Lobe   WL 307
Frontal Sinus   WV 350
Frostbite   WG 530
Frottage see Paraphilias
Frozen Foods   WA 710
Frozen Sections   QH 233
Frozen Semen see Semen Preservation
Fructose   QU 75
Fructose–Bisphosphate Aldolase   QU 139
Fructosediphosphate Aldolase see
Fructose–Bisphosphate Aldolase
Fructosediphosphates   QU 75
Fruit
As a dietary supplement in health or disease
WB 430
Plant culture   SB 354–399
Sanitation and other public health aspects   WA
703
Fruit, Citrus see Citrus
Fruit Flies see Drosophila
Frusemide see Furosemide
Frustration   BF 575.F7
Adolescence   WS 462
Child   WS 105.5.E5
Infant   WS 105.5.E5
FSH   WK 515
FSH–Releasing Hormone see Gonadorelin
Ftorafur see Tegafur
Fuchsin Dyes see Rosaniline Dyes
Fuchsins see Rosaniline Dyes
Fucidin see Fusidic Acid
Fucosyltransferases   QU 141
FUdR see Floxuridine
Fuel Oils
Chemical technology   TP 345–359
Toxicology   QV 633
Fuels
Chemical technology   TP 315–360
Energy conservation   TJ 163.3–163.5
Heating   WA 770
Pollution   WA 754
See also Gas Poisoning   QV 662, etc. and names
of other specific fuels
Fugue see Dissociative Disorders
Full Dentures see Denture, Complete
Fumigation see Sterilization
Function Tests see Heart Function Tests; Kidney
Function Tests; Liver Function Tests; Ovarian
Function Tests; Pituitary–Adrenal Function Tests;
Pituitary Function Tests; Placental Function
Tests; Respiratory Function Tests; Thyroid

Function Tests; Vestibular Function Tests; See
also names of specific tests
Functional Heart Disease see Neurocirculatory
Asthenia and names of other functional disorders
Functional Psychoses see Psychotic Disorders
Functionally-Impaired Elderly see Frail Elderly
Fund Raising
    Hospitals   WX 157
    Other special topics, by subject
Funding, Capital see Capital Financing
Fundus Fluorescence Photography see Fluorescein
Angiography
Fundus Oculi   WW 270
Funduscopes see Ophthalmoscopes
Funeral Directors see Mortuary Practice
Funeral Rites
    Ethnology   GN 486
    Manners and customs   GT 3150–3390.5
    Psychology   BF 789.F8
Fungal Antigens see Antigens, Fungal
Fungal Spores see Spores, Fungal
Fungal Toxins see Mycotoxins
Fungal Vaccines   WC 450
Fungi
    As a cause of disease   QZ 65
    Non-pathogenic   QK 600–635
    Pathogenic   QW 180–180.5
Fungi imperfecti see Deuteromycetes
Fungicides, Industrial
    Agriculture   SB 951.3
    Public health aspects   WA 240
    See also Antifungal Agents   QV 252
Fungicides, Therapeutic see Antifungal Agents
Fungus Diseases see Mycoses
Fungus Poisoning see Mycotoxicosis
Funnel Chest   WE 715
Furans
    Organic chemistry   QD 405
Furazosin see Prazosin
Furniture see Interior Design and Furnishings
Furocoumarins see Psoralens
Furosemide   QV 160
Furrow Keratitis see Keratitis, Dendritic
Fursemide see Furosemide
Furunculosis   WR 235
Fusarium   QW 180.5.D38
Fusidic Acid   QV 350
Fusobacterium   QW 133
Fusobacterium Infections   WC 200
    Veterinary   SF 809.F87
Futurology see Forecasting
F1 ATPase see H(+)-Transporting ATP Synthase
F1F0 ATPase Complex see H(+)-Transporting
ATP Synthase

G

G Force see Gravitation
G Periods see Interphase
G Phases see Interphase
G-Proteins   QU 55
GABA   QU 60
GABA Receptors see Receptors, GABA

GABA Transaminase see 4-Aminobutyrate
Transaminase
Gagging   WI 143
Gait   WE 103
Galactokinase   QU 141
Galactose   QU 75
Galactosemia   WD 205.5.C2
Galactosidases   QU 136
Galago   QL 737.P955
    As laboratory animals   QY 60.P7
    Diseases   SF 997.5.P7
Galanin   WL 104
Galantamin see Galanthamine
Galanthamine   QV 124
Gallbladder   WI 750
Gallbladder Diseases   WI 750
Gallbladder Neoplasms   WI 765
Gallium
    Organic chemistry   QD 181.G2
    Pharmacology   QV 290
Gallodesoxycholic Acid see Chenodeoxycholic Acid
Gallopamil   QV 150
Gallstones see Cholelithiasis
Gallstones, Common Bile Duct see Common Bile
Duct Calculi
Galvanic Skin Response
    Psychiatric test   WM 145
    Reflex test (general)   WL 106
Galvanism, Oral see Electrogalvanism, Intraoral
Galvanosurgery see Electrosurgery
Galvanotherapy see Electric Stimulation Therapy
Gamasoidiasis see Mite Infestations
Gambling
    As an impulse control disorder   WM 190
    See also Risk-Taking   BF 637.R57
Game Theory   QA 269–272
    In leadership development   HM
    Other uses with the area being studied, e.g.,
      doctor/nurse relations   WY 87
Games see Physical Education and Training; Play
and Playthings; Sports; Recreation
Games, Experimental   QA 269
Gamete Intrafallopian Transfer
    Human   WQ 208
Gametogenesis   WQ 205
Gamma-Aminobutyric Acid see GABA
gamma-Aminobutyric Acid Receptors see
Receptors, GABA
gamma-Benzene Hexachloride see Lindane
Gamma Camera Imaging see Radionuclide Imaging
Gamma Globulin, 7S see IgG
Gamma Globulins   WH 400
    Clinical examination   QY 455
    Prophylactic   QW 806
    Used for treatment of particular disorder, with
      the disorder or system
gamma-Interferon see Interferon Type II
Gamma Rays   WN 105
Gammaphos see Amifostine
Ganciclovir   QV 268.5
Ganglia   WL 500
Ganglia, Autonomic   WL 600
Ganglia, Basal see Basal Ganglia

Ganglia, Parasympathetic   WL 610
Ganglia, Sympathetic   WL 610
Ganglion of Corti see Spiral Ganglion
Ganglioneuroma   QZ 380
   Localized, by site
Ganglionic Blockers   QV 132
Ganglionic Blocking Agents see Ganglionic Blockers
Ganglioplegic Agents see Ganglionic Blockers
Gangliosides   QU 85
Gangliosidoses   WD 205.5.L5
Gangrene   QZ 180
   Gas see Gas Gangrene   WC 375
Ganja see Cannabis
Garbage Disposal see Refuse Disposal
Gargoylism see Mucopolysaccharidosis I
Garlic
   As a dietary supplement in health or disease
   WB 430
   As a medicinal plant   QV 766
Gas Gangrene   WC 375
Gas Masks see Respiratory Protective Devices
Gas Poisoning   QV 662
   In industry   WA 465
Gases
   Analysis   QD 121
   As anesthetics   QV 81
   Asphyxiating see Lung irritants   QV 664 under
   Irritants
   Chemical technology   TP 242-244
   Description and properties   QC 161-168.86
   In air pollution see Air Pollutants   WA 754,
   etc.
   Inorganic chemistry   QD 162
   Irritant see Irritants   QV 666, etc.
   Lacrimator see Tear Gases   QV 665
   Paralysants   QV 667
   Pharmacology   QV 310-318
   Poisonous see Gas Poisoning   QV 662, etc.
   Vesicant see Irritants   QV 666, etc.
   War see Chemical Warfare Agents   QV 663-667
Gasoline
   Chemical technology   TP 692.2
   Handling and storage   TP 692.5
   Toxicology   QV 633
Gastrectomy   WI 380
   Child   WS 310
   Infant   WS 310
Gastric Acid   WI 302
Gastric Acidity Determination   QY 130
Gastric Antacid Drugs see Antacids
Gastric Antrum see Pyloric Antrum
Gastric Chief Cells see Chief Cells, Gastric
Gastric Contents see Analysis   QY 130 under
   Stomach
Gastric Emptying   WI 302
Gastric Fistula   WI 300
Gastric Fundus   WI 300
Gastric Hypothermia   WI 380
   Used for treatment of particular disorders, with
   the disorder
Gastric Juice   WI 302
   Clinical pathology   QY 130

Gastric Mucosa
   Cytology   WI 301
   Physiology   WI 302
Gastric Parietal Cells see Parietal Cells, Gastric
Gastric Ulcer see Stomach Ulcer
Gastric Varices see Esophageal and Gastric Varices
Gastrin Receptors see Receptors, Cholecystokinin
Gastrins   WK 170
Gastritis   WI 310
Gastroduodenal Ulcer see Peptic Ulcer
Gastroenteritis   WI 140
Gastroenteritis, Transmissible, of Swine   SF 977.T7
Gastroenterology   WI
   Child   WS 310-312
   Infant   WS 310-312
Gastroenterostomy   WI 900
Gastroesophageal Reflux   WI 250
Gastrointestinal Agents   QV 66
Gastrointestinal Diseases   WI 140
   Child   WS 310-312
   Infant   WS 310-312
   Nursing   WY 156.5
   Veterinary   SF 851
Gastrointestinal Hemorrhage   WI 143
   Particular types, by type
Gastrointestinal Hormone Receptors see Receptors,
   Gastrointestinal Hormone
Gastrointestinal Hormones   WK 170
Gastrointestinal Motility   WI 102
Gastrointestinal Neoplasms   WI 149
Gastrointestinal Surgical Procedures see Digestive
   System Surgical Procedures
Gastrointestinal System   WI
   Child   WS 310-312
   Drugs acting on see Gastrointestinal Agents
   QV 66
   Hormones see Gastrointestinal Hormones   WK
   170
   Infant   WS 310-312
   Manifestations of disease   WI 143
Gastroscopes see Endoscopes
Gastroscopy   WI 300
Gatekeepers, Health Service see Referral and
   Consultation
Gaucher's Disease   WD 205.5.L5
Gays see Homosexuality, Male
GB Hepatitis Agents see Hepatitis Agents, GB
GB Virus A see Hepatitis Agents, GB
GB Virus B see Hepatitis Agents, GB
GB Virus C see Hepatitis Agents, GB
Geese   QL 696.A52
   Culture   SF 505-505.63
   Diseases   SF 995.2
Gehrig's Disease see Amyotrophic Lateral Sclerosis
Geiger-Mueller Counters see Radiometry
Gel Diffusion Tests see Immunodiffusion
Gel Electrophoresis, Two-Dimensional see
   Electrophoresis, Gel, Two-Dimensional
Gel Precipitation Test see Immunodiffusion
Gelada Baboon see Theropithecus
Gelatin   QU 55
Gels   QV 785
Gelsemium   QV 766

Toxicology   QV 628
Gender see Sex
Gender Identity   HQ 1075
    Adolescence   WS 462
    Child   WS 105.5.P3
    Infant   WS 105.5.P3
    Psychological aspects   BF 692.2
        In men   BF 692.5
        In women   HQ 1206, etc.
Gender Role see Gender Identity
Gene Action Regulation see Gene Expression
    Regulation
Gene Activation see Gene Expression Regulation
Gene Amplification   QH 450.3
Gene Bank see Gene Library
Gene Clusters see Multigene Family
Gene Duplication   QH 447
Gene Expression   QH 450
Gene Expression Regulation   QH 450
Gene Expression Regulation, Bacterial   QW 51
Gene Expression Regulation, Enzymologic   QU
    135
Gene Expression Regulation, Neoplastic   QZ 202
Gene Expression Regulation, Viral   QW 160
Gene Fusion   QH 462.G46
Gene Library   QH 442.4
Gene Mapping see Chromosome Mapping
Gene Pool   QH 455
Gene Probes, DNA see DNA Probes
Gene Products see Proteins
Gene Products, Bacterial see Bacterial Proteins
Gene Products, Viral see Viral Proteins
Gene Proteins see Proteins
Gene Rearrangement   QW 541
    In antibodies   QW 575
Gene Therapy   QZ 50
    Genetic engineering aspects   QH 442
    Of a specific disease, with the disease
Gene Transfer see Transfection
General Adaptation Syndrome   QZ 160
General Paralysis see Paresis
General Practice see Family Practice
General Practice, Dental   WU 21
    Textbooks   WU 100
General Practitioners see Physicians, Family
General Systems Theory see Systems Theory
Generalists see Physicians, Family
Generalization (Psychology)   BD 235
    Stimulus   BF 319.5.S7
Generalized Radiation Sickness see Radiation
    Injuries
Generic Equivalency see Therapeutic Equivalency
Genes   QH 447–447.8
Genes, Bacterial   QW 51
Genes, Class I see Genes, MHC Class I
Genes, Class II see Genes, MHC Class II
Genes, H–2 Class I see Genes, MHC Class I
Genes, HLA Class I see Genes, MHC Class I
Genes, HLA Class II see Genes, MHC Class II
Genes, Homeobox   QH 447.8.H65
Genes, Ig see Genes, Immunoglobulin
Genes, Immune Response see Genes, MHC Class
    II

Genes, Immunoglobulin   QW 601
Genes, Immunoglobulin Heavy Chain see Genes,
    Immunoglobulin
Genes, Immunoglobulin Light Chain see Genes,
    Immunoglobulin
Genes, Immunoglobulin VH Germ Line see Genes,
    Immunoglobulin
Genes, MHC Class I
    In immunogenetics   QW 541
    Speical topics, by subject
Genes, MHC Class II
    In immunogenetics   QW 541
    Special topics, by subject
Genes, ras   QZ 202
Genes, Regulator   QH 450
    Genetic regulation   QH 450–450.6
Genes, Reiterated see Multigene Family
Genes, Spliced see DNA, Recombinant
Genes, Split see Genes
Genes, Suppressor, Tumor   QZ 202
Genes, Synthetic   QH 447
Genes, Viral   QW 160
Genetic...
    See also inverted headings, e.g., Transformation,
        Genetic QW 51
Genetic Carriers see Heterozygote
Genetic Carriers, Detection see Heterozygote
    Detection
Genetic Code   QH 450.2
Genetic Counseling   QZ 50
    In family planning   HQ 766
    Other special topics, by subject
Genetic Diversity see Variation (Genetics)
Genetic Engineering   QH 442–442.6
    Chemical technology   TP 248.6
    Special topics, by subject
Genetic Engineering of Proteins see Protein
    Engineering
Genetic Induction see Gene Expression Regulation
Genetic Intervention see Genetic Engineering
Genetic Markers   QZ 50
Genetic Predisposition see Genetic Predisposition to
    Disease
Genetic Predisposition to Disease   QZ 50
    To specific diseases, with the disease
Genetic Recombination see Recombination, Genetic
Genetic Screening   QZ 50
Genetic Skin Diseases see Genetic (General)   WR
    218 under Skin Diseases
Genetic Susceptibility see Genetic Predisposition to
    Disease
Genetic Techniques   QH 441
    Medical   QZ 50
    Social and moral aspects   QH 438.7
Genetic Toxicity Tests see Mutagenicity Tests
Genetic Translation see Translation, Genetic
Genetic Vectors   QH 442.2
Genetics   QH 426–470
    Animal (General)   QH 432
        Domestic animal breeding   SF 105
    Developmental   QH 453
    Plant   QK 981–981.7
    Veterinary genetics   SF 756.5

See also Cytogenetics   QH 605, etc.;
   Pharmacogenetics   QV 38
Genetics, Bacterial see Genetics, Microbial
Genetics, Behavioral   QH 457
Genetics, Biochemical
   For the biochemist   QU 4
   Genetic regulation   QH 450–450.6
   General works   QH 430
     Human   QH 431
   Works on the retarded child   WS 107.5.B4
   Special topics, by subject
Genetics, Human see Genetics; Genetics, Medical
Genetics, Medical   QZ 50
Genetics, Microbial   QW 51
Genetics, Molecular see Genetics, Biochemical
Genetics, Population · QH 455
   Physical anthropology   GN 289
Genetics, Radiation see Radiation Genetics
Geniculate Ganglion   WL 330
Genital Diseases, Female   WP
   General works   WP 140
   Child   WS 360
   Diagnosis   WP 140
   Infant   WS 360
   Nursing   WY 156.7
     See also Obstetrical Nursing   WY 157, etc.
   Surgery   WP 660
     See also Gynecologic Surgical Procedures
     WP 660
   Therapy   WP 650
   Urologic   WJ 190
   Veterinary   SF 871
Genital Diseases, Male   WJ 700
   Veterinary   SF 871
Genital Neoplasms, Female   WP 145
Genital Neoplasms, Male   WJ 706
Genitalia
   General works (male and female, combined)
   WJ 700
   Animals, Domestic   SF 871
   Child   WS 320
   Drugs affecting   QV 170–177
   Infant   WS 320
     See also Gonads   WK 900
Genitalia, Female   WP
   General works   WP 100
   Child   WS 360
   Infant   WS 360
   See also specific organs
Genitalia, Male   WJ 700–875
   Child   WS 320
   Infant   WS 320
Genitourinary Diseases see Urogenital Diseases
Genitourinary Neoplasms see Urogenital Neoplasms
Genitourinary System see Urogenital System
Genius see Child, Gifted; Creativeness; Intelligence
Genome, Human   QH 447
Genomic Library   QH 442.4
Genotype   QH 447
   Histocompatibility   WO 680
Gentamicins   QV 350.5.G3
Gentamycin see Gentamicins
Gentian see Plants, Medicinal

Gentian Violet
   As an anthelmintic   QV 253
   As an anti–infective agent   QV 235
Geographic Tongue see Glossitis, Benign Migratory
Geography
   Medical see Climate   WB 700–710;
     Epidemiology   WA 900, etc.; names of
     diseases in a particular area   WB 700–710, etc.
Geology   QE
   General works   QE 26–26.2
Geopathology see Climate; Disease Reservoirs;
   Environmental Health
Gerbillinae   QL 737.R666
   As laboratory animals   QY 60.R6
   As pets   SF 459.G4
Gerbils see Gerbillinae
Geriatric Assessment   WT 30
Geriatric Dentistry   WU 490
Geriatric Health Services see Health Services for
   the Aged
Geriatric Nursing   WY 152
Geriatric Ophthalmology see Aged   WW 620 under
   Ophthalmology
Geriatric Psychiatry   WT 150
   As a career   WT 150
Geriatrics   WT
   See also Aged
Germ Cells   WQ 205
   Animal   QL 964–966
Germ–Free Life
   Experimentation   QY 56
     Particular experiments, by subject
   Laboratory animals   QY 56
Germ–Line Cells see Germ Cells
Germ Line Theory see Antibody Diversity
Germ Theory of Disease see Pathogenesis   QZ 65
   under Disease
German Measles see Rubella
Germanium
   Inorganic chemistry   QD 181.G5
   Pharmacology   QV 290
Germinoblastoma see Lymphoma
Gerontology see Geriatrics
Gestalt Theory   BF 203
Gestalt Therapy   WM 420.5.G3
Gestation see Pregnancy
Gestational Age   WQ 210.5
Gestosis, EPH   WQ 215
Gestures
   Adolescence   WS 462
   Child   WS 105.5.C8
   Infant   WS 105.5.C8
   Psychology   BF 637.N66
   Social psychology   HM
Ghettos see Poverty Areas
Giant Cell Arteritis see Temporal Arteritis
Giant Cell Granuloma see Granuloma, Giant Cell
Giant Cell Tumors   QZ 340
   Bone   WE 258
   Localized, by site
Giardia   QX 70
Giardiasis   WC 700
Gibbons see Hylobates

ALWAYS CONSULT MAIN SCHEDULES. USE NUMBER ASSIGNED ONLY WHEN
SUBJECT REPRESENTS MAJOR EMPHASIS OF WORK BEING CLASSIFIED

Gibraltar Fever see Brucellosis
GIFT see Gamete Intrafallopian Transfer
Gifted Child see Child, Gifted
Gifts, Financial see Fund Raising
Gigantism   WK 550
Gilbert's Disease   WD 205.5.H9
Gilles de la Tourette's Disease see Tourette
   Syndrome
Ginger see Zingiberales
Gingiva   WU 240
Gingival Crevicular Fluid   WU 240
Gingival Diseases   WU 240
Gingival Exudate see Gingival Crevicular Fluid
Gingival Index see Periodontal Index
Gingivectomy   WU 240
Gingivitis   WU 240
Gingivitis, Necrotizing Ulcerative
   For the dentist   WU 240
   For the gastroenterologist   WI 200
Gingivosis see Gingival Diseases
Gingivostomatitis, Herpetic see Stomatitis, Herpetic
Ginkgo biloba
   As a medicinal plant   QV 766
   Botany   QK 494.5.G48
Ginkgophyta see Ginkgo biloba
Ginseng   QV 766
Glanders   WC 330
   Veterinary   SF 796
Glands see Endrocrine Glands; Exocrine Glands;
   names of specific glands
Glandula Carotica see Carotid Body
Glandular Fever see Infectious Mononucleosis
Glass
   Occupational medicine   WA 400–495
   Materials of engineering and construction   TA
   450
   Optical instruments   QC 375
Glass Ionomer Cements   WU 190
Glasses see Eyeglasses
Glaucoma   WW 290
Glaucoma, Angle-Closure   WW 290
Glaucoma, Closed-Angle see Glaucoma,
   Angle-Closure
Glaucoma, Open-Angle   WW 290
Glaucoma, Pigmentary see Glaucoma, Open-Angle
Glaucoma, Simple see Glaucoma, Open-Angle
Glaucoma Simplex see Glaucoma, Open-Angle
Glial Fibrillary Acidic Protein   QU 55
Glial Intermediate Filament Protein see Glial
   Fibrillary Acidic Protein
Gliclazide   WK 825
   Organic chemistry   QD 305.S6
Gliding Bacteria   QW 128
Gliobastoma see Astrocytoma
Glioblastoma   QZ 380
   Localized, by site
Glioblastoma-Derived T-Cell Suppressor Factor see
   Transforming Growth Factor beta
Glioblastoma Multiforme see Glioblastoma
Glioma   QZ 380
   Localized, by site
Global Warming see Greenhouse Effect
Globulins   QU 55

Globus Hystericus see Conversion Disorder
Globus Pallidus   WL 307
Glomangioma see Glomus Tumor
Glomerular Filtration Rate   QY 175
Glomerulonephritis   WJ 353
Glomerulonephritis, IGA   WJ 353
Glomerulonephritis, Lupus see Lupus Nephritis
Glomerulosclerosis, Diabetic see Diabetic
   Nephropathies
Glomus Caroticum see Carotid Body
Glomus Tumor   QZ 340
   Localized, by site
Glossalgia   WI 210
Glossectomy   WI 210
Glossina see Tsetse Flies
Glossitis   WI 210
Glossitis Areata Exfoliativa see Glossitis, Benign
   Migratory
Glossitis, Benign Migratory   WI 210
Glossodynia see Glossalgia
Glossopharyngeal Nerve   WL 330
Gloves, Surgical   WO 162
GLQ223 see Trichosanthin
Glucagon   WK 801
   Associated with hypoglycemia   WK 880
Glucagonoma   WK 885
Glucan Phosphorylase see Phosphorylase
Glucans   QU 83
Glucitol see Sorbitol
Glucocorticoid Analogs see Glucocorticoids,
   Synthetic
Glucocorticoid Receptors see Receptors,
   Glucocorticoid
Glucocorticoids   WK 755
Glucocorticoids, Synthetic   WK 757
Glucocorticoids, Topical   QV 60
Glucokinase   QU 141
Gluconeogenesis   QU 75
Glucosamine   QU 75
Glucose   QU 75
   Dietary supplement   WB 427
   Infusion technique   WB 354
   Pharmacology   QU 75
Glucose, Blood see Blood Glucose
Glucose Infusion see Glucose; Infusions, Parenteral
Glucose Oxidase   QU 140
Glucose Solution, Hypertonic   QU 75
   Infusion   WB 354
Glucose Tolerance Test   QY 470
Glucose-6-Phosphatase   QU 136
Glucose-6-Phosphatase Deficiency see Glycogen
   Storage Disease Type I
Glucose-6-Phosphate Dehydrogenase see
   Glucosephosphate Dehydrogenase
Glucosephosphatase see Glucose-6-Phosphatase
Glucosephosphatase Deficiency see Glycogen
   Storage Disease Type I
Glucosephosphate Dehydrogenase   QU 140
Glucosephosphate Dehydrogenase Deficiency
   WH 170
Glucosides   QU 75
Glucosiduronates see Glucuronates
Glucosyltransferases   QU 141

Glucuronates   QU 84
   Organic chemistry   QD 321
Glucuronidase   QU 136
Glucuronides see Glucuronates
Glue Sniffing see Substance-Related Disorders
Glues see Adhesives
Glutamate-Ammonia Ligase   QU 138
Glutamate Dehydrogenase   QU 140
Glutamates   QU 60
Glutamic-Oxaloacetic Transaminase see Aspartate
   Transaminase
Glutamic-Pyruvic Transaminase see Alanine
   Transaminase
Glutaminase   QU 136
Glutamine   QU 60
Glutamine Synthetase see Glutamate-Ammonia
   Ligase
Glutaminyl-Peptide Gamma-Glutamyltransferase
   see Protein-Glutamine
   gamma-Glutamyltransferase
Glutaraldehyde-Stabilized Grafts see Bioprosthesis
Glutathione   QU 68
Glutathione Peroxidase   QU 140
Glutathione Reductase   QU 140
Gluteal Region see Buttocks
Gluten   QK 898.G49
Gluten Enteropathy see Celiac Disease
Glutethimide   QV 85
Glybutamide see Carbutamide
Glycans see Polysaccharides
Glycerides   QU 85
Glycerin see Glycerol
Glycerites see Solutions
Glycerol
   Biochemistry   QU 75
   In blood preservation   WH 460
   In tissue culture   QS 525
   Organic chemistry   QD 305.A4
   Pharmacology   QV 82
Glycerophosphates   QU 93
Glyceryl Trinitrate see Nitroglycerin
Glycine Max see Soybeans
Glycoconjugates   QU 75
Glycogen   QU 83
Glycogen Phosphorylase see Phosphorylase
Glycogen Storage Disease   WD 205.5.C2
Glycogen Storage Disease Type I   WD 205.5.C2
Glycogen Synthase   QU 136
Glycogen Synthetase see Glycogen Synthase
Glycogenosis see Glycogen Storage Disease
Glycogenosis 1 see Glycogen Storage Disease Type
   I
Glycolates   QU 98
   Organic chemistry
     Aliphatic compounds   QD 305.A2
Glycolipids   QU 85
Glycols
   Organic chemistry   QD 305.A4
   Pharmacology   QV 82
Glycolysis   QU 75
Glyconeogenesis see Gluconeogenesis
Glycophorin
Glycoprotein Sialyltransferases see Sialyltransferases

Glycoproteins   QU 55
Glycosidases see Glycoside Hydrolases
Glycoside Antibiotics see Antibiotics,
   Aminoglycoside
Glycoside Hydrolases   QU 136
Glycosides   QU 75
   Cardiac see Cardiac Glycosides   QV 153
Glycosuria   WK 870
Glycosylation
   Of proteins   QU 55
Glycyrrhetic Acid see Glycyrrhetinic Acid
Glycyrrhetinic Acid
   As a dermatologic agent   QV 60
   As a gastrointestinal agent   QV 66
Glycyrrhiza   QV 766
Glyoxylates   QU 98
   Organic chemistry
     Aliphatic compounds   QD 305.A2
Gnathostoma   QX 203
Gnotobiotics see Germ-Free Life
GnRH see Gonadorelin
Goals   BF 505.G6
   As a philosopical concept   B 105.G63
Goat Diseases   SF 968-969
Goat Fever see Brucellosis
Goats
   Culture   SF 380-388
Goggles see Eye Protective Devices
Goiter   WK 259
   Veterinary   SF 768.3
Goiter, Endemic   WK 259
Goiter, Exophthalmic see Graves' Disease
Goiter, Intrathoracic see Goiter, Substernal
Goiter, Substernal   WK 259
Goitrogens see Thyroid Antagonists
Gold
   Dental application   WU 180
   In organic chemistry   QD 181.A9
   Pharmacology   QV 296
   Used for treatment of particular disorders, with
     the disorder or system
Gold Alloys
   Analytical chemistry   QD 137.G6
   Dentistry   WU 180
Gold Anti-Inflammatory Agents see Antirheumatic
   Agents, Gold
Gold Antiarthritic Agents see Antirheumatic Agents,
   Gold
Gold Colloid, Radioactive   WN 420
   Nuclear physics   QC 796.A9
   See also special topics under Radioisotopes
Gold Isotopes
   Inorganic chemistry   QD 181.A9
   Pharmacology   QV 296
Gold Salts, Anti-Rheumatic see Antirheumatic
   Agents, Gold
Gold Thioglucose see Aurothioglucose
Goldfish   SF 458.G6
   As laboratory animals   QY 60.F4
Golf   QT 260.5.G6
Golgi Apparatus   QH 603.G6
Gonadal Disorders   WK 900
   See also Ovarian Diseases   WP 320-322

See also Testicular Diseases   WJ 800–875
Gonadal Dysgenesis   QS 677
Gonadal Dysgenesis, 45,X see Turner's Syndrome
Gonadal Dysgenesis, 45,XO see Turner's Syndrome
Gonadoliberin see Gonadorelin
Gonadorelin   WK 515
Gonadotropin-Releasing Hormone see Gonadorelin
Gonadotropins   WK 900
Gonadotropins, Chorionic   WK 920
Gonadotropins, Chorionic, Human see
    Gonadotropins, Chorionic
Gonadotropins, Human Menopausal see Menotropins
Gonadotropins, Pituitary   WK 515
Gonads   WK 900
    See also Ovary   WP 320–322, etc.
    Testis   WJ 830, etc.; Castration   WJ 868, etc.
Gonioscopy   WW 210
Goniotomy see Trabeculectomy
Gonococcus see Neisseria gonorrhoeae
Gonorrhea   WC 150
    Female   WP 157
Gonosomes see Sex Chromosomes
Gonyaulax see Dinoflagellida
Gordius see Helminths
Gossypium see Cotton
Gout   WE 350
    Drugs for see Gout Suppressants   QV 98
Gout Suppressants   QV 98
Governing Board
    Hospitals   WX 150
    Of other organizations and institutions, in the
        administration number for the agency or lacking
        that, in the general number, e.g., governing
        board of the American Medical Association
        WB 1
Government   J
    Agencies (General), with the country in J
        schedule
    Medical practice   W 94
        See also Institutional Practice   W 96, etc.;
        Veterinary Service, Military   UH 650–655
    Nursing service   WY 130
        See also Military Nursing   WY 130; Public
        Health Nursing   WY 108, etc.; Specialties,
        Nursing   WY 130, etc.
Government Agencies   JF 1501–1525
    Public health   WA 540–546
    See also Hospitals, Veterans   UH 460–485;
        names of particular types of agencies
Government Nursing Services see Military Nursing;
    Public Health Nursing
Government Programs   J
    Programs in particular areas, by subject, e.g.,
        National Health Programs   WA 540
    Other special topics, by subject
Government Publications
    Administrative serials   W2
    Bibliography   Z 7164.G7
        Of individual countries   Z 1201–4980
    Statistical serials   W2
    Subject oriented publications
        Monographs, by subject
        Serials (Medicine and related fields)   W1

Government Regulations see Legislation; names of
    products or specialties being regulated, e.g. Drug
    and Narcotic Control
Government-Sponsored Programs see Government
    Programs
Government, State see State Government
Graafian Follicle see Ovarian Follicle
Graduate Education see Education, Medical,
    Graduate; names of other branches of graduate
    education
Graduate Records Examination see Educational
    Measurement
Graffi Virus see Leukemia Viruses, Murine
Graffi's Chloroleukemic Strain see Leukemia
    Viruses, Murine
Graft Occlusion, Vascular   WG 170
Graft Rejection   WO 680
Graft-Versus-Host Disease see Graft vs Host
    Disease
Graft vs Host Disease   WD 300
    Transplantation complication   WO 680
Graft vs Host Reaction   WO 680
Grafting, Bone see Bone Transplantation
Grafting, Bone Marrow see Bone Marrow
    Transplantation
Grafting, Brain Tissue see Brain Tissue
    Transplantation
Grafting, Heart see Heart Transplantation
Grafting, Heart-Lung see Heart-Lung
    Transplantation
Grafting, Islets of Langerhans see Islets of
    Langerhans Transplantation
Grafting, Kidney see Kidney Transplantation
Grafting, Liver see Liver Transplantation
Grafting, Lung see Lung Transplantation
Grafting of Tissue see Transplantation
Grafting, Organ see Organ Transplantation
Grafting, Pancreas see Pancreas Transplantation
Grafting, Skin see Skin Transplantation
Grafting, Tissue see Tissue Transplantation
Grafts see Transplants
Grain see Cereals
Gram-Negative Aerobic Bacteria   QW 131
Gram-Negative Anaerobic Bacteria   QW 133
Gram-Negative Bacteria   QW 131
Gram-Negative Chemolithotrophic Bacteria   QW
    135
Gram-Negative Facultatively Anaerobic Rods
    QW 137–141
Gram-Positive Asporogenous Rods   QW 142.5.A8
Gram-Positive Bacteria   QW 142–142.5
Gram-Positive Cocci   QW 142.5.C6
Gram-Positive Organisms see Bacteria
Gramicidin   QV 350
Graminea see Grasses
Grammar see Philology; "phrase books" under
    specialties, e.g., Medicine
Grana see Chloroplasts
Grand Mal Attacks see Epilepsy, Tonic-Clonic
Grants and Subsidies, Educational see Training
    Support
Grants and Subsidies, Government see Financing,
    Government

ALWAYS CONSULT MAIN SCHEDULES.   USE NUMBER ASSIGNED ONLY WHEN
SUBJECT REPRESENTS MAJOR EMPHASIS OF WORK BEING CLASSIFIED

Grants and Subsidies, Health Planning see Health Planning Support

Grants and Subsidies, Research see Research Support

Granulocyte Colony-Stimulating Factor WH 200

Granulocytes WH 200

Granulocytic Leukemia see Leukemia, Myeloid

Granulocytic Leukemia, Chronic see Leukemia, Myeloid, Chronic

Granulocytopenia see Agranulocytosis

Granuloma QZ 140
    Eosinophilic see Eosinophilic Granuloma WH 650, etc.
    Fungoides see Mycosis Fungoides WR 500

Granuloma, Eosinophilic see Eosinophilic Granuloma

Granuloma Gangraenescens see Granuloma, Lethal Midline

Granuloma, Giant Cell
    Gingiva WU 240
    Jaws WU 140.5

Granuloma, Giant Cell Reparative see Granuloma, Giant Cell

Granuloma, Hodgkin see Hodgkin Disease

Granuloma Inguinale WC 180

Granuloma, Lethal Midline WV 300

Granuloma, Malignant see Hodgkin Disease

Granuloma, Periapical see Periapical Granuloma

Granuloma, Reparative Giant Cell see Granuloma, Giant Cell

Granuloma, Respiratory Tract WF 140
    See also names of specific diseases, e.g.,
        Rhinoscleroma WV 300; Wegener's
        Granulomatosis WF 600

Granuloma Sarcomatodes see Mycosis Fungoides

Granuloma Venereum see Granuloma Inguinale

Granulomatosis, Wegener's see Wegener's Granulomatosis

Granulomatous Disease, Chronic QW 690

Granulosa Cell Tumor WP 322

Grapes see Rosales

Graphite
    Pharmacology QV 138.C1
    Inorganic chemistry QD 181.C1

Grasses
    As allergens QW 900
    Cultivation SB 197-202

Grave Robbing WZ 320

Graves' Disease WK 265

Gravitation QC 178
    Aviation medicine WD 720
    Physiological effects QT 162.G7
    Space medicine WD 752

Gravity see Gravitation

Grawitz Tumor see Carcinoma, Renal Cell

Graylings see Salmonidae

Green Monkey see Cercopithecus aethiops

Greenhouse Effect
    On environmental health WA 30
    Physics QC 912.3
        Global warming QC 981.8.G56
    Special topics, by subject

Grenz Rays see X-Rays

Grief BF 575.G7
    Adolescence WS 462
    Child WS 105.5.E5
    Infant WS 105.5.E5

Grievances, Employee see Employee Grievances

Grippe see Influenza

Grivet Monkey see Cercopithecus aethiops

Grommet Insertion see Middle Ear Ventilation

Groundnuts see Peanuts

Group Health Insurance see Insurance, Health

Group Health Organizations, Prepaid see Health Maintenance Organizations

Group Hospitalization see Insurance, Hospitalization

Group Identification see Social Identification

Group Practice W 92

Group Practice, Dental WU 79

Group Practice, Prepaid W 92

Group Processes HM
    Psychotherapy WM 430
    Small groups HM
    Sensitivity training groups WM 430.5.S3 etc.
    Special topics, by subject

Group Psychotherapy see Psychotherapy, Group

Group Structure HM

Group Therapy see Psychotherapy, Group

Growth
    General growth of child WS 103
    Mental growth see Child Development WS 105, etc.
    Physical WS 103
    Tables WS 16

Growth Disorders
    Child WS 104
    Congenital WE 250
    Endocrine WK 550
    Infant WS 104
    Manifestation of disease QZ 190
    Pathogenesis QZ 45

Growth Factor, Mast-Cell see Interleukin-3

Growth Factors see Growth Substances

Growth Hormone see Somatotropin

Growth Hormone, Pituitary see Somatotropin

Growth Hormone Receptors see Receptors, Somatotropin

Growth Inhibitors QU 107
    See also Growth Disorders WE 250, etc.

Growth Plate WE 200

Growth Retardation, Intrauterine see Fetal Growth Retardation

Growth Substances QU 107
    Plant see Plant Growth Regulators QK 745

GTP-Binding Proteins QU 55

GTP-Regulatory Proteins see G-Proteins

GTP-Regulatory Proteins see GTP-Binding Proteins

Guanacos see Camelids, New World

Guanidines QU 61
    Organic chemistry QD 305.A8

Guanine Nucleotide Regulatory Proteins see G-Proteins

Guanine Nucleotide Regulatory Proteins see GTP-Binding Proteins

Guanosine Cyclic Monophosphate see Cyclic GMP

Guanosine Cyclic 2',3'-Monophosphate see Cyclic
   GMP
Guanosine Cyclic 3',5'-Monophosphate see Cyclic
   GMP
Guanylyl Imidodiphosphate   QU 57
Guerin–Stern Syndrome see Arthrogryposis
Guest Relations see Hospital–Patient Relations
Guided Imagery see Imagery (Psychotherapy)
Guidelines for Health Planning see Health Planning
   Guidelines
Guillain–Barre Syndrome see Polyradiculoneuritis
Guilt   BF 575.G8
   Adolescence   WS 462
   Child   WS 105.5.E5
   Infant   WS 105.5.E5
Guinea Pigs   QL 737.R634
   As laboratory animals   QY 60.R6
Guinea Worm see Dracunculus
Gulf War Syndrome see Persian Gulf Syndrome
Gums see Gingiva
Gunshot Wounds see Wounds, Gunshot
Gymnastics   QT 255
   Medical   WB 541
Gymnodinium see Dinoflagellida
Gymnotid see Electric Fish
Gynecologic Diseases see Genital Diseases, Female
Gynecologic Neoplasms see Genital Neoplasms,
   Female
Gynecologic Surgical Procedures   WP 660
Gynecology   WP
   Pediatrics   WS 360
   Physiology   WP 505
   Urology   WJ 190
   Surgery   WP 660
      See also Gynecologic Surgical Procedures
      WP 660
Gynecomastia   WP 840
Gypsies see Transients and Migrants   WA 300, etc.
Gypsum see Calcium Sulfate
Gypsum Dressings see Calcium Sulfate
Gyrectomy see Psychosurgery

H

H(+)ATPase Complex see H(+)-Transporting
   ATP Synthase
H–D Antibodies see Antibodies, Heterophile
H(+)-Transporting ATP Synthase   QU 136
H(+)-Transporting ATPase see H(+)-Transporting
   ATP Synthase
H–Y Antigen   WO 680
H–2 Antigens   WO 680
   See also Mice as laboratory animals   QY 60.R6
H 93–26 see Metoprolol
Ha–ras Genes see Genes, ras
Habilitation see Rehabilitation
Habit Disturbances see Habits
Habitations see Housing
Habits   BF 335
Habituation (Psychophysiology)   WL 103
Haem Oxygenase see Heme Oxygenase
   (Decyclizing)
Haemophilus   QW 139

Haemophilus ducreyi   QW 139
Haemophilus Infections   WC 200
   See also Chancroid   WC 155
Haemophilus influenzae   QW 139
Haemophilus pertussis see Bordetella pertussis
Hafnium
   Inorganic chemistry   QD 181.H5
   Pharmacology   QV 290
Hair   WR 450–465
Hair Balls see Bezoars
Hair Cells   WV 250
Hair Color   WR 450
Hair Colorants see Hair Dyes
Hair Diseases   WR 450
Hair Dyes   WR 465
   Pharmacology   QV 235
Hair Follicle   WR 450
Hair Follicle Diseases see Hair Diseases
Hair Preparations   WR 465
   See also Barbering   WA 744, etc.
Hair Removal   WR 450
Hairy Cell Leukemia see Leukemia, Hairy Cell
Halfway Houses
   For criminal offenders   HV 9081–9920.5
   For psychiatric patients   WM 29
Halitosis   WI 143
Hallucinations   WM 204
Hallucinogens   QV 77.7
Hallux   WE 835
Hallux Abductovalgus see Hallux Valgus
Hallux Valgus   WE 883
Halogenated Hydrocarbons see Hydrocarbons,
   Halogenated
Halogens   QV 280
   Antiseptics   QV 231
Haloperidol   QV 77.9
Halothane   QV 81
Halsted Mastectomy see Mastectomy, Radical
Hamadryas see Papio
Hamman–Rich Syndrome see Pulmonary Fibrosis
Hamsters
   As laboratory animals   QY 60.R6
Hamsters, Armenian see Cricetulus
Hamsters, Chinese see Cricetulus
Hamsters, Golden see Mesocricetus
Hamsters, Golden Syrian see Mesocricetus
Hamsters, Grey see Cricetulus
Hamsters, Syrian see Mesocricetus
Hand   WE 830
   Infections   WE 832
      See also Hand Dermatoses   WR 140
Hand Deformities   WE 830
Hand Deformities, Acquired   WE 830
Hand Deformities, Congenital   WE 830
Hand Dermatoses   WR 140
   See also Infections   WE 832 under Hand
Hand Injuries   WE 830
Hand–Schueller–Christian Syndrome   WH 650
Hand–Shoulder Syndrome see Reflex Sympathetic
   Dystrophy
Handbooks
   (Form number 39 in any NLM schedule where
   applicable)

ALWAYS CONSULT MAIN SCHEDULES. USE NUMBER ASSIGNED ONLY WHEN
SUBJECT REPRESENTS MAJOR EMPHASIS OF WORK BEING CLASSIFIED

Anesthesiology   WO 231
Animal poisoning   WD 401
Aviation and space medicine   WD 701
Dentistry   WU 49
Diseases and injuries caused by physical agents
    WD 601
Embryology   QS 629
Forensic medicine and dentistry   W 639
Histology   QS 529
History of medicine   WZ 39
Hospital personnel
    Manuals for general staff and for
      non-professional personnel   WX 159
    Manuals for professional staff only   WX 203
Immunologic diseases. Hypersensitivity.
  Collagen diseases   WD 301
Immunology   QW 539
Medical secretaries   W 80
Medicine   W 49
Metabolic diseases   WD 200.1
Nursing   WY 49
Nutrition disorders   WD 101
Pharmacy   QV 735
Physiology   QT 29
Plant poisoning   WD 501
Psychiatry   WM 34
Toxicology   QV 607
See also Manuals   WX 159, etc.
Handedness see Laterality
Handicapped see Disabled
Handicapped Children see Disabled Children
Handwashing
    In hospitals   WX 165
    In preventive medicine   WA 240
Handwriting
    Graphology   BF 889–905
    Paleography   Z 105–115.5
    Used for diagnostic purposes, with the disorder
Hanganutziu–Deicher Antibodies see Antibodies,
  Heterophile
Hansen's Disease see Leprosy
Hantaan Virus   QW 168.5.B9
Hantavirus   QW 168.5.B9
Haplorhini   QL 737.P925–737.P965
    Diseases   SF 997.5.P7
    As laboratory animals   QY 60.P7
Happiness   BF 575.H27
    Adolescence   WS 462
    Child   WS 105.5.E5
    Infant   WS 105.5.E5
Haptoglobins   WH 400
    Clinical examination   QY 455
Harassment, Non–Sexual see Social Behavior
Harbor Porpoises see Porpoises
Hard of Hearing Persons see Hearing Impaired
  Persons
Hardware, Computer see Computers
Harelip see Cleft Lip
Harvest Mites see Mites
Hashish see Cannabis
Hashish Abuse see Marijuana Abuse
Hashish Smoking see Marijuana Smoking
Hate   BF 575.H3

Adolescence   WS 462
    Child   WS 105.5.E5
    Infant   WS 105.5.E5
Haverhill Fever see Rat–Bite Fever
Hawks see Raptors
Hay Fever   WV 335
Hazardous Chemicals see Hazardous Substances
Hazardous Materials see Hazardous Substances
Hazardous Substances
    Environment   WA 670–788
    Occupational   WA 400–495
    Radioactive   WN 615
    Other specific conditions, by subject
Hazardous Waste   WA 788
Hazardous Waste, Radioactive see Radioactive
  Waste
Hazardous Waste Sites see Hazardous Waste
Hazards, Equipment see Equipment Safety
HBAg see Hepatitis B Antigens
HBeAg see Hepatitis B e Antigens
HBsAg see Hepatitis B Surface Antigens
HCB see Hexachlorobenzene
HCG see Gonadotropins, Chorionic
HDL Cholesterol see Lipoproteins, HDL
  Cholesterol
Head   WE 705–707
    See also Scalp   WR 450
Head and Neck Neoplasms   WE 707
Head Banging see Stereotypic Movement Disorder
Head Injuries   WE 706
    See also Skull Fractures   WL 354
Head Nurses see Nursing, Supervisory
Head Protective Devices
    In industry   WA 485
Headache   WL 342
    See also Migraine   WL 344
Healing, Mental see Mental Healing
Healing of Wounds see Wound Healing
Healing, Religious see Mental Healing
Health
    Developing countries   WA 395
    Occupational see Occupational Health   WA
      400–495
    Maintenance of personal health   QT 255
    Mental see Mental Health   WM 105, etc.
    Oral see Oral Health   WU 113
    Public see Public Health   WA, etc.
    Rural see Rural Health   WA 390
    Statistics   WA 900
    Students see School Health Services   WA 350,
      etc.; Student Health Services   WA 351, etc.
    Suburban see Suburban Health   WA 300
    Urban see Urban Health   WA 380
    See also Hygiene   QT 180–275, etc.; Physical
      Fitness   QT 255
Health and Welfare Planning see Health Planning
Health Behavior   W 85
    Special topics, by subject
Health Benefit Plans, Employee   W 100–275
Health Benefits see Insurance Benefits
Health Care see Delivery of Health Care
Health Care Coalitions   WA 525–546
    In special fields, by subject

**ALWAYS CONSULT MAIN SCHEDULES. USE NUMBER ASSIGNED ONLY WHEN
SUBJECT REPRESENTS MAJOR EMPHASIS OF WORK BEING CLASSIFIED**

Health Care Costs
    General   W 74
    For providing particular types of care, by subject,
        if specific; if general, in economics number
        where applicable
Health Care Delivery see Delivery of Health Care
Health Care Evaluation Mechanisms
    General works   W 84
    Hospitals   WX 153
    Private practice   WB 50
    Public health   WA 525–546
    Special topics, by subject
Health Care Market see Health Care Sector
Health Care Rationing   WA 525–546
Health Care Reform   WA 525–546
Health Care Research see Health Services Research
Health Care Sector
    Economics (General)   W 74
    Special topics, by subject
Health Care Seeking Behavior see Patient
    Acceptance of Health Care
Health Care Surveys   W 84.3
Health Care Systems see Delivery of Health Care
Health Care Team see Patient Care Team
Health Centers, Ambulatory see Ambulatory Care
    Facilities
Health Centers, Ambulatory, Non–Hospital see
    Ambulatory Care Facilities
Health Clubs see Fitness Centers
Health Diaries see Medical Records
Health Education
    Informal   WA 590
    Physical see Physical Education and Training
        QT 255
    School texts   QT 200–215
    See also Patient Education   W 85, etc.
Health Education, Dental   WU 113
Health Expenditures   W 74
Health Facilities   WX
    General works   WX 27
    Special types of facilities, with the specialty for
        which designed
    See also names of types of facilities, e.g.,
        Maternal–Child Health Centers   WA 310;
        Rehabilitation Centers   WM 29, etc.
Health Facility Administrators   WX 155
    Directories   WX 22
Health Facility Conversion see Health Facility
    Planning
Health Facility Planning   WX 140
    Facility planning in the specialties, with the
        specialty, e.g., Coronary Care Units   WG
        27–28
Health Facility Size   WX 140
    Special types of facility, with the specialty for
        which designed
Health Fairs   WA 590
    Special topics, by subject
Health Food
    Nutritive value   QU 145.5
    Public health aspects   WA 695–722
Health Insurance see Insurance, Health

Health Insurance for Aged and Disabled, Title 18
    see Medicare
Health Insurance Reimbursement see Insurance,
    Health, Reimbursement
Health Insurance, Voluntary see Insurance, Health
Health Legislation see Legislation
Health Maintenance Organizations   W 132
Health Manpower   W 76
    Excluding physicians   W 21.5
    In specialties see Manpower in the economics
        number under the specialty, e.g., Dentistry
        WU 77, etc. or lacking that in the number for
        the career, e.g., manpower in otolaryngology
        WV 21
Health Occupations   W 21
    Specialties, with the field, e.g., Surgery   WO
        21
    Types of medical practice   W 87
    See also names of particular occupations, e.g.,
        Allied Health Occupations   W 21.5, etc.;
        Mortuary Practice   WA 840–847
Health Occupations Manpower see Health
    Manpower
Health Occupations Schools see Schools, Health
    Occupations
Health Personnel   W 21
    For the availability and distribution of health
        personnel see Health Manpower   W 76
    See also names of specific types of personnel,
        e.g., Allied Health Personnel   W 21.5
Health Physics   WN 110
Health Plan Implementation   WA 525–546
    Special topics, by subject
Health Planning
    Government   WA 525–546
    Of health services   W 84
    Of other special topics, by subject
Health Planning Councils   WA 525–546
    With special topics, class by subject
Health Planning Guidelines
    Government   WA 525–546
    Special topics, by subject
Health Planning Organizations   WA 23
    In special fields, by subject, e.g., WW 23 for
        ophthalmology institutes
Health Planning Support   WA 525–546
Health Plans, Accountable see Managed Competition
Health Policy
    Government   WA 525–546
    Special topics, by subject
Health Priorities   WA 525–546
    In special areas by subject
Health Professions see Health Occupations
Health Promotion
    Government   WA 525–546
    Through education   WA 590
    Special topics, by subject
Health Records, Personal see Medical Records
Health Resorts   WB 760
    History   WB 760
Health Resources   W 74
    Hospital financial management   WX 157
    Specific purposes, by subject

**ALWAYS CONSULT MAIN SCHEDULES. USE NUMBER ASSIGNED ONLY WHEN
SUBJECT REPRESENTS MAJOR EMPHASIS OF WORK BEING CLASSIFIED**

Health Risk Appraisal see Health Status Indicators
Health Service Area see Catchment Area (Health)
Health Services W 84–84.8
    Community see Community Health Services
      WA 546
    Emergency see Emergency Medical Services
      WX 215, etc.
      See also Emergency Service, Hospital WX
      215
    For children see Child Health Services WA
      320, etc.
    For the aged WT 31
    For the indigent W 250
      See also Medical Indigency W 250, etc.
    Occupational see Occupational Health Services
      WA 412
    Maternal see Maternal Health Services WA 310
    Mental see Community Mental Health Services
      WM 30; Mental Health Services WM 30,
      etc.
    Organization & administration see Health Services
      Administration W 84, etc.
    Personal see Personal Health Services W 84
    Private practice WB 50
    Public see Preventive Health Services WA 108;
      Public Health Administration WA 525–590
    School see School Health Services WA 350,
      etc.; Student Health Services WA 351, etc.
    Supply & distribution W 76
    See also names of specific services, e.g., Home
      Care Services WY 115, etc.
Health Services Accessibility W 76
    Special population groups WA 300–395
Health Services Administration
    General W 84
    Public health see Public Health Administration
      WA 525–546
Health Services for the Aged WT 31
Health Services, Indigenous
    General W 84
    Private practice WB 50
    Special population groups WA 300–395
Health Services Marketing see Marketing of Health
Services
Health Services Misuse W 84–84.8
    Special topics, by subject
Health Services Needs and Demand
    In a particular population or community, by
    subject
Health Services Research W 84.3
    In special areas, by subject
Health Status WB 141.4
Health Status Index see Health Status Indicators
Health Status Indicators WA 900
    Special topics, by subject
Health Surveys WA 900
    Chronic disease WT 30
    Dental see Dental Health Surveys WU 30
    Diet see Nutrition Surveys QU 146
    Geriatric WT 30
    Hospital surveys WX 27
    Nursing surveys WY 31
    Public health WA 900

Sanitary WA 672
    Of special population groups WA 300, etc.
Health Systems Agencies WA 525–546
Health Systems Plans WA 540–546
Health Transition
    Epidemiology WA 105
    Statistics WA 900
    Special population groups WA 300–395
Health Visitors see Community Health Nursing
Healthcare Industry see Health Care Sector
Healthcare Surveys see Health Care Surveys
Hearing WV 270–280
    Conservation WV 276
Hearing Aids WV 274
Hearing Disorders WV 270
    Child WV 271
    Infant WV 271
    See also Hearing Impaired Persons WV
      270–280, etc.; Rehabilitation of Hearing
      Impaired WV 270–280, etc.
Hearing Impaired Persons
    Education HV 2417–2500
    Rehabilitation
      Physical & medical WV 270–280
      Social HV 2353–2990.5
      See also Rehabilitation of Hearing Impaired
      WV 270–280, etc.
    Special topics, by subject
    See also Deafness WV 270–280; Hearing
      Disorders WV 270; and terms for specific
      hearing disorders
Hearing Impaired Rehabilitation see Rehabilitation
of Hearing Impaired
Hearing Loss, Bilateral WV 270
Hearing Loss, Conductive WV 270
Hearing Loss, Extreme see Deafness
Hearing Loss, Functional WV 270
Hearing Loss, Noise–Induced WV 270
    Industrial WA 470
    Veterinary SF 891
Hearing Loss, Nonorganic see Hearing Loss,
Functional
Hearing Loss, Partial WV 270
Hearing Loss, Sensorineural WV 270–276
Hearing Protective Devices see Ear Protective
Devices
Hearing Tests WV 272
    See also Acoustic Impedance Tests WV 272;
      Audiometry WV 272; names of other specific
      tests
Heart WG
    Beat
      Disorders WG 330
      Physiology WG 202
      See also Heart Rate WG 106; Pulse WB
      282, etc.; Tachycardia WG 330
    Child WS 290
    Drugs affecting QV 150
      See also specific drugs
    Fetal see Fetal heart WQ 210.5
    Infant WS 290
    Radiography WG 141.5.R2
    Radionuclide imaging WG 141.5.R3

**ALWAYS CONSULT MAIN SCHEDULES. USE NUMBER ASSIGNED ONLY WHEN
SUBJECT REPRESENTS MAJOR EMPHASIS OF WORK BEING CLASSIFIED**

Sounds see Heart Auscultation   WG 141.5.A9;
   Phonocardiography   WG 141.5.P4
   Tomography   WG 141.5.T6
Heart Abnormalities see Heart Defects, Congenital
Heart Aneurysm   WG 300
Heart Arrest   WG 205
Heart, Artificial   WG 169.5
Heart-Assist Devices   WG 169.5
Heart Atrium   WG 201–202
Heart Auscultation   WG 141.5.A9
   See also Phonocardiography   WG 141.5.P4
Heart Block   WG 330
Heart Catheterization   WG 141.5.C2
   Veterinary   SF 811
Heart Conduction System   WG 201–202
Heart Contractility see Myocardial Contraction
Heart Defects, Congenital   WG 220
   Child   WS 290
   Infant   WS 290
Heart Disease, Ischemic see Myocardial Ischemia
Heart Diseases   WG 210
   Child   WS 290
   Infant   WS 290
   Ischemic see Myocardial Ischemia   WG 300
   Pick's disease see Pericarditis, Constrictive   WG
      275
   Pulmonary see Pulmonary Heart Disease   WG
      420
   Rheumatic see Rheumatic Heart Disease   WG
      240
   Veterinary   SF 811
Heart Enlargement see Heart Hypertrophy
Heart Failure, Congestive   WG 370
   Popular works   WG 113
   See also Adverse effects   WO 245 under
      Anesthesia
Heart Function Tests   WG 141.5.F9
   See also names of specific tests
Heart Hypertrophy   WG 210
Heart Injuries   WG 210
   Surgery   WG 169
Heart-Lung Machine   WG 169.5
Heart-Lung Transplantation   WG 169
Heart Massage   WG 205
Heart, Mechanical see Heart-Lung Machine
Heart Rate   WG 106
Heart Rate, Fetal   WQ 210.5
   Monitoring   WQ 209
Heart Rupture, Traumatic see Heart Injuries
Heart Septal Defects   WG 220
Heart Septal Defects, Atrial   WG 220
Heart Septal Defects, Ventricular   WG 220
Heart Sounds
   Physiology   WG 106
   See also Heart Auscultation   WG 141.5.A9;
      Phonocardiography   WG 141.5.P4
Heart Transplantation   WG 169
Heart Valve Diseases   WG 260–269
Heart Valve Prosthesis   WG 169
Heart Valve Prosthesis Implantation   WG 169
Heart Valves   WG 260–269
Heart Ventricle   WG 201–202
Heart Ventricle, Artificial see Heart-Assist Devices

Heart Volume see Cardiac Volume
Heartburn   WI 145
Heartworm Disease see Dirofilariasis
Heat
   As a cause of disease   QZ 57
   Body see Body Temperature   WB 270, etc.; Skin
      Temperature   WR 102
   Control in industry   WA 450
   Prostration see Heat Exhaustion   WD 610
   Therapeutic use   WB 469
   See also Desert Climate   QT 150, etc.;
      Temperature   WB 700, etc.
Heat Cramps see Heat Stress Disorders
Heat Exhaustion   WD 610
   See also Sunstroke   WD 610
Heat Loss see Body Temperature Regulation
Heat Production see Body Temperature Regulation
Heat-Shock Protein 70 see Heat-Shock Proteins
Heat-Shock Protein 90 see Heat-Shock Proteins
Heat-Shock Proteins   QU 55
Heat-Shock Reaction see Heat-Shock Response
Heat-Shock Response   QT 120
   See also Heat-Shock Proteins   QU 55
Heat Stress Disorders   WD 610
Heat Stress Syndromes see Heat Stress Disorders
Heat Stroke   WD 610
   See also Sunstroke   WD 610
Heat Waves see Infrared Rays
Heating   WA 770
   In industry   WA 450
Heatstroke see Heat Exhaustion
Heavy Ions   WN 415–450
   General physics   QC 702.7.H42
   Health physics   WN 110
Heavy Metals see Metals, Heavy
Hebephrenic Schizophrenia see Schizophrenia,
   Disorganized
Hedgehogs   QL 737.I53
Hedonism see Philosophy
Heel   WE 880
Height see Body Height
Height-Weight-Growth Tables see Tables   WS 16
   under Birth Weight, Body Height, Body Weight,
   Growth
Hela Cells   QH 585
Helicobacter Infections   WC 200
   In specific diseases, with the disease
Helicobacter pylori   QW 154
Helicopters see Aircraft
Heliotherapy
   General medical   WB 480
   For treating pulmonary tuberculosis   WF 330
Heliotrope see Valerian
Helium   QV 318
   Inorganic chemistry   QD 181.H4
Hellebore see Veratrum
Helmets see Head Protective Devices
Helminth Antigens see Antigens, Helminth
Helminthiasis   WC 800–890
   Veterinary See Helminthiasis, Animal   SF
      810.H44
Helminthiasis, Animal   SF 810.H44

Helminths   QX 200–442
    See also Anthelmintics   QV 253
Helping Behavior   BF 637.H4
Helplessness, Learned   WM 165
Hemadsorption Virus 2 see Parainfluenza Virus 1,
    Human
Hemagglutinating Virus of Japan see Paramyxovirus
Hemagglutination   QW 640
Hemagglutination Inhibition Tests   QY 265
    Used for special purposes by subject
Hemagglutination Tests
    Used for special purposes, by subject
Hemagglutinins, Plant see Lectins
Hemangioma   QZ 340
    Localized, by site
Hemangioma, Cavernous   QZ 340
    Localized, by site
Hemangiopericytoma   QZ 340
    Localized, by site
Hemarthrosis   WH 325
Hematemesis   WI 146
    Related to a particular disease, with the disease
Hematin see Heme
Hematinics   QV 181
Hemato–Encephalic Barrier see Blood–Brain Barrier
Hematoblast see Blood Cells
Hematochezia see Gastrointestinal Hemorrhage
Hematocrit   QY 408
    Apparatus   QY 26
Hematologic Agents
    General works   QV 180
    See also names of specific agents, e.g.,
        Anticoagulants   QV 193; Coagulants   QV
        195; Hematinics   QV 181
Hematologic Diseases   WH
    General works   WH 120
    Child   WS 300
    In pregnancy see Pregnancy Complications,
        Hematologic   WQ 252, etc.
    Infant   WS 300
    Nursing   WY 152.5
    Veterinary   SF 769.5
Hematologic Malignancies see Hematologic
    Neoplasms
Hematologic Neoplasms   WH 525
    Clinical pathology   QZ 350
Hematologic Tests   QY 400–415
    See also names of specific tests
Hematology   WH
    Blood (Clinical analysis)   QY 400–490
    Child   WS 300
    Infant   WS 300
    In nursing   WY 152.5
Hematoma   WH 312
Hematoma, Epidural   WL 355
Hematoma, Subdural   WL 200
Hematopoiesis   WH 140
Hematopoietic Agents see Hematinics
Hematopoietic Cell Growth Factors   WH 140
Hematopoietic Neoplasms see Hematologic
    Neoplasms
Hematopoietic Stem Cells   WH 380
Hematopoietic System   WH 140
    Child   WS 300

    Infant   WS 300
        Drugs affecting   QV 180
Hematopoietins see Hematopoietic Cell Growth
    Factors
Hematoporphyria see Porphyria
Hematoporphyrin Photoradiation   WB 480
Hematuria   WJ 344
Heme   WH 190
Heme Oxygenase (Decyclizing)   QU 140
Hemeproteins   WH 190
    Clinical examination   QY 455
Hemeralopia see Vision Disorders
Hemianopsia   WW 276
Hemic System see Hematology
Hemicrania see Migraine
Hemifacial Spasm   WE 705
Hemin   WH 190
Hemiparesis see Hemiplegia
Hemiplegia   WL 346
    Specific etiological factors, by cause, e.g.,
        Cerebrovascular Disorders   WL 355
Hemiptera   QX 503
Hemispheres, Cerebral see Brain
Hemisporosis see Sporotrichosis
Hemochromatosis   WR 267
Hemocuprein see Superoxide Dismutase
Hemocyanin   WH 190
    Clinical examination   QY 455
Hemocytes   WH 140
Hemodialysis   WJ 378
    Nursing   WY 164
Hemodialysis, Home   WJ 378
Hemodilution   WG 166
    In blood transfusion   WB 356
    In hypothermia   WD 670
    In microculation   WG 104
    For other purposes, by subject
Hemodynamics   WG 106
Hemoencephalic Barrier see Blood–Brain Barrier
Hemofiltration
    Speicial topics, by subject
Hemofiltration, Continuous Arteriovenous see
    Hemofiltration
Hemoglobin A   WH 190
    Clinical examination   QY 455
Hemoglobin A, Glycosylated   WH 190
Hemoglobin C   WH 190
    Clinical examination   QY 455
Hemoglobin F see Fetal Hemoglobin
Hemoglobin Substitutes see Blood Substitutes
Hemoglobinopathies   WH 190
Hemoglobins   WH 190
    Clinical examination   QY 455
Hemoglobins, Abnormal   WH 190
Hemoglobinuria   WJ 344
Hemoglobinuria, Bacillary   WJ 344
Hemoglobinuria, Paroxysmal   WJ 344
Hemoglobinuric Fever see Malaria
Hemolymph   WH 400
Hemolysins   QW 660
Hemolysis
    Erythrocyte destruction   WH 150
    Immunology   QW 660

**ALWAYS CONSULT MAIN SCHEDULES.   USE NUMBER ASSIGNED ONLY WHEN
SUBJECT REPRESENTS MAJOR EMPHASIS OF WORK BEING CLASSIFIED**

Hemolytic Anemias see Anemia, Hemolytic
Hemolytic Disease of Newborn see Erythroblastosis, Fetal
Hemoperfusion   WG 168
Hemopericardium see Pericardial Effusion
Hemoperitoneum   WI 575
Hemophilia see Hemophilia A
Hemophilia A   WH 325
Hemophilia B   WH 325
Hemophilia, Vascular see von Willebrand Disease
Hemophilus see Haemophilus
Hemophilus Infections see Haemophilus Infections
Hemophthalmos see Eye Hemorrhage
Hemopneumothorax   WF 746
Hemoptysis   QY 120
    Associated with a particular disease, with the disease
Hemorrhage   WO 700
    Cerebral see Cerebral Hemorrhage   WL 355
    Drugs checking   QV 195
    In labor   WQ 330
    Nasal see Epistaxis   WV 320
    Ovarian   WP 320
    Peptic ulcer see Peptic Ulcer Hemorrhage   WI 350
    Retinal see Retinal Hemorrhage   WW 270
    Subarachnoid see Subarachnoid Hemorrhage   WL 200
    Uterine see Uterine Hemorrhage   WP 440
    Veterinary   SF 811
    Vulva   WP 200
    See also Menorrhagia   WP 555
Hemorrhage, Cerebral see Cerebral Hemorrhage
Hemorrhage, Eye see Eye Hemorrhage
Hemorrhage, Gastrointestinal see Gastrointestinal Hemorrhage
Hemorrhage, Oral see Oral Hemorrhage
Hemorrhage, Peptic Ulcer see Peptic Ulcer Hemorrhage
Hemorrhage, Postoperative see Postoperative Hemorrhage
Hemorrhage, Postpartum see Postpartum Hemorrhage
Hemorrhage, Retinal see Retinal Hemorrhage
Hemorrhage, Subarachnoid see Subarachnoid Hemorrhage
Hemorrhage, Surgical see Blood Loss, Surgical
Hemorrhage, Uterine see Uterine Hemorrhage
Hemorrhagic Diathesis see Hemorrhagic Disorders
Hemorrhagic Disease of Newborn   WS 421
Hemorrhagic Disorders   WH 312-325
    See also names of specific disorders
Hemorrhagic Fever, American   WC 534
Hemorrhagic Fever, Argentinian see Hemorrhagic Fever, American
Hemorrhagic Fever, Bolivian see Hemorrhagic Fever, American
Hemorrhagic Fever, Crimean   WC 534
Hemorrhagic Fever, Dengue see Dengue Hemorrhagic Fever
Hemorrhagic Fever, Ebola   WC 534
Hemorrhagic Fever, Epidemic see Hemorrhagic Fever with Renal Syndrome

Hemorrhagic Fever, Korean see Hemorrhagic Fever with Renal Syndrome
Hemorrhagic Fever, Omsk   WC 534
Hemorrhagic Fever Virus, Epidemic see Hantaan Virus
Hemorrhagic Fever Virus, Korean see Hantaan Virus
Hemorrhagic Fever Virus, Omsk see Encephalitis Viruses, Tick-Borne
Hemorrhagic Fever with Renal Syndrome   WC 534
    Veterinary   SF 809.H45
Hemorrhagic Fever with Renal Syndrome Virus see Hantaan Virus
Hemorrhagic Fevers, Viral   WC 534
Hemorrhagic Nephroso-Nephritis see Hemorrhagic Fever with Renal Syndrome
Hemorrhagic Nephroso-Nephritis Virus see Hantaan Virus
Hemorrhoids   WI 605
Hemosiderin   QV 183
Hemosiderosis   WD 200.5.I7
    Localized, by site
Hemosorption see Hemoperfusion
Hemostasis   WH 310
Hemostasis, Surgical   WO 500
    Complications   WO 184
    See also Embolization, Therapeutic   WH 310, etc.
Hemostatic Techniques   WH 310
    See also· Embolization, Therapeutic   WH 310, etc.
Hemostatics   QV 195
Hemothorax   WF 746
Hemotoxins see Hemolysins
Hemp see Cannabis
Heparin   QV 193
Heparin-Clearing Factor see Lipoprotein Lipase
Heparin Cofactor see Antithrombin III
Heparin, Low-Molecular-Weight   QV 193
Heparinic Acid see Heparin
Heparinoids   QV 193
Hepatectomy   WI 770
Hepatic Amebiasis see Liver Abscess, Amebic
Hepatic Artery   WG 595.H3
    See also Blood Supply   WI 702 under Liver; Liver Circulation   WI 702
Hepatic Cirrhosis see Liver Cirrhosis
Hepatic Coma see Hepatic Encephalopathy
Hepatic Duct, Common   WI 750
Hepatic Encephalopathy   WI 700
Hepatic Entamoebiasis see Liver Abscess, Amebic
Hepatic Failure, Fulminant see Hepatic Encephalopathy
Hepatic Transplantation see Liver Transplantation
Hepatic Veins   WG 625.H3
    See also Blood Supply   WI 702 under Liver; Liver Circulation   WI 702
Hepatitis   WI 715
    Veterinary see Hepatitis, Animal   SF 851
    See also specific names of hepatitis, e.g., Hepatitis, Viral, Human   WC 536
Hepatitis A   WC 536
Hepatitis A Virus see Hepatovirus

Hepatitis Agents, GB   QW 170
Hepatitis, Alcoholic   WI 715
Hepatitis, Animal   SF 851
Hepatitis, Autoimmune   WI 715
Hepatitis B   WC 536
Hepatitis B Antigens   WC 536
Hepatitis B e Antigens   WC 536
Hepatitis B Surface Antigens   WC 536
Hepatitis B Vaccines   WC 536
Hepatitis B Virus   QW 170
Hepatitis C   WC 536
Hepatitis C, Chronic   WC 536
Hepatitis, Chronic
   General or unspecified   WI 715
   See also specific names of hepatitis, e.g., Hepatitis
    C, Chronic   WC 536
Hepatitis D   WC 536
Hepatitis D Virus see Hepatitis Delta Virus
Hepatitis, Delta see Hepatitis D
Hepatitis Delta Virus   QW 170
Hepatitis E   WC 536
Hepatitis G Virus see Hepatitis Agents, GB
Hepatitis, Homologous Serum see Hepatitis B
Hepatitis, Infectious see Hepatitis A
Hepatitis, Toxic   WI 715
Hepatitis, Viral, Human   WC 536
Hepatitis, Viral, Non-A, Non-B,
   Enterically-Transmitted see Hepatitis E
Hepatitis, Viral, Non-A, Non-B,
   Parenterally-Transmitted see Hepatitis C
Hepatitis, Viral, Vaccines see Viral Hepatitis
   Vaccines
Hepatitis Virus, Homologous Serum see Hepatitis B
   Virus
Hepatitis Virus, Infectious see Hepatovirus
Hepatitis Virus, Marmoset see Hepatitis Viruses
Hepatitis Viruses   QW 170
Hepatitis, Water-Borne see Hepatitis E
Hepatocellular Carcinoma see Carcinoma,
   Hepatocellular
Hepatolenticular Degeneration   WI 740
Hepatology see Gastroenterology
Hepatoma see Carcinoma, Hepatocellular
Hepatoma, Experimental see Liver Neoplasms,
   Experimental
Hepatoma, Morris see Liver Neoplasms,
   Experimental
Hepatoma, Novikoff see Liver Neoplasms,
   Experimental
Hepatomegaly   WI 700
Hepatorenal Glycogen Storage Disease see
   Glycogen Storage Disease Type I
Hepatovirus   QW 170
Herbal Teas see Beverages
Herbalism see Medicine, Herbal
Herbicides
   Plant culture   SB 951.4
   Public health aspects   WA 240
Herbs   QV 767
Herbs, Medicinal see Plants, Medicinal
Hereditary Diseases   QZ 50
   Child   WS 200
   Infant   WS 200

   Prenatal diagnosis   QZ 50
   Veterinary genetics   SF 756.5
   See also names of specific diseases
Hereditary Multiple Exostoses see Exostoses,
   Multiple Hereditary
Hereditary Nonpolyposis Colorectal Neoplasms see
   Colorectal Neoplasms, Hereditary Nonpolyposis
Hereditary Spinal Sclerosis see Friedreich's Ataxia
Hereditary Type I Motor and Sensory Neuropathy
see Charcot-Marie Disease
Heredity see Genetics
Hermaphroditism   WJ 712
Hernia   WI 950
   Vaginal   WP 250
   See also names of specific hernias, e.g., Hernia,
    Diaphragmatic   WF 810, etc.
Hernia, Abdominal see Hernia, Ventral
Hernia, Cerebral see Encephalocele
Hernia, Diaphragmatic   WF 810
Hernia, Diaphragmatic, Traumatic   WF 810
Hernia, Femoral   WI 965
Hernia, Hiatal   WI 250
Hernia, Inguinal   WI 960
Hernia, Umbilical   WI 940
Hernia, Ventral   WI 955
Heroin   QV 92
   Dependence see Heroin Dependence   WM 288
Heroin Dependence   WM 288
Herpes Genitalis   WC 578
Herpes labialis Virus see Simplexvirus
Herpes Simplex   WC 578
   Veterinary   SF 809.H47
Herpes Simplex, Genital see Herpes Genitalis
Herpes Simplex, Oral see Stomatitis, Herpetic
Herpes Simplex Virus see Simplexvirus
Herpes Zoster   WC 575
Herpes Zoster, Ocular see Herpes Zoster
   Ophthalmicus
Herpes Zoster Ophthalmicus   WW 160
Herpes zoster Virus see Herpesvirus 3, Human
Herpesviridae   QW 165.5.H3
Herpesviridae Infections   WC 571
   Veterinary   SF 809.H47
Herpesvirus hominis see Simplexvirus
Herpesvirus Infections see Herpesviridae Infections
Herpesvirus platyrhinae see Simplexvirus
Herpesvirus saimiri see Herpesvirus 2, Saimirine
Herpesvirus varicellae see Herpesvirus 3, Human
Herpesvirus 1, Bovine   QW 165.5.H3
Herpesvirus 1, Saimirine see Simplexvirus
Herpesvirus 1, Suid   QW 165.5.H3
Herpesvirus 2, Saimirine   QW 165.5.H3
Herpesvirus 3, Human   QW 165.5.H3
Herpesvirus 4, Human   QW 165.5.H3
Herpesvirus 5 (beta), Human see Cytomegalovirus
Herpesvirus 5, Human see Cytomegalovirus
Hertzian Waves see Radio Waves
HESW see High-Energy Shock Waves
Hetastarch
   Plasma Substitute   WH 450
   Biochemistry   QU 83
HETE see Hydroxyeicosatetraenoic Acids
Heteroantibodies see Antibodies, Heterophile

**ALWAYS CONSULT MAIN SCHEDULES. USE NUMBER ASSIGNED ONLY WHEN
SUBJECT REPRESENTS MAJOR EMPHASIS OF WORK BEING CLASSIFIED**

Heterochromatin   QU 56
Heterochromic Cyclitis see Iridocyclitis
Heterocyclic Compounds
    Associated with amino acid biochemistry   QU 65
    Organic chemistry   QD 399–406
    Used for special purposes, by subject
    See also names of specific compounds
Heterocyclic N-Oxides see Cyclic N-Oxides
Heterograft see Transplantation, Heterologous
Heterograft Bioprosthesis see Bioprosthesis
Heterograft Dressings see Biological Dressings
Heterologous Antibodies see Antibodies, Heterophile
Heterophile Antibodies see Antibodies, Heterophile
Heterophoria see Strabismus
Heterophyes see Heterophyidae
Heterophyidae   QX 353
Heteroptera   QX 503
Heterosexuality   HQ 23
Heterotropia see Strabismus
Heterozygote   QH 447
    Histocompatibility   WO 680
Heterozygote Detection
    Of a particular trait, with the trait
Hexachlorobenzene
    Toxicology   QV 633
Hexachlorocyclohexane see Lindane
Hexachlorophene   QV 233
Hexadecadrol see Dexamethasone
Hexadecanoic Acid see Palmitic Acids
Hexamethonium Compounds   QV 140
Hexamethylenamine see Methenamine
Hexamethylenetetramine see Methenamine
Hexamine see Methenamine
Hexanes
    Microbial chemistry   QW 52
    Toxicology   QV 633
Hexanoates see Caproates
Hexestrol   WP 522
Hexobarbital   QV 81
Hexokinase   QU 141
Hexose Monophosphate Shunt see Pentosephosphate Pathway
Hexosephosphates   QU 75
Hexoses   QU 75
Hexylresorcinol   QV 253
Heymann Nephritis see Glomerulonephritis
HFRS see Hemorrhagic Fever with Renal Syndrome
HFRS Virus see Hantaan Virus
Hiatal Hernia see Hernia, Hiatal
Hibernation   QL 755
Hibernation, Artificial see Hypothermia, Induced
Hiccup   WF 805
Hidradenoma see Adenoma, Sweat Gland
Hidrotic Ectodermal Dysplasia see Ectodermal Dysplasia
Hierarchy, Social   HM
    Special topics, by subject
High-Cost Technology see Technology, High-Cost
High-Energy Shock Waves
    Therapeutic use   WB 480
    Used for special purposes, by subject
    See also Lithotripsy   WJ 166, etc.

High-Frequency Currents see Electric Stimulation Therapy; Electricity
High-Frequency Jet Ventilation   WF 145
High Mobility Protein 20 see Ubiquitin
High Performance Computing see Computing Methodologies
Higher Nervous Activity   WL 102
Highway Accidents see Accidents, Traffic
Hill-Burton Act see Financing, Government
Hindbrain see Cerebellum; Pons; Medulla Oblongata
Hindlimb   QL 950.7
Hip   WE 855
Hip Contracture   WE 855
Hip Dislocation   WE 860
Hip Dislocation, Congenital   WE 860
Hip Dysplasia, Canine   SF 992.H56
Hip Dysplasia, Congenital see Hip Dislocation, Congenital
Hip Fractures   WE 855
Hip Joint   WE 860
Hip Prosthesis   WE 860
Hip Prosthesis Implantation see Arthroplasty, Replacement, Hip
Hip Replacement, Total see Arthroplasty, Replacement, Hip
Hippocampus   WL 314
Hippocratic Oath   W 50
Hippurates   QU 62
    Organic chemistry   QD 341.A7
    In human urine   WJ 303
    In urinalysis   QY 185
Hirschsprung Disease   WI 528
Hirsutism   WR 455
Hirudinea see Leeches
His-Werner Disease see Trench Fever
Hispanic Americans   E 184.S75
    Special topics, by subject
    See also special topics under Ethnic Groups
Histaminase see Amine Oxidase (Copper-Containing)
Histamine   QV 157
    Biochemistry   QU 61
Histamine Antagonists   QV 157
Histamine Binding Sites see Receptors, Histamine
Histamine H1 Antagonists   QV 157
Histamine H1 Receptor Antagonists see Histamine H1 Antagonists
Histamine H1 Receptor Blockaders see Histamine H1 Antagonists
Histamine H2 Antagonists   QV 157
Histamine H2 Receptor Antagonists see Histamine H2 Antagonists
Histamine H2 Receptor Blockaders see Histamine H2 Antagonists
Histamine H2 Receptors see Receptors, Histamine H2
Histamine Liberation see Histamine Release
Histamine Receptors see Receptors, Histamine
Histamine Release
    In anaphylaxis and hypersensitivity   QW 900
    Special topics, by subject
Histapyridamine see Pheniramine
Histidine   QU 60

Histiocytes   WH 650
  In phagocytosis   QW 690
Histiocytic Lymphoma see Lymphoma, Large–Cell
Histiocytosis, Langerhans–Cell   WH 650
Histiocytosis, Lipid see Niemann–Pick Disease
Histiocytosis X see Histiocytosis, Langerhans–Cell
Histochemistry see Histocytochemistry
Histocompatibility   WO 680
  Blood bank procedures   WH 460
Histocompatibility Antigens   QW 573.5.H6
  Transplantation immunology   WO 680
Histocompatibility Antigens Class II   QW 573.5.H6
  Transplantation immunology   WO 680
Histocompatibility Complex see Major
  Histocompatibility Complex
Histocompatibility Testing   WO 680
Histocytochemistry
  Cytology   QH 613
  Histology   QS 531
Histological Techniques   QS 525
Histologists, Directories see Directories   QS 22
  under Histology
Histology   QS 504–539
  Dental   WU 101
  Directories   QS 522
  Experimental   QS 530
  Pathological   QZ 4
  Veterinary medicine   SF 757.3
  See also special topics under Anatomy
Histology, Comparative   QS 504
  Animal only   QL 807
Histomoniasis see Protozoan Infections
Histones   QU 56
Histopathology see Pathology   QZ 4 under
  Histology
Histoplasmosis   WC 465
Historical Cohort Studies see Cohort Studies
Historiography   D 13–15
  Medical   WZ 345
History of Dentistry   WU 11
History of Medicine   WZ
  By locality   WZ 70
  For special groups   WZ 80–80.5
  General works   WZ 40
  Symbols see Emblems and insignia   WZ 334
  See also form number 11 in any NLM schedule
    where applicable
History of Medicine, Ancient   WZ 51
History of Medicine, Medieval   WZ 54
History of Medicine, Modern   WZ 55
History of Medicine, 15th Cent.   WZ 56
History of Medicine, 16th Cent.   WZ 56
History of Medicine, 17th Cent.   WZ 56
History of Medicine, 18th Cent.   WZ 56
History of Medicine, 19th Cent.   WZ 60
History of Medicine, 20th Cent.   WZ 64
History of Nursing   WY 11
History Taking see Medical History Taking
Histrionic Personality Disorder   WM 173
HIV   QW 168.5.H6
HIV Antibodies   QW 575
HIV Antibody Positive see HIV Seropositivity
HIV–Associated Antibodies see HIV Antibodies

HIV–Associated Enteropathy see HIV Enteropathy
HIV–Associated Nephropathy see AIDS–Associated
  Nephropathy
HIV Dementia see AIDS Dementia Complex
HIV Encephalopathy see AIDS Dementia Complex
HIV Enteropathy   WC 503.5
HIV Infections   WC 503–503.7
HIV Seroconversion see HIV Seropositivity
HIV Serodiagnosis see AIDS Serodiagnosis
HIV Seronegativity   WC 503–503.7
HIV Seropositivity   WC 503–503.7
HIV Seroprevalence   WC 503.4
HIV Wasting Disease see HIV Wasting Syndrome
HIV Wasting Syndrome   WC 503.5
HIV–1   QW 168.5.H6
HIV–2   QW 168.5.H6
Hives see Urticaria
HLA Antigens   QW 573.5.H7
  Transplantation immunology   WO 680
HLA–D Antigens   QW 573.5.H7
  Transplantation immunology   WO 680
HLA–Dw Antigens see HLA–D Antigens
HMG CoA Reductases see Hydroxymethylglutaryl
  CoA Reductases
HMG–20 see Ubiquitin
HMN Distal Type I see Charcot–Marie Disease
HMO see Health Maintenance Organizations
HMSN Type I see Charcot–Marie Disease
Hoarseness   WV 510
Hobbies   QT 250
Hock see Hindlimb
Hockey   QT 260.5.H6
Hodgkin Disease   WH 500
HOE 766 see Buserelin
Hog Cholera   SF 973
Holidays   GT 3925–4995
Holistic Health   W 61
  Medical ethics   W 50
  Medical philosophy   W 61
  Veterinary   SF 745.5
Holistic Nursing
  General   WY 86.5
Holocaine Hydrochloride see Anesthetics, Local
Holography
  Acoustic (Physics)   QC 244.5
  Applied   TA 1540–1555
  Physical optics   QC 449–449.3
Holter Monitoring see Electrocardiography,
  Ambulatory
Home Accidents see Accidents, Home
Home Blood Glucose Monitoring see Blood Glucose
  Self–Monitoring
Home Care Agencies   WY 115
Home Care, Non–Professional see Home Nursing
Home Care Services   WY 115
  Mental patients   WM 35
  Tuberculous patients   WF 315
  See also Popular works   WB 120 under
    Medicine; Self Medication   WB 120
Home Childbirth   WQ 155
Home Health Agencies see Home Care Agencies
Home Health Care Agencies see Home Care
  Agencies

**ALWAYS CONSULT MAIN SCHEDULES. USE NUMBER ASSIGNED ONLY WHEN
SUBJECT REPRESENTS MAJOR EMPHASIS OF WORK BEING CLASSIFIED**

Home Hemodialysis see Hemodialysis, Home
Home Medicine see Popular works   WB 120 under
  Medicine; Self Medication
Home Nursing   WY 200
    See also Nursing, Practical   WY 195
    Home care services   WY 115, etc.
Home Range see Homing Behavior
Homeless Persons   HV 4480–4630
    Special topics, by subject, e.g., Health problems
      of homeless persons   WA 300–305
Homeopathy   WB 930
    Child   WS 366
    History   WB 930
    In treatment of particular diseases or system with
      the disease or system
    Infant   WS 366
    Veterinary medicine   SF 746
Homeostasis   QT 120
Homes for the Aged   WT 27–28
Homicide
    Criminology   HV 6499–6535
    Juvenile   HV 9067.H6
    Medicolegal aspects   W 860
Homing Behavior   QL 751
    See also Territoriality   QL 756.2
Hominidae   GN 51–289
Hominids see Hominidae
Homo sapiens see Hominidae
Homocystinuria   WD 205.5.A5
Homograft see Transplantation, Homologous
Homograft Dressings see Biological Dressings
Homologous Sequences, Nucleic Acid see Sequence
  Homology, Nucleic Acid
Homologous Wasting Disease see Graft vs Host
  Disease
Homosexuality   HQ 75–76.8
  Psychiatric aspects   WM 611
Homosexuality, Ego-Dystonic see Homosexuality
Homosexuality, Female   HQ 75.3–75.6
  Psychiatric aspects   WM 611
Homosexuality, Male   HQ 75.7–76.2
  Psychiatric aspects   WM 611
Homozygote   QH 447
  Histocompatibility   WO 680
Honey
    Dietary supplement in health or disease   WB
    447
    Pharmaceutical preparation   QV 785
Hoof and Claw   QL 942
    Domestic animals   SF 761–768
Hookworm Infections   WC 890
    Veterinary   SF 810.N4
Hookworm, New World see Necator
Hookworm, Old World see Ancylostoma
Hookworms see Ancylostomatoidea
Hordeolum   WW 205
Horehound see Lamiaceae
Hormone Analogs see Hormones, Synthetic
Hormone Antagonists   WK 102
    See also names of specific antagonists
Hormone-Dependent Neoplasms see Neoplasms,
  Hormone-Dependent
Hormone Replacement Therapy   WK 190

    For specific disorders, with the disorder
    See also Estrogen Replacement Therapy   WP
      522; and names of specific hormones
Hormone Replacement Therapy, Post-Menopausal
  see Estrogen Replacement Therapy
Hormones   WK
    Analysis   QY 330–335
    Female see Sex Hormones   WP 520–530, etc.;
      and names of specific hormones
    General works   WK 102
    Male see Sex Hormones   WJ 875, etc.; and
      names of specific hormones
    Renal   WK 180
    Secretion   WK 102
    Steroid   WK 150
    Therapeutic use   WK 190
      See also Hormone Replacement Therapy
      WK 190; Estrogen Replacement Therapy
      WP 522; and names of specific hormones
    See also names of specific hormones
Hormones, Ectopic   WK 185
    Neoplastic etiology   QZ 202
Hormones, Invertebrate see Invertebrate Hormones
Hormones, Synthetic   WK 187
    See also names of specific hormones
Hornets see Wasps
Horse Diseases   SF 951–959
Horseradish Peroxidase   QU 140
Horses   SF 277–360.4
    Anatomy   SF 765
    Horseshoeing   SF 907
    Military   UC 600–695
Horseshoe Crabs   QX 460
Hospice Care   WB 310
    Child   WS 200
    Infant   Ws 200
    Nursing   WY 152
    Of patients with a particular disease, with the
      disease
Hospice Programs see Hospice Care
Hospices   WX 28.6–28.62
Hospital-Addiction Syndrome see Munchausen
  Syndrome
Hospital Administration   WX 150–190
    As a career   WX 155
    Of specialty hospitals (Form number 27–28 in any
      NLM schedule where applicable)
    Of wards
      General hospitals   WX 159
      Psychiatric hospitals   WM 30
Hospital Administrators   WX 155
Hospital Admission Tests see Diagnostic Tests,
  Routine
Hospital Admissions Office see Admitting
  Department, Hospital
Hospital Admitting Department see Admitting
  Department, Hospital
Hospital Ancillary Services see Ancillary Services,
  Hospital
Hospital Anesthesia Department see Anesthesia
  Department, Hospital
Hospital Anesthesia–Resuscitation Department see
  Anesthesia Department, Hospital

Hospital Auxiliaries   WX 159.5
Hospital Bed Capacity   WX 140
Hospital Care see Hospitalization
Hospital Central Supply see Central Supply, Hospital
Hospital Chaplaincy Service see Chaplaincy Service,
   Hospital
Hospital Communication Systems   WX 150
   In disaster   WX 185
Hospital Dental Service see Dental Service, Hospital
Hospital Dental Staff see Dental Staff, Hospital
Hospital Departments   WX 200-225
   See also names of various hospital departments,
      e.g., Psychiatric Department, Hospital   WM
      27-28
Hospital Design and Construction   WX 140
   In specialty fields (Form number 27-28 in any
      NLM schedule where applicable)
Hospital Distribution Systems   WX 165
Hospital Diversification see Hospital Restructuring
Hospital Drug Distribution Systems see Medication
   Systems, Hospital
Hospital Economics see Economics, Hospital
Hospital Emergency Service see Emergency Service,
   Hospital
Hospital Engineering see Maintenance and
   Engineering, Hospital
Hospital Equipment and Supplies see Equipment and
   Supplies, Hospital
Hospital Financial Management see Financial
   Management, Hospital
Hospital Food Service see Food Service, Hospital
Hospital Gift Shops see Hospital Shops
Hospital Groundskeeping see Maintenance and
   Engineering, Hospital
Hospital Housekeeping see Housekeeping, Hospital
Hospital Incident Reporting see Risk Management
Hospital Infections see Cross Infection
Hospital Information Systems   WX 26.5
   In particular fields (Form number 26.5 in any
      NLM schedule where applicable)
Hospital Insurance Program, Medicare see Medicare
   Part A
Hospital Jurisprudence see Jurisprudence
Hospital Laboratories see Laboratories, Hospital
Hospital Laundry Service see Laundry Service,
   Hospital
Hospital Licensure see Licensure, Hospital
Hospital Maintenance see Maintenance and
   Engineering, Hospital
Hospital Materials Management see Materials
   Management, Hospital
Hospital Medical Records Department see Medical
   Records Department, Hospital
Hospital Medical Staff see Medical Staff, Hospital
Hospital Medication Systems see Medication
   Systems, Hospital
Hospital Nuclear Medicine Department see Nuclear
   Medicine Department, Hospital
Hospital Nurseries see Nurseries, Hospital
Hospital Nursing Service see Nursing Service,
   Hospital
Hospital Nursing Staff see Nursing Staff, Hospital
Hospital Obstetrics and Gynecology Department see
Obstetrics and Gynecology Department, Hospital
Hospital Occupational Therapy Department see
   Occupational Therapy Department, Hospital
Hospital Organization and Administration see
   Hospital Administration
Hospital Outpatient Clinics see Outpatient Clinics,
   Hospital
Hospital-Patient Relations   WX 158.5
Hospital Personnel see Personnel, Hospital
Hospital Personnel Administration see Personnel
   Administration, Hospital
Hospital Pharmacy Service see Pharmacy Service,
   Hospital
Hospital Physical Therapy Department see Physical
   Therapy Department, Hospital
Hospital-Physician Joint Ventures   WX 150
Hospital Planning   WX 140
   Mental hospitals   WM 30
   Other special hospitals (Form number 27-28 in
      any NLM schedule where applicable)
Hospital Psychiatric Department see Psychiatric
   Department, Hospital
Hospital Purchasing see Purchasing, Hospital
Hospital Radiology Department see Radiology
   Department, Hospital
Hospital Readmission see Patient Readmission
Hospital Records   WX 173
Hospital Recovery Room see Recovery Room
Hospital Referral see Referral and Consultation
Hospital Renovation see Hospital Design and
   Construction
Hospital Reorganization see Hospital Restructuring
Hospital Respiratory Therapy Department see
   Respiratory Therapy Department, Hospital
Hospital Restructuring   WX 150
Hospital Services, Centralized see Centralized
   Hospital Services
Hospital Shared Services   WX 150
Hospital Shops   WX 161
Hospital Social Work Department see Social Work
   Department, Hospital
Hospital Surgery Department see Surgery
   Department, Hospital
Hospital Units   WX 200-218
   Self-care units   WX 200
   Wards   WX 200
Hospital Urology Department see Urology
   Department, Hospital
Hospital Volunteers   WX 159.5
   Mental hospitals   WM 30.5
   Nursing   WY 193
Hospitalists   WX 203
   See also names of specific types of hospitals
Hospitalization   WX 158-158.5
   Anecdotes about   WZ 305.5
      Children see Child, Hospitalized   WS
         105.5.H7
   Insurance see Insurance, Hospitalization   W 160
   Tuberculosis   WF 330
Hospitalization Insurance see Insurance,
   Hospitalization
Hospitalized Child see Child, Hospitalized
Hospitals   WX

Administrative serial reports (all types of hospitals)   WX 2
Directories (Form number 22 in any NLM schedule where applicable)
Disasters   WX 185
Food service see Food Service, Hospital   WX 168
Libraries see Libraries, Hospital   Z 675.H7
Medical record libraries see Medical Records, Medical Record Administrators   WX 173, etc.
Safety measures   WX 185
Social service   W 322
Standards   WX 15
Surveys   WX 27
Veterinary see Hospitals, Animal   SF 604.4-604.7
See also Accreditation   WX 15, etc.; Hospitals, Military   UH 460-485; Utilization Review WX 153
Hospitals, Air Force see Hospitals, Military
Hospitals, Animal   SF 604.5
Hospitals, Army see Hospitals, Military
Hospitals, Cancer see Cancer Care Facilities
Hospitals, Community   WX 27-28
    Administration and organization   WX 150-190
    Architectural planning and construction   WX 140
Hospitals, Convalescent   WX 27-28
    Administration and organization   WX 150-190
    Architectural planning and construction   WX 140
Hospitals, General   WX 27-28
    Administration and organization   WX 150-190
    Architectural planning and construction   WX 140
Hospitals, Maternity   WQ 27-28
Hospitals, Military   UH 460-485
    Naval   VG 410-450
Hospitals, Navy see Hospitals, Military
Hospitals, Private, Not-for-Profit see Hospitals, Voluntary
Hospitals, Psychiatric   WM 27-28
    Administration   WM 30
    Directories   WM 22
    For children only   WS 27-28
    Practices in care of mental patients   WM 35
    See also Psychiatric Department, Hospital   WM 27-28, etc.
Hospitals, Public   WX 27-28
    See also special topics under Hospitals
Hospitals, Special
    (Form number 27-28 in any NLM schedule where applicable)
    Cancer   QZ 23-24
    Hospices   WX 28.6-28.62
    Isolation   WC 27-28
    Leprosaria   WC 27-28
    Maternity   WQ 27-28
    Quarantine   WC 27-28
    Tuberculosis   WF 27-28
Hospitals, Teaching   WX 27-28
    For specific curriculum, in hospital number of appropriate schedule

Hospitals, Veterans   UH 460-485
    Administration   UH 460-465
    Nursing   WY 130
    Special topics, by subject
Hospitals, Veterinary see Hospitals, Animal
Hospitals, Voluntary see Hospitals   WX 27-28, etc.
Host-Parasite Relations   QX 45
Hostility   BF 575.H6
    Adolescence   WS 462
    Child   WS 105.5.E5
    Infant   WS 105.5.E5
Hostility Catharsis see Abreaction
Hot Climate
    Physiological effect   QT 150
Hot Flashes   WP 580
Hotlines
    Special topics, by subject, e.g., Emergency Services, Psychiatric   WM 401
House Calls   WB 50
House Staff see Internship and Residency
Houseflies   QX 505
Household Articles
    Accidents from   WA 288
    Safety control
        Home measures   WA 288
        Regulatory measures   WA 288
Household Equipment see Household Articles
Household Medicine see Popular works   WB 120, etc. under Medicine
Household Products
    As a cause of accidents   WA 288
    Ocular toxicity   WW 100
    Safety control
        Home measures   WA 288
        Regulatory measures   WA 288
    See also names of specific products
Household Supplies see Household Products
Housekeeping
    Building operations and housekeeping   TX 955-985
    Home economics   TX 301-323
    Plant housekeeping   TS 193
    See also Self Help Devices   WB 320
Housekeeping, Hospital   WX 165
Housing
    Design for the disabled   WA 795
        See also Architecture   WA 795, etc.
            Architectural Accessibility   WA 795-799
    For the elderly   WT 30
    Real estate   HD 251-1395
    Repairs and maintenance   TH 4817
    Rural   HD 7289
    Sanitation   WA 795
    See also Public Housing   HD 7288-7288.78
Housing, Animal   SF 91
    Laboratory animals   QY 56
    Of particular animals, by animal
Housing for the Elderly   WT 30
HPLC see Chromatography, High Pressure Liquid
HSAN Type III see Dysautonomia, Familial
HTLV-BLV Infections   WC 502
HTLV-BLV Viruses   QW 168.5.R18
HTLV-I   QW 168.5.R18

ALWAYS CONSULT MAIN SCHEDULES.   USE NUMBER ASSIGNED ONLY WHEN SUBJECT REPRESENTS MAJOR EMPHASIS OF WORK BEING CLASSIFIED

HTLV–I Infections   WC 502
HTLV–III see HIV
HTLV–III Antibodies see HIV Antibodies
HTLV–III Infections see HIV Infections
HTLV–III–LAV Antibodies see HIV Antibodies
HTLV–III–LAV Infections see HIV Infections
HTLV–III Seroconversion see HIV Seropositivity
HTLV–III Serodiagnosis see AIDS Serodiagnosis
HTLV–III Serology see AIDS Serodiagnosis
HTLV–III Seronegativity see HIV Seronegativity
HTLV–III Seropositivity see HIV Seropositivity
HTLV Infections see HTLV–BLV Infections
HTLV–IV see HIV–2
HTLV Viruses see HTLV–BLV Viruses
Human Anatomy see Anatomy
Human Class II Antigens see HLA–D Antigens
Human Cloning see Cloning, Organism
Human Development   BF 713
    Aging process   WT 104
    Physical development   WS 103
Human Engineering   TA 166–167
    Special topics, by subject, e.g., Biomedical
        Engineering   QT 36, etc.; Space Flight   WD
        750–758
Human Experimentation   W 20.55.H9
    Special topics, by subject, e.g., in drug research
        QV 20.5
Human Figure in Art see Anatomy, Artistic
Human Forefoot see Forefoot, Human
Human Genome see Genome, Human
Human Growth Hormone see Somatropin
Human Immunodeficiency Virus–Associated
    Nephropathy see AIDS–Associated Nephropathy
Human Immunodeficiency Virus Type 1 see HIV–1
Human Immunodeficiency Virus Type 2 see HIV–2
Human Immunodeficiency Viruses see HIV
Human–Pet Bonding see Bonding, Human–Pet
Human Physiology see Physiology
Human Reproduction see Reproduction
Human Resources Development see Staff
    Development
Human Rights
    Constitutional law (United States)   KF
        4741–4786
    Right to education   KF 4151–4155
    Political theory   JC 571–628
    Special topic by subject, e.q., Advocacy of Child
        Health Services   WA 320
    See also Civil Rights   WM 30–32, etc.; Women's
        Rights   HQ 1236–1236.5
Human T–Cell Leukemia–Lymphoma Viruses see
    HTLV–BLV Viruses
Human T–Cell Leukemia Virus I see HTLV–I
Human T–Cell Leukemia Viruses see HTLV–BLV
    Viruses
Human T–Cell Lymphotropic Virus Type III see
    HIV
Human T–Lymphotropic Virus Type III see HIV
Human T–Lymphotropic Virus Type IV see HIV–2
Humanism
    In medical ethics   W 50
    In medical philosophy   W 61
    Modern   B 821

    Renaissance   B 778
    In other areas, by subject
Humanities   CB, AZ
    And religion   BL 65.H8
    And science   AZ 361, etc.
    Education (Humanistic)   LC 1001–1024
        Renaissance   LA 106–108
    Other special topics, by subject
Humeral Fractures   WE 810
Humeral Fractures, Proximal see Shoulder Fractures
Humerus   WE 810
Humic Acids
    Geochemistry   QE 516–516.5
    Soil acidity (agriculture)   S 592.57–592.575
Humidity
    Control   WA 774
        In industry   WA 450
    Hygienic aspects   QT 230
        Hot climates   QT 150
    Meteorology   QC 915–917
    Physiological effects (General)   QT 162.H8
Humor see Wit and Humor
Hunger
    Malnutrition   WD 100
    Nutrition surveys   QU 146
    Physiology   WI 102
    Prevention   WA 695
Huntington Chorea see Huntington's Disease
Huntington's Disease   WL 390
Hurler–Scheie Syndrome see Mucopolysaccharidosis
    I
Hurler's Syndrome see Mucopolysaccharidosis I
Hurricanes see Natural Disasters
Hutchinson's Teeth see Syphilis, Congenital
HY Antigen see H–Y Antigen
Hyaline Membrane Disease   WS 410
Hyaluronic Acid   QU 83
Hybrid Cells   QH 425
Hybridization   QH 421–425
    Animals   QH 425
    Plants   QK 982
        See also Animals   SF 105–109 and Plants
        under Breeding   SB 123–123.5
Hybridomas
    As fused cells   QH 451
    In the production of monoclonal antibodies   QW
        575.5.A6
Hydantoins   QV 85
Hydatid see Echinococcus
Hydatid Cyst see Echinococcosis
Hydatid Cyst, Hepatic see Echinococcosis, Hepatic
Hydatid Cyst, Pulmonary see Echinococcosis,
    Pulmonary
Hydatidiform Mole   WP 465
    Malignant see Hydatidiform Mole, Invasive   WP
        465, etc.
    Pathology   QZ 310
Hydatidiform Mole, Invasive   WP 465
    Pathology   QZ 310
Hydatidosis see Echinococcosis
Hydatidosis, Hepatic see Echinococcosis, Hepatic
Hydatidosis, Pulmonary see Echinococcosis,
    Pulmonary

Hydralazine   QV 150
Hydrallazin see Hydralazine
Hydrarthrosis   WE 304
Hydrated Alumina see Aluminum Hydroxide
Hydrazines
    As antiparkinson agents   QV 80
    Biochemistry   QU 60
    Organic chemistry
        Aliphatic compounds   QD 305.A8
    Neoplasm etiology   QZ 202
    See also Phenylhydrazines   QD 341.A8, etc.
Hydrocarbons
    Organic chemistry
        Aliphatic compounds   QD 305.H5–H9
        Aromatic compounds   QD 341.H9
    Toxicology   QV 633
Hydrocarbons, Chlorinated
    As anesthetics   QV 81
    Organic chemistry   QD 305.H5
        Aliphatic   QD 305.H5
        Aromatic   QD 341.H9
    Toxicology   QV 633
Hydrocarbons, Fluorinated
    Organic chemistry
        Aliphatic compounds   QD 305.H5
        Aromatic compounds   QD 341.H9
    Toxicology   QV 633
Hydrocarbons, Halogenated
    As anesthetics   QV 81
    As carcinogens   QZ 202
    Organic chemistry
        Aliphatic   QD 305.H5
        Aromatic   QD 341.H9
    Toxicology   QV 633
Hydrocarbons, Polycyclic see Polycyclic
  Hydrocarbons
Hydrocele   WJ 800
Hydrocephalus   WL 350
Hydrochloric Acid   QD 181.C5
    Gastric see Gastric Juice   WI 302, etc.
    Toxicology   QV 612
Hydrochloric Acid, Gastric see Gastric Acid
Hydrochlorothiazide   QV 160
Hydrocortisone   WK 755
    Deficiency   WK 760
        As a cause of a particular disorder, with the
        disorder
Hydrocortisone, Topical   QV 60
Hydrocyanic Acid see Hydrogen Cyanide
Hydroelectric Power Plants see Power Plants
Hydrogels
    As biocompatible materials (General)   QT
    37.5.P7
    As dosage form   QV 785
    Biochemisty   QU 133
    Used for special purposes, by subject
Hydrogen
    Inorganic chemistry   QD 181.H1
    Pharmacology   QV 275
Hydrogen Acceptors see Oxidation–Reduction
Hydrogen Bonding   QD 464.H1
Hydrogen Chloride see Hydrochloric Acid
Hydrogen Cyanide   QV 632

Hydrogen–Ion Concentration
    Electrochemistry   QD 562.H93
    Disorders of body fluids   WD 220
    In body fluids   QU 105
Hydrogen Ions see Protons
Hydrogen Peroxide   QV 229
Hydrogen Sulfide
    Inorganic chemistry   QD 181.S1
    Toxicology   QV 662
Hydrogenation   QD 281.H8
Hydrogenomonas see Pseudomonas
Hydrogymnastics see Hydrotherapy
Hydrolases   QU 136
Hydrolysis
    Organic chemistry   QD 281.H83
    Physical chemistry   QD 501
Hydronephrosis   WJ 300
Hydrophobia see Rabies
Hydrophthalmos   WW 290
Hydrops see Edema
Hydroquinones
    As dermatologic agents   QV 60
    Organic chemistry   QD 341.P5
Hydrostatic Pressure
    Physiological adaptation   WD 650
Hydrotherapy   WB 520–525
Hydroxamic Acids   QU 61
    Organic chemistry   QD 305.A8
Hydroxides   QV 280
Hydroxy Acids   QU 98
    Organic chemistry
        Aliphatic compounds   QD 305.A2
        Aromatic compounds   QD 341.A2
Hydroxyampicillin see Amoxicillin
Hydroxyapatites
    Of bone in general   WE 200
    Of teeth   WU 101
Hydroxybutyrates
    In diabetic acidosis   WK 830
    Organic chemistry   QD 305.A2
Hydroxychlorobenzenes see Chlorophenols
Hydroxychlorochin see Hydroxychloroquine
Hydroxychloroquine   QV 256
Hydroxycholecalciferols   QU 173
Hydroxycorticosteroids   WK 755
Hydroxycorticosteroids, Synthetic see
  Glucocorticoids, Synthetic
Hydroxyeicosatetraenoic Acids   QU 90
Hydroxyethyl Starch see Hetastarch
Hydroxyethylrutoside   QU 220
Hydroxyimino Compounds see Oximes
Hydroxylamines   QU 61
    Inorganic chemistry   QD 181.N1
Hydroxylases   QU 140
Hydroxylation
    Organic chemistry   QD 281.H85
Hydroxymethoxyphenylglycol see
  Methoxyhydroxyphenylglycol
Hydroxymethylglutaryl CoA Reductases   QU 140
Hydroxymethyltestosterone   WJ 875
Hydroxynaphthalenes see Naphthols
Hydroxyphenylbutazone see Oxyphenbutazone
Hydroxyproline   QU 60

Hydroxyquinolines
  As anti–infective agents QV 250
  Organic chemistry QD 401
Hydroxysteroid Dehydrogenases QU 140
Hydroxytetracycline see Oxytetracycline
Hydroxytyramine see Dopamine
Hydroxyvitamins D see Hydroxycholecalciferols
Hygiene QT 180–275
  Adolescence WS 460
  Aged WT 120
  Child WS 113
  Cleanliness QT 240
  Dental see Dental Prophylaxis WU 113
    See also Preventive Dentistry WU 113
  In cardiovascular diseases WG 113
  In gastrointestinal diseases WI 113
  Infant WS 113
  Pregnancy WQ 150
    Prenatal care WQ 175
  Industrial see Occupational Health WA 400–495
  Mental see Mental Health WA 495, etc.
  Military see Military Hygiene UH 600–629.5
  Naval VG 470–475
    See also Naval Medicine VG 470–475
  Of cold climates QT 160
  Of eyes WW 113
  Of hot climates QT 150
  Of school children WA 350
  Of students WA 350
  Oral see Oral Hygiene WU 113, etc.
  Prisons HV 8833–8841
  Public see Public Health WA, etc.
  Rural see Rural Health WA 390, etc.
  Surgery WO 113
  Tropical QT 150
    See also Tropical Medicine WC 680, etc.
Hygienists, Dental see Dental Hygienists
Hylobates QL 737.P96
  Diseases SF 997.5.P7
  As laboratory animals QY 60.P7
Hymen WP 250
Hymenolepis QX 400
Hymenoptera QX 565
Hyoid Bone WE 705
Hyoscine see Scopolamine
Hyoscyamine see Atropine
Hyoscyamus see Atropine
Hyperactive Child see Hyperkinesis
Hyperactivity, Motor see Hyperkinesis
Hyperaldosteronism WK 770
Hyperalimentation, Parenteral see Parenteral
  Nutrition, Total
Hyperbaric Oxygenation WF 145
  Used in general therapeutics WB 342
  For treatment of other special conditions, by
    subject
Hyperbilirubinemia WI 703
Hyperbilirubinemia, Hereditary WD 205.5.H9
Hyperbilirubinemia, Neonatal see Jaundice, Neonatal
Hypercalcemia WD 200.5.C2
Hypercapnia WF 140
Hypercholesteremia see Hypercholesterolemia

Hypercholesterolemia WD 200.5.H8
Hypercorticism see Adrenal Gland Hyperfunction
Hyperemesis Gravidarum WQ 215
Hyperemia QZ 170
  Localized, by site
Hyperesthesia WL 710
  Of skin WR 280
  Of the vagina WP 250
  Other localities, by site
Hyperglycemia WK 880
Hyperglycemic Hyperosmolar Nonketotic Coma
  WK 830
Hyperhidrosis WR 400
Hyperhomocysteinemia WD 205.5.A5
Hyperinsulinemia WK 880
Hyperinsulinism WK 880
Hyperkeratosis Linguae see Tongue, Hairy
Hyperkeratosis Palmaris et Plantaris see
  Keratoderma, Palmoplantar
Hyperkinesis WM 197
  Adolescence WS 463
  Child WS 350.8.H9
  Infant WS 350.8.H9
Hyperkinetic Heart Syndrome see Neurocirculatory
  Asthenia
Hyperkinetic Syndrome see Attention Deficit
  Disorder with Hyperactivity
Hyperlipemia see Hyperlipidemia
Hyperlipidemia WD 200.5.H8
Hyperlipidemia, Essential Familial see
  Hyperlipidemia
Hyperlipoproteinemia WD 205.5.L5
Hyperlipoproteinemia Type IV WD 205.5.L5
Hypermedia
  In medicine (General) W 26.55.S6
  In other special fields (Form number 26.5 in any
    NLM schedule where applicable)
Hypermenorrhea see Menorrhagia
Hypermetropia see Hyperopia
Hypermobility, Joint see Joint Instability
Hypernatremia WD 220
Hypernephroma see Carcinoma, Renal Cell
Hyperopia WW 300
Hyperostosis Corticalis Generalisata see
  Osteochondrodysplasias
Hyperostosis Frontalis Interna WE 705
Hyperparathyroidism WK 300
Hyperphagia WM 175
Hyperpipecolic Acidemia see Peroxisomal Disorders
Hyperpituitarism WK 550
Hyperplasia QZ 190
Hyperprebetalipoproteinemia see
  Hyperlipoproteinemia Type IV
Hyperprolactinemia WD 200.5.H9
Hypersensitivity
  Allergenic substances see Allergens QW 900
  Diseases (General) WD 300–330
  Drug see Drug Hypersensitivity WD 320
  Eye WW 160
  Food see Food Hypersensitivity WD 310
  Immunology QW 900
  Light see Photosensitivity Disorders WR 160
  Respiratory see Respiratory Hypersensitivity

WF 150
Skin   WR 160–190
Veterinary   SF 757.2
See also other specific diseases or disease groups
    associated with hypersensitivity, e.g., Collagen
    Diseases   WD 375
Hypersensitivity, Atopic see Hypersensitivity,
    Immediate
Hypersensitivity, Contact see Dermatitis, Contact
Hypersensitivity, Delayed   WD 300–330
    General works   WD 300
    Immunologic factors   QW 900
Hypersensitivity, Drug see Drug Hypersensitivity
Hypersensitivity, Environmental see Environmental
    Illness
Hypersensitivity, Food see Food Hypersensitivity
Hypersensitivity, Immediate   WD 300–305
    General works   WD 300
    Immunological factors   QW 900
Hypersensitivity Pneumonitis, Avian see Bird
    Fancier's Lung
Hypersensitivity, Respiratory see Respiratory
    Hypersensitivity
Hypersensitivity, Tuberculin–Type see
    Hypersensitivity, Delayed
Hypersensitivity, Type I see Hypersensitivity,
    Immediate
Hypersensitivity, Type III see Immune Complex
    Diseases
Hypersensitivity, Type IV see Hypersensitivity,
    Delayed
Hypersomnia   WM 188
Hypersomnia with Periodic Respiration see Sleep
    Apnea Syndromes
Hypersplenism   WH 600
Hypertelorism   WE 705
Hypertensinogen see Angiotensinogen
Hypertension   WG 340
Hypertension–Edema–Proteinuria Gestosis see
    Gestosis, EPH
Hypertension, Goldblatt see Hypertension,
    Renovascular
Hypertension, Malignant   WG 340
Hypertension, Portal   WI 720
Hypertension, Pulmonary   WG 340
Hypertension, Pulmonary, of Newborn, Persistent
    see Persistent Fetal Circulation Syndrome
Hypertension, Renal   WG 340
Hypertension, Renovascular   WG 340
Hypertext see Hypermedia
Hyperthermia see Fever
Hyperthermia, Induced   WB 469
    In mental disorders   WM 405
Hyperthermia, Local see Hyperthermia, Induced
Hyperthermia, Therapeutic see Hyperthermia,
    Induced
Hyperthyroidism   WK 265
Hypertonic Glucose Solution see Glucose Solution,
    Hypertonic
Hypertonic Saline Solution see Saline Solution,
    Hypertonic
Hypertonic Solution, Glucose see Glucose Solution,
    Hypertonic

Hypertonic Solution, Saline see Saline Solution,
    Hypertonic
Hypertonic Solutions   QV 786
Hypertrichosis   WR 455
Hypertriglyceridemia   WD 200.5.H8
Hypertriglyceridemia, Familial see
    Hyperlipoproteinemia Type IV
Hypertrophic Arthritis see Osteoarthritis
Hypertrophy   QZ 190
    See also Cervix Hypertrophy   WP 470; Gingival
        Hypertrophy   WU 240; Heart Hypertrophy
        WG 210; Myocardial Diseases, Primary   WG
        280; Prostatic Hyperplasia   WJ 752
Hypertropia see Strabismus
Hyperventilation   WF 143
Hyphomycetes   QW 180.5.D38
Hypnosis
    Parapsychology   BF 1111–1156
    Psychiatric therapy   WM 415
    Self Hypnosis   WM 415
    Surgery see Hypnosis, Anesthetic   WO 200
Hypnosis, Anesthetic   WO 200
Hypnosis, Dental   WO 460
Hypnotics and Sedatives   QV 85–88
Hypoactive Sexual Desire Disorder see Sexual
    Dysfunctions, Psychological
Hypobaropathy see Altitude Sickness
Hypocalcemia   WD 200.5.C2
    Veterinary   SF 910.H86
Hypochlorhydria see Achlorhydria
Hypocholesteremic Agents see Anticholesteremic
    Agents
Hypochondriasis   WM 178
Hypochromic Anemias see Anemia, Hypochromic
Hypodermic Medication see Infusions, Parenteral;
    Injections, Subcutaneous
Hypodermoclysis see Infusions, Parenteral; names of
    solutions or agents used, e.g., Sodium Chloride
Hypodermyiasis   WC 900
Hypodontia see Anodontia
Hypogalactia see Lactation Disorders
Hypogammaglobulinemia see Agammaglobulinemia
Hypogastric Plexus   WL 600
Hypoglossal Nerve   WL 330
Hypoglycemia   WK 880
Hypoglycemic Agents   WK 825
Hypogonadism   WK 900
Hypohidrosis   WR 400
    Drugs for   QV 122
Hypokalemia   WD 220
Hypokinesia see Immobilization
Hypomenorrhea see Menstruation Disorders
Hyponatremia   WD 220
Hypoparathyroidism   WK 300
Hypopharyngeal Neoplasms   WV 410
Hypophysectomy   WK 590
Hypophysectomy, Chemical   WK 590
Hypophysis see Pituitary Gland
Hypophysis Cerebri see Pituitary Gland
Hypopituitarism   WK 550
Hypopotassemia see Hypokalemia
Hypoprothrombinemias   WH 322
Hyposalivation see Xerostomia

ALWAYS CONSULT MAIN SCHEDULES.   USE NUMBER ASSIGNED ONLY WHEN
SUBJECT REPRESENTS MAJOR EMPHASIS OF WORK BEING CLASSIFIED

Hyposensitization Therapy see Desensitization,
　Immunologic
Hyposomnia see Insomnia
Hypospadias　WJ 600
Hypotension　WG 340
Hypotension, Controlled　WO 350
Hypotension, Orthostatic　WG 340
Hypotension, Postural see Hypotension, Orthostatic
Hypothalamic Diseases　WL 312
Hypothalamic Hormones　WL 312
Hypothalamo-Hypophyseal System　WK 501-502
Hypothalamus　WL 312
Hypothalamus, Infundibular see Hypothalamus,
　Middle
Hypothalamus, Medial see Hypothalamus, Middle
Hypothalamus, Middle　WL 312
Hypothermia　WD 670
　Pathogenesis　QZ 57
　Physiological adaptation　QT 160
Hypothermia, Induced　WO 350
　For extending life for future therapy　WO 350
　Veterinary　SF 914
　See also Cryogenic Surgery　WO 510; Gastric
　　Hypothermia　WI 380; Surgery of particular
　　organs or systems, by part, e.g., Hypothermia
　　in neurosurgery　WL 368
Hypothyroidism　WK 250
Hypoventilation, Central Alveolar see Sleep Apnea
　Syndromes
Hypovolemic Shock see Shock
Hypoxemia see Anoxemia
Hypoxia see Anoxia
Hypoxia, Cellular see Cell Hypoxia
Hypsarrhythmia see Spasms, Infantile
Hysterectomy　WP 468
Hysterectomy, Vaginal　WP 468
Hysteria　WM 173-173.7
Hysteria, Conversion see Conversion Disorder
Hysteria, Dissociative see Dissociative Disorders
Hysterical Neuroses see Hysteria
Hysterical Personality see Histrionic Personality
　Disorder
Hysterosalpingography　WP 141
Hysteroscopy　WP 440
　Used in surgical interventions　WP 468
Hystrix see Rodentia

I

Ia Antigens see Histocompatibility Antigens Class
　II
Ia-Like Antigens see Histocompatibility Antigens
　Class II
Ia-Like Antigens, Human see HLA-D Antigens
IAP Pertussis Toxin see Pertussis Toxins
Iatrogenic Disease　QZ 42
IBR-IPV Virus see Herpesvirus 1, Bovine
Ibuprofen　QV 95
　As an enzyme inhibitor　QU 143
Ice
　Physical geography　GB 2401-2598
　Sanitation　WA 675

Ice Cream
　As a dietary supplement in health or disease
　　WB 428
　Sanitary control　WA 715
Ichthyosis　WR 500
ICI-46474 see Tamoxifen
ICI 66082 see Atenolol
ICSH see LH
Icterus see Jaundice
Icterus Gravis Neonatorum see Erythroblastosis,
　Fetal
Id　WM 460.5.U6
IDDM see Diabetes Mellitus, Insulin-Dependent
Identification of Persons see Forensic medicine　W
　786, etc. and names of special means of
　identification, e.g., Dermatoglyphics
Identification (Psychology)
　Adolescence　WS 462
　Child　WS 105.5.P3
　Infant　WS 105.5.P3
　Personality development (General)　BF 698
　Psychoanalysis　WM 460.5.I4
Identification, Social see Social Identification
Identity Crisis　BF 697
　Adolescence　WS 463
　Child　WS 350.8.I3
　In psychoanalysis　WM 460.5.P3
Idiocy see Mental Retardation
Idiopathic Hypercatabolic Hypoproteinemia see
　Protein-Losing Enteropathies
Idiosyncrasy, Drug see Pharmacology
Idiotypes, Immunoglobulin see Immunoglobulin
　Idiotypes
Iditol Dehydrogenase　QU 140
Ifosfamide
　As an antineoplastic agent　QV 269
　As an immunosuppressive agent　QW 920
IGA Glomerulonephritis see Glomerulonephritis,
　IGA
IGA Nephropathy see Glomerulonephritis, IGA
IgE　QW 601
IGF-I see Insulin-Like Growth Factor I
IGF-II see Insulin-Like Growth Factor II
IgG　QW 601
IL-1 see Interleukin-1
IL-2 see Interleukin-2
IL-2 Receptors see Receptors, Interleukin-2
IL-3 see Interleukin-3
IL-8 see Interleukin-8
Ileal Neoplasms　WI 512
Ileitis　WI 512
Ileitis, Regional see Crohn Disease
Ileitis, Terminal see Crohn Disease
Ileocecal Valve　WI 512
Ileocolitis see Crohn Disease
Ileostomy　WI 512
Ileum　WI 512
Ileus see Intestinal Obstruction
Iliac Artery　WG 595.I5
Iliac Vein　WG 625.I5
Ilizarov Technique
　Bone lengthening　WE 168
　Fracture fixation　WE 185

See also names of particular bones, joints, or conditions
Illegitimacy   HQ 998–999
   Adolescents   WS 462, etc.
   Child psychology   WS 105.5.A8
   Maternal welfare   WA 310
   Paternity   W 791
   Unwed parents
     Relationship to children   WS 105.5.F2
Illicit Drug Testing see Substance Abuse Detection
Illicit Drugs see Street Drugs
Illiteracy see Educational Status
Illness Behavior see Sick Role
Illuminating Gas Poisoning see Carbon Monoxide Poisoning
Illumination see Lighting
Illusions   BF 491–493
   Optical   WW 105
   Psychotic   WM 204
Illustrated Books see Books, Illustrated
Illustration, Medical see Medical Illustration
Illustrations, Surgical see Medical Illustration
Image Analysis, Computer-Assisted see Image Processing, Computer-Assisted
Image Enhancement
   Photoelectronic devices   TK 8316
   Photography
     Treatment of negatives   TR 299
     Treatment of positives   TR 335
   Specific objects, by subject
   See also Radiographic Image Enhancement WN 160
Image Intensifiers see Image Enhancement
Image Interpretation, Computer-Assisted
   General   WB 141
   For particular disorders, with the disorder
Image Processing, Computer-Assisted
   In particular fields (Form number 26.5 in any NLM schedule where applicable)
   Used for special purposes, by subject
Image Reconstruction see Image Processing, Computer-Assisted
Imagery, Guided see Imagery (Psychotherapy)
Imagery (Psychotherapy)   WM 420.5.I3
Imagination
   Adolescence   WS 462
   Child   WS 105.5.C7
   Infant   WS 105.5.C7
   Creative processes   BF 408–426
   Mental imagery (General)   BF 367
   See also Fantasy   BF 408–411, etc.
Imaging, Diagnostic see Diagnostic Imaging
Imaging, Medical see Diagnostic Imaging
Imaging Techniques see Diagnostic Imaging
Imbecility see Mental Retardation
Imidazoles   QU 65
   Organic chemistry   QD 401
Imidazolidinethione see Ethylenethiourea
Imidobenzyle see Imipramine
Imines   QU 54
   Organic chemistry
     Aliphatic compounds   QD 305.I6
     Aromatic compounds   QD 341.I6

Imipemide see Imipenem
Imipenem   QV 350
Imipramine   QV 77.5
Imitative Behavior   BF 357
   Child   WS 105.5.S6
   Infant   WS 105.5.S6
Imizin see Imipramine
Immaturity Syndromes see Personality Disorders
Immediate Recall see Memory, Short-Term
Immersion
   As a cause of accident or disease   QZ 57
   Special conditions resulting, with the condition, e.g., Hypothermia   WD 670, etc.
Immersion Foot   WG 530
Immigration see Emigration and Immigration
Immobilization   WE 168
   Used for special purposes, by subject
Immobilized Cells see Cells, Immobilized
Immobilized Cells see Cells, Immobilized
Immobilized Enzymes see Enzymes, Immobilized
Immotile Cilia Syndrome see Ciliary Motility Disorders
Immune-Associated Antigens see Histocompatibility Antigens Class II
Immune-Associated Antigens, Human see HLA-D Antigens
Immune Body see Antibodies
Immune Complex Diseases   WD 308
Immune Monitoring see Monitoring, Immunologic
Immune Precipitates see Precipitins
Immune Response Antigens see Histocompatibility Antigens Class II
Immune-Response Antigens, Human see HLA-D Antigens
Immune-Response-Associated Antigens see Histocompatibility Antigens Class II
Immune Response-Associated Antigens, Human see HLA-D Antigens
Immune Response Genes see Genes, MHC Class II
Immune Response, Mucosal see Immunity, Mucosal
Immune RNA Manipulation see Immunization, Passive
Immune Sera   QW 815
Immune System   QW 504
Immune Tolerance   QW 504
   Transplantation immunology   WO 680
Immunity   QW 540–949
   Acquired   QW 551
   Artificial   QW 551
   As affected by stress   QZ 160
   Child   WS 135
   Infant   WS 135
   Local   QW 563
   Preparations producing   QW 800–815
Immunity, Active   QW 552
Immunity, Cellular   QW 568
Immunity, Humoral see Antibody Formation
Immunity, Mucosal
   General   QW 563
Immunity, Natural   QW 541
Immunity, Non-Specific see Immunity, Natural
Immunity, Passive   QW 553

Immunization   QW 800–815
   Child   WS 135
   Infant   WS 135
   Public health aspects   WA 110
   Veterinary   SF 757.2
   For a particular disease, with the disease
Immunization, Active see Vaccination
Immunization, Booster see Immunization, Secondary
Immunization, Passive   QW 945
   Of a particular disease, with the disease
Immunization Programs   WA 110
   Child   WS 135
   Infant   WS 135
   For prevention of specific diseases, by disease
Immunization Schedule   QW 800–815
   Child   WS 135
   Infant   WS 135
Immunization, Secondary   QW 800–815
   Child   WS 135
   Infant   WS 135
Immunoactivators see Adjuvants, Immunologic
Immunoadjuvants see Adjuvants, Immunologic
Immunoadsorbents see Immunosorbents
Immunoassay
   General   QW 525.5.I3
   Assay of hormones   QY 330
   Used for diagnostic, monitoring, or evaluation
     tests in special fields, with the field
Immunoassay, Enzyme see Immunoenzyme
Techniques
Immunoblastic Lymphadenopathy   WH 700
Immunoblotting   QW 525.5.I32
   Used for diagnostic, monitoring, or evaluation
     tests in special fields, with the field
Immunoblotting, Western see Blotting, Western
Immunochemistry   QW 504.5
Immunocompetence   QW 568
Immunocompromised Host   QW 504
Immunocontraception see Contraception,
   Immunologic
Immunocytochemistry see Immunohistochemistry
Immunodeficiency Syndrome, Acquired see
   Acquired Immunodeficiency Syndrome
Immunodiagnosis see Immunologic Tests
Immunodiagnostic Tests see Immunologic Tests
Immunodiffusion   QY 265
Immunoelectroblotting see Immunoblotting
Immunoelectroosmophoresis see
   Counterimmunoelectrophoresis
Immunoelectrophoresis   QY 250–275
   Assay of hormones   QY 330
   Veterinary   SF 774
   Used for diagnostic monitoring, or evaluation
     tests in special-fields, with the field
Immunoelectrophoresis, Countercurrent see
   Counterimmunoelectrophoresis
Immunoelectrophoresis, Crossover see
   Counterimmunoelectrophoresis
Immunoenzyme Techniques   QW 525.5.I34
   In immunodiagnostic tests   QY 250
Immunofluorescence Microscopy see Microscopy,
   Fluorescence
Immunofluorescence Technique see Fluorescent
   Antibody Technique

Immunofluorometric Assay see Fluoroimmunoassay
Immunogenetics   QW 541
Immunogens, Synthetic see Vaccines, Synthetic
Immunoglobulin Allotypes   QW 575
Immunoglobulin Genes see Genes, Immunoglobulin
Immunoglobulin Idiotypes   QW 601
Immunoglobulin–Producing Cells see
   Antibody–Producing Cells
Immunoglobulin–Secreting Cells see
   Antibody–Producing Cells
Immunoglobulin Therapy see Immunization, Passive
Immunoglobulins   QW 601
Immunoglobulins, alpha–Chain   QW 601
Immunoglobulins, mu–Chain   QW 601
Immunogold–Silver Techniques see
   Immunohistochemistry
Immunogold Techniques see Immunohistochemistry
Immunohistochemistry   QW 504.5
Immunohistocytochemistry see
   Immunohistochemistry
Immunolabeling Techniques see
   Immunohistochemistry
Immunologic Accessory Cells see
   Antigen–Presenting Cells
Immunologic Competence see Immunocompetence
Immunologic Deficiency Syndrome, Acquired see
   Acquired Immunodeficiency Syndrome
Immunologic Deficiency Syndromes   WD 308
Immunologic Diseases   WD 300–330
Immunologic Factors   QW 568
Immunologic Markers see Biological Markers
Immunologic Monitoring see Monitoring,
   Immunologic
Immunologic Receptors see Receptors, Immunologic
Immunologic Stimulation see Immunization
Immunologic Surveillance   QW 568
Immunologic Techniques   QW 525
   Immunodiagnostic tests   QY 250–275
   See also names of particular tests and procedures,
     e.g., Immunoassay   QW 525.5.I3, etc.
Immunologic Tests
   Used in diagnosis   QY 250–275
   Techniques   QW 525
   See also names of specific tests
Immunologists see Biography   WZ 112.5.I5 and
   Directories   QW 522 under Immunology
Immunology see Allergy and Immunology
Immunology, Transplantation see Transplantation
   Immunology
Immunomodulators see Adjuvants, Immunologic
Immunoperoxidase Techniques see Immunoenzyme
   Techniques
Immunophenotyping   QW 525.5.I36
Immunopotentiators see Adjuvants, Immunologic
Immunoscintigraphy, Radiolabeled see
   Radioimmunodetection
Immunosorbents
   In antigen–antibody complex   QW 570
Immunostimulants see Adjuvants, Immunologic
Immunostimulation see Immunization
Immunosuppressed Host see Immunocompromised
   Host
Immunosuppression   QW 920

Immunosuppression (Physiology) see Immune
Tolerance
Immunosuppressive Agents   QW 920
Immunosurveillance see Monitoring, Immunologic
Immunotherapy   QW 940-949
Of a particular disease, with the disease
Immunotherapy, Active   QW 949
Veterinary   SF 919
Of a particular disease, with the disease
Immunotherapy, Adoptive   QW 940
Immunotherapy, Allergen see Desensitization,
Immunologic
Immunotherapy, Passive see Immunotherapy,
Adoptive
Immunotoxins   QW 630.5.I3
Impedance Tests, Acoustic see Acoustic Impedance
Tests
Impedance, Transthoracic see Cardiography,
Impedance
Impetigo   WR 225
Impetigo Contagiosa see Impetigo
Implant Radiotherapy see Brachytherapy
Implant-Supported Dental Prosthesis see Dental
Prosthesis, Implant-Supported
Implantable Catheters see Catheters, Indwelling
Implantable Infusion Pumps see Infusion Pumps,
Implantable
Implantation, Blastocyst see Ovum Implantation
Implantation, Dental see Dental Implantation
Implantation, Ovum see Nidation
Implantation, Ovum, Delayed see Ovum
Implantation, Delayed
Implants, Artificial see Prostheses and Implants
Implants, Cochlear see Cochlear Implants
Implants, Dental see Dental Implants
Implosive Therapy   WM 425.5.D4
Impotence   WJ 709
Impregnation, Artificial see Insemination, Artificial
Impulse Control Disorders   WM 190
Impulse-Ridden Personality see Personality
Disorders
Impulsive Behavior   BF 575.I46
In Situ Hybridization   QH 452.8
Inadequate Personality see Personality Disorders
Inanition see Deficiency Diseases
Inborn Errors of Metabolism see Metabolism, Inborn
Errors
Inbreeding
Animal   SF 105
Physical anthropology   GN 252
Social pathology   HV 4981
Incentive Reimbursement see Reimbursement,
Incentive
Incentives see Motivation
Incest   WM 610
Incidence Studies see Cohort Studies
Incident Reporting, Hospital see Risk Management
Incipient Schizophrenia see Schizotypal Personality
Disorder
Incisor   WU 101
Inclusion Bodies   QH 603.I49
Inclusion Disease see Cytomegalovirus Infections

Income
Economic theory   HB 522-715
Labor   HD 4906-5100.7
Of dentists   WU 77
Of nurses   WY 77
Of physicians   W 79
Of other specialties, by type
Income Tax   HJ 4621-4824
Incompatibility of Drugs see Drug Incompatibility
Incontinentia Pigmenti Achromians see Pigmentation
Disorders
Incubation Period see Time Factors; Carrier State
Incubators
(Form number 26 in any NLM schedule where
applicable)
Used in experimental histology   QS 530; in
microbiology   QW 26
Incubators, Infant
Catalogs   W 26
Description   WS 26
Usage   WS 410-421
Incunabula   Z 240-241
Medical   WZ 230
Incus   WV 230
Indans
Organic chemistry   QD 341.H9
Special topics, by subject
Indapamide   QV 160
Indazoles   QV 95
Organic chemistry   QD 401
Indenes
As anti-arrhythmia agents   QV 150
As anti-inflammatory analgesics   QV 95
Organic chemistry   QD 341.H9
Independent Living see Activities of Daily Living
Independent Practice Associations   W 130
Index Medicus see MEDLARS
Indexes
Of subjects represented in NLM's classification,
appropriate classification number preceded by
the letter Z
Of other subjects, LC's Z schedule
Indexing see Abstracting and Indexing
Indian Nursing Service see Public Health Nursing
Indians, Central American   F 1434-1435
See also special topics under Ethnic Groups
Indians, North American   E 75-99
As physicians
Collective biography   WZ 150
History   WZ 80.5.I3
Individual biography   WZ 100
See also special topics under Ethnic Groups
Mexico   F 1219-1220
Indians, South American   F 2229-2230.2 etc.
As physicians
Collective biography   WZ 150
History   WZ 80.5.I3
Individual biography   WZ 100
See also special topics under Ethnic Groups
Indicator Dilution Techniques   WG 141
Blood volume   WG 106
See also Dye Dilution Technique   WG 141, etc.;
Radioisotope Dilution Technique   WG 141,
etc.

**ALWAYS CONSULT MAIN SCHEDULES. USE NUMBER ASSIGNED ONLY WHEN
SUBJECT REPRESENTS MAJOR EMPHASIS OF WORK BEING CLASSIFIED**

etc.

Indicators and Reagents
    Analytical chemistry   QD 77
    Pharmaceutical chemistry   QV 744
    See also Dyes   QV 240, etc.
Indigency see Poverty
Indigency, Medical see Medical Indigency
Indigent Care see Medical Indigency
Indigents, Medical Care see Medicaid; Medical
    Indigency
Indigestion see Dyspepsia; Heartburn
Indium
    Inorganic chemistry   QD 181.I5
    Pharmacology   QV 290
Indium Radioisotopes   WN 415–450
    Used for special purposes, by subject
Individual Differences see Individuality
Individual Practice Associations see Independent
    Practice Associations
Individuality
    Psychology   BF 697
    Sociology   HM
Individuation   WM 460.5.I5
    In personality development   BF 697
        Adolescence   WS 462
        Child   WS 105.5.P3
        Infant   WS 105.5.P3
Indocyanine Green   QV 240
Indoleacetic Acids   QK 753.I5
    In amino acid metabolism   QU 65
Indoleamine 2,3–Dioxygenase see Tryptophan
    Oxygenase
Indoles
    As antidepressive agents   QV 77.5
    As hallucinogens   QV 77.7
    As tranquilizers   QV 77.9
    Organic chemistry   QD 401
Indolylethylamines see Tryptamines
Indomethacin   QV 95
Indoor Air Pollution see Air Pollution, Indoor
Indoor Air Quality see Air Pollution, Indoor
Indoprofen   QV 95
Indri see Strepsirhini
Indriidae see Strepsirhini
Induction of Labor see Labor, Induced
Industrial Accidents see Accidents, Occupational
Industrial Arts see Technology
Industrial Bacteriology see Bacteriology
Industrial By–Products in Air Pollution see Air
    Pollutants
Industrial Chemistry see Chemistry
Industrial Dentistry see Occupational Dentistry
Industrial Dermatoses see Dermatitis, Occupational
Industrial Diseases see Occupational Diseases
Industrial Health see Occupational Health
Industrial Hygiene see Occupational Health
Industrial Medical Departments see Occupational
    Health Services
Industrial Medicine see Occupational Medicine
Industrial Mental Health see Mental Health
Industrial Microbiology   QW 75
Industrial Nursing see Occupational Health Nursing

Industrial Oils
    Biochemistry   QU 86
    Chemical technology   TP 670–699
    Public health aspects   WA 722
Industrial Ophthalmology see Ophthalmology
Industrial Poisoning see Poisoning
Industrial Surgery see Surgery
Industrial Toxicology see Occupational Medicine;
    Poisons; Toxicology
Industrial Waste   WA 788
    See also names of specific types of waste, e.g.
        Air Pollutants   WA 450, etc.
Industry   HD 2321–4730.9
Inert Gas Narcosis
    Aviation and space medicine   WD 715
    Submarine medicine   WD 650
Infant   WS
    Anesthesia   WO 440
    General   WS 430
    Nursing see Pediatric Nursing   WY 159
    Radiography   WN 240
    Surgery   WO 925
    Welfare see Child Welfare   WA 310–320
    See also Birth Injuries   WS 405, other headings
        beginning with Birth.
Infant Care   WS 113
Infant Food   WS 115–125
Infant Health Services see Child Health Services
Infant, Low Birth Weight   WS 420
Infant Mortality   HB 1323.I4
    Including causes of death   WA 900
    See also Fetal Death   WQ 225, etc.
Infant, Newborn   WS 420
    Legal establishment of life   W 789
    Nursing see Neonatal Nursing   WY 157.3
    Resuscitation   WQ 450
Infant, Newborn, Diseases   WS 421
Infant, Newborn, Intensive Care see Intensive Care,
    Neonatal
Infant, Newborn, Screening see Neonatal Screening
Infant Nutrition
    Feeding   WS 120–125
    Requirements   WS 115
Infant Nutrition Disorders   WS 120
Infant, Premature   WS 410
Infant, Premature, Diseases   WS 410
Infant Psychology see Child Psychology
Infant Radiant Warmers see Incubators, Infant
Infant, Small for Gestational Age   WS 420
Infant Welfare
    Public health aspects   WA 310–320
    Social aspects   HV 697–700
Infanticide
    Criminology   HV 6537–6541
    Medicolegal aspects   W 867
Infantile Paralysis see Poliomyelitis
Infantile Refsum Disease see Peroxisomal Disorders
Infantilism   WK 900
    See also Dwarfism   WE 250
Infantilism, Genital see Hypogonadism
Infantilism, Sexual see Hypogonadism
Infanto Sexuality see Paraphilias
Infarction   QZ 170

Coronary see Coronary Disease   WG 300, etc.;
   Myocardial Infarction   WG 300
   Pulmonary see Pulmonary Embolism   WG 420
Infection
   Bacteriological aspects   QW 700
   Eye   WW 160   .
   Disease process   WC 195
   Surgical see Surgical Wound Infection   WO 185
   Veterinary   SF 781
   Wound see Wound infection   WC 255
   Localized, by site
   See also Cross Infection   WC 195, Focal
     Infection   WC 230, etc.; Laboratory Infection
      WC 195; names of other specifc types of
     infection
Infection Control   WC 195
   In dentistry   WU 29
   In hospitals   WX 167
Infection Control, Dental   WU 29
Infectious Bovine Rhinotracheitis Virus see
   Herpesvirus 1, Bovine
Infectious Bronchitis Virus, Avian   QW 168.5.C8
Infectious Bronchitis Virus of Birds
   Infectious Bronchitis Virus, Avian
Infectious Disease Contact Tracing see Contact
   Tracing
Infectious Diseases see Communicable Diseases;
   names of particular infectious diseases
Infectious Human Wart Virus see Papillomavirus,
   Human
Infectious Keratoconjunctivitis see
   Keratoconjunctivitis, Infectious
Infectious Mononucleosis   WC 522
Infectious Mononucleosis–Like Syndrome, Chronic
see Fatigue Syndrome, Chronic
Infectious Mononucleosis Virus see Herpesvirus 4,
   Human
Infectious Pustular Vulvovaginitis Virus see
   Herpesvirus 1, Bovine
Inferiority Complex see Personality Disorders
Inferiority, Constitutional Psychopathic see
   Antisocial Personality Disorder
Infertility   WP 570
   Veterinary   SF 871
Infertility, Female   WP 570
Infertility, Male   WJ 709
Infibulation see Circumcision, Fcmale
Infiltration anesthesia see Anesthesia, Local
Inflammation   QZ 150
   Immunological aspects   QW 700
   Localized, by site
Inflammatory Bowel Diseases   WI 420
Inflation, Economic
   By subject, in economics number where
     applicable
Influenza   WC 515
Influenza A Virus, Avian   QW 168.5.O7
Influenza A Virus, Porcine   QW 168.5.O7
Influenza, Asian see Influenza
Influenza D Virus see Parainfluenza Virus 1, Human
Influenza Vaccine   WC 515
Influenza Virus, Avian see Influenza A Virus, Avian
Influenza Virus, Porcine see Influenza A Virus,

   Porcine
Influenza Viruses see Orthomyxoviridae
Information Display see Data Display
Information Dissemination see Information Services
Information Management
   General works   Z 665+
   Special topics, by subject
Information Processing, Automatic see Automatic
   Data Processing
Information Processing, Human see Mental
   Processes
Information Retrieval see Information Storage and
   Retrieval
Information Retrieval Systems see Information
   Systems
Information Science   Z 665–718.8
   Information theory   Q 350–390
   Special topics, by subject
Information Services   Z 674.2–674.5
   Services in particular fields, by subject
Information Storage and Retrieval   Z 699
   By subject   Z 699.5.A–Z
   In medicine (General)   W 26.55.I4
   In other special fields (Form number 26.5 in any
     NLM schedule where applicable)
Information Systems   Z 699
   By subject   Z 699.5.A–Z
   In medicine (General)   W 26.55.I4
   In other special fields (Form number 26.5 in any
     NLM schedule where applicable)
   See also Automatic Data Processing   W
     26.55.A9, etc.; Computers   W 26.55.C7, etc.;
     MEDLARS   W 26.55.I4
Information Theory   Q 350–390
   Special applications, by subject
Informed Consent
   In human experimentation   W 20.55.H9
   Legal aspects   W 32–33
   Other special topics, by subject, e.g., in drug
     research   QV 20.5
Infrared Detectors see Instrumentation   WB 26
   under Infrared Rays
Infrared Rays   QC 457
   Diagnostic use   WB 288
   General medical use   WB 117
   Instrumentation   WB 26
   Technology (Applied optics)   TA 1570
   Therapeutic use   WB 480
   See also Spectrophotometry, Infrared   QC 457,
     etc.
Infrared Spectroscopy see Spectrophotometry,
   Infrared
Infusion see Drug Compounding
Infusion Pumps   WB 354
Infusion Pumps, External see Infusion Pumps
Infusion Pumps, Implantable   WB 354
Infusions, Intra–Arterial   WB 354
Infusions, Intravenous   WB 354
Infusions, Parenteral   WB 354
   Glucose   WB 354
   Saline   WB 354
   See also Sodium Chloride   WB 354, etc.
Infusions, Regional Arterial see Infusions,
   Intra–Arterial

**ALWAYS CONSULT MAIN SCHEDULES. USE NUMBER ASSIGNED ONLY WHEN
SUBJECT REPRESENTS MAJOR EMPHASIS OF WORK BEING CLASSIFIED**

Infusors see Infusion Pumps
Inguinal Hernia see Hernia, Inguinal
Inhalation see Respiration
Inhalation Anesthesia see Anesthesia, Inhalation
Inhalation Burns see Burns, Inhalation
Inhalation Devices see Nebulizers and Vaporizers
Inhalation Drug Administration see Administration, Inhalation
Inhalation Injury, Smoke see Smoke Inhalation Injury
Inhalation of Drugs see Administration, Inhalation
Inhalation Provocation Tests see Bronchial Provocation Tests
Inhalation Therapy see Respiratory Therapy
Inhalators see Nebulizers and Vaporizers
Inhalers see Nebulizers and Vaporizers
Inhibin   WK 900
    Female   WP 520
    Male   WJ 875
Inhibition, Neural see Neural Inhibition
Inhibition (Psychology)   BF 335–337
    Child   WS 350.8.I4
    Infant   WS 350.8.I4
Injections   WB 354
    Hypodermic   WB 354
    Saline   WB 354
    See also Enema   WB 344
Injections, Intra–Arterial   WB 354
Injections, Intradermal   WB 354
Injections, Intramuscular   WB 354
Injections, Intravenous   WB 354
Injections, Jet   WB 354
Injections, Sclerosing see Sclerosing Solutions
Injections, Subcutaneous   WB 354
Injured, Transportation see Transportation of Patients
Injuries see Wounds and Injuries
Injuries, Multiple see Multiple Trauma
Ink
    Paleography   Z 112
    Toxicology   QV 627
Ink Blot Tests   WM 145.5.I5
Inlays   WU 360
Innate Behavior see Instinct
Innominate Artery see Brachiocephalic Trunk
Innominate Veins see Brachiocephalic Veins
Innovation Diffusion see Diffusion of Innovation
Inoculation see Vaccination
Inoculation Lymphoreticulosis see Cat–Scratch Disease
Inorganic Carbon Compounds see Carbon Compounds, Inorganic
Inorganic Chemicals
    Inorganic chemistry   QD 146–197
Inorganic Chemistry see Chemistry, Inorganic
Inorganic Ions see Ions
Inorganic Poisons see Poisons
Inorganic Substances, Biochemistry see Biochemistry
Inosine
    Biochemistry   QU 57
    Pharmacology   QV 185

Inosine Phosphorylase see Purine–Nucleoside Phosphorylase
Inositol   QU 87
Inositol Hexaphosphate see Phytic Acid
Inositol Phosphates   QU 75
Inositol Phosphoglycerides see Phosphatidylinositols
Inotropic Agents, Positive Cardiac see Cardiotonic Agents
Inotropism see Muscle Contraction
Inotropism, Cardiac see Myocardial Contraction
Inpatients   WX 158.5
    With specific disabilities, with the disability
    See also Patients
Inproquone   QV 269
    Cancer chemotherapy   QZ 267
Insanity see Mental Disorders
Insanity Defense   W 740
    Legislation   WM 32–33
Insect Bites and Stings   WD 430
Insect Control   QX 600
Insect Growth Regulators see Juvenile Hormones
Insect Poisons see Insect Bites and Stings
Insect Repellents
    Pest control in agriculture   SB 951.5–951.54
    Public health aspects   WA 240
Insect Sterilization see Insect Control
Insect Vectors   QX 650
    Preventive medicine   WA 110
Insect Viruses   QW 162
Insecticide Resistance
    Agriculture   SB 957
    Chemically induced mutations   QH 465.C5
    Insect control (Parasitology)   QX 600
    Public health aspects   WA 240
Insecticides
    Agriculture   SB 951.5–951.54
    Public health   WA 240
Insecticides, Carbamate
    Agriculture   SB 952.C3
    Public health   WA 240
Insecticides, Organochlorine
    Agriculture   SB 952.C44
    Public health   WA 240
Insecticides, Organophosphate
    Agriculture   SB 952.P5
    Public health   WA 240
Insecticides, Organophosphate, Antagonists see Cholinesterase Reactivators
Insecticides, Organothiophosphate, Antagonists see Cholinesterase Reactivators
Insectivora   QL 737.I5–737.I58
Insects
    Diseases   SB 942
    Parasitology   QX 500–650
    Poisoning   WD 430
Insemination   WQ 205
Insemination, Artificial   WQ 208
    Sociological aspects   HQ 761
    Veterinary   SF 105.5
Insemination, Artificial, Heterologous   WQ 208
Insemination, Artificial, Homologous   WQ 208
Insemination, Artificial, Human Donor see Insemination, Artificial, Heterologous

Insemination, Artificial, Husband see Insemination, Artificial, Homologous
Insertion Elements, DNA see DNA Transposable Elements
Insertion Sequence Elements see DNA Transposable Elements
Inservice Training   HF 5549.5.T7
   In hospitals   WX 159
   For particular jobs, by subject, e.g. as a nurses' aide   WY 193
Insignia see Emblems and Insignia
Insomnia   WM 188
Inspection, Sanitary see Sanitation
Inspiratory Positive-Pressure Ventilation see Intermittent Positive-Pressure Ventilation
Instability, Joint see Joint Instability
Instillation, Bladder see Administration, Intravesical
Instillation, Rectal see Administration, Rectal
Instinct
   Animal   QL 781
   Psychology   BF 685
   Social psychology   HM
Institutes see Academies and institutes
Institutional Liability see Liability, Legal
Institutional Nursing see Nursing   WY 125 under Institutional Practice; Specialties, Nursing
Institutional Personnel Licensure see Licensure
Institutional Practice   W 96
   Nursing   WY 125
Institutional Review Board see Professional Staff Committees
Institutional Tax see Taxes
Institutionalization   W 84.7
   Geriatrics   WT 31
   See also Hospitals, Psychiatric   WM 27-28, etc.; Hospitalization   WX 158-158.5, etc.
Institutionalized Child see Child, Institutionalized
Institutions see Organizations
Instructional Technology see Educational Technology
Instrumental Learning see Conditioning, Operant
Instruments see Equipment and Supplies; Surgical instruments; Catalogs, Commercial   W 26, etc. and names of particular instruments
Insufflation Anesthesia see Anesthesia, Inhalation
Insufflation Radiography see Pneumoradiography
Insula of Reil see Cerebral Cortex
Insular Tissue, Pancreas see Islets of Langerhans
Insulin   WK 820
   Shock see Hypoglycemia   WK 880
   Shock Therapy see Shock Therapy, Insulin   WM 410
Insulin Antibodies   QW 575
Insulin Coma Therapy see Convulsive Therapy
Insulin Infusion Systems   WK 820
Insulin, Lente   WK 820
Insulin-Like Growth Factor I
   As a growth substance   QU 107
Insulin-Like Growth Factor II
   As a growth substance   QU 107
Insulinoma   WK 885
Insuloma see Insulinoma
Insurance   HG 8016-9999

Insurance, Accident   W 100-250
   Medicolegal aspects   W 900
Insurance Audit see Insurance Claim Review
Insurance Benefits
   Life insurance rates   HG 8751-9295
   Medical, etc. service plans   W 100-275
   For particular disabilities, by subject
Insurance Carriers
   Of health insurance   W 100-275
Insurance Case Management see Managed Care Programs
Insurance Claim Reporting
   Related to health insurance in general   W 100-275
   Special topics, by subject
Insurance Claim Review   W 100-275
   For particular disorder, by subject
Insurance Claims Processing see Insurance Claim Review
Insurance Coverage
   General   HG 8011-9343
   Health insurance   W 100-275
   See also names of specific types of insurance, e.g., Medicare   WT 31
Insurance, Dental   W 260
Insurance, Disability   HD 7105.2-7105.25
   Medicare   WT 31
Insurance, Health   W 100-275
   Medicolegal aspects   W 900
   Surgical   W 100-275
Insurance, Health, Catastrophic see Insurance, Major Medical
Insurance, Health, for Aged and Disabled see Medicare
Insurance, Health, Reimbursement   W 100-275
Insurance, Hospitalization   W 160
Insurance, Liability   HG 9990
   (Form number 33 or 33.1 in any NLM schedule where applicable and practical)
Insurance, Life   HG 8751-9271
Insurance, Long-Term Care   W 160
   For the aged   WT 31
Insurance, Major Medical   W 160
Insurance, Medigap   WT 31
Insurance, Nursing Services   W 255
Insurance, Old Age see Medicare; Social Security
Insurance, Pharmaceutical Services   W 265
Insurance, Physician Services   W 100-275
Insurance, Psychiatric   W 270
Insurance Status see Insurance Coverage
Insurance, Surgical   W 100-275
Insurers see Insurance Carriers
Integral Membrane Proteins see Membrane Proteins
Integrase   QU 141
Integrated Delivery Systems see Delivery of Health Care, Integrated
Integrated Health Care Systems see Delivery of Health Care, Integrated
Integration, Prophage see Lysogeny
Integumentary System see Skin
Intellectual Property
   Copyright   Z 551-656
   Patents   T 201-342

Intelligence   BF 431–433
  Child   WS 105
  Genius   BF 412–426
  Infant   WS 105
  See also Educational Measurement   LB 3051;
    Psychological Tests   BF 176, etc.
Intelligence Tests   BF 431–433
  Child   BF 432.C48
  Infant   BF 432.C48
Intensive Care   WX 218
  Child   WS 366
  Infant   Ws 366
  Nursing   WY 154
    Pediatric   WY 159
  Of a particular disease or in a particular field
    General, with the disease or field
    Nursing, with the nursing specialty
Intensive Care, Neonatal   WS 421
Intensive Care Nursing see Nursing   WY 154 under
  Intensive Care
Intensive Care, Surgical see Intensive Care
Intensive Care Units   WX 218
  Coronary see Coronary Care Units   WG 27–28
  Respiratory see Respiratory Care Units   WF
    27–28
  Special fields, form numbers 27–28 where
    applicable
  See also Critical Care   WX 218, etc.
Interagency Relations see Interinstitutional Relations
Interbrain see Diencephalon
Intercalated Neurons see Interneurons
Intercarotid Ganglion see Carotid Body
Intercellular Junctions   QH 603.C4
Intercellular Space see Extracellular Space
Intercostal Muscles   WE 715
Interdigitating Cells see Dendritic Cells
Interdisciplinary Health Team see Patient Care Team
Interface, User Computer see User–Computer
  Interface
Interferometry, Microscopic see Microscopy,
  Interference
Interferon Alfa, Recombinant
  Immunology   QW 800
  As an antiviral agent   QV 268.5
  As an antineoplastic agent   QV 269
Interferon Alfa-2c see Interferon Alfa, Recombinant
Interferon–gamma see Interferon Type II
Interferon, Immune see Interferon Type II
Interferon Inducers
  Immunology   QW 800
  Pharmacology   QV 268.5
Interferon Type I
  Immunology   QW 800
  As an antiviral agent   QV 268.5
  As an antineoplastic agent   QV 269
Interferon Type I, Recombinant see Interferon Alfa,
  Recombinant
Interferon Type II
  Immunology   QW 800
  As an antiviral agent   QV 268.5
  As an antineoplastic agent   QV 269
Interferons
  Immunology   QW 800

  Pharmacology   QV 268.5
Interinstitutional Relations
  Hospitals   WX 160
  Other types of institutions, by subject
Interior Design and Furnishings
  In health facilities   WX 140
    For the specialties (Form number 27–29 in any
      NLM schedule where applicable)
  Hospital departments   WX 200–225
  Public health aspects of houses and public
    buildings   WA 795–799
Interior Furnishings see Interior Design and
  Furnishings
Interleukin–1
  Cellular immunity   QW 568
  As a growth substance   QU 107
Interleukin–2
  Cellular immunity   QW 568
  As a growth substance   QU 107
Interleukin–2 Receptors see Receptors, Interleukin–2
Interleukin–3
  Cellular immunity   QW 568
  As a growth substance   QU 107
Interleukin–8
  Cellular immunity   QW 568
  As a growth substance   QU 107
Interleukins
  Cellular immunity   QW 568
  As growth substances   QU 107
Intermediary Body see Hemolysins
Intermediate Filaments   QH 603.C95
Intermedins see MSH
Intermetatarsal Joint see Tarsal Joint
Intermittent Claudication   WG 550
Intermittent Fever see Malaria
Intermittent Positive–Pressure Ventilation   WF 145
Internal Ear see Labyrinth
Internal–External Control
  Child development   WS 105.5.S6
  School management and discipline   LB 3011
  Training of will   BF 632
Internal Mammary–Coronary Artery Anastomosis
  WG 169
Internal Medicine   WB 115
  Directories   W 22
Internal Secretions see Body Fluids; Hormones;
  Intestinal Secretions   WI 400 and names of
  specific secretions
International Agencies   JX 1995
International Cooperation
  General works   JC 362
  Special area of cooperation, by subject
International Health Administration see World
  Health
International Health Problems see World Health
International System of Units   QC 90.8–94
  Pharmaceutical   QV 16
  In other special fields (Form number 16 in any
    NLM schedule where applicable)
Internet   TK 5105.875.I57
  In medicine (General)   W 26.5
  In other special fields (Form number 26.5 in any
    NLM schedule where applicable)

Interneurons   WL 102.5
Internists, Directories see Directories   W 22 under
   Internal Medicine
Internship and Residency
   Dental   WU 20
   Medical   W 20
      Hospital program   WX 203
   Nursing   WY 18.5
   Pharmacy   QV 20
Internship, Dental see Internship and Residency
Internship, Nonmedical
   Nursing   WY 18.5
   Pharmacy   QV 20
   Other fields, by subject
Interpersonal Relations   HM
   Adolescence   WS 462
   Child   WS 105.5.I5
   Infant   WS 105.5.I5
      Of the retarded child   WS 107.5.R4
   In hospitals   WX 160
   Of surgeons   WO 62
   See also specific relationships terms, e.g.,
      Dentist-Patient Relations   WU 61, etc.;
      Family Relations   WS 105.5.F2, etc.;
      Nurse-Patient Relations   WY 87, etc.;
      Physician-Nurse Relations   W 62, etc.;
      Physician-Patient Relations   W 62, etc.
Interphase   QH 605
Interprofessional Relations
   Dentists   WU 61
   In hospitals   WX 160
   Nurses   WY 87
   Physicians   W 62
   Surgeons   WO 62
   Others, with specialty primarily involved
   See also specific relationship terms, e.g.,
      Physician-Nurse Relations   W 62, etc.
Intersexuality see Hermaphroditism
Interstitial Cell-Stimulating Hormone see LH
Interstitial Fluid see Extracellular Space
Interstitial Lung Diseases see Lung Diseases,
   Interstitial
Intertarsal Joint see Tarsal Joint
Intertrochanteric Fractures see Hip Fractures
Intervertebral Disk   WE 740
   Of the lumbosacral region   WE 750
Intervertebral Disk Chemolysis   WE 740
Intervertebral Disk Displacement   WE 740
   Veterinary   SF 901
Interview, Psychological
   Applied psychology   BF 637.I5
   Child   WS 105
   Psychiatry   WM 141
Interviews
   For admission to schools (Form number 19 or
   20 in any NLM schedule where applicable)
   For hospital jobs   WX 159
   For nurses   WY 105
   Of physicians and specialists of medically related
   fields
      Collective   WZ 112-150
      Individual   WZ 100
   Other special topics, by subject

Intestinal Absorption   WI 402
Intestinal Amebiasis see Dysentery, Amebic
Intestinal Atresia   WI 412
Intestinal Diseases   WI 400-650
   General works   WI 400
   Child   WS 310-312
   Infant   WS 310-312
   Signs and symptoms   WI 405
   Veterinary   SF 851
Intestinal Diseases, Parasitic   WC 698
   Veterinary   SF 810.A3
Intestinal Fistula   WI 400
Intestinal Hormone Receptors see Receptors,
   Gastrointestinal Hormone
Intestinal Hormones see Gastrointestinal Hormones
Intestinal Motility see Gastrointestinal Motility
Intestinal Neoplasms   WI 435
   Localized, by site
Intestinal Obstruction   WI 460
   Veterinary   SF 851
   Volvulus   WI 450
   See also Stomach Volvulus   WI 300
Intestinal Perforation
   General   WI 400
   Localized, by site
Intestinal Polyps   WI 430
   Localized, by site
Intestinal Secretions   WI 400
Intestine, Large   WI 400
   See-also names of specific organs, e.g., Colon
   WI 520-529
Intestine, Small   WI 500-512
Intestines   WI 400-650
   See also specific organs, e.g., Rectum   WI
   600-650
Intoxication see Poisoning
Intoxication, Alcoholic see Alcoholic Intoxication
Intra-Abdominal Infusions see Infusions, Parenteral
Intra-Aortic Balloon Pumping   WG 168
Intra-Arterial Lines see Catheters, Indwelling
Intracaine see Benzocaine
Intracellular Adhesion Molecules see Cell Adhesion
   Molecules
Intracellular Fluid   QU 105
Intracellular Membranes   QH 601
Intracellular Second Messengers see Second
   Messenger Systems
Intracerebral Pressure see Intracranial Pressure
Intracoronal Attachment see Denture Precision
   Attachment
Intracranial Aneurysm see Cerebral Aneurysm
Intracranial Arteriovenous Malformations see
   Cerebral Arteriovenous Malformations
Intracranial Hypertension   WL 203
Intracranial Hypertension, Benign see Pseudotumor
   Cerebri
Intracranial Hypotension   WL 203
Intracranial Pressure   WL 203
Intraligamentous Pregnancy see Preganancy,
   Ectopic
Intramedullary Nailing see Fracture Fixation,
   Intramedullary
Intraocular Pressure   WW 103

Independent Practice Associations
Ipecac   QV 73
Ipecine see Emetine
IPPV see Intermittent Positive–Pressure Ventilation
Iproniazid   QV 77.5
Iproveratril see Verapamil
Ir Genes see Genes, MHC Class II
Iridium
    Inorganic chemistry   QD 181.I7
    Radioactive   WN 420
Iridocyclitis   WW 240
Iridodiagnosis see Eye Manifestations
Iridoviridae   QW 165.5.I6
Iridoviruses see Iridoviridae
Iris   WW 240
Iris Diseases   WW 240
Iritis   WW 240
Iron
    Pharmacology   QV 183
Iron Chelates see Iron Chelating Agents
Iron Chelating Agents
    Pharmacology   QV 183
    Physical chemistry   QD 474
Iron–Deficiency Anemia see Anemia,
    Iron–Deficiency
Iron, Dietary
    Biochemistry   QU 130.5
    Pharmacology   QV 183
Iron Isotopes
    Inorganic chemistry   QD 181.F4
    Pharmacology   QV 183
Iron Lung see Ventilators, Mechanical
Iron Metabolism Disorders   WD 200.5.I7
Iron Overload   WD 200.5.I7
Iron Salts see Iron; names of specific salts
Iron–Sulfur Proteins   QU 55
Irritable Bowel Syndrome see Colonic Diseases,
    Functional
Irritable Heart see Neurocirculatory Asthenia
Irritants   QV 65
    Gases   QV 666
      Lung irritants   QV 664
    Poisons other than gases   QV 618
    Therapeutic use   WB 371
IS Elements see DNA Transposable Elements
Ischemia   QZ 170
    Localized, by site
    See also Myocardial Ischemia   WG 300
Ischemia, Myocardial see Myocardial Ischemia
Ischemia–Reperfusion Injury see Reperfusion Injury
Ischemic Heart Disease see Myocardial Ischemia
Ischemic Optic Neuropathy see Optic Neuropathy,
    Ischemic
Ischemic Preconditioning   QZ 170
    Localized, by site
    See also Ischemic Preconditioning, Myocardial
    WG 300
Ischemic Preconditioning, Myocardial   WG 300
Islam   BP 1–253
    Birth control   HQ 766.37
    Psychological aspects   BP 175
    Special topics, by subject
Islamic Physicians see Physicians

Island Fever see Scrub Typhus
Island Flaps see Surgical Flaps
Islands of Langerhans see Islets of Langerhans
Islet–Activating Protein see Pertussis Toxins
Islet Cell Tumor see Adenoma, Islet Cell
Islet Cell Tumor, Ulcerogenic see Zollinger–Ellison
    Syndrome
Islets of Langerhans   WK 800–885
    Neoplasms   WK 885
Islets of Langerhans Transplantation   WK 800
Isoantibodies   QW 575
Isoantigens   QW 573
Isoaspartic Acid see Aspartic Acid
Isocyanates see Cyanates
Isocyanides see Cyanides
Isoelectric Focusing
    Analytical chemistry (General)   QD 79.E44
    Biochemistry   QU 25
    Clinical pathology   QY 25
    Microbiology   QW 25
    Parasitology   QX 25
    Used for special purposes, by subject
Isoelectric Focusing Agents see Ampholyte Mixtures
Isoenzymes   QU 135–141
Isoephedrine see Ephedrine
Isoflurane   QV 81
Isoflurophate   QV 124
Isofosfamide see Ifosfamide
Isohexanes see Hexanes
Isoimmunization, Rhesus see Rh Isoimmunization
Isolation Hospitals see Hospitals, Special; Patient
    Isolation
Isolation, Patient see Patient Isolation
Isolation Perfusion see Perfusion, Regional
Isolation Perfusion Therapy see Perfusion, Regional
Isolation, Social see Social Isolation
Isoleucine   QU 60
Isoleucyl, Leucyl Vasopressin see Oxytocin
Isomerases   QU 137
Isomerism   QD 471
Isometric Contraction   WE 500
Isometric Exercise see Exercise
Isoniazid   QV 268
Isonicotinic Acid Hydrazide see Isoniazid
Isonipecain see Meperidine
Isophosphamide see Ifosfamide
Isoprenaline see Isoproterenol
Isoprenoid Phosphate Sugars see Polyisoprenyl
    Phosphate Sugars
Isoprenoid Phosphates see Polyisoprenyl Phosphates
Isopropanol see 2–Propanol
Isopropyl Alcohol see 2–Propanol
Isopropylarterenol see Isoproterenol
Isoproterenol   WK 725
Isoquinolines
    As antihypertensive agents   QV 150
    In opium alkaloids   QV 90
    Organic chemistry   QD 401
Isotachophoresis see Electrophoresis
Isotonic Solutions   QV 786
Isotopes
    In organic chemistry   QD 181
    Physical chemistry   QD 466.5

**ALWAYS CONSULT MAIN SCHEDULES. USE NUMBER ASSIGNED ONLY WHEN
SUBJECT REPRESENTS MAJOR EMPHASIS OF WORK BEING CLASSIFIED**

Radioactive see Radioisotopes   WN 420, etc.
   Research in medicine, etc., by subject
Isotretinoin   QU 167
Isozymes see Isoenzymes
Itch see Scabies
Itch Mites see Sarcoptes scabiei
Itching see Pruritus
Ito Syndrome see Pigmentation Disorders
IUGR see Fetal Growth Retardation
Ivermectin   SF 918.I83
Ivy, Poison see Toxicodendron
Ixodoidea see Ticks

J

Jackknife Seizures see Spasms, Infantile
Jacksonian Seizure see Epilepsy, Partial
Jamestown Canyon Virus see California Group
   Viruses
Jansky–Bielschowsky Disease see Neuronal
   Ceroid–Lipofuscinosis
Japanese see Mongoloid Race
Japanese Americans see Asian Americans
Japanese Monkey see Macaca
Japanese River Fever see Scrub Typhus
Jaundice   WI 703
   Of the newborn see Jaundice, Neonatal   WH
   425
   Spirochetal see Weil's Disease   WC 420, etc.
Jaundice, Cholestatic see Cholestasis
Jaundice, Cholestatic, Extrahepatic see Bile Duct
   Obstruction, Extrahepatic
Jaundice, Chronic Idiopathic   WI 703
Jaundice, Hemolytic see Anemia, Hemolytic
Jaundice, Mechanical see Cholestasis
Jaundice, Neonatal   WH 425
   See also Erythroblastosis, Fetal   WH 425
Jaundice, Obstructive see Cholestasis
Jaundice, Obstructive, Extrahepatic see Bile Duct
   Obstruction, Extrahepatic
Jaundice, Spirochetal see Weil's Disease
Jaw
   Anatomy   WU 101
   Dislocation   WU 610
   Physiology   WU 102
Jaw Abnormalities   WU 101.5
Jaw Cysts   WU 140.5
Jaw Diseases   WU 140.5
Jaw, Edentulous, Partially   WU 140.5
Jaw Fixation Techniques   WU 610
Jaw Fractures   WU 610
Jaw Neoplasms   WU 280
Jealousy   BF 575.J4
   Adolescence   WS 462
   Child   WS 105.5.E5
   Infant   WS 105.5.E5
Jehovah's Witnesses see Christianity
Jejunum   WI 510
Jellyfish Venoms see Coelenterate Venoms
Jervell–Lange Nielsen Syndrome see Long QT
   Syndrome
Jews
   Cookery for the sick   WB 405

Dietary laws   BM 710
Diseases   WB 720
General works   DS 101–151
In medicine
   Collective biography   WZ 150
   History   WZ 80.5.J3
Religion see Judaism   BM
See also special topics under Ethnic Groups
Jimsonweed see Stramonium
Jird see Gerbillinae
Job Application
   Hospitals   WX 159
   Nursing   WY 29
   Medicine as a career   W 21
   Special fields, by subject
Job Description
   Hospitals   WX 159
   Dentistry   WU 21
   Medicine   W 21
   Nursing   WY 29
   Special fields, by subject
Job Ladders see Career Mobility
Job Satisfaction   HF 5549.5.J63
Jogging   QT 260.5.J6
Johne's Disease see Paratuberculosis
Joint Contracture see Contracture
Joint Diseases   WE 304–350
   General works   WE 304
   Child   WS 270
   Infant   WS 270
   Veterinary   SF 901
Joint Instability   WE 304
Joint Prosthesis   WE 312
Joint Prosthesis Implantation see Arthroplasty,
   Replacement
Joint Tuberculosis see Tuberculosis, Osteoarticular
Joint Ventures, Hospital–Physician see
   Hospital–Physician Joint Ventures
Joints   WE 300–350
   Localized, by site
Journalism   PN 4699–5650
   In medicine (General)   WZ 345
Journals see Periodicals
Judaism   BM
   And medicine   WZ 80.5.J3
     See also Religion and Medicine   W 50, etc.
   Medical ethics   W 50
   See also Jews   WZ 150, etc.
Judgment   BF 447
   Child   WS 105.5.D2
   Infant   WS 105.5.D2
Jugular Veins   WG 625.J8
   See also Blood Supply   WE 708 under Neck
Jungian Theory   WM 460
Juniper   QV 766
Jurisprudence
   Dental see Forensic Dentistry   W 705
   Hospital   WX 33
   Medical   W 32.5–32.6
   Nursing   WY 33
   Pharmaceutical   QV 33
   Psychiatric see Forensic Psychiatry   W 740, etc.
   Veterinary   K 3615–3617

**ALWAYS CONSULT MAIN SCHEDULES. USE NUMBER ASSIGNED ONLY WHEN
SUBJECT REPRESENTS MAJOR EMPHASIS OF WORK BEING CLASSIFIED**

See also Forensic Medicine   W 601–925, etc.
Jurisprudence, Psychiatric see Forensic Psychiatry
Juvenile Delinquency
    Legal problem (non–medical) U.S.   KF 184
    Parent and physician   WS 463, etc.
    Society   HV 9051–9230.7
Juvenile Hormones   SF 768.3
    Zoology   QL 868
Juxtaglomerular Apparatus   WJ 301

K

K Cells see Killer Cells
Kahn Test see Syphilis Serodiagnosis
Kainic Acid   QV 253
Kakke see Beriberi
Kala–Azar see Leishmaniasis, Visceral
Kallidin   QU 68
Kallikrein   QU 136
Kallikrein–Kinin System
    Enzymology   QU 136
    In regulating blood pressure   WG 106
    In water–electrolyte balance   QU 105
Kallikrein–Trypsin Inactivator see Aprotinin
Kanamycin   QV 268
Kandinsky Syndrome see Delirium, Dementia,
    Amnestic, Cognitive Disorders
Kangaroos   QL 737.M35
Kanner's Syndrome see Autistic Disorder
Kaolin   QV 71
Kaposi Disease see Xeroderma Pigmentosum
Kaposi Sarcoma see Sarcoma, Kaposi
Kappa Allotypes see Immunoglobulin Allotypes
Karwinskia see Rhamnus
Karyokinesis see Mitosis
Karyometry   QH 595
    Neoplasm diagnosis   QZ 241
Kawasaki Disease see Mucocutaneous Lymph Node
    Syndrome
Kedani Disease see Scrub Typhus
Kell Blood–Group System   WH 420
Keloid   WR 143
    Localized, by site
Kepone see Chlordecone
Keratan Sulfate   QU 83
Keratectomy, Excimer Laser see Keratectomy,
    Photorefractive, Excimer Laser
Keratectomy, Excimer Laser Photorefractive see
    Keratectomy, Photorefractive, Excimer Laser
Keratectomy, Photorefractive, Excimer Laser
    WW 220
Keratin   QU 55
Keratitis   WW 220
Keratitis, Dendritic   WW 220
Keratitis, Furrow see Keratitis, Dendritic
Keratitis, Ulcerative see Corneal Ulcer
Keratoconjunctivitis, Infectious
    Veterinary (General)   SF 891
    In cattle   SF 967.K47
    In sheep and goats   SF 969.K47
Keratoconjunctivitis, Vernal see Conjunctivitis,
    Allergic
Keratoconus   WW 220

Keratoderma, Palmoplantar   WR 500
Keratoma see Keratosis
Keratomalacia see Xerophthalmia
Keratomycosis Linguae see Tongue, Hairy
Keratosis   WR 500
Keratosis Palmaris et Plantaris see Keratoderma,
    Palmoplantar
Keratosis, Palmoplantar see Keratoderma,
    Palmoplantar
Keratosulfate see Keratan Sulfate
Keratotomy, Radial   WW 220
Kernicterus   WL 362
Kerosene
    Chemical technology   TP 692.4.K4
    Toxicology   QV 633
Kerosine see Kerosene
Ketamine   QV 81
Ketoacidosis, Diabetic see Diabetic Ketoacidosis
Ketoconazole   QV 252
Ketoglutaric Acids   QU 98
    Organic chemistry   QD 305.A2
Ketone Bodies
    Organic chemistry
        Aliphatic compounds   QD 305.K2
        Aromatic compounds   QD 341.K2
    Liver metabolism and physiology   WI 702
Ketones
    Organic chemistry
        Aliphatic compounds   QD 305.K2
        Aromatic compounds   QD 341.K2
    Used for special purposes, by subject
Ketoquinolines see Quinolones
Ketosis, Diabetic see Diabetic Ketoacidosis
Ketotifen   QV 157
Khellin   QV 150
Ki–ras Genes see Genes, ras
Kickbacks see Crime
Kidd Blood–Group System   WH 420
Kidnapping see Crime
Kidney   WJ 300–378
    Blood supply   WJ 301
        See also Renal Artery   WG 595.R3; Renal
        Veins   WG 625.R3
Kidney, Artificial   WJ 378
Kidney Bean Lectins see Phytohemagglutinins
Kidney Calculi   WJ 356
Kidney Calices   WJ 301
Kidney Circulation see Renal Circulation
Kidney Concentrating Ability   WJ 303
Kidney Cortex   WJ 301
Kidney, Cystic   WJ 358
Kidney Diseases   WJ 300–378
    General works   WJ 300
    Child   WS 320
    Infant   WS 320
    Veterinary   SF 871
Kidney Failure, Acute   WJ 342
Kidney Failure, Chronic   WJ 342
Kidney Function Tests   QY 175
Kidney Glomerulus   WJ 301
Kidney Insufficiency, Acute see Kidney Failure,
    Acute
Kidney Insufficiency, Chronic see Kidney Failure,
    Chronic

**ALWAYS CONSULT MAIN SCHEDULES. USE NUMBER ASSIGNED ONLY WHEN
SUBJECT REPRESENTS MAJOR EMPHASIS OF WORK BEING CLASSIFIED**

Kidney Medulla   WJ 301
Kidney Neoplasms   WJ 358
Kidney Papilla see Kidney Medulla
Kidney Papillary Necrosis   WJ 351
Kidney Pelvis   WJ 301
Kidney, Polycystic   WJ 358
Kidney Stones see Kidney Calculi
Kidney Transplantation   WJ 368
Kidney Tubular Transport, Inborn Errors see Renal
   Tubular Transport, Inborn Errors
Kidney Tubules   WJ 301
Kienboeck's Disease see Osteochondritis
Killer Cells   WH 200
   Cytotoxicity   QW 568
Killer Cells, Lymphokine-Activated   WH 200
   In cellular immunity   QW 568
Killer Cells, Natural   WH 200
   In cellular immunity   QW 568
Killer Phenotype see Phenotype
Kimmelstiel-Wilson Syndrome see Diabetic
   Nephropathies
Kinases see Phosphotransferases
Kindling (Neurology)   WL 102
Kinesics
   Adolescence   WS 462
   Child   WS 105.5.C8
   Infant   WS 105.5.C8
   Psychology   BF 637.N66
   Social psychology   HM
Kinesiology see Movement
Kinesiology, Applied   WB 890
   Used for particular disorders, with the disorder
Kinesitherapy see Exercise Therapy
Kinesthesis   WE 104
   See also Motion Perception   WW 105; Weight
    Perception   WE 104
Kinetics
   Biochemical techniques   QU 25
   Enzymology   QU 135
   Pharmacology   QV 38
   Physical chemistry   QD 502-502.2
   Special topics, by subject, e.g.; mechanokinetics
    in the nervous system   WL 102
Kinetics, Drug see Pharmacokinetics
Kinetocardiography   WG 141.5.K5
Kininase II Inhibitors see Angiotensin-Converting
   Enzyme Inhibitors
Kininogenase see Kallikrein
Kinins   QU 68
Kinship see Consanguinity
Kitchens, Hospital see Food Service, Hospital
Klebsiella   QW 138.5.K5
Klebsiella Infections   WC 260
   See also Pneumonia   WC 209, etc.
   Rhinoscleroma   WV 300
Kleptomania see Impulse Control Disorders
Klinefelter's Syndrome   QS 677
Kloramfenikol see Chloramphenicol
Knee   WE 870
   Blood supply   WE 870
    See also Popliteal Artery   WG 595.P6;
     Popliteal Vein   WG 625.P6

Knee Injuries   WE 870
Knee Prosthesis   WE 870
   See also Arthroplasty, Replacement, Knee   WE
    870
Knee Replacement, Total see Arthroplasty,
   Replacement, Knee
Knowledge Acquisition (Computer) see Artificial
   Intelligence
Knowledge, Attitudes, Practice
   Related to specific topics, by subject
   See also Attitude to Health   W 85
Knowledge Bases (Computer) see Artificial
   Intelligence
Knowledge of Results (Psychology)
   Incentive (Educational psychology)   LB 1065
   See also Motivation   BF 501-505, etc.; Feedback
    WL 102, etc.
Knowledge Representation (Computer) see Artificial
   Intelligence
KO 1173 see Mexiletine
Koehler's Disease see Osteochondritis
Korsakoff Psychosis see Alcohol Amnestic Disorder
Korsakoff Syndrome see Alcohol Amnestic Disorder
Korsakoff's Syndrome see Alcohol Amnestic
   Disorder
Koumiss see Milk
Kraurosis Vulvae   WP 200
Krause's End Bulbs see Thermoreceptors
Krebiozen see Quackery
Krebs Cycle see Citric Acid Cycle
Krill see Crustacea
Krypton
   Inorganic chemistry   QD 181.K6
   Pharmacology   QV 310
   Radioactive   WN 420
Kufs Disease see Neuronal Ceroid-Lipofuscinosis
Kunitz Pancreatic Trypsin Inhibitor see Aprotinin
Kupffer Cells   WH 650
   Localized, by site
Kuru   WC 540
Kwashiorkor   WS 115
Kyasanur Forest Disease Virus see Encephalitis
   Viruses, Tick-Borne
Kyasanur Forest Disease Virus see Flaviviruses
Kymography
   In cardiology   WG 141.5.K9
   Radiographic see Electrokymography   WN 100,
    etc.
   Used for diagnosis of particular disorders, with
    the disorder or system
Kymography, Radiographic see Electrokymography
Kynurenine   QU 60
Kyphosis   WE 735

L

L Cells (Cell Line)   QS 532.5.C7
L Cells (Intestine) see Endocrine Cells of Gut
L-Dopa see Levodopa
L Forms   QW 51
La Crosse Virus see California Group Viruses
Labeling, Drug see Drug Labeling
Labeling, Product see Product Labeling

Lagothrix see Cebidae
LAK Cells see Killer Cells, Lymphokine–Activated
lambda Phage see Bacteriophage lambda
Lamblia see Giardia
Lambliasis see Giardiasis
Lamiaceae   QV 767
Laminagraphy, X–Ray see Tomography, X–Ray
Laminar Air–Flow Areas see Environment,
   Controlled
Laminectomy   WE 725
Lampreys   QL 638.2–638.25
   As laboratory animals   QY 60.F4
LAN see Local Area Networks
Landau–Kleffner Syndrome   WL 340.5
Landscaping, Hospital see Maintenance and
   Engineering, Hospital
Langerhans–Cell Granulomatosis see Histiocytosis,
   Langerhans–Cell
Langerhans' Islands see Islets of Langerhans
Language   P 1–410
   Disorders   WL 340.2
   In psychoanalysis, psychoanalytic therapy, or
      psychoanalytic interpretation   WM 460.5.L2
   Psychology   BF 455–463
   Other special topics, by subject
   See also Communication   WM 460.5.C5, etc.
Language Comprehension Tests see Language Tests
Language Delay see Language Development
   Disorders
Language Development   WS 105.5.C8
   Formal education   LB 1139.L3
Language Development Disorders
   Neurologic   WL 340.2
   Psychogenic   WM 475
Language Disorders
   General   WL 340.2
   Child   WL 340.2, etc.
   Infant   WL 340.2, etc.
   Neurologic   WL 340.2
   Psychogenic   WM 475
   See also Speech Disorders   WM 475, etc.
Language Pathology see Speech–Language
   Pathology
Language Tests
   For aphasia of neurologic origin   WL 340.5
   For aphasia of psychogenic origin   WM 475.5
   For general and neurologic speech and language
      disorders   WL 340.2
   For psychogenic speech and language disorders
      WM 475
Language Therapy
   General   WL 340.2
   For disorders of neurologic origins   WL 340.2
   For disorders of psychogenic origins   WM 475
Language Training see Language Therapy
Langurs see Cercopithecidae
Lansing Virus see Polioviruses, Human 1–3
Lanthanides see Metals, Rare Earth
Lanthanum
   Inorganic chemistry   QD 181.L2
   Pharmacology   QV 290
Lanugo see Hair
Laparoscopes see Endoscopes

Laparoscopic Surgical Procedures see Surgical
   Procedures, Laparoscopic
Laparoscopy   WI 575
   Child   WS 310
   Gynecologic   WP 141
   Infant   WS 310
Laparotomy   WI 900
Laryngeal Cartilages   WV 500–501
Laryngeal Diseases   WV 500–540
   General works   WV 500
   Child   WV 500–540
   Infant   WV 500–540
   Nursing   WY 158.5
   Veterinary   SF 891
Laryngeal Edema   WV 500
Laryngeal Muscles   WV 500
Laryngeal Neoplasms   WV 520
Laryngeal Nerves   WL 330
   See also Innervation   WV 501 under Larynx
Laryngeal Paralysis see Vocal Cord Paralysis
Laryngeal Prosthesis see Larynx, Artificial
Laryngectomy   WV 540
Laryngismus   WV 500
   See also Adverse effects   WO 245 under
      Anesthesia
Laryngitis   WV 510
Laryngologists see Biography   WZ 112.5.08, etc.
   and Directories   WV 22 under Otolaryngology
Laryngology see Laryngeal Diseases;
   Otolaryngology
Laryngoscopy   WV 505
Laryngospasm see Laryngismus
Larynx   WV 500–540
   Innervation   WV 501
   Surgery   WV 540
Larynx, Artificial   WV 540
Laser Angioplasty see Angioplasty, Laser
Laser Coagulation   WO 198
   In ophthalmology   WW 168
   Used for treatment of a particular disorder, with
      the disorder or system
Laser Knife see Laser Surgery
Laser Scalpel see Laser Surgery
Laser Surgery   WO 511
Lasers
   Applied optics   TA 1671–1707
   Biomedical application   WB 117
   Diagnostic use   WB 288
   In dentistry (General)   WU 26
   In surgery (General)   WO 511
   Physics   QC 685–689.5
   Therapeutic use   WB 480
   Used for other purposes, by subject
   See also special topics under Radiation,
      Non–ionizing
Lassitude see Fatigue
Late Gene Transcription see Transcription, Genetic
Latency in Infection see Infection
Latency Period (Psychology)   WS 105.5.P3
Latent Schizophrenia see Schizotypal Personality
   Disorder
Lateral Cyst see Periodontal Cyst
Lateral Sclerosis see Amyotrophic Lateral Sclerosis

ALWAYS CONSULT MAIN SCHEDULES. USE NUMBER ASSIGNED ONLY WHEN
SUBJECT REPRESENTS MAJOR EMPHASIS OF WORK BEING CLASSIFIED

Laterality   WL 335
  Physical anthropology   GN 233
Latex
  Hypersensitivity see Latex Allergy   WD 300,
    etc.
  Phytochemistry   QK 898.L3
  Used for special purposes, by subject, e.g., in
    scanning electron microscopy   QH 212.S3
Latex Allergy
  General   WD 300
  Contact dermatitis   WR 175
  Occupational dermatitis   WR 600
Latex Hypersensitivity see Latex Allergy
Latex Rubber see Rubber
Lathyrism   WD 500
Lathyrus see Legumes
Latices see Latex
Latinos see Hispanic Americans
Latrines see Toilet Facilities
LATS Receptors see Receptors, Thyroid Hormone
Laughter   BF 575.L3
  Adolescence   WS 462
  Child   WS 105.5.E5
  Infant   WS 105.5.E5
Laundering
  Hygiene   QT 240-245
  See also Laundry Service, Hospital   WX 165
Laundries, Hospital see Laundering; Housekeeping,
  Hospital
Laundry Service, Hospital   WX 165
Laurence-Moon-Biedl Syndrome   QS 675
LAV Antibodies see HIV Antibodies
LAV-HTLV-III see HIV
LAV-2 see HIV-2
Lavender see Lamiaceae
Law and Psychiatry see Forensic Psychiatry;
  Legislation & jurisprudence   WM 32-33 under
  Psychiatry
Laws see Legislation
Laxatives see Cathartics
Laxity, Joint see Joint Instability
Laying-on-of-Hands see Therapeutic Touch
LDL Cholesterol see Lipoproteins, LDL Cholesterol
LDL Receptors see Receptors, LDL
LE Cells   WH 200
  In bone marrow   WH 380
  In lupus erythematosus   WR 152
Lead   QV 292
Lead Poisoning   QV 292
Leader Signal Peptides see Signal Peptides
Leadership   BF 637.L4
  Special topics, by subject
  See also Nursing, Supervisory   WY 105
Learned Helplessness see Helplessness, Learned
Learning
  Educational psychology   LB 1051-1091
  General psychology   BF 318
  Adolescence   LB 1603-1632
  Adult   LB 2300-2397
  Child
    Formal   LB 1051-1091
    Informal   WS 105.5.D2
  Kindergarten children   LB 1141-1489

  Informal   WS 105.5.D2
Preschool children
  Formal   LB 1140-1140.5
  Informal   WS 105.5.D2 and WS 113
Special topics, by subject
Learning Disorders
  Associated with poor vision   WW 480
  Educational aspects   LC 4704, etc.
  Medical aspects   WS 110
Lecithin Acyltransferase see
  Phosphatidylcholine-Sterol O-Acyltransferase
Lecithin Cholesterol Acyltransferase see
  Phosphatidylcholine-Sterol O-Acyltransferase
Lecithinase A1 see Phospholipases A
Lecithinase A2 see Phospholipases A
Lecithinases see Phospholipases
Lecithins see Phosphatidylcholines
Lectin, Castor Bean see Ricin
Lectin, Ricinus see Ricin
Lectins   QW 640
  See also Phytohemagglutinins   QW 640, etc.
Lectins, Kidney Bean see Phytohemagglutinins
Lectures see Form number 9 in any NLM schedule
  where applicable
Leeches   QX 451
  Poisoning   WD 420
Leeching see Bloodletting
Leeks see Onions
Left Ventricular Remodeling see Ventricular
  Remodeling
Leg   WE 850
  Artificial see Artificial Limbs   WE 172
  Blood supply   WE 850
  Lower   WE 870
  Upper   WE 855
  See also specific parts of the leg; Varicose Veins
    WG 620, etc.
Leg Bones   WE 850
Leg Dermatoses   WR 140
Leg Injuries   WE 850
  Lower leg   WE 870
  Upper leg   WE 855
Leg Length Inequality   WE 850
Leg Ulcer   WE 850
Legal Guardians
  Special topics, by subject
Legal Medicine see Forensic Medicine
Legg-Perthes Disease   WE 865
Legionella
  QW 131
Legionella pneumophila Infections see Legionnaires'
  Disease
Legionellosis   WC 200
Legionnaires' Disease   WC 200
Legislation
  (Form number 32-33 in any NLM schedule where
    applicable)
  Non-medical subjects, in general works number
    for subject (avoiding K schedules when
    possible)
  See also specific legislation terms, i.e., Legislation,
    Dental; Legislation, Drug; Legislation, Food;
    etc.

**ALWAYS CONSULT MAIN SCHEDULES. USE NUMBER ASSIGNED ONLY WHEN
SUBJECT REPRESENTS MAJOR EMPHASIS OF WORK BEING CLASSIFIED**

Legislation, Dental WU 32–44.1
Legislation, Drug QV 32–33
    Food and drug laws WA 697
Legislation, Food WA 697
Legislation, Hospital WX 32–33
Legislation, Medical W 32–44
Legislation, Nursing WY 32–44
Legislation, Pharmacy QV 732–733
Legislation, Veterinary K 3615–3617
Legumes
    As dietary supplement in health and disease
      WB 430
    As food plants SB 177.L45
    As medicinal plants QV 766
    Botany QK 495.L52
    Poisoning WD 500
Leiomyoblastoma see Leiomyoma, Epithelioid
Leiomyoma QZ 340
    Localized, by site, e.g., of the uterus WP 459
Leiomyoma, Epithelioid QZ 340
    Localized, by site, e.g., of the stomach WI 320
Leiomyosarcoma QZ 340
    Localized, by site
Leishmania QX 70
Leishmaniasis WR 350
Leishmaniasis, Mucocutaneous WR 350
Leishmaniasis, Visceral WC 715
Leisure Activities QT 250
    Special topics, by subject
Lemmings see Microtinae
Lemmus see Microtinae
Lemuriformes see Strepsirhini
Lemuroidea see Strepsirhini
Length of Life see Longevity
Length of Stay WX 158
    At specialized hospitals (Form number 27–28 in
      any NLM schedule where applicable)
Leninism see Communism
Lens, Crystalline WW 260
Lens Diseases WW 260
Lens Implantation, Intraocular WW 358
    For cataracts WW 260
Lens Opacities see Cataract
Lens Proteins see Crystallins
Lenses QC 385–385.2
    Ophthalmic see Contact Lenses WW 355;
      Eyeglasses WW 350–354
    See also Lenses, Intraocular WW 358, etc.
Lenses, Contact see Contact Lenses
Lenses, Contact, Hydrophilic see Contact Lenses,
    Hydrophilic
Lenses, Intraocular WW 358
    For cataracts WW 260
Lenticular Nucleus see Corpus Striatum
Lentiform Nucleus see Corpus Striatum
Lentiginosis see Lentigo
Lentigo WR 265
Lentils see Legumes
Lentinan QU 83
Leon Virus see Polioviruses, Human 1–3
Leontiasis Ossium see Hyperostosis Frontalis Interna
Leontideus see Callitrichinae
Leontopithecus see Callitrichinae

Leper Colonies WC 27–28
    See also Medical Missions, Official W 323
Leper Hospitals see Hospitals, Special
Lepidoptera QX 560
Leprosaria see Hospitals, Special; Leper Colonies
Leprostatic Agents QV 259
Leprosy WC 335
    Drugs affecting see Leprostatic Agents QV 259
    Hospitals see Hospitals, Special WC 27–28, etc.;
      Leper Colonies WC 27–28, etc.
Leptazole see Pentylenetetrazole
Leptoconops see Ceratopogonidae
Leptomeninges see Arachnoid; Pia Mater
Leptophos
    Agriculture SB 952.P5
    Public health WA 240
Leptospirosis WC 420
    Icterohemorrhagic see Weil's Disease WC 420
    Veterinary SF 809.L4
Leptospirosis, Icterohemorrhagic see Weil's Disease
Leptothrix QW 153
Leriche's Syndrome WG 410
Lesbianism see Homosexuality, Female
Lesch–Nyhan Syndrome WD 205.5.P8
LET see Energy Transfer
Lethal Midline Granuloma see Granuloma, Lethal
    Midline
Lethargy see Sleep Stages
LETS Proteins see Fibronectins
Leu Antigens see Antigens, Differentiation
Leu Antigens, B–Lymphocyte see Antigens,
    Differentiation, B–Lymphocyte
Leucine QU 60
Leucine Aminopeptidase see Leucyl Aminopeptidase
Leucokinin see Tuftsin
Leucosarcoma see Leukosarcoma
Leucotomy see Psychosurgery
Leucovorin QU 195
Leucyl Aminopeptidase QU 136
Leukapheresis WH 460
Leukemia WH 250
    Clinical pathology QZ 350
    Veterinary SF 910.L4
Leukemia, Granulocytic see Leukemia, Myeloid
Leukemia, Granulocytic, Chronic see Leukemia,
    Myeloid, Chronic
Leukemia, Hairy Cell WH 250
    Clinical pathology QZ 350
Leukemia, Lymphoblastic see Leukemia,
    Lymphocytic
Leukemia, Lymphoblastic, Acute see Leukemia,
    Lymphocytic, Acute
Leukemia, Lymphoblastic, Acute, L1 see Leukemia,
    Lymphocytic, Acute, L1
Leukemia, Lymphoblastic, Chronic see Leukemia,
    Lymphocytic, Chronic
Leukemia, Lymphocytic WH 250
    Clinical pathology QZ 350
Leukemia, Lymphocytic, Acute WH 250
    Clinical pathology QZ 350
Leukemia, Lymphocytic, Acute, L1 WH 250
    Clinical pathology QZ 350
Leukemia, Lymphocytic, Chronic WH 250

ALWAYS CONSULT MAIN SCHEDULES. USE NUMBER ASSIGNED ONLY WHEN
SUBJECT REPRESENTS MAJOR EMPHASIS OF WORK BEING CLASSIFIED

Clinical Pathology   QZ 350
Leukemia, Lymphoid see Leukemia, Lymphocytic
Leukemia, Monoblastic   WH 250
  Clinical pathology   QZ 350
Leukemia, Monocytic   WH 250
  Clinical pathology   QZ 350
Leukemia, Monocytic, Chronic   WH 250
  Clinical pathology   QZ 350
Leukemia, Myeloblastic   WH 250
  Clinical pathology   QZ 350
Leukemia, Myelocytic see Leukemia, Myeloid
Leukemia, Myelocytic, Chronic see Leukemia,
  Myeloid, Chronic
Leukemia, Myelogenous see Leukemia, Myeloid
Leukemia, Myelogenous, Chronic see Leukemia,
  Myeloid, Chronic
Leukemia, Myeloid   WH 250
  Clinical pathology   QZ 350
Leukemia, Myeloid, Chronic   WH 250
  Clinical Pathology   QZ 350
Leukemia, Radiation-Induced   WH 250
  Clinical pathology   QZ 350
Leukemia Virus, Avian see Avian Leukosis Viruses
Leukemia Virus, Bovine   QW 166
Leukemia Virus I, Human T-Cell see HTLV-I
Leukemia Viruses, Human T-Cell see HTLV-BLV
  Viruses
Leukemia Viruses, Murine   QW 166
Leukemic Reticuloendotheliosis see Leukemia, Hairy
  Cell
Leukemogenic Viruses see Leukoviruses
Leukemoid Reaction   WH 200
Leukocytapheresis see Leukapheresis
Leukocyte Adherence Inhibition Test   QW
  525.5.L6
Leukocyte Adhesion Inhibitor see Interleukin-8
Leukocyte Antigens see HLA Antigens
Leukocyte Count   QY 402
Leukocyte Count, Differential see Leukocyte Count
Leukocyte Differentiation Antigens, Human see
  Antigens, CD
Leukocyte Number see Leukocyte Count
Leukocyte Transfusion   WB 356
Leukocytes   WH 200
  In inflammation   QW 700
Leukocytes, Polymorphonuclear see Neutrophils
Leukocytopenia see Leukopenia
Leukocytosis   WH 200
  Veterinary   SF 769.5
Leukoderma see Vitiligo
Leukokeratosis see Leukoplakia
Leukokinin see Tuftsin
Leukokraurosis see Kraurosis Vulvae
Leukoma see Corneal Opacity; Leukoplakia, Oral
Leukopenia   WH 200
Leukopheresis see Leukapheresis
Leukoplakia   QZ 204
  Localized, by site, e.g., cervical   WP 470
Leukoplakia, Oral   WU 280
  For the gastroenterologist   WI 200
Leukorrhea   WP 255
Leukosarcoma   WH 525
  Clinical pathology   QZ 350

Leukosis, Avian see Avian Leukosis
Leukosis Virus, Avian   QW 166
Leukostasis   WH 200
Leukostasis Syndrome see Leukostasis
Leukotaxis see Chemotaxis, Leukocyte
Leukotomy see Psychosurgery
Leukotriene B4   QU 90
Leukotrienes   QU 90
Leukotrienes B see Leukotriene B4
Leukoviruses see Retroviridae
Leurocristine see Vincristine
Levarterenol see Norepinephrine
LeVeen Shunt see Peritoneovenous Shunt
Level of Health see Health Status
Levodopa   WK 725
Levomycetin see Chloramphenicol
Levonorepinephrine see Norepinephrine
Levulose see Fructose
Lewisite   QV 666
Lewy Body Disease see Parkinson Disease
LH   WK 515
LH-FSH Releasing Hormone see Gonadorelin
LH-Releasing Hormone see Gonadorelin
LHRH see Gonadorelin
Liability see Insurance, Liability; Malpractice
Liability, Legal   W 44
  General   W 44
  Dentistry   WU 44
  Nursing   WY 44
  (Form number 33 in any other NLM schedule
  where applicable)
Libido
  Psychoanalysis   WM 460.5.S3
Libman-Sacks Disease see Lupus Erythematosus,
  Systemic
Librarianship see Library Science
Libraries   Z 665-997.2
Libraries, Dental   Z 675.D3
Libraries, Health Science see Libraries, Medical
Libraries, Hospital   Z 675.H7
  Patients' libraries   Z 675.P27
Libraries, Medical   Z 675.M4
Libraries, Medical Record see Medical Records
Libraries, Nursing   Z 675.N8
  Nursing school   Z 675.N8
Library Administration   Z 678 678.88
Library Associations   Z 673
Library Automation   Z 678.9
Library Materials
  Acquisition and selection   Z 689-689.8
  Cataloging   Z 693-695.83
  Classification   Z 696-697
    Medicine   Z 697.M4
  Collection development   Z 687
  Library bookbinding   Z 700
  Preservation   Z 700.9-701.5
Library Schools   Z 668-669.5
Library Science   Z 665-718.8
Library Services   Z 665-997
  Circulation   Z 712-714
  Extension   Z 716
  Reference   Z 711-711.92
  Reports   Z 729-871

ALWAYS CONSULT MAIN SCHEDULES. USE NUMBER ASSIGNED ONLY WHEN
SUBJECT REPRESENTS MAJOR EMPHASIS OF WORK BEING CLASSIFIED

See also special types of service and specific types of libraries, e.g., Library technical services Z 688.5; Libraries, Medical Z 675.M4; also headings beginning with Book

Library Surveys Z 721–871
Library Technical Services Z 688.5
Lice QX 501–502
   Body lice QX 502
   Disinfestation WA 240
   Infestations see Lice Infestations WR 375
   Plant lice see Aphids QX 503, etc.
Lice Infestations WR 375
Lice, Plant see Aphids
Licenses see Licensure
Licensure
   Barbers, beauticians, etc. WA 32
   Dental hygienists WU 40
   Midwives WQ 32
   Other specialties, not listed here or below, by specialty
Licensure, Dental WU 40
Licensure, Hospital WX 15
Licensure, Institutional, Personnel see Licensure
Licensure, Medical W 40
Licensure, Nursing WY 21
Licensure, Pharmacy QV 29
Lichen Planus WR 215
Lichen Ruber Planus see Lichen Planus
Lichen Simplex Chronicus see Neurodermatitis
Lichens QK 580.7–597.7
Licorice see Glycyrrhiza
Lidocaine QV 115
Lidoflazine QV 150
Lie Detection HV 8078
Life
   Medical philosophy W 61
   See also Life (Biology) QH 501 under Biology
Life–Breath (Philosophy) see Ch'i
Life Care Centers, Retirement see Housing for the Elderly
Life Change Events
   Adolescence WS 462
   Aged WT 104
   Child WS 105
   Infant WS 105
   Special topics, by subject
Life Expectancy WT 116
   Actuarial science HG 8781–8793
   Tables WT 16
Life Experiences see Life Change Events
Life Insurance see Insurance, Life
Life Islands see Patient Isolators
Life, Legal Establishment see Biogenesis; Birth Certificates; Infant, Newborn; Physical Examination
Life Style
   Adolescents WS 462
   Aging WT 30
   Other special topics, by subject, e.g., Anthropology, Cultural GN 315, etc.; conduct of life BJ 1545–1697
Life Support Care WX 162
   Aged WT 31

   Ethical questions W 50
   Nursing WY 152
Life Support Systems WD 756
Life Support Systems, Regenerative see Ecological Systems, Closed
Life Table Analysis see Life Tables
Life Table Methods see Life Tables
Life Table Models see Life Tables
Life Tables
   Demography HB 1322
   Specific topics, by subject
   See also Actuarial Analysis
Ligament, Broad see Adnexa Uteri
Ligaments WE 300
   Localized, by site
Ligaments, Articular WE 300
   Localized, by site
Ligases QU 138
Ligation, Tubal see Sterilization, Tubal
Ligatures, Surgical see Sutures
Light
   Adverse effects (General) WD 605
   As cause of disease QZ 57
   Diagnostic use (General) WB 288
   General medical use WB 117
   Hygiene see Lighting QT 230, etc.; Sunlight QT 230, etc.
   Perception WW 105
   Photobiology QH 515
   Phototherapy WB 480
   Physics QC 350–467
   Physiological effects (General) QT 162.L5
Light Coagulation WW 166
   Used for specific disorders, by subject
Light, Luminescent see Luminescence
Light Metals see Metals, Light
Light, Visible see Light
Lighting
   Industrial health WA 470
   Private homes QT 230
   School buildings WA 350
   Vision conservation WW 113
Lightning
   Electric injuries WD 602
   Meteorology QC 966–966.7
Lignin
   Animal feed SF 98.L54
   Biochemistry QU 83
   Phytochemistry QK 898.L5
Lignocaine see Lidocaine
Limb Deformities, Congenital WE 800
   Of specific limb, with the limb
Limbic System WL 314
Limbs see Extremities
Limbs, Artificial see Artificial Limbs
Limitation of Activity, Chronic see Activities of Daily Living
Limulus see Horseshoe Crabs
Limulus Test QW 25
   Special topics, by subject
Lincolnensin see Lincomycin
Lincomycin QV 350

ALWAYS CONSULT MAIN SCHEDULES. USE NUMBER ASSIGNED ONLY WHEN SUBJECT REPRESENTS MAJOR EMPHASIS OF WORK BEING CLASSIFIED

Lindane
    As an insecticide   WA 240
    Toxicology   QV 633
Linear Accelerators see Particle Accelerators
Linear Energy Transfer see Energy Transfer
Linear Regression see Regression Analysis
Linens see Bedding and Linens
Lingua Geographica see Glossitis, Benign Migratory
Lingua Villosa Negra see Tongue, Hairy
Lingual Bone see Hyoid Bone
Linguistics   P 121-149
Liniments   QV 785
Linkage (Genetics)   QH 445.2-445.5
Linkage Mapping see Chromosome Mapping
Linseed Oil   QV 785
Liothyronine see Triiodothyronine
Lip   WI 200
    Cleft see Cleft Lip   WV 440
    For the dentist   WU 140
Lip Diseases   WI 200
    For the dentist   WU 140
Lip Neoplasms   WU 280
    For the gastroenterologist   WI 200
Lip Reading see Lipreading
Lipase   QU 136
Lipectomy   WO 600
Lipemia-Clearing Factor see Lipoprotein Lipase
Lipid Bilayers   QU 85
Lipid Emulsions, Intravenous see Fat Emulsions, Intravenous
Lipid Metabolism, Inborn Errors   WD 205.5.L5
    See also Xanthomatosis   WD 205.5.X2
Lipid Mobilization   QU 85
Lipid Peroxidation   QU 85
Lipid Peroxides
    Biochemistry   QU 85
Lipidosis see Lipoidosis
Lipids   QU 85-95
    Clinical analysis   QY 465
Lipoamide Dehydrogenase   QU 140
Lipocaic see Lipotropic Factors
Lipochondrodystrophy see Mucopolysaccharidosis I
Lipodystrophy
    Internal   WD 214
    Progressive   WD 214
Lipofuscin   QU 110
Lipoic Acid see Thioctic Acid
Lipoidosis   WD 205.5.L5
Lipoids   QU 85
Lipolysis   QU 85
Lipolysis, Suction see Lipectomy
Lipoma   QZ 340
    Localized, by site
Lipomatosis   WD 214
Lipopolysaccharides   QU 83
Lipoprotein LDL Receptors see Receptors, LDL
Lipoprotein Lipase   QU 136
Lipoproteins   QU 85
    In blood chemistry   QY 465
Lipoproteins, HDL Cholesterol   QU 95
Lipoproteins, LDL Cholesterol   QU 95
Liposarcoma   QZ 345

    Localized, by site
Liposomes   QU 93
Liposuction see Lipectomy
Lipotropic Agents   QU 87
Lipotropic Factors see Lipotropic Agents
Lipreading   HV 2487
Liquid Paraffin see Mineral Oil
Liquors see Alcoholic Beverages
Listeria   QW 142.5.A8
Listeria Infections   WC 242
    Veterinary   SF 809.L5
Listeria monocytogenes   QW 142.5.A8
Lisuride   QV 174
Literacy Programs see Education
Literature   P
    By physicians   WZ 350
    Chinese   PL 2250-3190
    General works   PN
    Influence on children   WS 105.5.E9
    Medicine in see Medicine in Literature   WZ 330, etc.
    Physicians in   WZ 330
    Psychiatry and literature   WM 49
    Psychotherapeutic Use see Bibliotherapy   WM 450.5.B5
    Other languages, in appropriate LC schedule
    Other special topics, by subject
        See also Psychoanalytic Interpretation   WM 460.7
Literature, Medieval
    History   PN 661-694
    Special topics, by subject, e.g., Dante e le scienze mediche   WZ 330
Literature, Modern   PN 695-779
    Special topics, by subject
Lithiasis   QZ 180
    Localized, by site
    See also Bladder Calculi   WJ 500; Calculi   QZ 180, etc.; Cholelithiasis   WI 755; Common Bile Duct Calculi   WI 755; Kidney Calculi   WJ 356; Salivary Duct Calculi   WI 230; Ureteral Calculi   WJ 400; Urinary Calculi   WJ 140
Lithium   QV 77.9
Litholapaxy see Lithotripsy
Lithospermum   QV 766
Lithotripsy
    For urinary calculi   WJ 166
    For special purposes, with subject
Litomosoides see Filarioidea
Little's Disease see Cerebral Palsy
Liver   WI 700-770
    Blood supply   WI 702
        See also Hepatic Artery   WG 595.H3; Hepatic Veins   WG 625.H3; Liver Circulation   WI 702
    Surgery   WI 770
    Tests   QY 140-147
        See also Liver Function Tests   QY 147
Liver Abscess   WI 730
Liver Abscess, Amebic   WI 730
Liver, Artificial   WI 770
Liver Cell Adhesion Molecules see Cell Adhesion Molecules

Liver Circulation   WI 702
　Disorders   WI 720
Liver Cirrhosis   WI 725
　Pigmentary   WR 267
　Veterinary   SF 851
　See also Hemochromatosis   WR 267
Liver Cirrhosis, Alcoholic   WI 725
Liver Diseases   WI 700–770
　General works   WI 700
　Child   WS 310
　Infant   WS 310
　Veterinary   SF 851
Liver Diseases, Alcoholic   WI 700
Liver Diseases, Parasitic   WI 700
　Veterinary   SF 851
Liver Extracts
　Pharmacology   QV 184
　Therapeutic use (General)   WB 391
　Used for treatment of particular disorders, with
　　the disorder or system
Liver Failure, Fulminant see Hepatic
　Encephalopathy
Liver Fibrosis see Liver Cirrhosis
Liver Function Tests   QY 147
Liver Glycogen   WI 704
Liver Microsomes see Microsomes, Liver
Liver Mitochondria see Mitochondria, Liver
Liver Neoplasms   WI 735
Liver Neoplasms, Experimental   WI 735
Liver Regeneration   WI 702
Liver Transplantation   WI 770
Livestock see Animals, Domestic
Living Donors   QS 523–524
　Of specific organs, with the organ
Living Space see Environment
Living Wills   W 85.5
Livor Mortis see Postmortem Changes
Lizards   QL 666.L2–666.L295
　Diseases   SF 997.5.R4
Llamas see Camelids, New World
LMWH see Heparin, Low-Molecular-Weight
Loa   QX 301
Loa loa see Loa
Lobar Pneumonia see Pneumonia, Pneumococcal
Lobbying
　Special topics, by subject
Lobectomy see Pneumonectomy; Psychosurgery
Lobotomy see Psychosurgery
Lobstein's Disease see Osteogenesis Imperfecta
Lobsters   QX 463
Local Anesthesia see Anesthesia, Local
Local Area Networks   TK 5105.7–5105.8
Local Immunity see Immunity
Localization of Function see Brain Mapping;
　Dominance, Cerebral
Localization of Infection see Infection
Location Directories and Signs
　In health facilities   WX 140
　　For the specialties (form number 27–29 in any
　　　NLM schedule where applicable)
　In hospital departments   WX 200–225
　Public health aspects in public buildings   WA
　　799

Lochia see Leukorrhea
Locked-In Syndrome see Quadriplegia
Lockjaw see Tetanus; Trismus
Locomotion   WE 103
Locomotion, Cell see Cell Movement
Locomotor Ataxia see Tabes Dorsalis
Locomotor System see Musculoskeletal System
Locus Coeruleus   WL 310
Locus of Control see Internal-External Control
Lofepramine   QV 77.5
Logic   BC
　Adolescents   WS 462
　Child   WS 105.5.D2
　Medical   W 61
Logotherapy   WM 460.5.E8
Loneliness   BF 575.L7
　Adolescence   WS 462
　Child   WS 105.5.E5
　Infant   WS 105.5.E5
Long QT Syndrome   WG 330
Long-Term Care   WX 162–162.5
　Aged   WT 31
　Nursing   WY 152
　Of mentally ill   WM 30
Long-Term Care Insurance see Insurance,
　Long-Term Care
Longevity   WT 116
　See also Life Expectancy   WT 116, etc.
Longitudinal Studies   WA 950
　Special topics, by subject, e.g., of characteristics,
　　etc. of medical school graduates   W 76
Loop Ileostomy see Ileostomy
Loperamide   QV 71
Lopramine see Lofepramine
Lordosis   WE 735
Loris, Slow see Lorisidae
Lorisidae   QL 737.P955
　Diseases   SF 997.5.P7
　As laboratory animals   QY 60.P7
Lorr's Inpatient Multidimensional Psychiatric Rating
　Scale see Psychiatric Status Rating Scales
Lotions see Cosmetics; Dermatologic Agents;
　Suspensions; Sunscreening Agents
Lou Gehrig's Disease see Amyotrophic Lateral
　Sclerosis
Loudness Perception   WV 272
Louping Ill Virus see Encephalitis Viruses,
　Tick-Borne
Lovastatin
　As an anticholesteremic agent   QU 95
Love
　Adolescent psychology   WS 462
　Child psychology   WS 105.5.E5
　Family   HQ 728–743
　Marriage   HQ 728–746
　Psychology (General)   BF 575.L8
　Sex behavior   HQ 19–25
Low Back Pain   WE 755
Low Cardiac Output see Cardiac Output, Low
Low-Income Population see Poverty
Low-Molecular-Weight Heparin see Heparin,
　Low-Molecular-Weight
Low Molecular Weight Nuclear RNA see RNA,

Small Nuclear
Low Sodium Diets see Diet, Sodium–Restricted
Lower Extremities see Extremities; names of
particular parts
Lower Extremity see Leg
LSD see Lysergic Acid Diethylamide
LTB4 see Leukotriene B4
Luciferase   QU 140
Ludwig's Angina   WI 200
Luliberin see Gonadorelin
Lumbago see Low Back Pain
Lumbar Manipulation see Manipulation, Spinal
Lumbar Puncture see Spinal Puncture
Lumbar Region see Lumbosacral Region
Lumbar Vertebrae   WE 750
Lumbosacral Plexus   WL 400
Lumbosacral Region   WE 750–755
Luminal see Phenobarbital
Luminescence
    Bioluminescence   QH 641
    Radiation physics (General)   QC 476.4–480.2
    Used for particular purposes, by subject, in the
    techniques number 25 in any NLM schedule
    where applicable, or comparable LC number
Luminescent Proteins   QU 55
Lumpy Skin Disease   WC 584
Lunar Cycle see Moon
Lunar Phases see Moon
Lundborg-Unverricht Syndrome see Epilepsy,
Myoclonic
Lung   WF 600–668
    Blood supply   WF 600
    Irritants   QV 664
    Radiography   WF 600
        See also Mass Chest X-Ray   WF 225
    Surgery   WF 668
        See also Pneumonectomy   WF 668;
        Pulmonary Surgical Procedures   WF 668
Lung Abscess   WF 651
Lung Capacities see Lung Volume Measurements
Lung Diseases   WF 600–668
    Child   WS 280
    Infant   WS 280
    Veterinary   SF 831
Lung Diseases, Fungal   WF 652
Lung Diseases, Interstitial   WF 600
Lung Diseases, Obstructive   WF 600
Lung Diseases, Parasitic   WF 600
Lung Function Tests see Respiratory Function Tests
Lung Irritants see Irritants
Lung Lavage see Bronchoalveolar Lavage
Lung Lavage Fluid see Bronchoalveolar Lavage
Fluid
Lung Neoplasms   WF 658
Lung Transplantation   WF 668
Lung Volume Measurements
    General diagnosis   WB 284
    Respiratory diseases   WF 141
Lupus   WR 245
Lupus Erythematosus, Chronic Cutaneous see Lupus
Erythematosus, Discoid
Lupus Erythematosus, Cutaneous   WR 152
Lupus Erythematosus, Cutaneous, Chronic see

Lupus Erythematosus, Discoid
Lupus Erythematosus, Cutaneous, Subacute see
Lupus Erythematosus, Cutaneous
Lupus Erythematosus, Discoid   WR 152
Lupus Erythematosus Disseminatus see Lupus
Erythematosus, Systemic
Lupus Erythematosus, Subacute Cutaneous see
Lupus Erythematosus, Cutaneous
Lupus Erythematosus, Systemic   WR 152
Lupus Glomerulonephritis see Lupus Nephritis
Lupus Nephritis   WJ 353
Lupus Vulgaris see Lupus
Lurcher Mice see Mice, Neurologic Mutants
Luteinizing Hormone see LH
Luteinizing Hormone-Releasing Hormone see
Gonadorelin
Luteinoma see Luteoma
Luteoma   WP 322
Luteotropin see Prolactin
Lutropin see LH
Lyases   QU 139
Lycine see Betaine
Lycoremine see Galanthamine
Lyell's Syndrome see Epidermal Necrolysis, Toxic
Lying see Deception
Lying-In Hospitals see Hospitals, Maternity
Lyme Borreliosis see Lyme Disease
Lyme Disease   WC 406
Lymph   WH 700
Lymph Node Excision   WH 700
    Localized, by site
Lymph Node Syndrome, Mucocutaneous see
Mucocutaneous Lymph Node Syndrome
Lymph Nodes   WH 700
    Tuberculosis see Tuberculosis, Lymph node
    WF 290
Lymphadenectomy see Lymph Node Excision
Lymphadenitis   WH 700
Lymphadenitis, Tuberculous see Tuberculosis,
Lymph Node
Lymphadenopathy-Associated Antibodies see HIV
Antibodies
Lymphadenopathy-Associated Virus see HIV
Lymphadenopathy, Immunoblastic see
Immunoblastic Lymphadenopathy
Lymphadenopathy Syndrome see AIDS-Related
Complex
Lymphangioendothelioma see Lymphangioma
Lymphangiography see Lymphography
Lymphangioma   QZ 340
    Localized, by site
Lymphangitis   WH 700
Lymphapheresis see Leukapheresis
Lymphatic Capillaries see Lymphatic System
Lymphatic Diseases   WH 700
    Child   WS 300
    Infant   WS 300
    Nursing   WY 152.5
    Veterinary   SF 769.5
    Localized, by site
Lymphatic Filariasis see Elephantiasis, Filarial
Lymphatic Metastasis   WH 700
    Of particular types of neoplasms, by site, e.g.,
    of the stomach   WI 320

Lymphatic Sarcoma see Lymphoma, Diffuse
Lymphatic System   WH 700
  Child   WS 300
  Infant   WS 300
  Tuberculosis see Tuberculosis, Lymph Node
  WF 290
Lymphedema   WH 700
  Secondary to filariasis   WC 880
  Veterinary   SF 769.5
  Localized, by site
Lymphoblast Transformation see Lymphocyte
Transformation
Lymphoblastic Leukemia see Leukemia,
  Lymphocytic
Lymphoblastic Leukemia, Acute see Leukemia,
  Lymphocytic, Acute
Lymphoblastic Leukemia, Acute, Childhood see
  Leukemia, Lymphocytic, Acute, L1
Lymphoblastic Leukemia, Acute, L1 see Leukemia,
  Lymphocytic, Acute, L1
Lymphoblastic Leukemia, Chronic see Leukemia,
  Lymphocytic, Chronic
Lymphocytapheresis see Leukapheresis
Lymphocyte-Activating Factor see Interleukin-1
Lymphocyte Activation see Lymphocyte
Transformation
Lymphocyte Cooperation
  Cellular immunity   QW 568
Lymphocyte Mediators see Lymphokines
Lymphocyte Mitogenic Factor see Interleukin-2
Lymphocyte Stimulation see Lymphocyte
Transformation
Lymphocyte Transformation
  Clinical pathology   QY 402
  Hematology   WH 200
  Transplantation immunology   WO 680
Lymphocyte Transfusion   WB 356
Lymphocytes   WH 200
  Cellular immunity   QW 568
Lymphocytic Choriomeningitis   WC 540
Lymphocytic Leukemia see Leukemia, Lymphocytic
Lymphocytic Leukemia, Acute see Leukemia,
  Lymphocytic, Acute
Lymphocytic Leukemia, Chronic see Leukemia,
  Lymphocytic, Chronic
Lymphocytic Leukemia, L1 see Leukemia,
  Lymphocytic, Acute, L1
Lymphocytopenia see Lymphopenia
Lymphocytosis   WH 200
Lymphocytotoxic Antibodies see Antilymphocyte
Serum
Lymphogranuloma Inguinale see Lymphogranuloma
Venereum
Lymphogranuloma, Malignant see Hodgkin Disease
Lymphogranuloma Venereum   WC 185
Lymphogranulomatosis Inguinalis see
  Lymphogranuloma Venereum
Lymphography   WH 700
Lymphoid Cells see Lymphocytes
Lymphoid Leukemia see Leukemia, Lymphocytic
Lymphoid Tissue   WH 700
Lymphokine-Activated Killer Cells see Killer Cells,

Lymphokine-Activated
Lymphokines
  Cellular immunity   QW 568
  Other special topics, by subject
Lymphoma   WH 525
  Clinical pathology   QZ 350
  See also Burkitt's Lymphoma   WH 525
Lymphoma, Burkitt see Burkitt Lymphoma
Lymphoma, Diffuse   WH 525
  Clinical pathology   QZ 350
Lymphoma, Follicular   WH 525
  Clinical pathology   QZ 350
Lymphoma, Giant Follicular see Lymphoma,
  Follicular
Lymphoma, Histiocytic see Lymphoma, Large-Cell
Lymphoma, Large-Cell   WH 525
  Clinical pathology   QZ 350
  Localized, by site
Lymphoma, Malignant see Lymphoma
Lymphoma, Nodular see Lymphoma, Follicular
Lymphoma, Non-Hodgkin   WH 525
  Clinical pathology   QZ 350
Lymphomatosis Virus, Avian see Leukosis Virus,
  Avian
Lymphopathia Venerea see Lymphogranuloma
  Venereum
Lymphopenia   WH 200
Lymphoproliferative Disorders
  General works   WH 700
  Child   WS 300
  Infant   WS 300
  Nursing   WY 152.5
  Veterinary   SF 769.5
  See also names of specific disorders, e.g.,
    Lymphoma   WH 525
Lymphosarcoma see Lymphoma, Diffuse
Lynch Syndrome see Colorectal Neoplasms,
  Hereditary Nonpolyposis
Lynestrenol   WP 530
  As a contraceptive   QV 177
Lyophilization see Freeze Drying
Lypressin   WK 520
Lysergic Acid Diethylamide   QV 77.7
Lysergide see Lysergic Acid Diethylamide
Lysine   QU 60
Lysine Vasopressin see Lypressin
Lysis see Bacteriolysis; Hemolysis; Lysogeny
Lysogeny   QW 660
Lysol see Cresols
Lysolecithins see Lysophosphatidylcholines
Lysophosphatidylcholines   QU 93
Lysosomes   QH 603.L9
Lysozyme see Muramidase
Lysuride Hydrogen Maleate see Lisuride
Lysyl Bradykinin see Kallidin

M

m-Dihydroxybenzenes see Resorcinols
M Phase see Mitosis
Macaca   QL 737.P93
  As laboratory animals   QY 60.P7
  Diseases   SF 997.5.P7

ALWAYS CONSULT MAIN SCHEDULES. USE NUMBER ASSIGNED ONLY WHEN
SUBJECT REPRESENTS MAJOR EMPHASIS OF WORK BEING CLASSIFIED

Macaca mulatta   QL 737.P93
  Diseases   SF 997.5.P7
  As laboratory animals   QY 60.P7
Macaca nemestrina   QL 737.P93
  Diseases   SF 997.5.P7
  As laboratory animals   QY 60.P7
Macaque see Macaca
Mace see omega–Chloroacetophenone
Maceration (Pharmacy) see Drug Compounding
Machiavellianism   BF 698.35.M34
Macrocytic Anemias see Anemia, Macrocytic
Macroglobulinemia see Waldenstrom
  Macroglobulinemia
Macromolecular Systems
  Polymers (General)
    Inorganic   QD 196
    Organic   QD 380–QD 388
    Polysaccharides   QU 83
    Proteins   QU 55
    Special topics, by subject
Macrophage Activation   QW 690
Macrophage-Granulocyte Inducer see
  Colony-Stimulating Factors
Macrophages   WH 650
  In phagocytosis   QW 690
Macula Lutea   WW 270
Macular Degeneration   WW 270
Madura Foot see Maduromycosis
Maduromycosis   WR 340
Maedi Virus see Visna–Maedi Virus
Maedi-Visna Virus see Visna–Maedi Virus
Magentas see Rosaniline Dyes
Maggot Infestations see Myiasis
Magic
  Medical   WZ 309
  Occult sciences   BF 1585–1628
Magnesium
  Metabolism   QU 130
  Pharmacology   QV 278
  Toxicology   QV 278
Magnesium Adenosinetriphosphatase see Ca(2+)
  Mg(2+)-ATPase
Magnesium ADP see Adenosine Diphosphate
Magnesium ATP see Adenosine Triphosphate
Magnesium ATPase see Ca(2+) Mg(2+)-ATPase
Magnesium Deficiency   WD 105
  Veterinary   SF 855.M34
Magnesium Hydroxide
  As an antacid   QV 69
Magnesium Sulfate   QV 75
Magnetic Fields see Magnetics
Magnetic Resonance see Nuclear Magnetic
  Resonance
Magnetic Resonance Imaging   WN 185
Magnetic Resonance Spectroscopy see Nuclear
  Magnetic Resonance
Magnetics
  And electricity collectively   QC 501–718.8
  Biophysics   QT 34
  Effect on cells   QH 656
  Physics   QC 750–766
  Physiological effects   QT 162.M3
Magnetism see Magnetics

Magnetism, Animal see Mental Healing
Magnetoencephalography   WL 141
Magnetometry see Magnetics
Maidenhair Tree see Ginkgo biloba
Maillard Reaction
  As pathogenesis of disease (General)   QZ 40
  Food processing technology   TP 372.55.M35
Mainstreaming (Education)
  General   LC 4015, LC 4031, etc.
  Of children with specific disabilities, with the
    disability
Maintenance
  Housing   WA 795–799
  Of special equipment, by subject
Maintenance and Engineering, Hospital   WX 165
Maize see Corn
Major Histocompatibility Complex   WO 680
Mal de Pinto see Pinta
Malabsorption Syndromes   WD 200.5.M2
  For the gastroenterologist   WI 500
  See also Celiac Disease   WD 175; Sprue   WD
  175
Malacosteon see Osteomalacia
Maladjustment see Personality Disorders
Malaria   WC 750–770
  Drugs for see Antimalarials   QV 256–258
  Prevention and control   WC 765
  Veterinary   SF 791
Malaria, Avian   SF 995.6.M3
Malaria, Hemolytic see Blackwater Fever
Malathion
  Carcinogenicity research   QZ 202
  Public health   WA 240
Male Fern see Plants, Medicinal
Male Genitalia see Genitalia, Male
Male Nurses see Nurses, Male
Male Pattern Baldness see Alopecia
Maleates   QU 98
  Organic chemistry
    Aliphatic compounds   QD 305.A2
Malformations, Congenital see Abnormalities;
  Arteriovenous Malformations; names of other
  specific malformations
Malfunction, Equipment see Equipment Failure
Malignant Carcinoid Syndrome   WI 435
Malignant Hypertension see Hypertension,
  Malignant
Malingering   W 783
Malleus   WV 230
Malnutrition see Nutrition Disorders
Malocclusion   WU 440
Malpractice   W 44
  General   W 44
  Dentistry   WU 44
  Gynecology   WP 34
  Nursing   WY 44
  Obstetrics   WQ 34
  (Form number 33 or 33.1 in any other NLM
    schedule where applicable and practical)
Malt
  As a dietary supplement in health or disease
    WB 431
  For alcoholic beverages   TP 587

**ALWAYS CONSULT MAIN SCHEDULES. USE NUMBER ASSIGNED ONLY WHEN
SUBJECT REPRESENTS MAJOR EMPHASIS OF WORK BEING CLASSIFIED**

Malta Fever see Brucellosis
Maltases see alpha–Glucosidases
Malthusianism see Population Dynamics
Maltose   QU 75
Mammae
   General   SF 890
   Wild animals   QP 188.M3
Mammals
   As laboratory animals   QY 60.M2
   Diseases   SF 600–1100
   Domestic   SF
   Wild   QL 700–739.3
Mammaplasty   WP 910
Mammary Arteries   WG 595.T4
Mammary Dysplasia see Fibrocystic Disease of
  Breast
Mammary Glands see Breast; Mammae; Udder
Mammary Glands, Animal see Mammae
Mammary Neoplasms, Experimental   WP 870
Mammography   WP 815
Mammotropic Hormone, Pituitary see Prolactin
Mammotropic Hormone, Placental see Placental
  Lactogen
Mammotropin see Prolactin
Man–Machine Systems   TA 167
   Biomedical engineering   QT 36
   Special topics, by subject
Managed Care Programs   W 130
Managed Competition
   Economic aspects   W 74
   Related to managed care   W 130
Managed Health Care Insurance Plans see Managed
  Care Programs
Management Information Systems   W 26.5
   Ambulatory Care Information Systems   WX
   26.5
   Clinical Laboratory Information Systems   QY
   26.5
   Database Management Systems   W 26.5
   Decision Support Systems, Management   W 26.5
   Hospital Information Systems   WX 26.5
   Office Automation   W 26.5
   Radiology Information Systems   WN 26.5
   In other areas, by subject
Management Quality Circles
   Hospitals   WX 159
   Nursing   WY 30
Mandatory Reporting
   Of child abuse   WA 320
     Legislation   WA 32–33
   Of elder abuse   WT 30
     Legislation   WT 32–33
Mandelic Acids   QV 243
Mandelonitrile beta Gentiobioside see Amygdalin
Mandible   WU 101
   See also special topics under Jaw
Mandibular Condyle   WU 101
   See also special topics under Jaw
Mandibular Diseases   WU 140.5
Mandibular Fractures   WU 610
Mandibular Injuries   WU 610
Mandibular Neoplasms   WU 280
Mandibular Nerve   WL 330

Mandibular Prosthesis   WU 600
Mandibular Ridge Augmentation see Alveolar Ridge
  Augmentation
Mandibulofacial Dysostosis   WU 101.5
Mandragora   QV 85
Mandrake, American see Podophyllum
Mandrake, European see Mandragora
Mandrake Root see Podophyllum
Mandrill see Papio
Manganese   QV 290
   Metabolism   QU 130.5
Mange see Mite Infestations
Mange, Sarcoptic see Scabies
Mania see Bipolar Disorder
Manic–Depressive Psychosis see Bipolar Disorder
Manic Disorder see Bipolar Disorder
Manic State see Bipolar Disorder
Manifestations of Disease see Disease; Eye
   Manifestations; Gastrointestinal System;
     Neurologic Manifestations; Oral Manifestations;
   Skin Manifestations
Manihot see Cassava
Manikins   QY 35
Manioc see Cassava
Manipulation, Chiropractic see Manipulation, Spinal
Manipulation, Orthopedic   WB 535
   Used for treatment of particular disorders, with
   the disorder
Manipulation, Psychological see Machiavellianism
Manipulation, Spinal   WB 535
   Used for treatment of particular disorders, with
   the disorder
Mannequins see Manikins
Mannitol   QV 160
Manpower see Health Manpower
Manslaughter see Homicide
Mantids see Orthoptera
Manual Communication   HV 2477–2480
   See also Sign Language   HV 2474–2476
Manuals
   Hospital staff
     Non–professional   WX 159
     Nursing   WY 105
     Pediatric   WS 29
     Ward manual   WX 203
     Other professional   WX 203
   Psychiatric   WM 30
   Others, by subject
   See also Handbooks   WO 231, etc.
Manuscripts   Z 6601–6625
Manuscripts, Medical
   Bibliography   Z 6611.M5
   Early western   WZ 220
   Other early   WZ 225
   Others, by subject
Mapharsen see Oxophenarsine
Maple Syrup Urine Disease   WD 205.5.A5
Maprotiline   QV 77.5
Maps   G
   Of diseases   WA 900
   See also Atlases   G
Marasmus see Protein–Energy Malnutrition
Marble Bone Disease see Osteopetrosis

Marchiafava–Micheli Syndrome see
  Hemoglobinuria, Paroxysmal
Marek's Disease   SF 995.6.M33
Marfan Syndrome   WD 375
Margarine
  As a dietary supplement in health or disease
    WB 425
  Biochemistry   QU 86
  Public health aspects   WA 722
Marguerite see Pyrethrum
Marie–Struempell Disease see Spondylitis,
  Ankylosing
Marihuana see Cannabis
Marijuana see Cannabis
Marijuana Abuse   WM 276
Marijuana Smoking
  Dependence   WM 276
  Pharmacological effect   QV 77.7
  Social pathology   HV 5822.M3
Marine Biology   QH 91–95.9
Marine Toxins   QW 630.5.M3
  See also Fish Venoms   WD 405
Marital Relationship see Marriage
Marital Therapy   WM 430.5.M3
Maritime Quarantine see Quarantine
Marker Antigens see Antigens, Differentiation
Markers, Biological see Biological Markers
Markers, DNA see Genetic Markers
Markers, Genetic see Genetic Markers
Markers, Laboratory see Biological Markers
Markers, Serum see Biological Markers
Markers, Surrogate see Biological Markers
Markers, Tumor see Tumor Markers, Biological
Marketing of Health Services   W 74
  Special topics, by subject
Marmoset Virus see Simplexvirus
Marriage   HQ 503–1058
  Counseling   WM 55
  Miscegenation   GN 254
  Statistics   HB 1111–1317
  See also Marital Therapy   WM 430.5.M3
Marriage Therapy see Marital Therapy
Marrow see Bone Marrow
Marsh Gas see Methane
Marsupialia   QL 737.M3–737.M39
Martial Arts   QT 260.5.M3
Marxism see Communism
Masks   WA 260
  In industry   WA 485
  In surgery   WO 162
Masochism   WM 610
Mass Behavior   HM
Mass Chest X-Ray   WF 225
Mass Media   P 87–96
  Special topics, by subject
Mass Screening   WA 245
  Child   WS 141
  Infant   WS 141
Mass Spectrometry see Spectrum Analysis, Mass
Mass Spectroscopy see Spectrum Analysis, Mass
Massage   WB 537
Mast-Cell Colony-Stimulating Factor see
  Interleukin-3

Mast Cells   QS 532.5.C7
Mastectomy   WP 910
Mastectomy, Modified Radical   WP 910
Mastectomy, Radical   WP 910
Mastication   WU 102
Masticatory Force see Bite Force
Masticatory Muscles
  Anatomy   WU 101
  Physiology   WU 102
Mastigophora   QX 70
Mastitis   WP 840
Mastitis, Cystic see Fibrocystic Disease of Breast
Mastocytosis, Bullous see Urticaria Pigmentosa
Mastocytosis, Diffuse Cutaneous see Urticaria
  Pigmentosa
Mastoid   WE 705
  Region of the middle ear   WV 233
Mastoiditis   WV 233
Mastomys see Muridae
Masturbation   HQ 447
  Psychiatric aspects   WM 611
Matched Case-Control Studies see Case-Control
  Studies
Materia Alba see Dental Deposits
Materia Medica   QV 760
Materials Management, Hospital   WX 147
Materials Testing
  General and mechanical   TA 410, etc.
  In special fields, with the field, i.e. in Dentistry
    WU 190
  Of biocompatible materials   QT 37
  Of specific materials, with the material
  Of specific property, with the property (e.g.,
    testing of impact strength   TA 418.34)
Maternal Age 35 and over
  Normal pregnancy   WQ 200
  Pregnancy complications   WQ 240–260
Maternal and Child Welfare see Child Welfare;
  Maternal Welfare
Maternal Behavior   WS 105.5.F2
Maternal-Child Health Centers see Health Facilities
  WA 310
Maternal-Child Nursing   WY 157.3
Maternal Deprivation   WS 105.5.D3
Maternal-Fetal Exchange   WQ 210.5
  Immunological factor   QW 553
Maternal Health see Maternal Welfare
Maternal Health Services   WA 310
  See also Prenatal Care   WQ 175; Postnatal Care
    WQ 500
Maternal Mortality   HB 1322.5
  Including causes of death   WA 900
Maternal Patterns of Care see Maternal Behavior
Maternal Welfare   WA 310
Maternity see Illegitimacy; Mothers; Parents;
  Pregnancy
Maternity Leave see Parental Leave
Maternity Nursing see Obstetrical Nursing
Mathematical Computing
  Special topics, by subject, e.g. Biological Models
    QH 324.8
Mathematics   QA
  Biomathematics

In general biological sciences   QH 323.5
In medicine and related fields   QT 35
In public health statistics   WA 950
Concept formation in children   WS 105.5.D2
Statistical methods (General)   QA 276–280
Used in various specialties
  (Form number 25 in any NLM schedule where
  applicable)
Mating Behavior, Animal see Sex Behavior, Animal
Matrix, Extracellular see Extracellular Matrix
Mattresses see Beds
Maxilla   WU
Maxillary Antrum see Maxillary Sinus
Maxillary Artery   WG 595.M2
Maxillary Diseases   WU 140.5
Maxillary Fractures   WU 610
Maxillary Neoplasms   WU 280
Maxillary Prosthesis see Maxillofacial Prosthesis
Maxillary Ridge Augmentation see Alveolar Ridge
  Augmentation
Maxillary Sinus   WV 345
Maxillary Sinus Neoplasms   WV 345
Maxillary Sinusitis   WV 345
Maxillofacial Abnormalities   WE 705
  Dental aspects   WU 101.5
Maxillofacial Development   WE 705
  Dental aspects   WU 101
Maxillofacial Injuries   WU 610
Maxillofacial Procedures see Oral Surgical
  Procedures
Maxillofacial Prosthesis   WU 600
Maxillofacial Prosthesis Implantation   WU 600
Maxillomandibular Fixation see Jaw Fixation
  Techniques
Maximal Expiratory Flow Rate   WF 102
  As a diagnostic test   WF 141
  General physical examination   WB 284
Maximal Expiratory Flow–Volume Curves   WF
  102
Maximum Allowable Concentration see Maximum
  Permissible Exposure Level
Maximum Permissible Exposure Level
  To industrial pollutants   WA 400–495
  To other specific conditions, by subject
May Apple see Podophyllum
McGill Pain Questionnaire see Pain Measurement
McNaughton Rule see Insanity Defense
MDA see 3,4–Methylenedioxyamphetamine
Meals on Wheels see Food Services
Measles   WC 580
Measles, German see Rubella
Measles Vaccine   WC 580
Measles Virus   QW 168.5.P2
Measles Virus, German see Rubella Virus
Meat
  As a dietary supplement in health or disease
  WB 426
  Butchering, packaging, etc.   TS 1960–1981
    Sanitation   WA 707
  Inspection   WA 707
Meat–Packing Industry   TS 1970–1973
  Occupational medicine   WA 400–495
  Industrial waste   WA 788

Meat inspection   WA 707
Meat Products
  As dietary supplement in health or disease   WB
  426
  Contamination   WA 701
  Preserved   WA 710
  Sanitation   WA 707
Meatus, External Auditory see Ear Canal
Meatus, Internal Auditory see Petrous Bone
Meballymal see Secobarbital
Mebubarbital see Pentobarbital
Mebumal see Pentobarbital
Mechanoreceptors   WL 102.9
Mechanotherapy see WB 535 for works including
  Exercise Therapy; Gymnastics; Manipulation,
  Orthopedic; Massage and/or other similar
  procedures treated together.
Mechlorethamine   QV 269
Mechlorethamine Oxide see Mechlorethamine
Meckel's Diverticulum   WI 412
Meclastine see Clemastine
Meclofenoxate
  Biochemistry   QU 98
  As an analeptic   QV 101
  As a plant growth regulator   QK 745
Mecloprodin see Clemastine
Meconium   WQ 210.5
Medex see Physician Assistants
Median Bar see Prostatic Diseases
Median Nerve   WL 400
  See also names of organs affected, e.g., Hand
  WE 830
Mediastinal Cyst   WF 900
Mediastinal Diseases   WF 900
Mediastinal Emphysema   WF 900
Mediastinal Neoplasms   WF 900
Mediastinitis   WF 900
Mediastinoscopy   WF 900
Mediastinum   WF 900
Medicaid
  W 250
Medical Assistance   W 100–275
Medical Assistance, Title 19 see Medicaid
Medical Audit   W 84
  Of a hospital   WX 153
Medical Botany see Plants, Medicinal
Medical Care see Health Services
Medical Care Costs see Health Care Costs
Medical Care Research see Health Services Research
Medical Care Team see Patient Care Team
Medical Centers see Health Facilities   WX and
  names of specific types of facilities
Medical Climatology see Climate; Weather
Medical Computer Science see Medical Informatics
Medical Curiosities see Abnormalities; Medicine
Medical Decision Making, Computer–Assisted see
  Decision Making, Computer–Assisted
Medical Device Design see Equipment Design
Medical Device Failure see Equipment Failure
Medical Device Safety see Equipment Safety
Medical Devices see Equipment and Supplies
Medical Dissertations see Dissertations, Academic
Medical Economics see Economics, Medical

Medical Education see Education, Medical

Medical Education, Continuing see Education, Medical, Continuing

Medical Education, Graduate see Education, Medical, Graduate

Medical Education, Undergraduate see Education, Medical, Undergraduate

Medical Emergencies see Emergencies; Emergency Medicine

Medical Errors
 In the practice of medicine (General)   WB 100
 In operative surgery   WO 500
 In particular areas, by subject
 See also Diagnostic Errors   WB 141; Medication Errors   QZ 42, etc.

Medical Ethics see Ethics, Medical

Medical Evidence see Forensic Medicine

Medical Examiners see Coroners and Medical Examiners

Medical Geography see Climate; Epidemiology; Weather; names of diseases involved

Medical Gymnastics see Exercise Therapy

Medical History Taking   WB 290
 See also Medical Records   WX 173

Medical Illustration   WZ 348
 (Form number 17 in any NLM schedule where applicable)
 Surgery   WO 517
 See also Anatomy, Artistic   NC 760–783.8; Medicine in Art   WZ 330; Photography   TR 708, etc.

Medical Imaging see Diagnostic Imaging

Medical Indigency   W 250
 See also Medicaid   W 250

Medical Informatics
 In particular fields (Form number 26.5 in any NLM schedules where applicable)
 Space medicine   WD 751.6
 Used for special purpose, by subject

Medical Informatics Applications
 In particular fields (Form number 26.5 in any NLM schedules where applicables)
 Used for special purpose, by subject

Medical Informatics Computing   W 26.5

Medical Information Science see Medical Informatics

Medical Insurance see Insurance, Health

Medical Jurisprudence see Jurisprudence

Medical Laboratory Technology see Technology, Medical Laboratory

Medical Literature Analysis and Retrieval System see MEDLARS

Medical Logic see Logic

Medical Missions, Official   W 323
 See also Missions and Missionaries   W 323, etc.

Medical Mistakes see Medical Errors

Medical Museums see Museums

Medical Oncology   QZ 200

Medical Philosophy see Philosophy, Medical

Medical Practice Management Services see Practice Management

Medical Profession see Medicine

Medical Psychology see Psychology, Medical

Medical Publishing see Publishing

Medical Record Administrators   WX 173

Medical Record Linkage   WX 173

Medical Records
 Medical record libraries   WX 173
 See also Hospital Records   WX 173; Medical History Taking   WB 290

Medical Records Department, Hospital   WX 173

Medical Records Librarians see Medical Record Administrators

Medical Records, Problem–Oriented   WX 173
 Hospital records   WX 173
 Specific topics, by subject

Medical Records Systems, Computerized
 Hospital Records   WX 173
 Specific topics, by subject

Medical Research see Research

Medical Savings Accounts
 Economic aspects   W 74
 Related to health insurance   W 100–275

Medical Schools see Schools, Medical

Medical Secretaries   W 80

Medical Service Plans see Insurance, Health

Medical Sociology see Sociology, Medical

Medical Staff   W 84
 Of industry
  Medical and dental   WA 412
  Mental health services   WA 495
 Of schools, colleges, universities
  Medical and dental   WA 350
   Elementary and secondary   WA 350
   University and college   WA 351
  Mental health services   WA 352
   Elementary and secondary   WA 352
   University and college   WA 353
 See also Medical Staff, Hospital   WX 203; names of specific types of hospitals
 See also Nursing Staff, Hospital   WY 125, etc. and other medical personnel
 See also Personnel, Hospital   WX 159; names of specific types of hospitals

Medical Staff, Hospital   WX 203
 See also Medical Staff   W 84; Personnel, Hospital   WX 159; names of specific types of hospitals

Medical Staff Privileges   WX 203

Medical Staff Privileges, Nonphysician see Medical Staff Privileges

Medical Symbols see Emblems and Insignia

Medical Technology see Technology, Medical

Medical Terminology see Nomenclature

Medical Topography see Topography, Medical

Medical Waste   WA 790

Medical Waste Disposal   WA 790

Medical Writing see Writing

Medically Underserved Area   W 76
 Developing countries   WA 395
 Rural areas   WA 390
 Urban areas   WA 380

Medicare   WT 31

Medicare Assignment   WT 31

Medicare Choice see Medicare Part C

Medicare Hospital Insurance Program see Medicare Part A

**ALWAYS CONSULT MAIN SCHEDULES. USE NUMBER ASSIGNED ONLY WHEN
SUBJECT REPRESENTS MAJOR EMPHASIS OF WORK BEING CLASSIFIED**

Membrane Fusion   QH 601
Membrane Glycoproteins   QU 55
Membrane Lipids   QU 85
Membrane Potentials
    Biophysics   QT 34
    Cytology   QH 601
    Metabolism   QU 120
    Physiology   QS 532.5.M3
Membrane Proteins   QU 55
Membrane Tympani see Tympanic Membrane
Membranes
    Cell see Cell Membrane   QH 601, etc.
    Fetal see Fetal Membranes   QS 645, etc.
    Histology   QS 532.5.M3
    Mucous see Mucous Membrane   QS 532.5.M8
    Periodontal   WU 240
    Synaptic see Synaptic Membranes   WL 102.8
    Synovial see Synovial Membrane   WE 300
Membranes, Artificial
    Chemical technology   TP 159.M4
    In dialysis (chemical engineering)   TP 156.D45
    In hemodialysis   WJ 378
    Saline water conversion   WA 687
    Used for other special purposes, by subject
Membranes, Intracellular see Intracellular
  Membranes
Memory   BF 370–387
    Child   WS 105.5.M2
    Infant   WS 105.5.M2
    Physiology   WL 102
    In psychoanalysis, psychoanalytic therapy, or
      psychoanalytic interpretation   WM 460.5.M5
Memory Disorders   WM 173.7
Memory for Designs Test see Neuropsychological
  Tests
Memory, Immediate see Memory, Short-Term
Memory, Photographic see Eidetic Imagery
Memory, Short-Term   BF 378.S54
Men
    Sexual life   HQ 36
    Other special topics, by subject
Menadione see Vitamin K
Menaquinone see Vitamin K
Menarche   WP 540
Mendel's Law see Genetics; Hybridization
Meniere's Disease   WV 258
Meniere's Syndrome see Meniere's Disease
Meningeal Arteries   WG 595.M3
Meningeal Neoplasms   WL 200
    Clinical pathology   QZ 380
Meninges   WL 200
Meningioma   QZ 380
    Localized, by site
Meningism   WL 340
Meningitis   WL 200
    Cerebral   WL 200
    Epidemic cerebrospinal see Meningitis,
      Meningococcal   WC 245
    Tuberculous see Tuberculosis, Meningeal   WL
      200
Meningitis, Listeria   WC 242
Meningitis, Meningococcal   WC 245
Meningitis, Tuberculous see Tuberculosis, Meningeal

Meningitis, Viral   WC 540
Meningocele   WL 200
Meningococcal Infections   WC 245
Meningococcal Meningitis see Meningitis,
  Meningococcal
Meningoencephalitis   WL 351
    Epidemic   WC 542
    Syphilitic see Paresis   WC 165, etc.
Meningomyelitis   WL 400
Meningomyelocele   WE 730
Menisci, Tibial   WE 870
Menopause   WP 580
Menorrhagia   WP 555
Menotropins   WK 515
Menstrual Cycle   WP 540
Menstrual Proliferative Phase see Menstrual Cycle
Menstrual Secretory Phase see Menstrual Cycle
Menstruation   WP 550–560
Menstruation Disorders   WP 550–560
    Hypomenorrhea   WP 552
    Oligomenorrhea   WP 552
    See also names of other specific disorders
Menstruation-Inducing Agents   QV 170
Menstruation, Retrograde see Menstruation
  Disorders
Mental Competency
    Competency to consent in the acceptance of
      health care   W 85
    Legal aspects   W 32–33
      Related to the mentally ill   WM 32–33
Mental Deficiency see Mental Retardation
Mental Disorders   WM
    General works   WM 140
    Adolescence   WS 463
    Aged   WT 150
    Case studies   WM 40
    Child   WS 350–350.8
    Diagnosis   WM 141
    Drug therapy   WM 402
    Environmental factors   WM 31
    In mental retardation   WM 307.M5
    Infant   WS 350–350.8
    Jurisprudence see Forensic Psychiatry   W 740,
      etc.
    Nursing see Psychiatric Nursing   WY 160
    Popular works (General)   WM 75
    Pregnancy   WQ 240
    Rehabilitation   WM 400–460.6
    Rehabilitation centers   WM 29
    Socioeconomic factors   WM 31
    Therapy   WM 400, etc.
    See also names of specific disorders
Mental Disorders, Organic see Delirium, Dementia,
  Amnestic, Cognitive Disorders
Mental Fatigue   WM 174
    Industrial   WA 495
Mental Healing   WB 880–885
    Faith cure   WB 885
    See also Christian Science   WB 885, etc.
Mental Health   WM 105
    Adolescence   WS 462
    Aged   WT 145
    Child   WS 105.5.M3

Environmental factors   WM 31
Infant   WS 105.5.M3
Occupational   WA 495
Military   UH 629–629.5
Popular works   WM 75
Rural   WA 390
School   WA 352
Socioeconomic factors   WM 31
Special population groups   WA 305
Women   WA 309
Mental Health Services   WM 30
Child   WM 30
In industry   WA 495
Infant   WM 30
Military   UH 629–629.5
School programs
Elementary and secondary   WA 352
University and college   WA 353
Special population groups   WA 305
Mental Health Services, Community see Community
Mental Health Services
Mental Hospitals see Hospitals, Psychiatric
Mental Hygiene see Mental Health
Mental Hygiene Services see Mental Health Services
Mental Processes   BF 441–449
Child   WS 105.5.D2
Infant   WS 105.5.D2
Mental Retardation   WM 300–308
Adolescence   WS 463
Complications   WM 300
Child   WS 107
Infant   WS 107
For infants and children   WS 107–105.5
Biographical accounts   WS 107.5.C2
Psychosocial problems   WS 107.5.P8
Rehabilitation   WS 107.5.R3
Mental disorders   WM 307.M5
Vocational guidance   HV 3005
See also Child, Exceptional   WS 105.5.C3, etc.;
Education of Mentally Retarded   LC
4601–4640.4, etc.
Mental Retardation, Psychosocial see Mental
Retardation
Mental Status Schedule   WM 141
Mental Tests see Intelligence Tests
Mentally Disabled see Mentally Disabled Persons
Mentally Disabled Persons
Education   LC 4815
See also Education of Mentally Retarded   LC
4601–4640.4, etc.
Medical apects   WM 300–308
Social aspects   HV 3004–3009
Transportation   HV 3005.5
Vocational guidance   HV 3005
See also Disabled Children   LC 4001–4806.5,
etc.; Mental Retardation   WM 300–308, etc.
Mentally Handicapped see Mentally Disabled
Persons
Menthol
Organic chemistry   QD 416
Pharmacology   QV 60
Menthyl Mercury Compounds   QV 293
As fungicides   WA 240, etc.

Mentors
In nursing education   WY 18–18.8
Special topics, by subject
Mentorships see Mentors
Menu Planning
In hospitals   WX 168
In schools
Elementary and secondary   WA 350
Universities and colleges   WA 351
Public health aspects in restaurants   WA 799
Mepacrine see Quinacrine
Meperidine   QV 89
Mepivacaine   QV 115
Meprobamate   QV 77.9
MER–29 see Triparanol
Mercaptamine see Cysteamine
Mercapto Compounds see Sulfhydryl Compounds
Mercaptoethanol   QV 84
Organic chemistry   QD 305.A4
Pharmacology   QV 84
Mercaptoethylamines   QU 61
Organic chemistry   QD 305.A8
Mercaptovaline see Penicillamine
Mercurial Diuretics see Diuretics, Mercurial
Mercuric Chloride
As an anti-infective agent   QV 231
Mercury   QV 293
For syphilis   QV 261
Mercury Dichloride see Mercuric Chloride
Mercury Isotopes
Inorganic chemistry   QD 181.H6
Pharmacology   QV 293
Mercury Poisoning   QV 293
Mercy Death see Euthanasia
Mercy Killing see Euthanasia
Meriones see Gerbillinae
Mescaline   QV 77.7
Used in North American Indian religion   E
98.R3
Mesencephalic Central Gray see Periaqueductal
Gray
Mesencephalon   WL 310
Mesenchyma see Connective Tissue
Mesenchyme see Mesoderm
Mesenchymoma   QZ 310
Localized, by site
Mesenteric Arteries   WG 595.M38
See also Blood supply   WI 500 under Mesentery
Mesenteric Circulation see Splanchnic Circulation
Mesenteric Cyst   WI 500
Mesenteric Lymphadenitis   WI 500
Mesenteric Vascular Occlusion   WI 500
Mesenteric Veins   WI 720
Mesentery   WI 500
Blood supply   WI 500
Neoplasms   WI 500
Pathology   QZ 340
Mesmerism see Hypnosis
Mesna   QV 76
Mesocolon   WI 500
Mesocricetus   QL 737.R666
As laboratory animals   QY 60.R6
As pets   SF 459.H3

**ALWAYS CONSULT MAIN SCHEDULES. USE NUMBER ASSIGNED ONLY WHEN
SUBJECT REPRESENTS MAJOR EMPHASIS OF WORK BEING CLASSIFIED**

Mesoderm   WQ 205
Mesonephroma   WP 322
Mesosigmoid see Mesocolon
Mesothelioma   QZ 340
Mesothelium see Epithelium
Messenger RNA see RNA, Messenger
Mestranol   WP 522
   As a contraceptive   QV 177
Mesylates   QU 98
   Organic chemistry   QD 305.S3
meta–Dihydroxybenzenes see Resorcinols
Metabolic Activation see Biotransformation
Metabolic Clearance Rate   QY 450
   Rate of particular substance, with the substance
Metabolic Detoxication, Drug   QV 38
Metabolic Diseases   WD 200–226
   General   WD 200
   Veterinary   SF 910.M48
   See also Calcium Metabolism Disorders   WD
   200.5.C2; Metabolism, Inborn errors   WD 205
   and other specific diseases
Metabolic Pump see Biological Transport, Active
Metabolism   QU
   Bacterial see Bacteria   QW 52
   Child   QU
   Disorders as a manifestation of disease   QZ 180
   General works   QU 120
   Infant   QU
   Radiation effects   WN 610
   Skin   WR 102
Metabolism and Endocrinology (Specialty) see
   Endocrinology
Metabolism, Basal see Basal Metabolism
Metabolism, Inborn Errors   WD 205–205.5
   See also names of specific disorders
Metabolite Markers, Neoplasm see Tumor Markers,
   Biological
Metaethics see Ethics
Metagonimiasis see Trematode Infections
Metagonimus see Heterophyidae
Metal Metabolism, Inborn Errors   WD 205.5.M3
Metal Plating see Electroplating
Metallo–Organic Compounds see Organometallic
   Compounds
Metalloproteases see Metalloproteinases
Metalloproteinases   QU 136
Metalloproteins   QU 55
Metallotherapy see Alternative Medicine
Metallothionein   QU 55
Metallurgy   TN 600–799
   Dental   WU 180
   Occupational medicine   WA 400–495
   Industrial waste   WA 788
Metals
   In dentistry   WU 180
   Inorganic chemistry   QD 171–172
   Metabolism   QU 130
     See also Metal Metabolism, Inborn Errors
     WD 205.5.M3
   Pharmacology and toxicology
     Alkaline earth metals   QV 275–278
     Heavy metals   290–298
   See also names of specific metals

Metals, Actinide see Metals, Actinoid
Metals, Actinoid   WN 420
Metals, Alkaline Earth
   Inorganic chemistry   QD 172.A42
   Pharmacology   QV 275
   Salts   QV 275
Metals, Heavy
   Pharmacology and toxicology   QV 290–298
   See also names of specific metals, e.g., Lead
   QV 292
Metals, Light   QV 275–278
   See also names of specific metals, e.g., Magnesium
   QV 278
Metals, Rare Earth
   Inorganic chemistry   QD 172.R2
   Pharmacology   QV 290
Metamizole see Dipyrone
Metamorphosis, Biological   QL 981
   Insects   QL 494.5
Metaphor
   In psychoanalysis   WM 460.5.D8
   In psychotherapy   WM 420
   In other specific subjects, with the subject
Metaphysical Healing see Mental Healing
Metaphysics   BD 100–131
Metaplasia   QZ 190
Metaproterenol see Orciprenaline
Metasqualene see Triparanol
Metastasis see Neoplasm Metastasis
Metatarsal Deformity see Foot Deformities
Metatarsus   WE 880
Metencephalon see Cerebellum
Meteorological Factors
   Climate and disease   WB 700–710
   Mental health   WM 31
   Public health   WA 30
   Other topics, by subject
Meteorology see Meteorological Factors; Weather
Metformin   WK 825
Methacholine Compounds   QV 122
Methadone   QV 89
   Dependence   WM 270
Methalamic Acid see Iothalamic Acid
Methaminodiazepoxide see Chlordiazepoxide
Methamphetamine   QV 102
   Dependence   WM 270
Methampyrone see Dipyrone
Methandienone see Methandrostenolone
Methandrostenolone   WJ 875
Methane
   Microbial chemistry   QW 52
   Toxicology   QV 662
Methanesulfonates see Mesylates
Methanobacteria see Methanogens
Methanogens   QW 50
Methanol
   Pharmacology   QV 83
Methantheline   QV 132
Methaqualone   QV 85
Methemoglobin   WH 190
Methemoglobinemia   WH 190
Methenamine   QV 243

Methicillin Resistance
  Bacteriology   QW 51
  Drug therapy   WB 330
  Pharmacology   QV 354
Methionine   QU 87
Methodologies, Computing see Computing
  Methodologies
Methodology Research, Nursing see Nursing
  Methodology Research
Methods   Q 180.55.M4
  In particular areas, by subject
Methofluranum see Methoxyflurane
Methohexital   QV 88
Methohexitone see Methohexital
Methotrexate
  Folic acid antagonist   QU 188
  In therapy of neoplasms   QZ 267
  Other special topics, by subject
Methoxsalen   QV 63
  Cosmetics   WA 744
Methoxyflurane   QV 81
Methoxyhydroxyphenylglycol   QV 82
Methoxyverapamil see Gallopamil
Methyl Chloride
  As an anesthetic   QV 115
  Organic chemistry
    Aliphatic compounds   QD 305.H5
  Toxicology   QV 633
Methyl Ethers   QV 81
  Organic chemistry   QD 305.E7
Methyl Violet see Gentian Violet
Methyl Viologen see Paraquat
Methyladenine Receptors see Receptors, Purinergic
Methylamines   QU 61
  Organic chemistry   QD 305.A8
Methylation   QD 281.M48
Methylcellulose
  Cathartic   QV 75
  Suspension agent   QV 787
Methylcephaeline see Emetine
Methylcholanthrene   QZ 202
Methyldopa   QV 150
Methyldopate see Methyldopa
Methylene Bichloride see Methylene Chloride
Methylene Bis(chloroaniline) see
  Methylenebis(chloroaniline)
Methylene Chloride
  Toxicology   QV 633
Methylene Dichloride see Methylene Chloride
Methylenebis(chloroaniline)
  As a carcinogen   QZ 202
  Toxicology   QV 633
Methylenesulfonates see Mesylates
Methylergol Carbamide see Lisuride
Methylglyoxal see Pyruvaldehyde
Methylhistamines   QV 157
Methylhydrazines
  Biochemistry   QU 60
  Neoplasm etiology   QZ 202
Methylhydroxyprogesterone see
  Medroxyprogesterone
Methylphenyl Ethers see Anisoles
Methylprednisolone   WK 757

Methylprednisolone Hemisuccinate   WK 757
Methylprednisolone Succinate see
  Methylprednisolone Hemisuccinate
Methylrosaniline Chloride see Gentian Violet
Methylxanthine Receptors see Receptors, Purinergic
Methypregnone see Medroxyprogesterone
Metindamide see Indapamide
Metipranolol see Trimepranol
Metolquizolone see Methaqualone
Metoprolol   QV 132
Metrazol see Pentylenetetrazole
Metric System   QC 90.8-94
  Used for special purposes, by subject
Metritis see Endometritis
Metrizamide
  As a contrast medium   WN 160
  Used for special purposes, by subject
Metronidazole   QV 254
Metrorrhagia   WP 555
Mevalonic Acid   QU 98
  Organic chemistry
    Aliphatic compounds   QD 305.A2
Mexiletine   QV 150
Mezcalin see Mescaline
MgADP see Adenosine Diphosphate
MgATP see Adenosine Triphosphate
MGI-1 see Colony-Stimulating Factors
MHC Class I Genes see Genes, MHC Class I
MHC Class II Genes see Genes, MHC Class II
MHPG see Methoxyhydroxyphenylglycol
Mianserin
  As an antidepressant   QV 77.5
Mice
  As laboratory animals   QY 60.R6
  Diseases   SF 997.5.M4
Mice, Athymic see Mice, Nude
Mice, House see Mice
Mice, Inbred Strains
  As laboratory animals   QY 60.R6
Mice, Laboratory see Mice
Mice, Mutant Strains
  As laboratory animals   QY 60.R6
Mice, Neurologic Mutants
  As laboratory animals   QY 60.R6
Mice, Nude
  As laboratory animals   QY 60.R6
Mice, Red-Backed see Microtinae
Mice, Transgenic
  As laboratory animals   QY 60.R6
  Genetic aspects   QH 442.6
Micelles
  Biochemistry   QU 133
Miconazole   QV 252
Micro-Organisms see Bacteria, Fungi, Rickettsia,
  Viruses
Microabrasion, Dental see Enamel Microabrasion
Microabrasion, Enamel see Enamel Microabrasion
Microangiopathy, Diabetic see Diabetic
  Angiopathies
Microbial Collagenase   QU 136
Microbial Sensitivity Tests   QW 25.5.M6
Microbiological Techniques   QW 25
  See also names of specific techniques and tests

**ALWAYS CONSULT MAIN SCHEDULES. USE NUMBER ASSIGNED ONLY WHEN
SUBJECT REPRESENTS MAJOR EMPHASIS OF WORK BEING CLASSIFIED**

Microbiology   QW
   Air see Air Microbiology   QW 82
   Dental   QW 65
   Food see Food Microbiology   QW 85
   Industrial   QW 75
   Plant   QW 60
   Soil see Soil microbiology   QW 60
   Veterinary medicine   QW 70
   Water see Water Microbiology   QW 80
   See also Microbiology under names of animals,
      organs, plants, diseases, etc., e.g., under Mouth
        QW 65; Bacteriology   QW; Virology   QW
      160, etc.
Microbodies   QH 603.M35
Microcapsules see Capsules
Microcephaly   QS 675
Microchemistry
   Analytical chemistry (General)   QD 79.M5
   Organic analysis (General)   QD 272.M5
   Qualitative analysis   QD 98.M5
   Quantitative analysis   QD 117.M5
Microcirculation   WG 104
Microclimate
   Of a particular area, with the area
   See also Climate
Microcomputers   QA 75.5–76.95
   As equipment in special fields
      In medicine (General)   W 26.55.C7
      (Form number 26.5 in any other NLM schedule
      where applicable)
   Computer engineering   TK 7885–7895
   See also Computers
Microcytotoxicity Tests see Cytotoxicity Tests,
Immunologic
Microelectrodes   QD 571
   Biomedical engineering   QT 36
   In electric stimulation therapy   WB 495
   In electrosurgery   WO 198
Microencapsulation see Drug Compounding
Microfilament Proteins   QU 55
Microfilaria   QX 301
Microfilming   TR 835
   In library science   Z 681
   In printing   Z 265
Microfluorometry see Cytophotometry
Microfluorometry, Flow see Flow Cytometry
Micrographic Surgery, Mohs see Mohs Surgery
Microinjections   WB 354
   Special topics, by subject
Microinterferometry see Microscopy, Interference
Micrometry see Weights and Measures
Micronutrients
   Biochemistry   QU 130.5
   Analytical chemistry   QD 139.T7
Microprocessors see Microcomputers
Micropunctures see Punctures
Microradiography   WN 100
Microscopy   QH 201–278.5
   Histology   QS 525
   Micrometry   QC 101–114
   Pathology   QZ 25
   Slit–lamp   WW 143
   Used for other special purposes, by subject

Microscopy, Electron   QH 212.E4
   In cytodiagnosis   QY 95
   Used for other special purposes, by subject
Microscopy, Electron, Scanning   QH 212.S3
   Used for special purposes, by subject, e.g., for
      examining dental pulp   WU 230
Microscopy, Electron, Transmission see Microscopy,
Electron
Microscopy, Electron, X–Ray Microanalysis see
Electron Probe Microanalysis
Microscopy, Fluorescence   QH 212.F55
   Used in diagnosis of pulmonary tuberculosis
      WF 300
   Used for other special purposes, by subject
Microscopy, Immunofluorescence see Microscopy,
Fluorescence
Microscopy, Interference   QH 212.I5
   Experimental histology   QS 530
   Used for other special purposes, by subject
Microscopy, Phase–Contrast   QH 212.P5
   Used for special purposes, by subject, e.g., in
      cytoscopic examination of urine   QY 185
Microscopy, Polarization   QH 212.P6
   Used for special purposes, by subject, e.g. in
      clinical pathology   QY 95
Microscopy, Polarized Light see Microscopy,
Polarization
Microscopy, Ultraviolet   QH 212.U48
Microsomes   QH 603.M4
Microsomes, Liver   WI 700
Microsurgery   WO 512
   Localized, by site
Microsurgery, Laser see Laser Surgery
Microsurgical Revascularization, Cerebral see
Cerebral Revascularization
Microtinae   QL 737.R666
   Diseases   SF 997.5.R3
   As laboratory animals   QY 60.R6
Microtines see Microtinae
Microtomy   QH 233
Microtrabecular Lattice see Cytoskeleton
Microtubule–Associated Proteins   QU 55
Microtubule Proteins   QU 55
Microtubules   QH 603.M44
Microtus see Microtinae
Microvascular Permeability see Capillary
Permeability
Microvilli   QH 601
Microwaves   TK 7876
   Diagnostic use   WB 141
   Therapeutic use   WB 510
Midazolam   QV 85
Midbrain see Mesencephalon
Midbrain Central Gray see Periaqueductal Gray
Middle Age
   Developmental psychology   BF 724.6
   Medical treatment   WT 100
   Special topics, by subject
Middle Ear see Ear, Middle
Middle Ear Ventilation   WV 232
Midges, Biting see Ceratopogonidae
Midges, Nonbiting see Chironomidae

Midwifery   WQ 160–165
  See also Nurse Midwives   WY 157
Mifepristone
  As an abortifacient agent   QV 175
  As a contraceptive agent   QV 177
  Special topics, by subject
Migraine   WL 344
Migrants see Transients and Migrants
Migration, Cell see Cell Movement
Migration, Internal see Transients and Migrants
Miliaria   WR 400
Miliaria Rubra see Miliaria
Miliary Tuberculosis see Tuberculosis, Miliary
Milieu Therapy   WM 440
  Adolescence   WS 463
  Child   WS 350.2
Military Dentistry   UH 430–435
  Aviation   WD 745
  Naval   VG 280–285
Military Hygiene   UH 600–629.5
Military Medicine   UH 201–570
  Biography
    Collective   WZ 112.5.M4
    Individual   WZ 100
  History   UH 215–324
    American Civil War   E 621–625
    World War I (U.S.)   D 629.U6, etc.
    World War II (U.S.)   D 807.U6, etc.
    See also other specific wars in LC schedules
    D–F.
  Surgery   WO 800
    History   WO 11
  Special topics, by subject
Military Nursing   WY 130
  Education   WY 18–18.5
  Veterans hospitals   WY 130
Military Personnel
  General topics   U 1–145
  Military life   U 750–773
  Veterans   UB 356–405
  See also special aspects of military life, e.g.
    Disabled Veterans   UB 360–366 under
    Rehabilitation
Military Physicians see Military Medicine; Physicians
Military Psychiatry   UH 629–629.5
  See also Combat Disorders   WM 184
Military Psychology see Psychology, Military
Military Science   U
  Air defense   UG 730
    Civil   UA 926–929
    Military
      Anti–aircraft guns   UF 625
      Military aeronautics   UG 623–1435
Military Surgeons see Military Medicine; Biography
  WZ 112.5.M4, etc. under Surgery
Military Surgery see Military Medicine; Military
  WO 800 under Surgery
Military Veterinary Service see Veterinary Service,
  Military
Milk
  Analysis
    Dairying   SF 251–262.5
    Public health   WA 716
  Bacteriology   QW 85

Dairying (General)   SF 221–275
  Public health aspects   WA 715–719
Diet (General)   WB 428
  Child   WS 120; WS 130
  Infant   WS 120; WS 130
  Preparation for use   SF 259
  Public health aspects   WA 715–719
  Pasteurization   WA 719
Milk–Alkali Syndrome see Hypercalcemia
Milk Fever, Animal see Parturient Paresis
Milk, Human
  Infant feeding   WS 125
  Secretion   WP 825
Milk Of Magnesia see Magnesium Hydroxide
Milk Proteins   WA 716
  Dairy science   SF 251
Milk Sickness   WD 530
Millipedes see Arthropods
Milroy's Disease see Lymphedema
Miltown see Meprobamate
Milzbrand see Anthrax
Mimetic Muscles see Facial Muscles
Minamata Disease see Mercury Poisoning
Mind–Body Relations (Metaphysics)
  In alternative medicine   WB 880
Mind–Body Relations (Non–Physiology) see
  Mind–Body Relations (Metaphysics)
Mineral Content of Food see Minerals
Mineral Fibers
  Biochemistry   QU 130
  As environmental air pollutants   WA 754
  Causing a specific disease, with the disease
Mineral Oil   QV 75
Mineral Waters   WB 442
Mineralocorticoids   WK 755
Minerals
  Biochemistry   QU 130
  Mineralogy   QE 351–399.2
  Of bone   WE 200
Miner's Anemia see Hookworm Infections
Minimal Access Surgical Procedures see Surgical
  Procedures, Minimally Invasive
Minimal Brain Dysfunction see Attention Deficit
  Disorder with Hyperactivity
Minimal Surgical Procedures see Surgical
  Procedures, Minimally Invasive
Minimally Invasive Surgical Procedures see Surgical
  Procedures, Minimally Invasive
Mining   TN
  Occupational accidents   WA 485
  Occupational medicine   WA 400–495
  See also Pneumoconiosis   WF 654 and other
  related disorders
Mink   QL 737.C25
  Culture   SF 405.M6
  Diseases   SF 997.5.M5
Mink Encephalopathy Virus see Prions
Minnesota Multiphasic Personality Inventory see
  MMPI
Minnows see Cyprinidae
Minocycline   QV 360
Minor Injuries see Wounds and Injuries
Minor Surgery see Surgical Procedures, Minor

ALWAYS CONSULT MAIN SCHEDULES. USE NUMBER ASSIGNED ONLY WHEN
SUBJECT REPRESENTS MAJOR EMPHASIS OF WORK BEING CLASSIFIED

Minority Groups
  Adolescents WS 462
  Representation JF 1061-1063
  Suffrage JF 879
  Special topics, by subject
  See also Ethnic Groups GN 301-673, etc. and
    specific ethnic groups
Minoxidil QV 150
Mint see Lamiaceae
Miopithecus talapoin see Cercopithecidae
Miotics QV 120
Mirex
  Agriculture SB 952.C44
  Public health WA 240
Mirror Writing see Dominance, Cerebral
Misarticulation see Articulation Disorders
Miscarriage see Abortion, Spontaneous
Miscegenation see Anthropology, Physical;
  Marriage; Racial Stocks
Missions and Missionaries W 323
  Biography (if medically related)
    Collective WZ 112-150
    Individual WZ 100
  See also Medical missions, Official W 323
Missions, Official Medical see Medical Missions,
  Official
Misuse, Equipment see Equipment Failure
Misuse of Health Services see Health Services
  Misuse
Mite-Borne Rickettsial Fevers see Rickettsia
  Infections; names of specific infections
Mite Control see Tick Control
Mite Infestations
  Disinfestation WC 900
  General WC 900
  Veterinary SF 810.M5
  See also Scabies WR 365, etc.
Mites
  General QX 473
  Sarcoptoidea QX 475
  See also names of specific mites, e.g., Sarcoptes
    Scabiei QX 475
Mithramycin see Plicamycin
Mitochondria QH 603.M5
Mitochondria, Liver WI 700
Mitochondria, Muscle WE 500
Mitogenic Factors, Lymphocyte see Interleukin-2
Mitogens QH 605.2
Mitogens, Endogenous see Growth Substances
Mitomycins QV 269
Mitosis QH 605.2
Mitoxantrone QV 269
Mitozantrone see Mitoxantrone
Mitral Click-Murmur Syndrome see Mitral Valve
  Prolapse
Mitral Incompetence see Mitral Valve Insufficiency
Mitral Regurgitation see Mitral Valve Insufficiency
Mitral Valve Incompetence see Mitral Valve
  Insufficiency
Mitral Valve Insufficiency WG 262
Mitral Valve Prolapse WG 262
Mitral Valve Stenosis WG 262
Mixed Connective Tissue Disease WD 375

Mixed Function Oxidases QU 140
Mixed Function Oxygenases see Mixed Function
  Oxidases
Mixtures see Dosage Forms
MK-421 see Enalapril
MMPI WM 145.5.M6
MN Sialoglycoprotein see Glycophorin
Mobile Emergency Units see Ambulances
Mobile Health Units WX 190
  In specialty fields (Form number 27-28 in any
    NLM schedule where applicable)
Models, Anatomic QY 35
Models, Biological QH 324.8
  Of a particular subject, by subject, e.g. of human
    gait WE 103
Models, Cardiovascular WG 20
  Of a particular subject, by subject
Models, Chemical QD 480
  Biochemistry QU 25 or in number for the item
    represented
Models, Computer see Computer Simulation
Models, Decision Support see Decision Support
  Techniques
Models, Dental see Dental Models
Models, Genetic
  Medical QZ 50
  Special topics, by subject
Models, Molecular QD 480
  Used for special purposes, by subject
Models, Neurological
  Research WL 20
  Study and teaching WL 18.2
Models, Nursing WY 20.5
  Specific topics, by subject
Models, Obstetrical see Models, Structural
Models, Psychological
  Experimental psychology BF 181-188
  Psychiatric
    Used in research WM 20
    Used in teaching WM 18.2
  Of specific subjects, by subject
Models, Statistical
  Used for special purposes, by subject
Models, Structural
  Construction QY 35
  Obstetrical WQ 26
  Other specific types, with the subject being
    illustrated
  Used in teaching (Form number 18.2 in any NLM
    schedule where applicable)
  See also Phantoms, Imaging WN 150
Models, Theoretical
  As an educational tool (Form number 18.2 in any
    NLM schedule where applicable)
  Model theory QA 9.7
  Used for special purposes, by subject
Mohammedanism see Islam
Mohs Surgery WR 500
Moire Topography TR 708
  Used for specific subjects, by subject
Molar WU 101
Molar, Third WU 101
  Abnormalities WU 101.5
  Extraction WU 605

Molasses
  As a dietary supplement in health or disease
    WB 447
Molds see Fungi
Molds (Casts) see Dental Models; Models, Structural
Molecular Biology   QH 506
Molecular Biology, Computational see
  Computational Biology
Molecular Cloning see Cloning, Molecular
Molecular Configuration see Molecular
  Conformation
Molecular Conformation   QC 179
Molecular Evolution see Evolution, Molecular
Molecular Genetics see Genetics, Biochemical
Molecular Models see Models, Molecular
Molecular Motors
  General   QU 55
  See also Cytoskeletal Proteins   QU 55;
    Cytoskeleton   QH 603.C96
Molecular Neurobiology see Neurobiology
Molecular Probes   QY 95
  Used for diagnosis of particular disorders, with
    the disorder or system
Molecular Radiobiology see Radiobiology
Molecular Sequence Data
  Of a specific substance, with the substance
Molecular Stereochemistry see Molecular
  Conformation
Molecular Structure   QD 461
Molecular Vaccines see Vaccines, Synthetic
Molecular Weight   QD 463-464
  Biochemistry   QU 25
Molestation, Sexual, Child see Child Abuse, Sexual
Mollities Ossium see Osteomalacia
Mollusca   QX 675
Molluscacides
  Agriculture   SB 951.65
  Public health   WA 240
Molluscum Contagiosum   WC 584
Molsidomine   QV 150
Molting Hormone see Ecdysone
Molybdenum
  Inorganic chemistry   QD 181.M7
  Metabolism   QU 130.5
  Pharmacology   QV 290
Mongolism see Down Syndrome
Mongoloid Race
  Anthropology   GN 548
  See also specific topics under Ethnic Groups
Monieziasis   SF 810.C5
Monilia see Candida
Moniliasis see Candidiasis
Moniliasis, Cutaneous see Candidiasis, Cutaneous
Moniliasis, Oral see Candidiasis, Oral
Monitoring, Ambulatory Electrocardiographic see
  Electrocardiography, Ambulatory
Monitoring, Environmental see Environmental
  Monitoring
Monitoring, Fetal see Fetal Monitoring
Monitoring, Holter see Electrocardiography,
  Ambulatory
Monitoring, Home Blood Glucose see Blood

Glucose Self–Monitoring
Monitoring, Immune see Monitoring, Immunologic
Monitoring, Immunologic   QW 525
Monitoring, Intraoperative   WO 181
Monitoring, Physiologic   WB 142
  Cardiovascular system   WG 140
  Drug utilization   WB 330
  In intensive care   WX 218, etc.
  Of particular function, by subject
  Of other systems, in the examination number,
    usually 141, in the schedule for the system
  See also Radiation Monitoring   WN 650
Monitoring, Radioimmunologic see Monitoring,
  Immunologic
Monitors, Blood Pressure see Blood Pressure
  Monitors
Monkey, African Green see Cercopithecus aethiops
Monkey, Capuchin see Cebus
Monkey, Colobus see Colobus
Monkey Diseases   SF 997.5.P7
Monkey, Green see Cercopithecus aethiops
Monkey, Grivet see Cercopithecus aethiops
Monkey, Japanese see Macaca
Monkey, Northern Night see Aotus trivirgatus
Monkey, Patas see Erythrocebus patas
Monkey, Pig–Tailed see Macaca nemestrina
Monkey, Red see Erythrocebus patas
Monkey, Rhesus see Macaca mulatta
Monkey, Ring–Tail see Cebus
Monkey, Spider see Cebidae
Monkey, Squirrel see Saimiri
Monkey, Talapoin see Cercopithecidae
Monkey, Vervet see Cercopithecus aethiops
Monkey, Woolly see Cebidae
Monkeypox Virus   QW 165.5.P6
Monkeys see Haplorhini
Monkeys, New World see Cebidae
Monkeys, Old World see Cercopithecidae
Monoacylglycerols see Glycerides
Monoamine Oxidase   QU 140
Monoamine Oxidase Inhibitors   QV 77.5
Monoblastic Leukemia see Leukemia, Monoblastic
Monoclonal Antibodies see Antibodies, Monoclonal
Monoclonal Gammopathies see Paraproteinemias
Monoclonal Gammopathies, Benign   WH 400
Monocytes   WH 200
  In phagocytosis   QW 690
Monocytic Angina see Infectious Mononucleosis
Monocytic Leukemia see Leukemia, Monocytic
Monocytic Leukemia, Chronic see Leukemia,
  Monocytic, Chronic
Mononucleosis, Infectious see Infectious
  Mononucleosis
Monorchidism see Abnormalities   WJ 840 under
  Testis
Monosaccharides   QU 75
Monosodium Glutamate see Sodium Glutamate
Monosomy, Partial see Chromosome Deletion
Monounsaturated Fatty Acids see Fatty Acids,
  Monounsaturated
Monsters   QS 675
Monte Carlo Method   QA 298
  Special topics, by subject

**ALWAYS CONSULT MAIN SCHEDULES. USE NUMBER ASSIGNED ONLY WHEN
SUBJECT REPRESENTS MAJOR EMPHASIS OF WORK BEING CLASSIFIED**

Mood see Affect
Mood Disorders   WM 171
   Adolescence   WS 463
   Child   WS 350.6
   Infant   WS 350.6
Moon
MOPEG see Methoxyhydroxyphenylglycol
Morale   BJ 45
   War   U 22
Morals
   Adolescence   WS 462
   Child   WS 105.5.M4
   Ethics   BJ 11–18
   Psychoanalysis   WM 460.5.R3
   Sex   HQ 32
   Sociology   HM
Moraxella   QW 131
Morbid Obesity see Obesity, Morbid
Morbidity   WA 900
Morbillivirus   QW 168.5.P2
Morgagni–Stewart–Morel Syndrome see
   Hyperostosis Frontalis Interna
Mormyrid see Electric Fish
Morning–After Pill see Contraceptives, Postcoital
Moronity see Mental Retardation
Morphea see Scleroderma, Circumscribed
Morphine   QV 92
Morphine Dependence   WM 286
Morphine Derivatives   QV 92
Morphogenesis
   General biology   QH 491
   Human embryology   QS 604
   Localized, by site
Morphology see Anatomy
Morquio's Disease see Mucopolysaccharidosis IV
Morsydomine see Molsidomine
Mortality   HB 1321–1528
   Child   HB 1323.C5
   Infant   HB 1323.I4
   Including causes of death   WA 900
   See also Fetal Death   WQ 225; Maternal
     Mortality   HB 1322.5, etc.
Mortuary Customs see Funeral Rites
Mortuary Practice   WA 840–847
   Burial   WA 846
   Cemeteries   WA 846
   Cremation   WA 847
   General works   WA 840
Mosaicism   QH 445.7
Mosquito Control   QX 600
   Malaria control   WC 765
Mosquitoes see Culicidae
Mosses   QK 534–549.5
Mother Cells see Stem Cells
Mother–Child Relations   WS 105.5.F2
Mothers   HQ 759–759.5
   Special topics, by subject
Mothers, Surrogate see Surrogate Mothers
Moths   QX 560
Motilin   WK 170
Motility, Cell see Cell Movement
Motion
   Aviation medicine   WD 720

Special effects, by subject
   See also Movement   WE 103
Motion Perception
   Visual   WW 105
   See also Kinesthesis   WE 104
Motion Pictures
   Catalogs and works about
     (Form number 18.2 in any NLM schedule
     where applicable)
   Influence on children   WS 105.5.E9
   Reels, etc., by subject
Motion Sickness   WD 630
Motivation   BF 501–504
   Adolescence   WS 462
   Child   WS 105.5.M5
   Infant   WS 105.5.M5
   Psychoanalysis   WM 460.5.M6
Motor Activity   WE 103
   Child   WE 103
   Infant   WE 103
   Perceptual motor learning   BF 295
Motor Cortex   WL 307
Motor Endplate   WL 102.9
Motor Epilepsy see Epilepsy
Motor Neuron Disease   WE 550
Motor Neurons   WL 102.7
Motor Neurons, Gamma   WL 102.7
Motor Skills   WE 103
   Child   WE 103
   Infant   WE 103
   Psychological aspects   WE 104
Motor Skills Disorders
   Developmental   WS 340
   Neurologic   WL 390
   Psychogenic   WM 197
Motor Vehicle Accidents see Accidents, Traffic
Motor Vehicles   TL 1–390
   Accidents   WA 275
   Air pollution   WA 754
   Human engineering in design   TL 250
   Noise hazard   WA 776
   See also specific type of vehicles, e.g.,
     Ambulances   WX 215, etc.
Mottled Enamel see Fluorosis, Dental
Moulages see Models, Anatomic
Mountain Sickness see Altitude Sickness
Mountaineering
   Accidents and illness   QT 260.5.M9
   Altitude sickness   WD 715
   First aid   WA 292
   Sports   QT 260.5.M9
Mourning see Grief
Mouse Leukemia Viruses see Leukemia Viruses,
   Murine
Mouse Thymic Virus see Herpesviridae
Mouse Tumor Viruses see Tumor Viruses, Murine
Mouth   WU
   General works for the dentist   WU 140
   General works for the gastroenterologist   WI
     200
   Injuries   WU 158
   Microbiology   QW 65
   Pathology   WU 140

Surgery   WU 600
See also Administration, Oral   WB 350
Mouth Abnormalities   WU 101.5
Mouth Breathing   WF 143
Special topics, by subject
Mouth Diseases
General works for the dentist   WU 140
Therapy   WU 166
General works for the gastroenterologist   WI 200
Therapy   WI 200
Mouth Dryness see Xerostomia
Mouth, Edentulous   WU 140
Dentures for   WU 530
Mouth Floor
Dentistry   WU 140
Gastroenterology   WI 200
Mouth Mucosa
For the dentist   WU 101
For the gastroenterologist   WI 200
Mouth Neoplasms   WU 280
Works for the gastroenterologist   WI 200
Mouth Rehabilitation   WU 140
Jaw injuries   WU 610
Oral and dental injuries   WU 158
Surgery   WU 600-640
Mouth-to-Mouth Resuscitation see
Cardiopulmonary Resuscitation
Mouth Ulcer see Oral Ulcer
Mouthwashes   WU 113
Pharmacology   QV 50
Movement   WE 103
Movement, Cell see Cell Movement
Movement disorder, Stereotypic see Stereotypic
Movement Disorder
Movement Disorders   WL 390
Child   WS 340
Infant   WS 340
Neuromuscular see Neuromuscular Diseases
WE 550-559
Psychomotor see Psychomotor Disorders   WM 197
Veterinary   SF 901
Localized, by site or disease involved
Moxalactam   QV 350
Moxibustion   WB 369
Moyamoya Disease   WL 355
MR Spectroscopy see Nuclear Magnetic Resonance
MR Tomography see Magnetic Resonance Imaging
MRI Scans see Magnetic Resonance Imaging
mRNA see RNA, Messenger
MSG see Sodium Glutamate
MSH   WK 515
mu Immunoglobulins see Immunoglobulins,
mu-Chain
Mucins   QU 55
Mucociliary Clearance   WF 102
Mucociliary Transport see Mucociliary Clearance
Mucocutaneous Lymph Node Syndrome   WH 700
Mucolytic Agents see Expectorants
Mucopolysaccharidosis I   WD 205.5.C2
Mucopolysaccharidosis IV   WD 205.5.C2
Mucopolysaccharidosis V see

Mucopolysaccharidosis I
Mucoproteins   QU 55
In blood chemistry   QY 455
Mucorales   QW 180.5.P4
Mucosal Immunity see Immunity, Mucosal
Mucous Membrane   QS 532.5.M8
Drugs affecting   QV 60-65
Mucoviscidosis see Cystic Fibrosis
Mucus   QS 532.5.M8
Mud Baths see Mud Therapy
Mud Therapy   WB 525
Mudminnows see Salmonidae
Multi-Hospital Information Systems see Hospital
Information Systems
Multi-Hospital Systems see Multi-Institutional
Systems
Multi-Infarct Dementia see Dementia, Multi-Infarct
Multi-Institutional Systems
Hospitals (General)   WX 157.4
In specific fields, by subject
Multiculturalism see Cultural Diversity
Multifactorial Inheritance see Polygenic Inheritance
Multigene Family   QH 447
Multilingualism
In language development   WS 105.5.C8
Multimedia
(Form number 18.2 in any NLM schedule where
applicable)
Special topics, by subject
Multimodal Treatment see Combined Modality
Therapy
Multiphasic Screening   WA 245
Multiple Epiphyseal Dysplasia see
Osteochondrodysplasias
Multiple Myeloma   WH 540
Multiple Organ Failure   QZ 140
In specific diseases, with the disease
Multiple Personality Disorder   WM 173.6
Multiple Pregnancy see Pregnancy, Multiple
Multiple Sclerosis   WL 360
Multiple Trauma   WO 700
Multiplication-Stimulating Activity see Insulin-Like
Growth Factor II
Multipotential Colony-Stimulating Factor see
Interleukin-3
Multivariate Analysis   QA 278
Special topics, by subject
Mumps   WC 520
Mumps Vaccine   WC 520
Munchausen Syndrome   WM 178
Mur-NAc-L-Ala-D-isoGln see
Acetylmuramyl-Alanyl-Isoglutamine
Muramidase   QU 136
Muramyl Dipeptide see
Acetylmuramyl-Alanyl-Isoglutamine
Murder see Homicide
Muridae   QL 737.R666
Diseases   SF 997.5.R64
As laboratory animals   QY 60.R6
Murids see Muridae
Murine Leukemia Viruses see Leukemia Viruses,
Murine
Murine Tumor Viruses see Tumor Viruses, Murine

Murine Typhus see Typhus, Endemic Flea–Borne
Murray Valley Encephalitis Virus see Flaviviruses
Mus see Muridae
Mus musculus see Mice
Musca domestica see Houseflies
Muscarinic Agents see Cholinergic Agents
Muscarinic Antagonists   QV 132
Muscarinic Receptors see Receptors, Muscarinic
Musci see Mosses
Muscle Contraction   WE 500
Muscle Contracture see Contracture
Muscle Cramp   WE 550
Muscle Denervation   WE 500
Muscle Dystonia see Dystonia
Muscle Neoplasms   WE 550
Muscle Proteins   WE 500
Muscle Relaxants, Central   QV 140
    In anesthesia   WO 297
Muscle Relaxants, Depolarizing see Neuromuscular
    Depolarizing Agents
Muscle Relaxants, Non–Depolarizing see
    Neuromuscular Nondepolarizing Agents
Muscle Relaxants, Polarizing see Neuromuscular
    Nondepolarizing Agents
Muscle Relaxation   WE 500
Muscle Rigidity   WE 550
Muscle, Smooth   WE 500
    Localized, by site
Muscle, Smooth, Vascular   WE 500
Muscle Spasticity   WE 550
    Child   WS 270
    Infant   WS 270
Muscle Spindles   WL 102.9
Muscle Tonus   WE 500
Muscle Weakness   WE 550
Muscles   WE 500–559
    Anatomy   WE 500
    Physiology   WE 500
    Localized, by site
Muscular Atrophy   WE 550
    Veterinary   SF 901
Muscular Atrophy, Spinal   WE 550
Muscular Diseases   WE 544–559
    General works   WE 550
    Child   WS 270
    Infant   WS 270
Muscular Dystrophy   WE 559
Musculocutaneous Nerve   WL 400
    See also names of organs innervated, e.g. Forearm
        WE 820
Musculoskeletal Abnormalities   WE 101
Musculoskeletal Diseases   WE 140
    Child   WS 270
    Infant   WS 270
    Nursing   WY 157.6
Musculoskeletal Physiology   WE 102
Musculoskeletal System   WE
    Child   WS 270
    Infant   WS 270
    Injuries (General)   WE 140
        See also Orthopedics   WE 168–190
    Neoplasms (General)   WE 140
        See also Muscle Neoplasms   WE 550;

    Neoplasms, Muscle Tissue   QZ 340
    Nursing care   WY 157.6
    Physiology see Musculoskeletal Physiology
        WE 102
    Trunk   WE 700
Museums
    (Form numbers 27–28 in QS–QT, QV–QZ, W,
        WA and WZ schedules)
    Art   N 405–3990
    General   AM
    Scientific   Q 105
Mushroom Poisoning   WD 520
Mushrooms
    Edible   QK 617
    Poisonous   QW 180.5.B2
Music   M
    Special topics, by subject, e.g., mouth instruments
        as a cause of malocclusion   WU 440
Music Therapy
    General   WB 550
    In psychiatry   WM 450.5.M8
Muskrats see Microtinae
Muslims see Islam
Mussels   QX 675
Mustard
    As a condiment plant   SB 307.M87
    As a skin irritant   QV 65
    Botany   QK 495.C9
Mustard Compounds
    As antineoplastics   QV 269
    Chemical warfare agent   QV 666
    Organic chemistry
        Aliphatic compounds   QD 305.H5
Mustard Gas
    As a carcinogen   QZ 202
    As a chemical warfare agent   QV 666
Mustard Plasters see Therapeutic use   WB 371
    under Irritants
Mustine see Mechlorethamine
Mutagen Screening see Mutagenicity Tests
Mutagenesis   QH 460–468
Mutagenesis, Oligonucleotide–Directed see
    Mutagenesis, Site–Directed
Mutagenesis, Site–Directed   QH 465.S5
Mutagenesis, Site–Specific see Mutagenesis,
    Site–Directed
Mutagenicity Tests   QH 465
Mutagens
    As a cause of congenital abnormalities   QS 679
    As air pollutants   WA 754
    General works on chemical mutagens   QH 460
    Industrial waste   WA 788
    Virology   QW 160
Mutases see Oxidoreductases
Mutation
    Evolution   QH 390
    Genetics   QH 460–468
    In specific organisms, with the organism
Mutational Analysis, DNA see DNA Mutational
    Analysis
Mutism
    Associated with deafness   WV 280
    Psychogenic   WM 475

Hysterical   WM 173.5
Other specific associations, by subject
See also Akinetic Mutism   WL 348;
   Deaf–Mutism   WV 280
Mutism, Akinetic see Akinetic Mutism
Myalgia, Epidemic see Pleurodynia, Epidemic
Myasthenia Gravis   WE 555
Myatonia Congenita see Neuromuscular Diseases
myb Genes see Oncogenes
Mycetoma see Maduromycosis
Mycobacteriaceae   QW 125.5.M9
Mycobacteriophages   QW 161.5.M9
Mycobacterium   QW 125.5.M9
Mycobacterium bovis   QW 125.5.M9
Mycobacterium Infections   WC 302
   See also Leprosy   WC 335; Paratuberculosis
   SF 809.J6; Tuberculosis   WF, etc.
Mycobacterium Infections, Atypical   WC 302
Mycobacterium leprae   QW 125.5.M9
Mycobacterium tuberculosis   QW 125.5.M9
Mycology
   Botany   QK 600–635
   Fungus diseases see Mycoses   WC 450–475
   Medical (General)   QW 180
      Dictionaries   QW 13
      Laboratory manuals   QW 25
   Methods in medical mycology   QY 110
   See also Fungi   QW 180, etc.
Mycoplasma   QW 143
Mycoplasma Infections   WC 246
   Veterinary   SF 809.M9
Mycoplasma Pneumonia see Pneumonia,
   Mycoplasma
Mycoplasmatales   QW 143
Mycoplasmatales Infections   WC 246
Mycoses   WC 450–475
   Veterinary   SF 780.7
   See also Dermatomycosis   WR 300–340, etc.;
      Lung Diseases, Fungal   WF 652; and names
      of specific fungal diseases
Mycosis Fungoides   WR 500
Mycotic Aneurysm see Aneurysm, Infected
Mycotic Lung Infections see Lung Diseases, Fungal
Mycotic Skin Infections see Dermatomycoses
Mycotoxicosis   WD 520
Mycotoxins   QW 630.5.M9
Mydriasis see Pupil   WW 240; Dilatation,
   Pathologic   WW 240, etc.
Mydriatics   QV 134
Myelencephalon see Embryology   WL 300 under
   Brain
Myelin Sheath   WL 102.5
Myelitis   WL 400
Myeloblastic Leukemia see Leukemia, Myeloblastic
Myelocele see Meningomyelocele
Myelocytic Leukemia see Leukemia, Myelocytic
Myelocytic Leukemia, Chronic see Leukemia,
   Myeloid, Chronic
Myelodysplasia see Neural Tube Defects
Myelodysplastic Syndromes   WH 380
Myelofibrosis   WH 380
Myelogenous Leukemia see Leukemia, Myeloid
Myelogenous Leukemia, Chronic see Leukemia,

Myeloid, Chronic
Myelography   WL 405
Myeloid Leukemia see Leukemia, Myeloid
Myeloid Leukemia, Chronic see Leukemia, Myeloid,
   Chronic
Myeloid Tissue see Bone Marrow
Myeloma, Plasma Cell see Multiple Myeloma
Myeloma Proteins   WH 540
Myelomeningocele see Meningomyelocele
Myelopathic Muscular Atrophy see Muscular
   Atrophy, Spinal
Myelophthisic Anemia see Anemia, Myelophthisic
Myeloproliferative Disorders   WH 380
   See also Anemia, Myelophthisic   WH 175;
      Leukemoid Reaction   WH 200; Polycythemia
      Vera   WH 180
Myelosclerosis see Myelofibrosis
Myenteric Plexus   WL 600
Myers–Briggs Type Indicator see Personality
   Inventory
Myiasis   WC 900
   Veterinary   SF 810.F5
Myoblastoma see Neoplasms, Muscle Tissue
Myocardial Contraction   WG 280
Myocardial Depressants see Anti–Arrhythmia
   Agents
Myocardial Diseases   WG 280
   Veterinary   SF 811
Myocardial Diseases, Primary see Myocardial
   Diseases
Myocardial Diseases, Secondary see Myocardial
   Diseases
Myocardial Infarction   WG 300
Myocardial Ischemia   WG 300
Myocardial Preconditioning see Ischemic
   Preconditioning, Myocardial
Myocardial Preinfarction Syndrome see Angina,
   Unstable
Myocardial Remodeling, Ventricular see Ventricular
   Remodeling
Myocardial Reperfusion   WG 280
Myocardial Reperfusion Injury   WG 280
Myocardial Revascularization   WG 169
Myocardial Stimulants see Cardiotonic Agents
Myocardiopathies see Myocardial Diseases
Myocarditis   WG 280
Myocardium   WG 280
   See also Myocardial Revascularization   WG 169
Myoclonia Epileptica see Epilepsy, Myoclonic
Myoclonic Epilepsy, Progressive see Epilepsy,
   Myoclonic
Myoclonic Jerking see Epilepsy, Myoclonic
Myoclonic Jerking, Massive see Spasms, Infantile
Myoclonus   WE 550
Myodystrophia Fetalis Deformans see
   Arthrogryposis
Myoepithelial Tumor see Myoepithelioma
Myoepithelioma   QZ 310
   Localized, by site
Myofascial Pain Dysfunction Syndrome,
   Temporomandibular Joint see
      Temporomandibular Joint Dysfunction Syndrome
Myofascial Pain Syndromes   WE 550

ALWAYS CONSULT MAIN SCHEDULES. USE NUMBER ASSIGNED ONLY WHEN
SUBJECT REPRESENTS MAJOR EMPHASIS OF WORK BEING CLASSIFIED

Myofibrils   WE 500
Myofunctional Therapy
    In dentistry (General)   WU 140-140.5
    For particular diseases, with the disease
Myoglobin   WH 190
    Clinical analysis   QY 455
Myoglobinuria   WJ 344
Myoinositol see Inositol
Myoma   QZ 340
    Uterine see Leiomyoma   WP 459; Uterine
      Neoplasms   WP 459, etc.
Myometrium   WP 400-460, 468
Myoneural Junction see Neuromuscular Junction
Myopathies see Muscular Diseases
Myopia   WW 320
Myositis   WE 544
Myotonia   WE 550
Myoxidae see Rodentia
Myringoplasty   WV 225
Mysticism   BV 5070-5095
    And alchemy   QD 23.3-26.5
    And hallucinogens   QV 77.7
Mythology   BL 300-325
    In medicine and related fields   WZ 309
Mytilus see Mussels
Myxedema   WK 252
Myxobacterales see Myxococcales
Myxococcales   QW 128
Myxoma   QZ 340
    Localized, by site
Myxoma Virus   QW 165.5.P6
Myxomatosis, Infectious   SF 997.5.R2
Myxomatosis Virus see Myxoma Virus
Myxomycetes   QW 180.5.M9
Myxomycota see Myxomycetes
Myxovirus Infections see Orthomyxoviridae
    Infections
Myxovirus influenzae-A suis see Influenza A Virus,
    Porcine
Myxovirus pestis galli see Influenza A Virus, Avian
Myxoviruses see Orthomyxoviridae

N

N-Formimidoylthienamycin see Imipenem
N-Methyl-D-Aspartate Receptors see Receptors,
    N-Methyl-D-Aspartate
N-ras Genes see Genes, ras
n-3 Fatty Acids see Fatty Acids, Omega-3
N(5)-Formyltetrahydrofolate see Leucovorin
Na(+)-K(+)-Exchanging ATPase   QU 136
Na(+)-K(+)-Transporting ATPase see
    NA(+)-K(+)-Exchanging ATPase
NAD   QU 135
NAD+ ADP-Ribosyltransferase   QU 141
NAD Diaphorase see Lipoamide Dehydrogenase
NADH Diaphorase see Lipoamide Dehydrogenase
Nadide see NAD
NADP   QU 135
Nail Biting   WM 172
    Adolescence   WS 463
    Child   WS 350.6
    Infant   WS 350.6

Nailing, Intramedullary see Fracture Fixation,
    Intramedullary
Nails   WR 475
Nails, Ingrown   WR 475
Naked DNA Vaccines see Vaccines, DNA
Nalbuphine   QV 92
Nalidixic Acid   QV 243
Nalidixin see Nalidixic Acid
Naltrexone   QV 89
Names
    Corporate names (cataloging)   Z 695.8
    Geographic names (General)   G 104-108
      Special country, in appropriate LC number
    Subject cataloging
      Personal names   Z 695.1.P4
Nanism see Dwarfism
NaN3 see Sodium Azide
Naphthalenediones see Naphthoquinones
Naphthalenes
    Organic chemistry   QD 391
    Pharmacology   QV 241
Naphthols   QV 241
Naphthoquinones
    As antiviral agents   QV 268.5
    Organic chemistry   QD 341.H9
Naproxen   QV 95
Narceine see Noscapine
Narcissism   WM 460.5.E3
Narcolepsy   WM 188
Narcosis, Therapeutic Use see Narcotherapy
Narcosynthesis see Narcotherapy
Narcotherapy   WM 402
Narcotic Abuse see Opioid-Related Disorders
Narcotic Addiction see Opioid-Related Disorders
Narcotic Analgesics see Analgesics, Opioid
Narcotic Antagonists   QV 89
Narcotic Control see Drug and Narcotic Control
Narcotic Dependence see Opioid-Related Disorders
Narcotic Laws see Legislation, Drug
Narcotics   QV 89
    Control see Drug and Narcotic Control   QV
      32, etc.
    Legislation see Legislation, Drug   QV 32-33
    Public health aspects   WA 730
    See also Analgesics, Opioid   QV 89-92, etc.
Narcotine see Noscapine
Nasal Accessory Sinuses see Paranasal Sinuses
Nasal Bone   WV 301
Nasal Cavity   WV 301
Nasal Decongestants   QV 150
Nasal Fossae see Nasal Cavity
Nasal Polyps   WV 300
Nasal Provocation Tests
    Used in the diagnosis of nasal hypersensitivity
      WV 335
Nasal Septum   WV 320
Nasal Sinuses see Paranasal Sinuses
Nasopharyngeal Diseases   WV 410
Nasopharyngeal Neoplasms   WV 410
Nasopharynx   WV 410
    In respiration   WF 490
National Ambulatory Medical Care Survey see
    Health Care Surveys

**ALWAYS CONSULT MAIN SCHEDULES.   USE NUMBER ASSIGNED ONLY WHEN
SUBJECT REPRESENTS MAJOR EMPHASIS OF WORK BEING CLASSIFIED**

National Council on Health Planning and
   Development see Health Planning Councils
National Health Insurance, Non-U.S. see National
   Health Programs
National Health Insurance, United States   W 275
National Health Policy see Health Policy
National Health Programs   WA 540
   Programs in particular areas, by subject, e.g.,
      Maternal Welfare   WA 310
National Health Service, British see State Medicine
National Health Service Corps see Medically
   Underserved Area
National Hospital Discharge Survey see Health Care
   Surveys
Nationality see Ethnic Groups
Native Americans see Indians, North American
Natriuresis   WJ 303
Natriuretic Factor see Natriuretic Hormone
Natriuretic Hormone   WK 185
Natriuretic Peptides, Atrial see Atrial Natriuretic
   Factor
Natural Childbirth   WQ 152
Natural Disasters
   Communicable disease control   WA 110
   Hospital emergency service   WX 215
   Medical emergencies   WB 105
   See also special topics under Disasters
Natural History of Drugs see Pharmacognosy
Natural Immunity see Immunity, Natural
Natural Killer Cells see Killer Cells, Natural
Natural Radiation see Background Radiation
Natural Resources see Conservation of Natural
   Resources   S 900–954, etc., and names of specific
   resources
Natural Selection   QH 375
Naturopathy   WB 935
Nausea   WI 146
Nautical Medicine see Naval Medicine
Naval Hygiene see Naval Medicine
Naval Medicine   VG 100–475
   Biography
      Collective   WZ 112.5.M4
      Individual   WZ 100
   Hygiene   VG 470–475
   Surgery   WO 800
Naval Nursing see Military Nursing
Naval Science   V
   General works   V 101–109
Naval Surgery see Naval Medicine; Naval   WO
   800 under Surgery
Nazism see Political Systems
Neamin see Neomycin
Neapolitan Fever see Brucellosis
Nearsightedness see Myopia
Nebramycin Factor 6 see Tobramycin
Nebulizers and Vaporizers   WB 342
Necator   QX 243
Necatoriasis   WC 890
Neck   WE 708
   Blood supply   WE 708
   Neoplasms see Head and Neck Neoplasms   WE
      707
Neck Injuries   WE 708

Neck Muscles   WE 708
Neck Neoplasms see Head and Neck Neoplasms
Neck Pain   WE 708
Neckache see Neck Pain
Necrobacillosis see Fusobacterium Infections
Necrophilia see Paraphilias
Necrosis   QZ 180
   Veterinary   SF 769
   Localized, by site
Necrotizing Arteritis see Polyarteritis Nodosa
Necrotizing Pyelonephritis see Kidney Papillary
   Necrosis
Need Certification, Health Care see Certificate of
   Need
Needle Biopsy see Biopsy, Needle
Needle Sharing
   Special topics, by subject
Needs Assessment   W 84.3
   In special areas, by subject
NEFA see Fatty Acids, Nonesterified
Nefopam   QV 95
Negative Contrast Radiography see
   Pneumoradiography
Negative Reinforcement see Reinforcement
   (Psychology)
Negatrons see Electrons
Negligence, Professional see Malpractice
Negotiating
   In business   HD 58.6
   Psychology   BF 637.N4
   Special topics, by subject
Negroes see Blacks
Negroid Race
   Anthropology   GN 645
   See also specific topics under Ethnic groups
Neisseria   QW 131
Neisseria gonorrhoeae   QW 131
Neisseriaceae   QW 131
Nelavane see Trypanosomiasis, African
Nemathelminthes see Acanthocephala; Nematoda
Nematoda   QX 203–301
Nematode Infections   WC 850–890
   Veterinary   SF 810.N4
Nematomorpha see Helminths
Nematomorpha Infections see Helminthiasis
Neoadjuvant Therapy   QZ 266–269
   For particular diseases, with the disease
Neoadjuvant Treatment see Neoadjuvant Therapy
Neoarsphenamine   QV 262
Neocaine see Procaine
Neomalthusianism see Population Dynamics
Neomycin   QV 350
Neomycin A see Neomycin
Neon
   Inorganic chemistry   QD 181.N5
   Pharmacology   QV 310
Neonatal Abstinence Syndrome   WS 421
Neonatal Intensive Care see Intensive Care, Neonatal
Neonatal Mortality see Infant Mortality
Neonatal Nursing   WY 157.3
Neonatal Screening
   For specific diseases, with the disease
Neonate see Infant, Newborn

Neonatology   WS 420
  See also Infant, Newborn   WS 420, etc.;
    Perinatology   WQ 210
Neophocaena see Porpoises
Neoplasm Antibodies see Antibodies, Neoplasm
Neoplasm Antigens see Antigens, Neoplasm
Neoplasm Antigens, Viral see Antigens, Viral,
  Tumor
Neoplasm Circulating Cells   QZ 202
Neoplasm DNA see DNA, Neoplasm
Neoplasm Invasiveness   QZ 202
Neoplasm Metastasis   QZ 202
Neoplasm Metastasis, Unknown Primary see
  Neoplasms, Unknown Primary
Neoplasm Proteins   QZ 200
Neoplasm Recurrence, Local   QZ 202
Neoplasm Regression, Spontaneous   QZ 202
Neoplasm Remission, Spontaneous see Neoplasm
  Regression, Spontaneous
Neoplasm RNA see RNA, Neoplasm
Neoplasm Staging   QZ 241
Neoplasm Stem Cell Assay see Tumor Stem Cell
  Assay
Neoplasm Transplantation   QZ 206
Neoplasm Vaccines see Cancer Vaccines
Neoplasms   QZ 200–380
  Adolescence (General)   QZ 275
  Child (General)   QZ 275
  Drug therapy   QZ 267
    See also Antineoplastic Agents   QV 269
  Infant (General)   QZ 275
  Nursing   WY 156
  Oncolysis   QZ 266
    Special topics, by subject
  Radiotherapy   QZ 269
  Surgery   QZ 268
  Therapy   QZ 266
  Veterinary   SF 910.T8
  Localized, by site
Neoplasms, Adipose Tissue   QZ 340
  Localized, by site
Neoplasms, Connective Tissue   QZ 340
Neoplasms, Dental Tissue see Odontogenic Tumors
Neoplasms, Embryonal and Mixed see Neoplasms,
  Germ Cell and Embryonal
Neoplasms, Experimental   QZ 206
Neoplasms, Germ Cell and Embryonal   QZ 310
Neoplasms, Glandular and Epithelial   QZ 365
Neoplasms, Hormone–Dependent   QZ 200
  Localized, by site
Neoplasms, Mesenchymal see Neoplasms,
  Connective Tissue
Neoplasms, Multiple Primary   QZ 200
Neoplasms, Muscle Tissue   QZ 340
  Localized, by site
Neoplasms, Nerve Tissue   QZ 380
Neoplasms, Occult Primary see Neoplasms,
  Unknown Primary
Neoplasms, Radiation–Induced   QZ 200
Neoplasms, Unknown Primary   QZ 202
Neoplasms, Vascular Tissue   QZ 340
Neoplastic Cells, Cultured see Tumor Cells, Cultured
Neoplastic Endocrine–Like Syndromes   QZ 200

  See also Hormones, Ectopic   QZ 202, etc.
Neoplastic Gene Expression Regulation see Gene
  Expression Regulation, Neoplastic
Neoplastic Processes   QZ 202
Neoplastic Transformation, Cell see Cell
  Transformation, Neoplastic
Neorickettsia see Rickettsiaceae
Neostigmine   QV 124
Neovascularization, Choroidal see Choroidal
  Neovascularization
Neovascularization, Pathologic   WG 500
Neovascularization, Physiologic   WG 500
Nephelometry and Turbidimetry
  Analytical chemistry   QD 79.P46
  Used for the diagnosis of particular disorder, with
    the disorder
Nephrectomy   WJ 368
  Veterinary   SF 871
Nephritis   WJ 353
  Veterinary   SF 871
Nephritis, Familial see Nephritis, Hereditary
Nephritis, Hereditary   WJ 353
  As a cause of deafness   WV 270
Nephritis, Lupus see Lupus Nephritis
Nephroblastoma   WJ 358
Nephrocalcinosis   WJ 356
Nephrolithiasis see Kidney Calculi
Nephrolithotomy, Percutaneous see Nephrostomy,
  Percutaneous
Nephrology   WJ 300–378
  Nursing   WY 164
Nephrons   WJ 301
Nephropathy, IGA see Glomerulonephritis, IGA
Nephrosis   WJ 340
Nephrostomy, Percutaneous   WJ 368
Nephrotic Syndrome   WJ 340
Neptunium   WN 420
  Nuclear physics   QC 796.N7
  See also special topics under Radioisotopes
Nerve Block
  Anesthetic uses   WO 300
  Diagnostic and therapeutic uses   WO 375
  See also Autonomic Nerve Block   WO 375
Nerve Block anesthesia see Anesthesia, Conduction
Nerve Cells see Neurons
Nerve Centers see Neurons
Nerve Compression Syndromes   WL 500
Nerve Conduction see Neural Conduction
Nerve Degeneration   WL 102.5
  Of a particular part, by subject, e.g., in the
    cerebellum   WL 320
Nerve Endings   WL 102.9
Nerve Endings, Sensory see Receptors, Sensory
Nerve Fibers   WL 102.5
Nerve Fibers, Myelinated   WL 102.5
Nerve Growth Factors   WL 104
Nerve Impulses see Physiology   WL 102 under
  Nervous System
Nerve Net   WL 102
Nerve Regeneration   WL 102
Nerve Roots see Spinal Nerve Roots
Nerve Tissue   WL 101–102
  Analysis   WL 104

Anatomy   WL 101
Histology   QS 532.5.N3
Neoplasms   QZ 380
Physiology   WL 102
Nerve Tissue Proteins   WL 104
Nerve Transmission see Synaptic Transmission
Nerve Transmitter Substances see Neurotransmitters
Nerves see Autonomic Nervous System; Nervous
   System; Peripheral Nervous System; Sympathetic
   Nervous System; names of specific nerves
Nervous Exhaustion see Neurasthenia
Nervous Mice see Mice, Neurologic Mutants
Nervous System
   Anatomy   WL 101
   Autonomic see Autonomic Nervous System
      WL 600–610
   Child   WS 340–342
   Drugs affecting   QV 76.5
      See also Analeptics   QV 101–107; Analgesics,
         Anti–Inflammatory   QV 95–98; Anesthetics
         QV 81, etc.; Anticonvulsants   QV 85;
         Autonomic Drugs   QV 120; Hypnotics and
         Sedatives   QV 85–88; Narcotics   QV 89;
         Neuromuscular Blocking Agents   QV 140;
         Neuromuscular Depolarizing Agents   QV
         140
   Infant   WS 340–342
   Neoplasms (General)   WL 160
   Parasympathetic see Parasympathetic Nervous
      System   WL 610
   Pathology   WL 140
   Physiology see Nervous System Physiology
      WL 102
   Surgery see Neurosurgical Procedures   WL 368
   Sympathetic see Sympathetic Nervous System
      WL 610
   See also Neoplasms, Nervous Tissue   QZ 380;
      Neuroanatomy (specialty only)   WL 101;
      Neurophysiology (specialty only)   WL 102;
      Neurosurgery (specialty only)   WL 368; names
      of specific nerves
Nervous System Diseases   WL 140–710
   Child   WS 340
   Diagnosis   WL 141
   ENT complications   WV 180
   Infant   WS 340
   Nursing   WY 160.5
   Surgery   WL 368
   Veterinary   SF 895
Nervous System Neoplasms   WL 160
Nervous System Physiology   WL 102
   See also Neurophysiology   WL 102
Nesidioblastoma see Adenoma, Islet Cell
Nesidioblastosis see Pancreatic Diseases
Nesidioblasts see Islets of Langerhans
Nested Case–Control Studies see Case–Control
   Studies
Nesting Behavior   QL 756
   Bird   QL 675
Netilmicin   QV 350
Nettle Rash see Urticaria
Network Communication Protocols see Computer
   Communication Networks

Neural Analyzers   WL 101–102
Neural Conduction   WL 102.7–102.8
Neural Crest   WL 101
   Animal   QL 938.N48
Neural Inhibition   WL 102.7–102.8
Neural Interconnections see Neural Pathways
Neural Networks (Anatomic) see Nerve Net
Neural Pathways   WL 102
   See also Pyramidal Tracts   WL 400; names of
      specific pathways
Neural Transmission see Synaptic Transmission
Neural Tube Defects   WL 101
   See also names of specific defects, e.g., Spinal
      Dysraphism   WE 730
Neuralgia   WL 544
   Cervico–brachial see Cervico–Brachial Neuralgia
      WL 400
   Facial see Facial Neuralgia   WL 544
   Trigeminal see Trigeminal Neuralgia   WL 544
Neuralgic Amyotrophy see Cervico–Brachial
   Neuralgia
Neuraminic Acids   QU 84
   Organic chemistry   QD 321
Neuraminidase   QU 136
Neurasthenia   WM 174
Neurasthenic Neuroses see Neurasthenia
Neurenteric Cyst see Spina Bifida Occulta
Neurilemmoma   QZ 380
   Localized, by site
Neurilemmoma, Acoustic see Neuroma, Acoustic
Neurinoma see Neurilemmoma
Neurinoma, Acoustic see Neuroma, Acoustic
Neurite Outgrowth Factor see Nerve Growth
   Factors
Neuritis   WL 544
   Endemic multiple see Beriberi   WD 122
   Optic see Optic Neuritis   WW 280
Neuritis, Experimental Allergic   WL 544
Neuro–Ophthalmology see Innervation   WW
   101–103 under Eye; Eye Movements; Oculomotor
   Muscles; Oculomotor Nerve; Optic Nerve
Neuroanatomy   WL 101
   See also Anatomy   WL 101 under Nervous
      System
Neurobiology   WL 100–102
Neuroblastoma   QZ 380
   Localized, by site
Neurochemistry   WL 104
   See also Analysis   WL 104 under Nerve Tissue
Neurocirculatory Asthenia   WG 320
Neurodegenerative Diseases   WL 359
Neurodermatitis   WR 280
Neurodermatitis, Atopic see Dermatitis, Atopic
Neurodermatitis, Circumscribed see Neurodermatitis
Neurodermatitis, Disseminated see Dermatitis,
   Atopic
Neurodermatitis, Localized see Neurodermatitis
Neuroeffector Junction   WL 102.9
Neuroendocrine System see Neurosecretory Systems
Neuroendocrinology   WL 105
Neurofibrils   WL 102.5
Neurofibroma   QZ 380
   Localized, by site

ALWAYS CONSULT MAIN SCHEDULES. USE NUMBER ASSIGNED ONLY WHEN
SUBJECT REPRESENTS MAJOR EMPHASIS OF WORK BEING CLASSIFIED

Neurotransmitters   QV 126
  See also names of specific neurotransmitters
Neurotropic Virus Infections see Virus Diseases
Neutron Activation Analysis   QD 606
  Of a particular substance, with the substance
Neutrons   WN 415–420
  In general nuclear physics   QC
    793.5.N462–793.5.N4629
  In health physics   WN 110
Neutropenia   WH 200
Neutrophil–Activating Peptide,
  Lymphocyte–Derived see Interleukin–8
Neutrophil–Activating Peptide, Monocyte–Derived
  see Interleukin–8
Neutrophil–Activating Peptides, Fibroblast–Derived
see Interleukin–8
Neutrophil–Derived Relaxant Factor see
  Endothelium–Derived Relaxing Factor
Neutrophils   WH 200
  In phagocytosis   QW 690
Nevus   WR 500
  Pathology   QZ 310
Nevus, Pigmented   WR 265
  Pathology   QZ 310
Nevus Syndrome, Dysplastic see Dysplastic Nevus
  Syndrome
Newborn see Infant, Newborn
Newborn Infant Screening see Neonatal Screening
Newcastle Disease   SF 995.6.N4
Newcastle Disease Virus   QW 168.5.P2
News Media Relations see Public Relations
Newsletters see Periodicals
Newspapers
  General bibliography   Z 6940–6967
  Medical and related areas   W1
    Bibliography   ZW 1
Niacin see Nicotinic Acids   QU 193
Niacinamide   QU 193
Nialamide   QV 77.5
Nicardipine   QV 150
Nickel
  Inorganic chemistry   QD 181.N6
  Pharmacology   QV 290
Nicolas–Favre Disease see Lymphogranuloma
  Venereum
Nicotiana see Tobacco
Nicotinamide see Niacinamide
Nicotinamide–Adenine Dinucleotide see NAD
Nicotinamide–Adenine Dinucleotide Phosphate see
  NADP
Nicotine   QV 137
  Dependence   WM 290
Nicotinic Acid see Niacin
Nicotinic Acids   QU 193
Nicotinic Agents see Cholinergic Agents
Nicotinic Receptors see Receptors, Nicotinic
Nidation see Ovum Implantation
Nidation, Delayed see Ovum Implantation, Delayed
NIDDM see Diabetes Mellitus,
  Non–Insulin–Dependent
Niemann–Pick Disease   WD 205.5.L5
Nifedipine   QV 150
Night Blindness   WD 110

Night Monkey, Northern see Aotus trivirgatus
Night Terrors see Sleep Disorders
Night Vision see Dark Adaptation
Nightmares see Dreams
NIH Consensus Development Conferences see
  Consensus Development Conferences, NIH
Nikethamide   QV 103
Nimodipine   QV 150
Niobium
  Inorganic chemistry   QD 181.N3
  Radioactive   WN 420
NIR Spectroscopy see Spectroscopy, Near–Infrared
Nisoldipine   QV 150
Nitrates   QV 156
  As caustics (e.g. when nitrates are used for nitric
    acid)   QV 612
Nitric Acid see Nitrates
Nitric Oxide
  As a neurotransmitter   QV 126
  As an air pollutant   WA 754
  Inorganic chemistry   QD 181.N1
Nitriles
  As antineoplastic agents   QV 269
  Organic chemistry
    Aliphatic compounds   QD 305.N7
    Aromatic compounds   QD 341.N7
Nitrites   QV 156
Nitrobacter   QW 135
Nitrobacteraceae   QW 135
Nitrobenzenes
  Organic chemistry   QD 341.H9
  Toxicology   QV 632
Nitrocellulose see Collodion
Nitroferricyanide see Nitroprusside
Nitrofural see Nitrofurazone
Nitrofurans   QV 243
Nitrofurazone   QV 243
  As a local anti–infective agent   QV 225
Nitrogen   QU 54
  Blood chemistry   QY 455
Nitrogen Dioxide
  As an air pollutant   WA 754
  Inorganic chemistry   QD 181.N1
Nitrogen Fixation   QU 70
  Chemical technology   TP 245.N8
  In plants   QK 898.N6
  In soil   QW 60
Nitrogen Isotopes   QU 54
  Inorganic chemistry   QD 181.N1
Nitrogen Mustard see Mechlorethamine; Mustard
  Compounds; Thio–Tepa; Triethylene Melamine
Nitrogen Mustard Compounds   QV 269
  As war gases   QV 666
Nitrogen Mustard N–Oxide see Mechlorethamine
Nitrogen Narcosis see Inert Gas Narcosis
Nitrogen Oxides
  As air pollutants   WA 754
  Inorganic chemistry   QD 181.N1
  Mineralogy   QE 389.5
Nitroglycerin   QV 156
  Toxicology   QV 632
Nitroprusside
  As a vasodilator agent   QV 156

Nitrosamines   QZ 202
Nitrosation
     As a metabolic phenomenon   QU 120
     Organic chemistry   QD 281.N5
Nitroso Compounds
     As carcinogens   QZ 202
     Organic chemistry
          Aliphatic compounds   QD 305.N8
          Aromatic compounds   QD 341.N8
Nitrosodiethylamine see Diethylnitrosamine
Nitrosomonas   QW 135
Nitrous Oxide   QV 81
Nizethamid see Nikethamide
NK Cells see Killer Cells, Natural
NMDA Receptor-Ionophore Complex see
     Receptors, N-Methyl-D-Aspartate
NMR Imaging see Magnetic Resonance Imaging
NMR Tomography see Magnetic Resonance
     Imaging
No-Fault Insurance see Insurance, Liability
No-Observed-Adverse-Effect Level   QV 602
     Of specific drugs, with the drug
No-Observed-Effect Level see
     No-Observed-Adverse-Effect Level
NOAEL see No-Observed-Adverse-Effect Level
Nobel Prize   AS 911
     Collective biography of winners
          Chemists   QD 21
          General   AS 911
          Physicians   WZ 112
          Physicists   QC 15
          Physiologists   WZ 112.5.P5
Nocardia Infections   WC 302
     Veterinary   SF 809.N63
     See also Maduromycosis   WR 340
Nociception Tests see Pain Measurement
Nociceptors   WL 102.9
Nodding Spasm see Spasms, Infantile
Nodulus Intercaroticus see Carotid Body
NOEL see No-Observed-Adverse-Effect Level
Noise   WA 776
     Abatement   WA 776
          In industry   WA 470
     Adverse effects   WV 270
          In aviation   WD 735
     Prevention & control
          General public health   WA 776
          In industry   WA 470
Noise-Induced Hearing Loss see Hearing Loss,
     Noise-Induced
Noise, Occupational see Noise   WA 470, etc.
Noise, Transportation see Noise   WA 776, etc.
Nomascus see Hylobates
Nomenclature
     (Form number 15 in any NLM schedule where
     applicable)
Nomifensine
     As an antidepressant   QV 77.5
     As an antiparkinson agent   QV 80
Non-Hodgkin Lymphoma see Lymphoma,
     Non-Hodgkin
Non-Steroidal Anti-Inflammatory Agents see
     Anti-Inflammatory Agents, Non-Steroidal

Nonagenarian see Aged, 80 and over
Nondirective Therapy   WM 420.5.N8
Nondisjunction, Genetic   QH 462.N65
Noninvasive Litholapaxy see Lithotripsy
Nonodontogenic Cysts   WU 280
Nonopioid Analgesics see Analgesics, Non-Narcotic
Nonprofit Organizations see Organizations,
     Nonprofit
Nonverbal Communication   HM
     Adolescence   WS 462
     Child   WS 105.5.C8
     Infant   WS 105.5.C8
     In speech disorders   WM 475
     Psychology   BF 637.N66
     See also Kinesics   WS 462, etc.; Manual
          Communication   HV 2477, etc.
Nootropic Drugs see Psychotropic Drugs
Noradrenaline see Norepinephrine
Noramidopyrine Methanesulfonate see Dipyrone
Norepinephrine   WK 725
Norethandrolone   WJ 875
Norethindrone   WP 530
     As a contraceptive   QV 177
Norethisterone see Norethindrone
Norethynodrel   WP 530
     As a contraceptive   QV 177
Norfloxacin   QV 250
Norgestrel   WP 530
     As a contraceptive   QV 177
Normal Range see Reference Values
Normal Serum Globulin Therapy see Immunization,
     Passive
Normal Values see Reference Values
Normethandrolone   WP 530
Normoblasts see Erythroblasts
Norpregneninolone see Norethindrone
Northern Blotting see Blotting, Northern
Nortropanes
     Organic chemistry   QD 401
Noscapine   QV 76
Nose   WV 300–335
     Innervation   WV 301
     Surgery   WV 300
          Plastic   WV 312
Nose Bleed see Epistaxis
Nose Diseases   WV 300–335
     General works   WV 300
     Child   WV 300–335
     Infant   WV 300–335
     Nursing   WY 158.5
     Veterinary   SF 891
Nose Neoplasms   WV 300
Nosebleed see Epistaxis
Nosocomial Infections see Cross Infection
Nosology see Classification
Nostrums   QV 772
Notifiable Diseases, Registration see Communicable
     Disease Control; Registries
Novelty-Seeking Behavior see Exploratory
     Behavior
Novocaine see Procaine
Nuclear Energy   WN 415
     Meteorology   QC 913.2.A8
     Nuclear physics   QC 770–798

Nuclear Envelope see Nuclear Membrane
Nuclear Magnetic Resonance   QC 762
  In biochemistry   QU 25
  Spectroscopy   QD 96.N8
  Other special topics, by subject
  See also Magnetic Resonance Imaging   WN 185
Nuclear Medicine   WN 440-450
Nuclear Medicine Department, Hospital   WN 27-28
Nuclear Membrane   QH 601.2
  See also Cell Membrane   QH 601, etc.
Nuclear Physics
  Biological sciences   WN 415
  Physical sciences   QC 770-798
Nuclear Pore see Nuclear Membrane
Nuclear Proteins   QU 55
Nuclear Radiology see Nuclear Medicine
Nuclear Reactors   QC 786.4-786.8
  Industrial hazard   WA 470
  Nuclear reactor engineering   TK 9202-9230
  Radioactive waste hazard   WA 788
  Special uses, by subject
Nuclear Warfare   WN 610
Nuclear Waste see Radioactive Waste
Nucleases see Phosphoric Diester Hydrolases; names of other specific nucleases, e.g., Deoxyribonucleases
Nucleases, DNA see Deoxyribonucleases
Nucleases, RNA see Ribonucleases
Nucleic Acid Conformation   QU 58
Nucleic Acid Hybridization   QU 58
Nucleic Acid Probes   QU 58
Nucleic Acid Synthesis Inhibitors   QU 58
Nucleic Acid Vaccines see Vaccines, DNA
Nucleic Acids   QU 58
  Derivatives
    Biochemistry   QU 58
    Pharmacology   QV 185
Nucleolar Organizer see Nucleolus Organizer Region
Nucleolar Proteins see Nuclear Proteins
Nucleolus Organizer Region   QH 600
Nucleolysis, Intervertebral Disk see Intervertebral Disk Chemolysis
Nucleoproteins   QU 56
Nucleoside Diphosphate Sugars
  Biochemistry   QU 57
  Pharmacology   QV 185
Nucleosides
  Biochemistry   QU 57
  Pharmacology   QV 185
    See also Hematopoiesis   WH 140
  See also names of specific nucleosides
Nucleosomes   QU 56
  Cytology   QH 599
Nucleotide Sequence see Base Sequence
Nucleotides
  Biochemistry   QU 57
  Pharmacology   QV 185
    See also Hematopoiesis   WH 140
  See also names of specific nucleotides
Nucleotides, Cyclic   QU 57

  Pharmacology   QV 185
Nucleus Accumbens   WL 314
Nucleus Dentatus see Cerebellar Nuclei
Nude Mice see Mice, Nude
Nudism   QT 245
Nuisances (Air Pollution) see Air Pollutants
Numerical Analysis, Computer-Assisted
  Special topics, by subject, e.g. Biological Models   QH 324.8
Numismatics   CJ 1-6661
  Medical   WZ 340
Nupercaine see Dibucaine
Nurse Administrators   WY 105
Nurse Anesthetists   WY 151
Nurse Clinicians   WY 128
Nurse Midwives   WY 157
  Directories   WY 22
  See also Obstetrical Nursing   WY 157, etc.; Midwifery   WQ 160-165
Nurse-Patient Relations   WY 87
  Child   WY 159
  Counseling   WY 87
  Education of patient   WY 87
  Infant   WY 159
Nurse-Physician Relations see Physician-Nurse Relations
Nurse Practitioners   WY 128
Nurseries   WA 320
Nurseries, Hospital   WX 200
Nursery Schools see Schools, Nursery
Nurses
  Biography
    Collective   WZ 112.5.N8
    Individual   WZ 100
  Directories   WY 22
  Employment   WY 29, etc.
  Liability   WY 44
    See also Insurance, Liability   WY 44, etc.
  Psychology   WY 87
Nurses' Aides   WY 193
  Psychiatric see Psychiatric Aides   WY 160
Nurses, Head see Nursing, Supervisory
Nurses' Instruction
  On specific topics, by subject
Nurses, Male   WY 191
Nurses Performance Evaluation see Employee Performance Appraisal
Nursing   WY
  Administration   WY 105
  Adolescence   WY 156.7
  AIDS/HIV   WY 153.5
  As a profession   WY 16
  Aviation   WY 143
  By country   WY 300
  Community health see Community Health Nursing   WY 106
  For infants and children see Pediatric Nursing   WY 159, WY 157.3, etc.
  Geriatric see Geriatric Nursing   WY 152
  Gynecological   WY 156.7
  History see History of Nursing   WY 11
  Holistic see Holistic Nursing   WY 86.5
  Home see Home Nursing   WY 200

Industrial see Occupational Health Nursing   WY 141
Military see Military Nursing   WY 130
Naval see Military Nursing   WY 130
Neurological   WY 160.5
Obstetrical see Obstetrical Nursing   WY 157
Office see Office Nursing   WY 109
Operating room see Operating Room Nursing   WY 162
Otolaryngological   WY 158.5
Pediatric see Pediatric Nursing   WY 159
Perioperative see Perioperative Nursing   WY 161–162
Psychiatric see Psychiatric Nursing   WY 160
Psychological aspects   WY 87
Rehabilitation see Rehabilitation Nursing   WY 150.5
Religious orders   WY 145
School see School Nursing   WY 113
Specialties see Specialties, Nursing   WY 101–164
Standards   WY 16
Statistics   WY 31
Surgical see Perioperative Nursing   WY 161–162
Surveys   WY 31
Transcultural see Transcultural Nursing   WY 107
Transportation nursing   WY 143
Veterinary   SF 774.5
See also names of diseases being treated or the specialty involved
Nursing Administration Research   WY 105
Nursing Assessment   WY 100.4
Nursing Audit   WY 100.5
Nursing Care
   General   WY 100
   In special field   WY 150–164
   Psychology (General)   WY 87
Nursing Care Plans see Patient Care Planning
Nursing Diagnosis   WY 100.4
Nursing Economics see Economics, Nursing
Nursing Education see Education, Nursing
Nursing Education, Associate see Education, Nursing, Associate
Nursing Education, Baccalaureate see Education, Nursing, Baccalaureate
Nursing Education, Continuing see Education, Nursing, Continuing
Nursing Education, Diploma Programs see Education, Nursing, Diploma Programs
Nursing Education, Graduate see Education, Nursing, Graduate
Nursing Education Research   WY 18
Nursing Ethics see Ethics, Nursing
Nursing Evaluation Research   WY 20.5
Nursing Faculty see Faculty, Nursing
Nursing, Holistic see Holistic Nursing
Nursing, Home see Home Nursing
Nursing Homes   WX 27–28
   Administration   WX 150
   Directories   WX 22
   For the aged   WT 27–28
      Directories   WT 22

For other purposes, by specialty
Nursing Libraries see Libraries, Nursing
Nursing, Maternal–Child see Maternal–Child Nursing
Nursing Methodology Research   WY 20.5
Nursing, Military and Naval see Military Nursing
Nursing Models see Models, Nursing
Nursing, Oncologic see Oncologic Nursing
Nursing Philosophy see Philosophy, Nursing
Nursing Pools see Employment; Nurses
Nursing, Practical   WY 195
   Education   WY 18.8
Nursing, Private Duty   WY 127
   Education   WY 18
Nursing Process   WY 100
   Specific activities, by subject
Nursing Program Evaluation see Nursing Evaluation Research
Nursing Protocols see Nursing Assessment
Nursing Records   WY 100.5
   See also Medical Records   WX 173, etc.
Nursing, Rehabilitation see Rehabilitation Nursing
Nursing Research   WY 20.5
Nursing Research, Administrative see Nursing Administration Research
Nursing Research, Clinical see Clinical Nursing Research
Nursing Research, Educational see Nursing Education Research
Nursing Schools see Schools, Nursing
Nursing Service, Hospital   WY 125 ·
   Administration   WY 105
Nursing Services   WY 100
Nursing Staff
   Of industry   WY 141
   Of schools   WY 113
Nursing Staff, Hospital   WY 125
   Administration   WY 105
Nursing, Supervisory   WY 105
   Of wards   WY 105
Nursing, Team   WY 125
   See also Patient Care Team   W 84.8, etc.
Nursing Theory   WY 86
Nursing, Transcultural see Transcultural Nursing
Nutcracker Esophagus see Esophageal Motility Disorders
Nutrition
   And oral health   WU 113.7
   General   QU 145
   Aged   WT 115
   In animals see Animal Nutrition   SF 95–99
   In children see Child Nutrition   WS 115, etc.
   In infants see Infant Nutrition   WS 115–125
   In sickness (General)   WB 400
   Pregnancy   WQ 175
   Tables   QU 145
      For children   WS 16
   See also Diet   QT 235; Parenteral Feeding   WB 410; other particular topics
Nutrition Assessment   QU 146
Nutrition Disorders   WD 100–175
   As a cause of disease   QZ 105
   Aged   WT 115

Child   WS 115, WS 130
Infant   WS 115
    See also Infant Nutrition Disorders   WS 120, etc.
Veterinary   SF 851
See also Obesity   WD 210-212
Nutrition Disorders, Child see Child Nutrition Disorders
Nutrition Disorders, Infant see Infant Nutrition Disorders
Nutrition, Enteral see Enteral Nutrition
Nutrition, Parenteral see Parenteral Nutrition
Nutrition Policy
    Nutrition   QU 145
    Public food supply   WA 695
Nutrition Surveys   QU 146
Nutrition, Total Parenteral see Parenteral Nutrition, Total
Nutritional Availability see Nutritive Value
Nutritional Requirements   QU 145
    Adolescence   WS 130
    Aged   WT 115
    For infants and children
        General   WS 115
        Child   WS 130
        Infant   WS 120-125
Nutritional Status   QU 145
Nutritive Value   QU 145.5
    Tables   QU 145.5
Nuts
    Diets for control of fats   WB 425
    Diets for control of protein   WB 426
Nux Vomica see Strychnine
Nyctalopia see Night Blindness
Nycticebus see Lorisidae
Nyctiphanes see Crustacea
Nyctohemeral Rhythm see Circadian Rhythm
Nylons
    Chemical technology   TP 1180.P55
    Used for special purposes, by subject, e.g., in plastic surgery   WO 640
Nymphae see Vulva
Nymphomania see Paraphilias
Nystagmus   WW 410
Nystagmus, Barany's see Nystagmus, Physiologic
Nystagmus, Caloric see Nystagmus, Physiologic
Nystagmus, Physiologic   WW 410
Nystagmus, Thermal see Nystagmus, Physiologic

O

o-Dihydroxybenzenes see Catechols
Oath, Hippocratic see Hippocratic Oath
Oats
    As a dietary supplement in health or disease   WB 431
    Cultivation   SB 191.O2
Obesity   WD 210-212
Obesity in Diabetes   WK 835
Obesity, Morbid   WD 210-212
Object Attachment   WM 460.5.O2
Object Relations see Object Attachment
Object Relationship see Object Attachment

Obligation, Social see Social Responsibility
Observation
    As a scientific method in research (Form number 20 or 20.5 in any NLM schedule where applicable)
    In specific topics, by subject
Obsessive Behavior   WM 176
Obsessive-Compulsive Disorder   WM 176
Obsessive-Compulsive Personality see Compulsive Personality Disorder
Obstetric Surgical Procedures   WQ 400-450
Obstetrical Forceps   WQ 425
Obstetrical Nursing   WY 157
    Education   WY 18-18.5
    See also Postnatal Nursing   WY 157.3
Obstetricians, Directories see Directories   WQ 22 under Obstetrics
Obstetrics   WQ
    Anesthesia see Anesthesia, Obstetrical   WO 450
    Cardiac problems   WQ 244
    Directories   WQ 22
    Nursing see Obstetrical Nursing   WY 157, etc.
    Urology   WJ 190
        Complications   WQ 260.
Obstetrics and Gynecology Department, Hospital   WQ 27-28
Obstruction, Intestinal see Intestinal Obstruction
Obturators, Palatal see Palatal Obturators
Occipital Lobe   WL 307
Occlusal Adjustment   WU 440
Occlusal Equilibration see Occlusal Adjustment
Occlusal Equilibration see Occlusal Adjustment
Occlusal Force see Bite Force
Occlusal Wear, Restoration see Dental Restoration Wear
Occlusion see Dental Occlusion
Occlusive Dressings   WO 167
Occult Blood   QY 160
Occult Primary Neoplasms see Neoplasms, Unknown Primary
Occult Spina Bifida see Spina Bifida Occulta
Occult Spinal Dysraphism see Spina Bifida Occulta
Occultism
    Medical superstitions   WZ 309
Occupational Accidents see Accidents, Occupational
Occupational Air Pollutants see Air Pollutants, Occupational
Occupational Dentistry   WA 412
Occupational Dermatitis see Dermatitis, Occupational
Occupational Diseases   WA 400-495
    Medicolegal aspects   W 925
    Mental disorders (General)   WA 495
    Nursing see Occupational Health Nursing   WY 141
    Ophthalmological   WW 505
    Prevention & control   WA 440-475
    See also Disability Evaluation   W 925, etc.;
        Workers' Compensation   HD 7103.6-7103.65, etc.
Occupational Exposure   WA 400-495
    See also Environmental Exposure
Occupational Health   WA 400-495

Special topics, by subject
Occupational Health Nursing   WY 141
   Education   WY 18-18.5
Occupational Health Services   WA 412
   Mental health   WA 495
     See also Mental Health Services   WM 30,
     etc.
Occupational Hygiene see Occupational Health
Occupational Medicine   WA 400-495
Occupational Mobility see Career Mobility
Occupational Neuroses see Occupational Diseases;
   Mental Health
Occupational Noise see Noise, Occupational
Occupational Nursing see Occupational Health
   Nursing
Occupational Safety see Occupational Health
Occupational Therapy   WB 555
   Hospital department   WX 225
   Adolescence   WS 463
   For infants and children
     For mentally disabled   WS 350.2
     For physically disabled   WS 368
   In psychiatry   WM 450.5.O2
   See also Rehabilitation, Vocational   HD
   7255-7256
Occupational Therapy Department, Hospital   WX
225
Occupational Toxicology see Poisons; Toxicology
Occupations
   Statistics and demographic discussions   HB
   2581-2787
   Specific occupations, by type, e.g., Surgery   WO
   21
   See also Vocational Guidance   HF
   5381-5382.67, etc.
Oceanography   GC
   General works   GC 10.9-11.2
Ochronosis   WR 267
Octadecenoic Acids see Oleic Acids
Octodon see Rodentia
Octogenarian see Aged, 80 and over
Ocular Accommodation see Accommodation,
   Ocular
Ocular Adaptation see Adaptation, Ocular
Ocular Dominance see Vision
Ocular Fixation see Fixation, Ocular
Ocular Fluorophotometry see Fluorophotometry
Ocular Herpes zoster Virus see Herpesvirus 3,
   Human
Ocular Infections, Parasitic see Eye Infections,
   Parasitic
Ocular Motility see Eye Movements
Ocular Motility Disorders   WW 410
Ocular Physiology   WW 103
Ocular Prosthesis see Eye, Artificial
Ocular Refraction see Refraction, Ocular
Ocular Tension see Intraocular Pressure
Ocular Torticollis see Ocular Motility Disorders
Ocular Toxoplasmosis see Toxoplasmosis, Ocular
Ocular Tuberculosis see Tuberculosis, Ocular
Oculomotor Muscles   WW 400-460
   See also Eye Movements   WW 400-460
Oculomotor Nerve   WL 330

Oculomotor Paralysis see Ophthalmoplegia
Ocytocin see Oxytocin
Oddi's Sphincter   WI 750
Odontoblasts   WU 230
Odontogenic Cysts   WU 280
Odontogenic Tumors   WU 280
   Pathology of dental tissue   QZ 200
Odontometry   WU 141.5.O2
Odontostomatology see Mouth   WU, Tooth   WU
   and related headings
Odors
   Industrial control   WA 450
   Otolaryngology   WV 301
   Pollution   WA 754
Oedipus Complex   WM 460
Oesophagus see Esophagus
Offenses, Sexual see Sex Offenses
Office Automation   W 26.5
   In special areas, by subject
Office Management   W 80
   Dental   WU 77
   See also Dental Offices   WU 77 and names of
     specialties involved, e.g., Psychiatry   WM 30
Office Nursing   WY 109
Office Surgery see Ambulatory Surgical Procedures
Office Visits
   Made for special purpose, by subject
Offspring of Impaired Parents see Child of Impaired
   Parents
Ofloxacin   QV 250
Oils   QV 785
   Biochemistry   QU 86
   Public health aspects   WA 722
   See also names of specific oils
Oils, Essential see Oils, Volatile
Oils, Plant see Plant Oils
Oils, Unsaturated see Fats, Unsaturated
Oils, Vegetable see Plant Oils
Oils, Volatile   QV 785
   Biochemistry   QU 86
   Chemical technology   TP 958-959
Ointments   QV 785
OK-432 see Picibanil
Oka Varicella Vaccine see Chickenpox Vaccine
Okadaic Acid
   As an enzyme inhibitor   QU 143
Old Age see Aged   WT
Old Age Assistance   WT 30
   Social Security   HD 7090-7250
Old Age Homes see Homes for the Aged
Old Age Insurance see Medicare; Social Security
Oldest Old see Aged, 80 and over
Oleates see Oleic Acids
Olefins see Alkenes
Oleic Acids   QU 90
   Pharmaceutical agents   QV 785
Oleomargarine see Margarine
Oleoresins see Resins; specific resins or plants from
   which derived, e.g., Aspidium
Olfaction see Smell
Olfactory Cortex see Olfactory Pathways
Olfactory Mucosa   WV 301

**ALWAYS CONSULT MAIN SCHEDULES. USE NUMBER ASSIGNED ONLY WHEN
SUBJECT REPRESENTS MAJOR EMPHASIS OF WORK BEING CLASSIFIED**

Olfactory Nerve   WL 330
   See also Smell   WV 301
Olfactory Pathways   WL 314
Olfactory Sense see Smell
Olfactory Tract see Olfactory Pathways
Olfactory Tubercle see Olfactory Pathways
Oligemia see Anemia
Oligochaeta   QX 451
Oligochromemia see Anemia
Oligomenorrhea   WP 522
Oligonucleotide–Directed Mutagenesis see
   Mutagenesis, Site–Directed
Oligonucleotides   QU 57
Oligonucleotides, Antisense   QU 57
Oligopeptides   QU 68
Oligoribonucleotides   QU 57
Oligosaccharides   QU 83
omega–Chloroacetophenone   QV 665
Omega Protein see DNA Topoisomerase
Omega–3 Fatty Acids see Fatty Acids, Omega–3
Omentum   WI 575
Omeprazole   QV 69
OMP Proteins see Bacterial Outer Membrane
   Proteins
Omphalocele see Hernia, Umbilical
On–Line Systems see Online Systems
Onchocerca   QX 301
Onchocerciasis   WC 885
Oncogenes   QZ 202
Oncogenic Viruses   QW 166
Oncogens see Carcinogens
Oncologic Nursing   WY 156
Oncology, Medical see Medical Oncology
Oncolysis see Neoplasms
Ondatra see Microtinae
Ondine's Curse see Sleep Apnea Syndromes
Onions
   As dietary supplements in health and disease
    WB 430
   As medicinal plants   QV 766
   Botany   QK 495.L72
Onlays see Inlays
Online Systems   Z 699
   By subject   Z 699.5.A–Z
   In medicine (General)   W 26.55.I4
   In other special fields (Form number 26.5 in any
    NLM schedule where applicable)
Only Child   WS 105.5.F2
Ontogeny   QH 491
   Specific animal   QL
   Specific plant   QK
   See also names of organ or organism involved
Onychophagia see Nail Biting
Oocytes   WQ 205
Oophoritis   WP 320
Opacity, Vitreous see Vitreous Body
Opaque Media see Contrast Media
Open–Angle Glaucoma see Glaucoma, Open–Angle
Open Fractures see Fractures, Open
Operating Room Nursing   WY 162
   Education   WY 18–18.5
Operating Room Technicians   WY 162
Operating Rooms   WX 200
   Architectural planning and construction   WX

   140
Operations Research
   Industrial engineering   T 57.6–57.97
   Special topics, by subject
Operative Dentistry see Dentistry, Operative
Operative Obstetrics see Abortion, Induced;
   Cesarean Section; Delivery; Embryotomy; and
   other specific subjects
Operative Surgery see Surgery, Operative
Operon   QH 450.2
Ophthalmia see Endophthalmitis
Ophthalmia, Sympathetic   WW 525
Ophthalmic Artery   WG 595.07
   See also Blood supply   WW 101–103 under Eye
Ophthalmic Assistants   WW 21.5
Ophthalmic Nerve   WL 330
Ophthalmic Solutions   WW 166
Ophthalmologic Surgical Procedures   WW 168
   See also Surgery   WW 168 under Eye Diseases
Ophthalmologists see Biography   WZ 100, etc, and
   Directories   WW 22 under Ophthalmology
Ophthalmology   WW
   Biography
    Collective   WZ 112.5.O7
    Individual   WZ 100
   Aged   WW 620
   Child   WW 600
   Directories   WW 22
   Infant   WW 600
   Occupational   WW 505
   Instrumentation   WW 26
   Surgery   WW 168
    See also Ophthalmological Surgical Procedures
     WW 168
   Traumatic see Eye Injuries   WW 525
   See also Eye Diseases   WW 140, etc.
Ophthalmoplegia   WW 410
Ophthalmoscopes   WW 26
Ophthalmoscopy   WW 143
   Veterinary   SF 891
Opiate Addiction see Opioid–Related Disorders
Opiate Dependence see Opioid–Related Disorders
Opiates see Narcotics
Opiates, Endogenous see Opioid Peptides
Opioid Analgesics see Analgesics, Opioid
Opioid Peptides   QU 68
Opioid–Related Disorders   WM 284
   See also names of specific narcotics
Opioids see Narcotics
Opisthorchiasis   WC 805
Opisthorchis   QX 353
Opisthorchis felineus see Opisthorchis
Opisthorchis sinensis see Clonorchis sinensis
Opisthorchis viverrini see Opisthorchis
Opium
   Dependence   WM 286
    See also Heroin Dependence   WM 288;
     Morphine Dependence   WM 286
   Alkaloids   QV 90
Opossums   QL 737.M34
Oppenheim–Ziehen Disease see Dystonia
   Musculorum Deformans
Oppenheim's Disease see Neuromuscular Diseases

Opportunistic Infections
    General   WC 195
    Parasitic   WC 695
    Viral   WC 500
Opportunistic Infections, AIDS–Related see
    AIDS–Related Opportunistic Infections
Oppositional Defiant Disorder see Attention Deficit
    and Disruptive Behavior Disorders
Opsonins
    Antibodies   QW 601
    Clinical analysis   QY 455
    Derived from complement   QW 680
    See also Phagocytosis   QW 690
Optic Atrophy   WW 280
Optic Chiasm   WW 280
    For the neurologist   WL 330
Optic Lobe   WL 310
Optic Nerve   WW 280
    For the neurologist   WL 330
    See also Innervation   WW 101–103 under Eye;
       Vision   WW 103, etc.
Optic Nerve Diseases   WW 280
Optic Nerve Neoplasms   WW 280
Optic Neuritis   WW 280
Optic Neuropathy, Ischemic   WW 280
Optical Dispensing see Optometry
Optical Illusions   WW 105
Optical Instruments see Instrumentation   WW 26
    under Ophthalmology or Optometry;
    Instrumentation   QC 370.5–379 under Optics;
    names of particular instruments or procedures
Optical Readers see Automatic Data Processing
Optical Rotatory Dispersion
    Physical chemistry   QD 473
Opticians see Optometry
Optics   QC 350–467
    Instrumentation   QC 370.5–379
    Physiological see Optometry   WW 704, etc.;
       Vision   WW, etc.
    Stereoscopy   WN 100
Optometrists see Biography   WZ 112.5.07, etc., and
    Directories   WW 722 under Optometry
Optometry   WW 704–722
    Biography
       Collective   WZ 122.5.O7
       Individual   WZ 100
    Directories   WW 722
    Instrumentation   WW 26
    Optical dispensing   WW 350–355
    Opticianry   WW 350–358
    Opticians   WW 704–722
    See also names of functions of the optometrist,
       e.g., Orthoptics   WW 405
Oral Fistula
    General works for the dentist   WU 140
    General works for the gastroenterologist   WI
    200
Oral Health   WU 113
    Child   WU 113.6
    Infant   WU 113.6
    See also Nutrition and oral health   WU 113.7
Oral Hemorrhage   WU 140
Oral Hygiene   WU 113

Child   WU 113.6
    Infant   WU 113.6
Oral Hygiene Index   WU 30
Oral Manifestations   WU 290
    Of particular diseases, with the disease
Oral Medicine   WU 140
Oral Myotherapy see Myofunctional Therapy
Oral Rehydration Therapy see Fluid Therapy
Oral Surgery see Surgery, Oral
Oral Surgical Procedures   WU 600–640
    Atlases   WU 600.7
    Child   WU 480
    Infant   WU 480
    See also Surgery, Oral   WU 600–640, etc.
Oral Surgical Procedures, Preprosthetic   WU 500
Oral Tobacco see Tobacco, Smokeless
Oral Ulcer   WU 140
Orangutan see Pongo pygmaeus
Orbit   WW 202
Orbital Diseases   WW 202
Orbital Implants   WW 358
Orbital Neoplasms   WW 202
Orchidectomy see Orchiectomy
Orchiectomy   WJ 868
Orchitis   WJ 830
Orciprenaline   QV 129
Orderlies see Personnel, Hospital
Ordiflazine see Lidoflazine
Orf see Ecthyma, Contagious
Organ Banks see Tissue Banks
Organ Donors see Tissue Donors
Organ Failure, Multiple see Multiple Organ Failure
Organ Grafts see Transplants
Organ of Corti   WV 250
Organ Preservation   WO 665
    Of specific organs, with the organ
Organ regeneration see Regeneration
Organ Specificity   QW 700
    Special topics, by subject
Organ Temperature see Body Temperature
Organ Transplantation   WO 660–690
Organ Transplants see Transplants
Organelles   QH 591
Organic Brain Syndrome, Nonpsychotic see
    Delirium, Dementia, Amnestic, Cognitive
    Disorders
Organic Chemicals
    Organic chemistry   QD 241–441
Organic Food see Health Food
Organic Food see Health Food
Organic Mental Disorders see Delirium, Dementia,
    Amnestic, Cognitive Disorders
Organic Mental Disorders, Psychotic see Delirium,
    Dementia, Amnestic, Cognitive Disorders
Organic Mental Disorders, Substance–Induced see
    Substance–Related Disorders
Organic Poisons see Poisons
Organic Psychoses see Delirium, Dementia,
    Amnestic, Cognitive Disorders
Organisms, Transgenic   QH 442.6
Organization and Administration
    Health services see Health Services
    Administration   W 84, etc.

ALWAYS CONSULT MAIN SCHEDULES. USE NUMBER ASSIGNED ONLY WHEN
SUBJECT REPRESENTS MAJOR EMPHASIS OF WORK BEING CLASSIFIED

Hospital see Hospital Administration   WX 150–190
Hospital personnel see Personnel Administration, Hospital   WX 159–159.5
Library see Library Administration   Z 678–678.88
Medicine   W 88
Neurology   WL 30
Nursing   WY 105
Nursing schools   WY 20
Pharmacy see Pharmacy Administration   QV 737
Psychiatry   WM 30
Public health see Public Health Administration   WA 525–590
Organization and Administration, Hospital see Hospital Administration
Organizational Change see Organizational Innovation
Organizational Decision Making see Decision Making, Organizational
Organizational Innovation
Hospital Administration   WX 150–190
Nursing Service   WY 105
Public Health Administration   WA 525–590
Specific types of organization, by organization
Organizations   HM
See also names of specific types of organizations, e.g. Voluntary Health Agencies   WA 1, etc.; names of specialties
Organizations, Nonprofit
(Form number 1 in any NLM schedule where applicable)
Non–medical   HD 2769.15–2769.2
Organochlorine Insecticides see Insecticides, Organochlorine
Organoids   QH 581–581.2
Organometallic Compounds
Biochemistry   QU 131
Organic chemistry   QD 410–412.5
Pharmacology   QV 290
Organophosphorus Compounds
Biochemistry   QU 131
Organic chemistry   QD 305.P6; QD 406
Toxicology   QV 627
See also Insecticides, Organophosphate   WA 240, etc.
Organoplatinum Compounds
Biochemistry   QU 131
Pharmacology   QV 290
Organotherapy   WB 391
Organothiophosphorus Compounds
Biochemistry   QU 131
Organic chemistry   QD 412.P1
Toxicology   QV 627
See also Insecticides, Organothiophosphate   WA 240, etc.
Orgasm   HQ 19–25
Orgasmic Disorder see Sexual Dysfunctions, Psychological
Oriental Medicine, Traditional see Medicine, Oriental Traditional

Orientation
Animal   QL 782.5
Aviation   WD 730
Bird navigation and migration   QL 698.8–698.9
Outer space   WD 754
Psychophysiology   WL 103
Reflex   WL 106
Spatial   WV 255
Visual see Adaptation, Ocular   WW 109
See also Adaptation, Psychological   WD 730, etc.
Orientation Programs, Employee see Inservice Training
Origin of Life see Biogenesis
Ormond's Disease see Retroperitoneal Fibrosis
Ornithine   QU 60
Ornithine Carboxy–lyase see Ornithine Decarboxylase
Ornithine Decarboxylase   QU 139
Ornithosis   WC 660
Orosomucoid   WH 400
Clinical examination   QY 455
Orotic Acid
In nucleic acid biosynthesis and metabolism   QU 58
Organic chemistry   QD 401
Oroya Fever see Bartonella Infections
Orphan Drug Production   QV 736
Orphanages   HV 959–1420.5
ortho–Dihydroxybenzenes see Catechols
Orthodontia see Orthodontics
Orthodontic Appliances   WU 426
Orthodontic Appliances, Activator see Activator Appliances
Orthodontic Wires   WU 426
Orthodontics   WU 400–440
See also Dental Occlusion   WU 440; Malocclusion   WU 440
Orthodontics, Corrective   WU 400–440
Orthodontics, Preventive   WU 400
Orthomolecular Therapy   WB 330
In psychiatry   WM 402
Orthomyxoviridae   QW 168.5.O7
Orthomyxoviridae Infections   WC 512
Orthomyxovirus Infections see Orthomyxoviridae Infections
Orthomyxovirus Type A, Avian see Influenza A Virus, Avian
Orthomyxovirus Type A, Porcine see Influenza A Virus, Porcine
Orthopantomography see Radiography, Panoramic
Orthopedic Equipment   WE 26
See also Prosthesis   WE 172, etc.; Specific types of equipment, e.g., Bone Plates   WE 185
Orthopedic Fixation Devices   WE 185
Orthopedic Nursing   WY 157.6
Orthopedic Procedures   WE 168–190
General works   WE 168
Child   WS 270
Infant   WS 270
Nursing   WY 157.6
Reconstructive orthopedic procedures   WE 190
Veterinary   SF 910.5

See also names of particular bones, joints, or
  procedures; Orthopedics   WE 168–190, etc.
Orthopedic Surgery see Orthopedics
Orthopedics   WE 168 190
  General works   WE 168
  Animals   SF 910.5
  Child   WS 270
  Infant   WS 270
  Nursing   WY 157.6
  Reconstructive orthopedics   WE 190
  See also Orthopedic Procedures   WE 168–190,
    etc.
Orthopsychiatry
  Adolescence   WS 463
  Child   WS 350.6
  Infant   WS 350.6
  Social Behavior Disorders   WM 600
    Child   WS 350.8.S6
    Infant   WS 350.8.S6
Orthoptera   QX 570
Orthoptics   WW 405
Orthoses see Orthotic Devices
Orthotic Devices   WE 26
Ortonal see Methaqualone
Oryza see Rice
Oscillators, Endogenous see Biological Clocks
Oscillometry
  Biophysics   QT 34
  Circulation studies   WG 106
Osgood–Schlatter Disease see Osteochondritis
OSHA see Legislation   WA 32–33 under Accidents,
  Occupational, Occupational Medicine, or
  Occupational Diseases
Osler–Rendu Disease see Telangiectasia, Hereditary
  Hemorrhagic
Osler–Vaquez Disease see Polycythemia Vera
Osler's Disease see Polycythemia Vera;
  Telangiectasia, Hereditary Hemorrhagic
Osmium
  Inorganic chemistry   QD 181.07
  Pharmacology   QV 290
Osmolality see Osmolar Concentration
Osmolar Concentration   QD 541
  Pharmaceutical chemistry   QV 744
Osmolarity see Osmolar Concentration
Osmoregulation see Water-Electrolyte Balance
Osmosis
  Biochemical phenomena   QU 34
  Cytology   QH 615
  Inorganic chemistry   QD 543
  Plant physiology   QK 871
Osmotic Diuretics see Diuretics, Osmotic
Osmotic Pressure   QD 543
Osseointegration   WE 200
Ossicular Prosthesis   WV 230
Ossicular Prosthesis Implantation see Ossicular
  Replacement
Ossicular Replacement   WV 230
Ossification, Heterotopic   QZ 180
  Localized, by site
Ossification of Posterior Longitudinal Ligament
  WE 725
Ossification, Pathologic see Ossification, Heterotopic

Ossification, Physiologic see Osteogenesis
Osteitis   WE 251
Osteitis Deformans   WE 250
Osteitis Fibrosa Cystica   WK 300
Osteitis Fibrosa Disseminata see Fibrous Dysplasia
  of Bone
Osteoarthritis   WE 348
  Localized, by site
    Veterinary   SF 901
Osteoarthritis, Hip   WE 860
Osteoarthritis, Knee   WE 870
Osteoarthrosis see Osteoarthritis
Osteoarthrosis Deformans see Osteoarthritis
Osteoblastoma   WE 258
  Localized, by site
Osteochondritis   WE 259
  Localized, by site
Osteochondrodysplasias   WE 250
Osteochondromas, Multiple see Exostoses, Multiple
  Hereditary
Osteochondromatosis   WE 250
Osteochondrosis see Osteochondritis
Osteoclastic Bone Loss see Bone Resorption
Osteocytes   WE 200
Osteogenesis   WE 200
Osteogenesis, Distraction   WE 168
  In oral surgery   WU 600
  Localized, by site
Osteogenesis Imperfecta   WE 250
Osteology see Bone and Bones
Osteolysis   WE 200
Osteoma   QZ 340
  Localized, by site
Osteoma, Giant Osteoid see Osteoblastoma
Osteoma, Osteoid   WE 258
  Localized, by site
Osteomalacia   WD 145
Osteomyelitis   WE 251
Osteopathic Manipulation see Manipulation,
  Orthopedic
Osteopathic Medicine   WB 940
Osteopathy see Osteopathic Medicine
Osteopenia see Bone Diseases, Metabolic
Osteopetrosis   WE 250
Osteophytosis, Spinal see Spinal Osteophytosis
Osteoporosis   WE 250
Osteoporosis, Age-Related see Osteoporosis
Osteoporosis, Post-Traumatic see Sudeck's Atrophy
Osteoporosis, Postmenopausal   WE 250
Osteoporosis, Senile see Osteoporosis
Osteoradionecrosis   WE 250
Osteosarcoma   WE 258
  Localized, by site
Osteosclerosis   WE 250
Osteosclerosis Fragilis see Osteopetrosis
Osteosclerotic Anemia see Anemia, Myelophthisic
Osteosynthesis, Fracture see Fracture Fixation,
  Internal
Osteosynthesis, Fracture, Intramedullary see
  Fracture Fixation, Intramedullary
Osteotomy   WE 168
Osteotomy, Le Fort   WU 610

Ostomy
    General works   WI 900
      See also specific kind of ostomy, e.g.,
        Enterostomy, Gastrostomy, etc.
Otalgia see Ear Diseases
OTC Drugs see Drugs, Non-Prescription
Otitic Barotrauma see Otitis Media
Otitis   WV 200
Otitis Externa   WV 220
Otitis Interna see Labyrinthitis
Otitis Media   WV 232
Otitis Media, Purulent see Otitis Media, Suppurative
Otitis Media, Secretory see Otitis Media with
   Effusion
Otitis Media, Serous see Otitis Media
Otitis Media, Suppurative   WV 232
Otitis Media with Effusion   WV 232
Otolaryngologists see Biography   WZ 112.5.O8,
   etc., and Directories   WV 22 under
   Otolaryngology
Otolaryngology   WV
   Biography
      Collective   WZ 112.5.O8
      Individual   WZ 100
   Child   WV
   Directories   WV 22
   Infant   WV
   Surgery   WV 168
      See also Otorhinolaryngologic Surgical
        Procedures   WV 168
Otologic Surgical Procedures   WV 200
   See also Surgery   WV 200 under Ear
Otology see Otolaryngology
Otorhinolaryngologic Diseases   WV 140
   Disability evaluation   WV 32
   In various age groups   WV 140
   Intracranial complications   WV 180
   Nursing   WY 158.5
   Signs and symptoms   WV 150
   Surgery   WV 168
Otorhinolaryngologic Neoplasms   WV 190
Otorhinolaryngologic Surgical Procedures   WV
   168
   See also Surgery   WV 168 under
      Otorhinolaryngologic Diseases
Otorhinolaryngology see Otolaryngology
Otosclerosis   WV 265
Otoscopes   WV 26
Otospongiosis see Otosclerosis
Outbreaks see Disease Outbreaks
Outcome and Process Assessment (Health Care)
   W 84
   Of particular treatments, by subject, e.g.,
      Psychotherapy   WM 420
Outdoor Games see Recreation; Sports
Outer Membrane Proteins, Bacterial see Bacterial
   Outer Membrane Proteins
Outlines
   (Form number 18.2 in any NLM schedule where
      applicable)
Outpatient Care see Ambulatory Care
Outpatient Clinics see Ambulatory Care Facilities
Outpatient Clinics, Hospital   WX 205

   Specialty hospitals (Form numbers 27-28 in any
      NLM schedule where applicable)
Outpatient Health Services see Ambulatory Care
Outpatient Surgery see Ambulatory Surgical
   Procedures
Outpatients   WX 205
   Patient with a particular disease, with the disease
   See also Ambulatory Care
Outsourced Services
   In medicine (General)   W 74
   Other topics, class by subject if specific; if general,
      in economics number where available
   See also Contract Services   W 74, etc.
Outsourcing see Outsourced Services
Ovarian Cycle see Menstrual Cycle
Ovarian Cysts   WP 322
Ovarian Diseases   WP 320-322
Ovarian Follicle   WP 320
Ovarian Function Tests   WP 520
Ovarian Neoplasms   WP 322
Ovary   WP 320-322
   Endocrine function   WP 520-530
      General works   WP 520
      See also Corpus Lateum   WP 320, etc.;
        Ovarian Follicle   WP 320; names of
        hormones produced
   Ovarian function   WP 540
   In pregnancy in see Pregnancy, Ectopic   WQ
      220
Over-the-Counter Drugs see Drugs,
   Non-Prescription
Overdenture see Denture, Overlay
Overdose
   Adverse effects   QZ 42
   Drug action   QV 38
   Medication errors   QZ 42
   Particular drug, with the drug
Overeating see Hyperphagia
Overpopulation see Population Density
Overuse Syndrome see Cumulative Trauma
   Disorders
Overutilization of Health Services see Health
   Services Misuse
Oviducts
   Domestic animals   SF 871
   Human see Fallopian Tubes   WP 300, etc.
   Wild animals   QL 881
Oviducts, Mammalian see Fallopian Tubes
Ovine Catarrhal Fever Virus see Bluetongue Virus
Ovocytes see Oocytes
Ovulation   WP 540
   Animal   SF 871
   See also Contraception   WP 630, etc.
Ovulation Detection   WP 540
Ovulation Induction   WP 540
Ovum
   Animal   QL 965
   Development   WQ 205
Ovum Implantation   QS 645
Ovum Implantation, Delayed   WQ 205
Ovum Proteins see Egg Proteins
Ovum-Sperm Interactions see Sperm-Ovum
   Interactions

**ALWAYS CONSULT MAIN SCHEDULES. USE NUMBER ASSIGNED ONLY WHEN
SUBJECT REPRESENTS MAJOR EMPHASIS OF WORK BEING CLASSIFIED**

Oxalates
　As disinfectants　QV 220
　Biochemistry　QU 98
　Toxicology　QV 632
Oxalic Acid
　Biochemistry　QU 98
　Toxicology　QV 632
Oxandrolone　WJ 875
Oxazoles　QV 95
Oxidants, Photochemical　WA 754
Oxidases see Oxidoreductases
Oxidation see Metabolism
Oxidation-Reduction
　Organic chemistry　QD 281.O9
　Metabolism　QU 125
Oxidative Phosphorylation　QU 125
Oxides　QV 312
Oxidizing Antiseptics see Anti-Infective Agents,
　Local; Hydrogen Peroxide; Potassium
　Permanganate
Oxidoreductases　QU 140
Oximes　QV 124
Oximetry　QY 480
Oximetry, Transcutaneous see Blood Gas
　Monitoring, Transcutaneous
Oxine see Oxyquinoline
Oxoglutarates see Ketoglutaric Acids
Oxophenarsine　QV 254
Oxopropanal see Pyruvaldehyde
Oxoquinolines see Quinolones
Oxycephaly see Craniosynostoses
Oxychlorochin see Hydroxychloroquine
Oxychloroquine see Hydroxychloroquine
Oxygen　QV 312
　Deficiency see Anoxia　WD 715, etc.
Oxygen Compounds　QV 312
Oxygen Consumption　WF 110
Oxygen Deficiency see Anoxia
Oxygen Inhalation Therapy　WF 145
Oxygen Partial Pressure Determination,
　Transcutaneous see Blood Gas Monitoring,
　Transcutaneous
Oxygenases　QU 140
Oxygenation, Hyperbaric see Hyperbaric
　Oxygenation
Oxygenators　WO 162
　Used for special purposes, by subject, e.g., during
　　open heart surgery　WG 168
Oxygenators, Membrane　WO 162
　Used for special purposes, by subject, e.g., during
　　postoperative care　WO 184, etc.
Oxyneurine see Betaine
Oxyntic Cells see Parietal Cells, Gastric
Oxyphenbutazone　QV 95
Oxyproline see Hydroxyproline
Oxyquinol see Oxyquinoline
Oxyquinoline
　As an anti-infective agent　QV 250
Oxytetracycline　QV 360
Oxytocics　QV 173-174
Oxytocin　QV 173
Oxyuriasis　WC 860
Oxyuroidea　QX 271

Oysters　QX 675
Ozena see Rhinitis, Atrophic
Ozone　QV 312

P

p-Aminohippuric Acid　QU 62
P-B Antibodies see Antibodies, Heterophile
P-Cell Stimulating Factor see Interleukin-3
p-Dihydroxybenzenes see Hydroquinones
p-Dimethylaminoazobenzene　QZ 202
P. P. Factor see Nicotinic Acids
Pacemaker, Artificial　WG 26
　See also Cardiac Pacing, Artificial　WG 168
Pacemakers, Biological see Biological Clocks
Pachymeninges see Dura Mater
Pacifiers see Infant Care
Pacing, Cardiac, Artificial see Cardiac Pacing,
　Artificial
Package Inserts see Product Labeling
Package Inserts, Drug see Drug Labeling
Packaging, Drug see Drug Packaging
Packaging of Drugs see Drug Packaging; Drug
　Labeling
Packed Red-Cell Volume see Hematocrit
Paclitaxel
　Pharmacology　QV 269
　Therapeutic use　QZ 267
PACS (Radiology) see Radiology Information
　Systems
Padutin see Kallikrein
PAF-Acether see Platelet Activating Factor
Paget's Disease of Bone see Osteitis Deformans
PAH see p-Aminohippuric Acid
PAI-3 see Protein C Inhibitor
Pain　WL 704
　Nursing (General)　WY 160.5
　Signs and symptoms　WB 176
　Localized, by site
　See also Abdominal Pain　WI 147; Pelvic Pain
　　WP 155
Pain Assessment see Pain Measurement
Pain, Facial see Facial Pain
Pain, Intractable　WL 704
Pain Measurement　WL 704
　In specific diseases, with the disease
Pain, Postoperative　WO 184
Pain Receptors see Nociceptors
Paint
　Chemical technology　TP 934-944
　Occupational health hazards, etc.　WA 400-495
　Lead poisoning　QV 292
Paintings
　Related to medicine　WZ 330
　Related to psychiatry　WM 49
Paired-Associate Learning　LB 1064
Palatal Neoplasms　WU 280
　For the otolaryngologist　WV 410
Palatal Obturators　WV 440
Palate　WV 410
　Cleft see Cleft Palate　WV 440
　Dentistry　WU 140
　Gastroenterology　WI 200

**ALWAYS CONSULT MAIN SCHEDULES.　USE NUMBER ASSIGNED ONLY WHEN
SUBJECT REPRESENTS MAJOR EMPHASIS OF WORK BEING CLASSIFIED**

Neoplasms see Palatal Neoplasms   WU 280, etc.
Palatine Tonsil see Tonsil
Palatopharyngeal Incompetence see Velopharyngeal
Insufficiency
Paleodontology   GN 209
Paleography   Z 105–115.5
Paleontology
Animal and plant   QE 701–996.5
Human   GN 282–286.7
Paleopathology   QZ 11.5
In veterinary medicine   SF 758
Paleostriatum see Globus Pallidus
Palladium
Dental chemistry and metallurgy   WU 180
Inorganic chemistry   QD 181.P4
Pharmacology   QV 290
Palliative Care   WB 310
Palliative Treatment see Palliative Care
Palm of Hand see Hand
Palmitic Acids   QU 90
Organic chemistry   QD 305.A2
Palmoplantar Keratoderma see Keratoderma,
Palmoplantar
Palmoplantaris Pustulosis see Psoriasis
Palpation   WB 275
Palsy see Cerebral Palsy; Facial Paralysis; Paralysis
Palsy, Progressive Supranuclear see Supranuclear
Palsy, Progressive
Paludism see Malaria
Pamphlets
Collections   W6 P3
Works about   Z 691
Others, by subject
Pan paniscus   QL 737.P96
As laboratory animals   QY 60.P7
Diseases   SF 997.5.P7
Pan troglodytes   QL 737.P9
As laboratory animals   QY 60.P7
Diseases   SF 997.5.P7
Panax see Ginseng
Pancoast's Syndrome   WF 658
Pancreas   WI 800–830
Surgery (General)   WI 830
See also Cystic Fibrosis   WI 820; Islets of
Langerhans   WK 800–885
Pancreas, Artificial   WI 830
Pancreas, Artificial Endocrine see Insulin Infusion
Systems
Pancreas, Endocrine see Islets of Langerhans
Pancreas Transplantation   WI 830
Pancreatectomy   WI 830
Pancreatic Alpha Cells see Islets of Langerhans
Pancreatic Beta Cells see Islets of Langerhans
Pancreatic Cyst   WI 810
Pancreatic Cystic Fibrosis see Cystic Fibrosis
Pancreatic Delta Cells see Islets of Langerhans
Pancreatic Diseases   WI 800–830
General works   WI 800
Pancreatic Ducts   WI 802
Pancreatic Extracts
Pharmacology   QV 370
Therapeutic use (General)   WB 391
Used for treatment of particular disorders, with

the disorder or system
Pancreatic Fistula   WI 800
Pancreatic Function Tests   WI 802
Pancreatic Hormones   WK 801
See also Glucagon   WK 801; Insulin   WK 820
Pancreatic Islets Transplantation see Islets of
Langerhans Transplantation
Pancreatic Juice   WI 802
Pancreatic Neoplasms   WI 810
Pancreatitis   WI 805
Pancreatitis, Alcoholic   WI 805
Pancreozymin see Cholecystokinin
Pancreozymin Receptors see Receptors,
Cholecystokinin
Paneth Cells   WI 500
Panic   WM 172
Panic Attacks see Panic Disorder
Panic Disorder   WM 172
Panniculitis, Nodular Nonsuppurative   WR 140
Panophthalmitis   WW 140
Panoramic Radiography see Radiography,
Panoramic
Panotitis see Otitis
Pantomography see Radiography, Panoramic
Pantothenic Acid   QU 195
Papain   QU 136
Papanicolaou Smear see Vaginal Smears
Papaver   QV 90
As a medicinal plant   QV 766
See also Opium   QV 90, etc.
Papaveretum see Opium
Paper
Industrial waste   WA 778
Printing   Z 237, Z 247
Papillary Muscles   WG 201–202
Papilledema   WW 280
Papilloma   QZ 365
Localized, by site
Papilloma, Shope see Tumor Virus Infections
Papillomavirus   QW 165.5.P2
Papillomavirus, Human   QW 165.5.P2
Papio   QL 737.P93
As laboratory animals   QY 60.P7
Diseases   SF 997.5.P7
Papovaviridae   QW 165.5.P2
PAPP-D see Placental Lactogen
Pappataci Fever see Phlebotomus Fever
Papulosquamous Dermatoses see Skin Diseases
para–Aminohippuric Acid see p–Aminohippuric
Acid
para–Dihydroxybenzenes see Hydroquinones
Parabiosis
Immunology   QW 504
Twins, Conjoined   QS 675
Other special topics, by subject
Paracentesis   WB 373–377
See also Punctures   WB 373–377, etc.
Parachuting   WD 700
Accidents   WD 740
Paracoccidioidomycosis   WC 460
Paracusis see Auditory Perception
Paradentium see Periodontium
Paradoxical Sleep see Sleep, REM

Paraffin   QV 800
　　Plastic surgery   WO 640
Paraganglia, Chromaffin
　　In sympathetic ganglia   WL 610
　　In other organs, with the organ
Paraganglia, Nonchromaffin   WL 600
Paraganglioma   QZ 380
　　Localized, by site
Paraganglioma, Extra–Adrenal   QZ 380
　　Localized, by site
Paraganglioma, Nonchromaffin see Paraganglioma,
　　Extra–Adrenal
Paragonimiasis   WC 805
Paragonimus   QX 353
Paraimmunoglobulinemias see Paraproteinemias
Parainfluenza see Paramyxoviridae Infections
Parainfluenza Virus Infections see Paramyxoviridae
　　Infections
Parainfluenza Virus 1, Human   QW 168.5.P2
Parainfluenza Virus 3, Bovine see Paramyxovirus
Parakeratosis Variegata see Parapsoriasis
Paralysants see Chemical Warfare Agents
Paralysins see Agglutinins
Paralysis   WL 346
　　Agitans see Parkinsonism   WL 359
　　Cervical sympathetic   WL 610
　　Divers'   WD 712
　　Facial see Facial paralysis   WL 330
　　General see Paresis   WC 165, etc.
　　Infantile see Poliomyelitis   WC 555, etc.
　　Ocular muscles see Oculomotor paralysis   WW
　　410
　　Respiratory see Respiratory Paralysis   WF 140
　　Vocal cord see Vocal Cord Paralysis   WV 535
　　See also Hemiplegia   WL 346; Paraplegia
　　　　WL 346; Quadriplegia   WL 346
Paralysis Agitans see Parkinson Disease
Paralysis, Bulbar   WL 310
Paralysis, Familial Periodic   WD 205.5.P2
Paralysis, General see Paresis
Paralysis, Obstetric   WS 405
Paralysis, Pseudobulbar see Paralysis
Paralysis, Spastic see Muscle Spasticity
Paramagnetic Resonance see Electron Spin
　　Resonance Spectroscopy
Paramecium   QX 151
Paramedical Personnel see Allied Health Personnel
Paramedics see Allied Health Personnel
Paramedics, Emergency see Emergency Medical
　　Technicians
Parametritis   WP 275
Paramyoclonus Multiplex see Myoclonus
Paramyxoviridae   QW 168.5.P2
Paramyxoviridae Infections   WC 518
Paramyxovirus   QW 168.5.P2
Paramyxovirus Infections   WC 518–520
　　Veterinary   SF 809.P37
　　See also Measles   WC 580
Paranasal Sinuses   WV 340–358
　　See also Ethmoid Sinus   WV 355; Frontal Sinus
　　　　WV 350; Maxillary Sinus   WV 345;
　　　　Sphenoid Sinus   WV 358
Paranoia see Paranoid Disorders

Paranoid Behavior   WM 205
Paranoid Disorder, Shared see Shared Paranoid
　　Disorder
Paranoid Disorders   WM 205
Paranoid Psychoses see Paranoid Disorders
Paranoid Schizophrenia see Schizophrenia, Paranoid
Paraphilias   WM 610
Paraphimosis   WJ 790
Paraphrenia, Involutional see Depression,
　　Involutional
Paraplegia   WL 346
Paraplegia, Spastic see Paraplegia
Paraproteinemias   WH 400
　　See also Amyloidosis   WD 205.5.A6; Multiple
　　　　Myeloma   WH 540
Paraproteins   QW 601
　　See also Bence Jones Protein   WH 540;
　　　　Myeloma Proteins   WH 540
Parapsoriasis   WR 204
Parapsoriasis en Plaques see Parapsoriasis
Parapsychology   BF 1009–1389
　　Occult sciences   BF 1405–1999
Paraquat
　　Public health aspects   WA 240
Parasite–Host Relations see Host–Parasite Relations
Parasites   QX
　　Animal parasites
　　　　As a cause of disease   QZ 85
　　　　Zoology   QL 757
　　Communicable disease control   WA 240
Parasitic Diseases   WC 695–900
　　Veterinary see Parasitic Diseases, Animal   SF
　　　　810.A3
Parasitic Diseases, Animal   SF 810.A3
Parasitic Eye Infections see Eye Infections, Parasitic
Parasitic Skin Diseases see Skin Diseases, Parasitic
Parasiticides see Antiparasitic Agents
Parasitology   QX
　　Nursing texts   QX 4
　　Veterinary medicine   SF 810.A3
　　See also Parasitic Diseases   WC 695–900, etc.
Parasympathetic–Blocking Agents see
　　Parasympatholytics
Parasympathetic Ganglia see Ganglia,
　　Parasympathetic
Parasympathetic Nervous System   WL 610
　　Child   WS 340
　　Infant   WS 340
Parasympatholytics   QV 132
Parasympathomimetics   QV 122
Parathion
　　Agriculture   SB 952.P3
　　Public health   WA 240
Parathyroid Diseases   WK 300
Parathyroid Glands   WK 300
Parathyroid Hormones   WK 300
Parathyroid Neoplasms   WK 300
Paratopes see Binding Sites, Antibody
Paratuberculosis   SF 809.J6
Paratyphoid Fever   WC 266
　　Veterinary   SF 809.S24
Paratyphoid Vaccine see Typhoid–Paratyphoid
　　Vaccines

ALWAYS CONSULT MAIN SCHEDULES. USE NUMBER ASSIGNED ONLY WHEN
SUBJECT REPRESENTS MAJOR EMPHASIS OF WORK BEING CLASSIFIED

Paravertebral Anesthesia see Anesthesia,
   Conduction; Nerve Block
Parent–Child Relations   WS 105.5.F2
Parent, Single see Single Parent
Parental Leave
   General works   HD 6065–6065.5
Parenteral Feeding see Parenteral Nutrition
Parenteral Hyperalimentation see Parenteral
   Nutrition, Total
Parenteral Infusions see Infusions, Parenteral
Parenteral Nutrition   WB 410
Parenteral Nutrition, Total   WB 410
Parenterally–Transmitted Non–A, Non–B Hepatitis
   see Hepatitis C
Parents   HQ 755.7–759.92
   And illegitimacy   HQ 998–999
   Special topics, by subject
Paresis   WC 165
   Veterinary (Milk fever) see Parturient Paresis
   SF 967.M5
Paresthesia   WR 280
Parietal Cells, Gastric
   Cytology   WI 301
   Physiology   WI 302
Parietal Lobe   WL 307
Parkinson Disease   WL 359
   Drugs for see Antiparkinson agents   QV 80
Parodontitis see Periodontitis
Parodontosis see Periodontal Diseases
Paronychia   WR 475
Parotid Gland   WI 230
Parotid Neoplasms   WI 230
Parotitis   WI 230
   See also Mumps   WC 520
Parovarian Cyst   WP 275
Paroxysmal Dyspnea see Dyspnea, Paroxysmal
Paroxysmal Tachycardia see Tachycardia,
   Paroxysmal
Parrot Fever see Ornithosis
Parrots   QL 696.P7
   Diseases   SF 994.2.P37
   As laboratory animals   QY 60.B4
Parsonage–Turner Syndrome see Cervico–Brachial
   Neuralgia
Parthenogenesis   QH 487
Partial Denture see Denture, Partial
Partial Monosomy see Chromosome Deletion
Particle Accelerators   QC 787.P3
   In neoplasm radiotherapy   QZ 269
   Nuclear engineering   TK 9340
Particle–Induced X–Ray Emission Spectrometry see
   Spectrometry, X–Ray Emission
Particle Size
   Air pollutants   WA 754, etc.
   Determination   TA 418.8, etc.
   Dosage form   QV 785
   Particle technology (Chemical engineering)   TP
   156.P3
Partner Notification see Contact Tracing
Partnership Practice   W 92
Partnership Practice, Dental   WU 79
Parturient Paresis   SF 967.M5
Parturition see Labor

Parvoviridae   QW 165.5.P3
Parvoviridae Infections   WC 500
Parvovirus   QW 165.5.P3
Parvovirus Infections see Parvoviridae Infections
Passive Addiction, Neonatal see Neonatal
   Abstinence Syndrome
Passive–Aggressive Personality Disorder   WM 190
Passive Antibody Transfer see Immunization, Passive
Passive–Dependent Personality see Dependent
   Personality Disorder
Passive Immunity see Immunity, Passive
Passive Transfer of Immunity see Immunization,
   Passive
Pastes see Ointments
Pasteurella   QW 140
Pasteurella Infections   WC 200
   Veterinary   SF 809.P37
Pasteurellosis see Pasteurella Infections
Pastoral Care   WM 61
   See also Religion and Medicine   W 50, etc.;
      Religion and Psychology   WM 61, etc.;
      Chaplaincy Service, Hospital   WX 187
Pastoral Psychiatry see Pastoral Care
Pastoral Psychology see Pastoral Care
Patas Monkey see Erythrocebus patas
Patch Tests   QY 260
Patella   WE 870
Patent Medicines see Drugs, Non–prescription
Patents   T 201–342
   Chemicals   TP 210
   Drugs   QV 736
   Medical instruments (Form number 26 in any
      NLM schedule where applicable)
Paternal Behavior   WS 105.5.F2
Paternal Deprivation   WS 105.5.D3
Paternity
   Medicolegal aspects   W 791
   See also headings beginning with Father and
      Paternal
Paternity Leave see Parental Leave
Pathogenesis of Disease see Disease
Pathogenic Fungi see Fungi
Pathogens, Blood–Borne see Blood–Borne
   Pathogens
Pathological Waste see Medical Waste
Pathologists see Biography   WZ 112.5.P2, etc., and
   Directories   QZ 22 under Pathology
Pathology   QZ
   Biography
      Collective   WZ 112.5.P2
      Individual   WZ 100
   Cardiovascular system   WG 142
   Child   WS 200
   Clinical   QY
   Comparative   QZ 33
   Dental see Pathology, Oral   WU 140 and
      subheading Pathology   WU 140 under Tooth
   Dermatology   WR 105
   Directories   QZ 22
   Infant   WS 200
   Nursing texts   QZ 4, etc.
      Clinical pathology   QY 4, etc.
   Physiological   QZ 140

**ALWAYS CONSULT MAIN SCHEDULES. USE NUMBER ASSIGNED ONLY WHEN
SUBJECT REPRESENTS MAJOR EMPHASIS OF WORK BEING CLASSIFIED**

I–194

See also the general works numbers for parts of
the body, diseases, or systems
Pathology, Clinical   QY
Pathology Department, Hospital   WX 207
Pathology, Oral   WU 140
See also Pathology under Mouth   WU 140 and
Tooth   WU 140
Pathology, Surgical   WO 142
Pathology, Veterinary   SF 769
Pathomimesis see Malingering
Patient Acceptance of Health Care   W 85
In the hospital   WX 158.5
Special areas of health care, by area
Patient Admission   WX 158
Patient Advocacy   W 85
Special topics, by subject
Patient Agent see Proxy
Patient Appointments see Appointments and
Schedules
Patient Care   W 84–84.8
Of hospital patients   WX 162–162.5
See also names of specific types of care, e.g.,
Nursing Care   WY 100, etc.
Patient Care Management   W 84.7
In nursing   WY 100
Of hospital patients   WX 162–162.5
Special topics, by subject
Patient Care Planning   W 84.7
In nursing   WY 100
Of hospital patients   WX 162–162.5
Patient Care Team   W 84.8
Hospital team   WX 162.5
See also Nursing, Team   WY 125
Patient Compliance   W 85
In hospitals   WX 158.5
In mental hospitals   WM 29.5
Special areas of compliance, by subject
Patient Cooperation see Patient Compliance
Patient Credit and Collection
Dental administration   WU 77
Hospital administration   WX 157
Medical administration   W 80
Nursing administration   WY 77
Pharmacy administration   QV 736
In other specific fields, by subject
Patient Data Privacy see Confidentiality
Patient Discharge   WX 158
Patient Education
General   W 85
See also Health Education   WA 590, etc.
In hospitals   WX 158.5
In mental institutions   WM 29.5
For specific conditions, with the condition
Patient–Family Lodging see Housing
Patient Isolation   WX 167
Patient Isolators   WX 147
Patient Monitoring see Monitoring, Physiologic
Patient Ombudsmen see Patient Advocacy
Patient Participation   WX 158.5
Patient Readmission   WX 158
Patient Representatives see Patient Advocacy
Patient Satisfaction
With health services, medical treatment, etc.

W 85
With hospitals   WX 158.5
With mental hospitals   WM 29.5
With other services or products, by subject
See also Patient Acceptance of Health Care
W 85
Patient Schedules see Appointments and Schedules
Patients   W 85
In hospitals   WX 158.5
In mental institutions   WM 29.5
With specific disabilities, with the disability
Patients' Libraries see Libraries, Hospital
Patients' Rights see Patient Advocacy
Pattern Recognition
Computer engineering   TK 7882.P3
(Form number 26.5 in any NLM schedule where
applicable)
Pattern Recognition, Visual   WW 105
Paul–Bunnell Antibodies see Antibodies, Heterophile
Pavor Nocturnus see Sleep Disorders
PCBs see Polychlorinated Biphenyls
PCP see Phencyclidine
PCP Abuse see Phencyclidine Abuse
PCR see Polymerase Chain Reaction
Peak Expiratory Flow Rate   WF 102
As a diagnostic test   WF 141
General physical examination   WB 284
Peanuts
Diets for control of fats   WB 425
Diets for control of protein   WB 426
Peas
As dietary supplement in health and disease
WB 430
Cultivation   SB 343
Peat   S 592.85
Soils   S 592.85
See also Mud Therapy   WB 525; Soil
Microbiology   QW 60
Peat Therapy see Mud Therapy
Pecten Oculi see Retinal Vessels
Pectins   QV 71
Pectoral Nerves see Thoracic Nerves
Pectoralis Muscles   WE 715
Pectus Excavatum see Funnel Chest
Pederasty see Paraphilias
Pediatric Dentistry   WU 480
See also special topics, e.g., Children   WU 113.6
under Oral hygiene
Pediatric Nursing   WY 159
Education   WY 18–18.5
Pediatric Ophthalmology see Child   WW 600;
Infant   WW 600
Pediatric Psychology see Child Psychology
Pediatricians, Directories see Directories   WS 22
under Pediatrics
Pediatrics   WS
Anesthesia   WO 440
Dentistry see Pediatric Dentistry   WU 480
Directories   WS 22
Diseases (General)   WS 200
Nursing see Pediatric Nursing   WY 159
Oncology   QZ 275
Ophthalmology   WW 600

Otolaryngology   WV
Radiology   WN 240
Surgery   WO 925
Pediculosis see Lice Infestations
Pediculus   QX 502
Pedodontics see Pediatric Dentistry
Pedophilia   WM 610
PEEP see Positive–Pressure Respiration
Peer Group
Adolescence   WS 462
Child   WS 105.5.I5
See also names of particular groups, e.g.
Physicians   W 21; persons with diabetes under
Diabetes mellitus   WK 810
Peer Review
(Form number 21 in any NLM schedule where
applicable, except Nursing   WY 16)
Peer Review Organizations see Professional Review
Organizations
Pelizaeus–Merzbacher Disease see Cerebral
Sclerosis, Diffuse
Pellagra   WD 126
Pelvic Bones   WE 750
Pelvic Exenteration   WE 750
Pelvic Infection see Adnexitis
Pelvic Inflammations see Adnexitis
Pelvic Inflammatory Disease see Adnexitis
Pelvic Neoplasms   WE 750
Pelvic Pain   WP 155
Pelvimetry   WQ 320
Pelvis
Gynecology   WP 155
Obstetrics   WQ 320
Pemphigus   WR 200
Neonatorum see Impetigo   WR 225
Pemphigus Vulgaris see Pemphigus
Penicillamine   QV 354
Penicillanic Acid   QV 354
Penicillin, Aminobenzyl see Ampicillin
Penicillin G   QV 354
Penicillin G, Benzathine   QV 354
Penicillin Resistance
Bacteriology   QW 51
Drug therapy   WB 330
Pharmacology   QV 354
Penicillinase   QU 136
Penicillins   QV 354
Penicillium   QW 180.5.D38
Penile Erection   WJ 790
Penile Implantation   WJ 790
For the treatment of impotence   WJ 709
Penile Neoplasms   WJ 790
Penile Prosthesis Implantation see Penile
Implantation
Penis   WJ 790
Pensions   HD 7105–7105.45
For particular groups of people, by group, e.g.,
for occupational health nurses   WY 141; for
nurses in general   WY 77
Pentachlorophenol
As an anti–infective agent   QV 223
Pentamethylenetetrazole see Pentylenetetrazole
Pentanoates see Valerates

Pentazocine   QV 89
Pentetrazole see Pentylenetetrazole
Penthiobarbital see Thiopental
Pentobarbital   QV 88
Pentose Phosphate Shunt see Pentosephosphate
Pathway
Pentose Shunt see Pentosephosphate Pathway
Pentosephosphate Pathway   QU 75
Pentoses   QU 75
Pentothal see Thiopental
Pentoxifylline   QV 107
Pentylenetetrazole   QV 103
In shock therapy   WM 410
People with Disabilities see Disabled Persons
Pepsin see Pepsin A
Pepsin A
Enzymology   QU 136
Gastric physiology   WI 302
Pepsinogens
Enzymology   QU 142
Gastric physiology   WI 302
Peptic Ulcer   WI 350–370
Peptic Ulcer Hemorrhage   WI 350
Peptic Ulcer Perforation   WI 350
Peptidase Inhibitors see Protease Inhibitors
Peptide Hormones see Hormones
Peptide Hydrolase Inhibitors see Protease Inhibitors
Peptide Hydrolases   QU 136
Peptide Peptidohydrolase Inhibitors see Protease
Inhibitors
Peptides   QU 68
Peptide hormones   WK 185
See also Oxytocin   QV 173
Peptococcus   QW 142.5.C6
Perception
Auditory see Auditory Perception   WV 272
Child   WS 105.5.D2
Color see Color Perception   WW 150
Depth see Depth Perception   WW 105
Distance see Distance Perception   WW 105
Form see Form Perception   WW 105
Infant   WS 105.5.D2
Motion see Kinesthesis   WE 104; Motion
Perception   WW 105
Neurophysiology   WL 705
Psychology   BF 311, etc.
Self see Self Concept   BF 697, etc.
Size see Size Perception   WW 105
Social see Social Perception   HM
Space see Space Perception   WW 105, etc.
Speech see Speech Perception   WV 272
Time see Time Perception   BF 468, etc.
Visual see Visual Perception   WW 105
Weight see Weight Perception   WE 104
Perception, Social see Social Perception
Perceptual Defense   WM 193.5.P3
Adolescence   WS 463
Child   WS 350.8.D3
Infant   WS 350.8.D3
Perceptual Disorders
General and psychotic   WM 204
Neurologic manifestation   WL 340
Specific sensory disorder, with the organ
involved

**ALWAYS CONSULT MAIN SCHEDULES. USE NUMBER ASSIGNED ONLY WHEN
SUBJECT REPRESENTS MAJOR EMPHASIS OF WORK BEING CLASSIFIED**

Perceptual Distortion   WL 705
Perceptual Motor Performance see Psychomotor
   Performance
Perchloroethylene see Tetrachloroethylene
Percussion   WB 278
Percutaneous Administration see Administration,
   Cutaneous
Percutaneous Electric Nerve Stimulation see
   Transcutaneous Electric Nerve Stimulation
Percutaneous Nephrolithotomy see Nephrostomy,
   Percutaneous
Percutaneous Nephrostomy see Nephrostomy,
   Percutaneous
Percutaneous Transluminal Angioplasty see
   Angioplasty, Balloon
Percutaneous Transluminal Coronary Angioplasty
   see Angioplasty, Transluminal, Percutaneous
   Coronary
Percutaneous Ultrasonic Lithotripsy see Lithotripsy
Performance Appraisal, Employee see Employee
   Performance Appraisal
Perfume   WA 744
   Chemical technology   TP 983.A1-983.Z5
Perfusion
   Organ preservation   WO 665
   Specific organs, with the organ
Perfusion, Pulsatile see Pulsatile Flow
Perfusion Pumps see Infusion Pumps
Perfusion Pumps, Implantable see Infusion Pumps,
   Implantable
Perfusion, Regional   QZ 267
   Localized, by site
Perhexiline   QV 150
Periadenitis Mucosa Necrotica Recurrens see
   Stomatitis, Aphthous
Perianeurysmal Fibrosis, Inflammatory see
   Retroperitoneal Fibrosis
Periaortitis, Chronic see Retroperitoneal Fibrosis
Periapical Abscess   WU 230
Periapical Cyst see Radicular Cyst
Periapical Diseases   WU 230
Periapical Granuloma   WU 240
Periapical Periodontitis, Chronic Nonsuppurative see
   Periapical Granuloma
Periapical Periodontitis, Suppurative see Periapical
   Abscess
Periaqueductal Gray   WL 310
Periarteritis Nodosa see Polyarteritis Nodosa
Periarthritis   WE 344
Pericardial Cyst see Mediastinal Cyst
Pericardial Effusion   WG 275
   Clinical examination   QY 210
Pericardial Fluid see Secretion under Pericardium
Pericarditis   WG 275
Pericarditis, Constrictive   WG 275
Pericardium   WG 275
   Secretion
      Clinical examination   QY 210
      General   WG 275
      In general diagnosis   WB 373
Pericementitis see Periodontitis
Pericytes   WG 700

Peridinium see Dinoflagellida
Perilymph   WV 250
Perilymphatic Duct see Cochlear Aqueduct
Perimenopausal Bone Loss see Osteoporosis,
   Postmenopausal
Perimetry   WW 145
Perinatal Medicine see Perinatology
Perinatal Mortality see Infant Mortality
Perinatal Nursing see Neonatal Nursing
Perinatology   WQ 210-211
   See also Neonatology   WS 420
Perineum   WE 750
   Injuries
      General   WE 750
      In the female   WP 170
Periodic Acid   QV 180
   Inorganic chemistry   QD 181.I1
Periodic Disease   WB 720
Periodic Health Examination see Physical
   Examination
Periodicals   W1
   Bibliography of medical and medically related
      ZW 1
   Government administrative reports and statistics
      W2
   Hospital administrative reports and statitics   WX
      2
   See also Newspapers   W1, etc.
Periodicity
   Animal behavior   QL 753-755.5
   Animal physiology   QP 84.6
   General biology   QH 527
   Human physiology   QT 167
   Menstrual cycle   WP 540
   Plants   QK 761
Periodontal Bone Loss see Alveolar Bone Loss
Periodontal Cyst   WU 240
Periodontal Cyst, Apical see Radicular Cyst
Periodontal Diseases   WU 240-242
   Periodontoclasia   WU 242
   Periodontosis   WU 242
   Pyorrhea alveolaris   WU 242
Periodontal Index   WU 240
Periodontal Pocket   WU 242
Periodontal Prosthesis   WU 240
Periodontal Resorption see Alveolar Bone Loss
Periodontal Splints   WU 240
Periodontics   WU 240-242
Periodontitis   WU 242
Periodontitis, Apical, Chronic Nonsuppurative see
   Periapical Granuloma
Periodontitis, Apical, Suppurative see Periapical
   Abscess
Periodontium   WU 240-242
Perioperative Care   WO 178
   See also Perioperative Nursing   WY 161, etc.
Perioperative Nursing   WY 161-162
   Education   WY 18-18.5
   See also Operating Room Nursing   WY 162;
      Perioperative Care   WO 178; Nursing   WY
      154, etc. under Critical Care
Peripheral Angiopathies see Peripheral Vascular
   Diseases

Peripheral Catheterization see Catheterization, Peripheral

Peripheral Nerve Diseases see Peripheral Nervous System Diseases

Peripheral Nerve Neoplasms   WL 500
   Localized, by site

Peripheral Nerves   WL 500–544
   See also Cranial Nerves   WL 330; Spinal Nerves
     WL 400

Peripheral Nervous System   WL 500–544

Peripheral Nervous System Agents   QV 76.5

Peripheral Nervous System Diseases   WL 500–544
   Child   WS 340
   Infant   WS 340
   Localized, by site
   Veterinary   SF 895

Peripheral Resistance see Vascular Resistance

Peripheral Vascular Diseases   WG 500–700
   General works   WG 500
     Child   WS 290
     Infant   WS 290
   Veterinary   SF 811

Periphlebitis see Phlebitis

Perissodactyla   QL 737.U6

Peristalsis   WI 102
   Intestinal   WI 402

Peristaltic Pumps, Implantable see Infusion Pumps, Implantable

Peritoneal Cavity   WI 575

Peritoneal Dialysis   WJ 378
   As treatment for diseases other than those of the kidney, by site or disease

Peritoneal Dialysis, Continuous Ambulatory   WJ 378

Peritoneal Diseases   WI 575

Peritoneal Effusion see Ascitic Fluid

Peritoneal Fluid see Ascitic Fluid

Peritoneal Infusions see Infusions, Parenteral

Peritoneal Neoplasms   WI 575

Peritoneoscopy see Laparoscopy

Peritoneovenous Shunt
   In the treatment of intractable ascites   WI 575

Peritoneum   WI 575

Peritonitis   WI 575

Peritonitis, Tuberculous see Tuberculosis, Peritoneal

Perkinism see Alternative Medicine

Permeability
   Capillary see Capillary Permeability   WG 700
   Cells see Cell Membrane Permeability   QH 601, etc.
   Magnetic induction   QC 754.2.P4
   Other special topics, by subject

Permeability, Capillary see Capillary Permeability

Permeability, Cell Membrane see Cell Membrane Permeability

Permeability, Microvascular see Capillary Permeability

Pernicious Anemia see Anemia, Pernicious

Pernio see Frostbite

Perodicticus potto see Lorisidae

Peroperative Care see Intraoperative Care

Peroperative Complications see Intraoperative Complications

Peroperative Period see Intraoperative Period

Peroxidase–Antiperoxidase Complex Technique see Immunoenzyme Techniques

Peroxidase–Labeled Antibody Technique see Immunoenzyme Techniques

Peroxidases   QU 140

Peroxide, Hydrogen see Hydrogen Peroxide

Peroxides
   Inorganic chemistry   QD 181.O1
   Organic chemistry   QD 305.E7
   Pharmacology   QV 60

Peroxisomal Disorders   WD 205.5.L5

Peroxisome Proliferators
   As carcinogens (General)   QZ 202
   Causing liver neoplasms   WI 735

Peroxisomes see Microbodies

Persian Gulf Syndrome
   Veterans' broad health care issues   UB 368–369.5
   Psychological aspects   WM 170–184
   Particular disorders, with the disorder

Persistent Common Atrioventricular Canal see Endocardial Cushion Defects

Persistent Fetal Circulation Syndrome   WS 421

Persistent Ostium Primum see Endocardial Cushion Defects

Persistent Pulmonary Hypertension of Newborn see Persistent Fetal Circulation Syndrome

Persistent Vegetative State   WB 182

Personal Expenditures see Financing, Personal

Personal Health Services   W 84

Personal Hygiene see Hygiene

Personal Liability see Liability, Legal

Personal narratives
   Physicians and specialists of medically related fields
     Collective   WZ 112–150
     Individual   WZ 100
   Special topics, by subject

Personal Satisfaction
   Job satisfaction   HF 5549.5.J63
   Success (General)   BJ 1611–1618
   Special topics, by subject

Personal Space
   Anthropogeography   GF 51
   Psychology   BF 469

Personality   BF 698–698.9
   Dependency   BF 575.D34
   In psychoanalysis   WM 460.5.P3
   See also Antisocial Personality Disorder   WM 190; Dual Personality   WM 173.6; Hysterical Personality   WM 173; Schizoid Personality   WM 203

Personality Assessment
   Psychiatric interview   WM 141
   Psychiatric testing   WM 145
   Psychological   BF 698.4–698.8

Personality Development   BF 698
   Adolescence   WS 462
   Child   WS 105.5.P3
   Infant   WS 105.5.P3

Personality Disorder, Antisocial see Antisocial Personality Disorder

Personality Disorder, Borderline see Borderline
   Personality Disorder
Personality Disorder, Compulsive see Compulsive
   Personality Disorder
Personality Disorder, Dependent see Dependent
   Personality Disorder
Personality Disorder, Histrionic see Histrionic
   Personality Disorder
Personality Disorder, Passive–Aggressive see
   Passive–Aggressive Personality Disorder
Personality Disorder, Schizoid see Schizoid
   Personality Disorder
Personality Disorder, Schizotypal see Schizotypal
   Personality Disorder
Personality Disorders
   General   WM 190
   Adolescence   WS 463
   Child   WS 350.8.P3
   Infant   WS 350.8.P3
Personality, Hysterical see Histrionic Personality
   Disorder
Personality Inventory
   Psychology   BF 698.5–698.8
   Psychiatry   WM 145
Personality Tests
   Psychology   BF 698.5–698.8
   Psychiatry   WM 145
Personality Type A see Type A Personality
Personnel Administration, Hospital   WX 159–159.8
   In psychiatric hospitals   WM 30
   In special hospitals, with the hospital
Personnel Discipline see Employee Discipline
Personnel Downsizing   HF 5549.5.D55
   Hospitals   WX 159
   Nursing   WY 30
   In special areas, by subject
Personnel, Hospital   WX 159–159.8
   See also names of specific types of personnel,
      e.g., Operating Room Technicians   WY 162
Personnel, Hospital, Organization and
   Administration see Personnel Administration,
   Hospital
Personnel Management   HF 5549.A2–5549.5
   Hospitals   WX 159
   Nursing   WY 30
   Special fields, by subject, e.g., Nursing,
      Supervisory   WY 105
Personnel Recruitment see Personnel Selection
Personnel Selection   HF 5549.5.S38
   Special fields, by subject
Personnel Staffing and Scheduling
   Hospitals   WX 159
   Nursing   WY 30
   Psychiatry   WM 30
Personnel Turnover
   Hospitals   WX 159
   Nursing   WY 30
   Psychiatry   WM 30
   Specific profession, by subject
Personnel Work see Personnel Management
Persons with Disabilities see Disabled Persons
Persons With Hearing Impairments see Hearing
   Impaired Persons

Perspiration see Sweat
Perspiratory Glands see Sweat Glands
Persuasion see Persuasive Communication
Persuasive Communication   BF 637.P4
Perthes Disease see Legg Perthes Disease
Pertussigen see Pertussis Toxins
Pertussis see Whooping Cough
Pertussis Toxins   WC 340
Pertussis Vaccine   WC 340
Pervasive Child Development Disorders see Child
   Development Disorders, Pervasive
Perversion, Sex see Paraphilias
Pes Cavus see Foot Deformities
Pes Planus see Flatfoot
Pessaries, Intracervical see Intrauterine Devices
Pessaries, Intrauterine see Intrauterine Devices
Pest Control   WA 240
   Agriculture   SB 950–990.5
   See also Insect Control   QX 600
Pest Control, Biological
   Agriculture   SB 975–978
   General public health   WA 240
   See also Insect Control   QX 600; names of other
      specific types of pest control
Pesticide Residues   WA 240
Pesticides
   Agriculture   SB 951–970.4
      Industrial poisoning   WA 465
   Public health   WA 240
   Toxicology   WA 240
Pet–Human Bonding see Bonding, Human–Pet
PET Scan see Tomography, Emission–Computed
Petechiae see Purpura
Pethidine see Meperidine
Petit Mal Epilepsy see Epilepsy, Absence
Petrolatum, Liquid see Mineral Oil
Petroleum
   Chemical technology   TP 690–699
   Toxicology   QV 633
Petrous Bone   WV 230
Petrous Pyramid see Petrous Bone
Pets see Animals, Domestic
Peyote see Mescaline
Pfaundler–Hurler Syndrome see
   Mucopolysaccharidosis I
PGE1 see Alprostadil
PGF2 see Dinoprost
PGF2alpha see Dinoprost
pH see Hydrogen–Ion Concentration
Phacoemulsification   WW 260
Phage lambda see Bacteriophage lambda
Phage Receptors see Receptors, Virus
Phage Typing see Bacteriophage Typing
Phages see Bacteriophages
Phages T see T–Phages
Phagocyte Bactericidal Dysfunction   QW 690
Phagocytes   QW 690
   See also Histiocytes   WH 650, etc.;
      Macrophages   WH 650, etc.; Monocytes
      WH 200, etc.; Neutrophils   WH 200, etc.
Phagocytosis   QW 690
Phanerochaete   QW 180.5.B2
   Botany   QK 629.C785

ALWAYS CONSULT MAIN SCHEDULES.   USE NUMBER ASSIGNED ONLY WHEN
SUBJECT REPRESENTS MAJOR EMPHASIS OF WORK BEING CLASSIFIED

Phantom Limb WE 170
Phantoms, Imaging WN 150
Phantoms, Radiographic see Phantoms, Imaging
Phantoms, Radiologic see Phantoms, Imaging
Pharmaceutic Aids QV 800
Pharmaceutical Chemistry see Chemistry,
   Pharmaceutical
Pharmaceutical Ethics see Ethics, Pharmacy
Pharmaceutical Preparations
   Administration & dosage QV 748
   Administrative methods WB 340–356
     See also Administration, Intranasal WB 342;
      Administration, Oral WB 350;
      Administration, Topical WB 340; Dosage
      Forms QV 785; Drug Administration
      Schedule WB 340; Injections WB 354;
      Perfusion, Regional QZ 267; Respiratory
      Therapy WF 145, etc., and particular
      diseases being treated
   Adverse effects QZ 42
   Analysis QV 25
   Autonomic see Autonomic Agents QV 120
   Catalogs see Catalogs, Drug QV 772
   General works QV 55
   Legislation see Legislation, Drug QV 32–33
   Metabolism QV 38
   Military supplies UH 420–425
   Mucopolysaccharidosis IV WD 205.5.C2
   Packaging QV 825
   Patent medicines see Drugs, Non–Prescription
   QV 772
   Preservation QV 754
    Public health aspects WA 730
   Proprietary QV 772
   Public health aspects WA 730
   Quack see Nostrums QV 722
   Receptors see Receptors, Drug QV 38
   Standards QV 771
   Supply & distribution QV 736
   See also Iatrogenic Disease QZ 42; names of
    specific drugs and types of drugs
Pharmaceutical Services QV 737
   Hospital see Pharmacy Service, Hospital WX
   179
   Insurance see Insurance, Pharmaceutical Services
    W 265, etc.
   Military
    General UH 420–425
    Navy VG 270–275
Pharmaceutical Solutions QV 786
   Used for specific purposes, by subject
   See also specific solution terms, e.g., Contact
    Lense Solutions WW 355; Hypertonic
    Solutions QV 786; Isotonic Solutions QV
    786; Ophthalmic Solutions WW 166
Pharmaceutics see Drugs
Pharmacies QV 737
   Directories QV 722
   Public health aspects WA 730
   See also Pharmacy Service, Hospital WX 179
Pharmacists
   Biography
    Collective WZ 112.5.P4

    Individual WZ 100
   Career books QV 21
   Directories QV 22
   Interprofessional and public relations QV 21
   Registration QV 29
Pharmacists' Aides QV 21.5
Pharmacoepidemiology QZ 42
   Special topics, by subject
Pharmacogenetics QV 38
Pharmacognosy QV 752
Pharmacokinetics QV 38
Pharmacology QV
   Dental QV 50
   Drug action QV 38
   Experimental QV 34
   Nursing texts QV 4, etc.
   Veterinary SF 915
   See also Psychopharmacology QV 77, etc.
Pharmacology, Arabic see Medicine, Arabic;
   Pharmacology
Pharmacology, Clinical QV 38
   See also Drug Therapy WB 330, etc.
Pharmacopoeias QV 738
Pharmacopoeias, Homeopathic WB 930
Pharmacotherapy see Drug Therapy
Pharmacy QV 701–835
   Instrumentation QV 26
   Military UH 420–425
   Naval VG 270–275
   Nursing texts QV 704, etc.
   Public health aspects WA 730
   Veterinary SF 915
Pharmacy Administration QV 737
   Veterinary medicine SF 915
   See also Pharmacy Service, Hospital WX 179
Pharmacy Education see Education, Pharmacy
Pharmacy Education, Continuing see Education,
   Pharmacy, Continuing
Pharmacy Education, Graduate see Education,
   Pharmacy, Graduate
Pharmacy Schools see Schools, Pharmacy
Pharmacy Service, Clinical see Pharmacy Service,
   Hospital
Pharmacy Service, Hospital WX 179
Pharyngeal Arches see Branchial Region
Pharyngeal Diseases WV 400–440
   General works WV 400
   Child WV 400–440
   Infant WV 400–440
   Nursing WY 158.5
Pharyngeal Region see Names of organs located in
   the region: Adenoids; Nasopharynx; Palate;
   Pharynx; Tonsil; Uvula
Pharyngitis WV 410
Pharynx WV 410
   In respiration WF 490
Phase–Contrast Microscopy see Microscopy,
   Phase–Contrast
Phaseolus see Legumes
Phaseolus vulgaris Lectins see Phytohemagglutinins
Phenacaine see Anesthetics, Local
Phenacetin QV 95
Phenadone see Methadone

Phenanthrenes   QV 138.C1
   Organic chemistry   QD 395
Phenanthridines
    As antineoplastic agents   QV 269
    Organic chemistry   QD 401
Phenantoin see Phenytoin
Phencyclidine   QV 77.7
Phencyclidine Abuse   WM 270
Phenemal see Phenobarbital
Phenethylamines   QU 61
   Organic chemistry   QD 341.A8
Phenformin   WK 825
Pheniramine   QV 157
Phenobarbital   QV 88
Phenobarbitone see Phenobarbital
Phenolphthaleins   QV 75
Phenols
    As anti-infective agents   QV 223
    Organic chemistry   QD 341.P5
Phenomenon see Anaphylaxis; Arthus Reaction;
   Shwartzman Phenomenon
Phenothiazine Antipsychotic Agents see
   Antipsychotic Agents, Phenothiazine
Phenothiazine Tranquilizers see Antipsychotic
   Agents, Phenothiazine
Phenothiazines   QV 253
    In veterinary pharmacology   SF 918.P5
    Organic chemistry   QD 401
Phenotype
    Human genetics   QH 431
    Human variation   GN 62.8-263
      Hereditary aspects   GN 247
    See also Somatotypes   GN 66.5
Phenoxybenzamine   QV 132
Phentanyl see Fentanyl
Phenyl Ethers
    Organic chemistry   QD 341.E7
    Used for special purposes, by subject
Phenylacetates   QU 98
    Organic chemistry   QD 341.A2
Phenylalanine   QU 60
Phenylamines see Aniline Compounds
Phenylbarbital see Phenobarbital
Phenylbutazone   QV 95
Phenylenediamines   QU 61
    Carcinogenicity research   QZ 202
Phenylethylamines see Phenethylamines
Phenylglycolic Acid see Mandelic Acids
Phenylhydrazines   QV 180
    Organic chemistry   QD 341.A8
Phenylketonuria   WD 205.5.A5
Phenylmethylamine see Benzylamines
Phenylthiocarbamide see Phenylthiourea
Phenylthiourea
    In goiter experiments   WK 259
    In taste experiments   WI 210
    Organic chemistry   QD 305.T45
Phenytoin   QV 85
Pheochromocytoma   QZ 380
    Localized, by site
Pheresis see Blood Component Removal
Pheromones
    Communication   QL 776

Secretion   QP 190
Phialophora   QW 180.5.D38
Philanthropic Funds see Fund Raising
Philately   HE 6187-6228
   Medical   WZ 340
Philocytase see Bacteriolysis; Hemolysins
Philology   P
   Chinese   PL 1001-2245
   General works   P
   English   PE
    Modern grammar   PE 1097-1400
   French   PC 2011-3761
   Latin   PA 2011-2915
   Modern (General)   PB 6-431
   Other languages in appropriate P schedule
   Special topics, by subject
   See also "phrase books" under specialty headings,
    e.g., Medicine, and names of language groups
    below
Philology, Classical   PA 1-2915
   Grammars for physicians and pharmacists   PA
   2092
   See also subheading, e.g., Latin   PA 2011-2915
   under Philology
Philology, Oriental   PJ-PL
   General works   PJ 10-187
   See also names of specific oriental languages
    under Philology, e.g., Chinese   PL 1001-2245
Philology, Romance   PC
   General works   PC 6-400
   See also language subheadings, e.g., French   PC
   2011-3761 under Philology
Philosophy   B-BD
   General works   B 69-5739
   Of science   Q 174-175.3
   Scientology   BP 605.S2
   See also names of specific philsophies, e.g.,
    Existentialism   B 105.E8 etc.; Humanism   B
   821
Philosophy, Medical   W 61
Philosophy, Nursing   WY 86
Phimosis   WJ 790
Phlebitis   WG 610
    Pyelophlebitis   WJ 351
    Other localities, by site
Phlebography   WG 600
    Localized, by site or disease
Phlebonarcosis see Anesthesia, Intravenous
Phlebothrombosis see Venous Thrombosis
Phlebotomus Fever   WC 526
Phlebotomy
    As therapy   WB 381
    As a diagnostic procedure   QY 25
Phlegmasia Alba Dolens see Thrombophlebitis
Phlegmon see Cellulitis
Phobia, School see Phobic Disorders
Phobia, Social see Phobic Disorders
Phobias see Phobic Disorders
Phobic Disorders   WM 178
Phobic Neuroses see Phobic Disorders
Phocoena see Porpoises
Phocoenidae see Porpoises
Phocoenoides see Porpoises

Phonation   WV 501
Phonation Disorders see Voice Disorders
Phonetics   P 215–240
  General   P 221
  Physiological aspects   WV 501
Phonocardiography   WG 141.5.P4
Phorbol Esters
  As carcinogens   QZ 202
Phorbol Myristate Acetate see
  Tetradecanoylphorbol Acetate
Phorias see Strabismus
Phosgene   QV 664
Phosphamidon
  Agriculture   SB 952.P5
  Public health   WA 240
Phosphatases see Phosphoric Monoester Hydrolases
Phosphates   QV 285
Phosphates, Inorganic see Phosphates
Phosphates, Organic see Organophosphorus
  Compounds
Phosphatidal Compounds see Plasmalogens
Phosphatidate Phosphatase   QU 136
Phosphatidate Phosphohydrolase see Phosphatidate
  Phosphatase
Phosphatides see Phospholipids
Phosphatidylcholine–Sterol O–Acyltransferase
  QU 141
Phosphatidylcholines   QU 93
Phosphatidylethanolamines   QU 93
Phosphatidylinositols   QU 93
Phosphines
  As pesticides   WA 240
  Inorganic chemistry   QD 181.P1
Phosphocreatine   WE 500
Phosphodiesterases see Phosphoric Diester
  Hydrolases
Phosphohydrolases see Phosphoric Monoester
  Hydrolases
Phosphoinositides see Phosphatidylinositols
Phospholipase A1 see Phospholipases A
Phospholipase A2 see Phospholipases A
Phospholipases   QU 136
Phospholipases A   QU 136
Phospholipids   QU 93
Phosphomonoesterases see Phosphoric Monoester
  Hydrolases
Phosphonic Acids
  Inorganic chemistry   QD 181.P1
  Pharmacology   QV 138.P4
Phosphonomycin see Fosfomycin
Phosphopeptides   QU 68
Phosphoprotein Phosphatase   QU 136
Phosphoprotein Phosphohydrolase see
  Phosphoprotein Phosphatase
Phosphoranes
  Inorganic chemistry   QD 181.P1
  Pharmacology   QV 138.P4
Phosphorescence see Luminescence
Phosphoric Acids   QD 181.P1
  Pharmacology   QV 138.P4
Phosphoric Diester Hydrolases   QU 136
Phosphoric Monoester Hydrolases   QU 136

Phosphorus
  Inorganic chemistry   QD 181.P1
  Metabolism   QU 130
  Of bone   WE 200
  Pharmacology   QV 138.P4
  Toxicology
    As an irritant poison   QV 618
    Organic poison   QV 627
Phosphorus Isotopes
  Inorganic chemistry   QD 181.P1
  Metabolism   QU 130
  Micro–organism metabolism   QW 52
  Of bone   WE 200
  Pharmacology   QV 138.P4
Phosphorus Metabolism Disorders   WD 200.5.P4
Phosphorus Poisons, Organic see Toxicology   QV
  627 under Organophosphorus Compounds
Phosphorus Radioisotopes   WN 420
  Nuclear physics   QC 796.P1
  See also special topics under Radioisotopes
Phosphorylase   QU 141
Phosphorylation   QD 281.P46
Phosphorylcholine, Acetyl Glyceryl Ether see
  Platelet Activating Factor
Phosphotransferases   QU 141
Phosphotransferases, ATP see Phosphotransferases
Phosvel see Leptophos
Photoaging of Skin see Skin Aging
Photobacterium   QW 141
Photobiology see Light
Photochemistry   QD 701–731
  Industrial   TP 249.5
  Other special topics, by subject
Photochemotherapy   WB 480
Photochemotherapy, Hematoporphyrin see
  Hematoporphyrin Photoradiation
Photocoagulation see Light Coagulation
Photodermatitis see Photosensitivity Disorders
Photodynamic Therapy see Photochemotherapy
Photofluorography   WN 220
  Used for diagnosis of particular disorders, with
    the disorder
Photogrammetry   TR 693–696
  For specific subjects, by subject
Photography   TR
  Dental   TR 708
  Fluorescent screen see Fluoroscopy   WN 220
  In psychotherapy   WM 450.5.P5
  Instrumentation   TR 570
  Medical   TR 708
  Roentgen–ray see Radiography   WN 200, etc.
  Used for specific subjects, by subject
Photokeratectomy see Keratectomy,
  Photorefractive, Excimer Laser
Photokymography see Electrokymography
Photometry
  Analytical chemistry (General)   QD 79.P46
  Optics   QC 391
  Quantitative analysis   QD 117.P5
  Used for diagnosis of particular disorders, with
    the disorder or system
Photomicrography   QH 251

Photons
  Physics   QC 793.5.P42–793.5.P429
  Radiation effects of   WN 600–630
  Special topics, by subject
Photoproteins see Luminescent Proteins
Photoradiation see Light
Photoradiation, Hematoporphyrin see
  Hematoporphyrin Photoradiation
Photoradiation Therapy see Phototherapy
Photoreceptors   WL 102.9
Photoreceptors, Invertebrate   QL 364
Photoreceptors, Vertebrate   WW 270
  See also Rods and Cones   WW 270
Photosensitivity Disorders   WR 160
Photosynthesis   QK 882
Phototherapy   WB 480
Phototrophic Bacteria   QW 145
Phrase Books see Medicine
Phrenic Nerve   WL 400
Phrenology   BF 866–885
  As a diagnostic technique   WB 365
Phthalein Dyes   QV 240
Phthalic Acids   QU 98
  Organic chemistry   QD 341.A2
  Toxicology   QV 612
Phthalic Anhydrides   QU 98
  Toxicology   QV 612
Phthalidyl Ampicillin see Talampicillin
Phthiraptera see Lice
Phthiriasis see Lice Infestations
Phthiroptera   QX 501
Phthisis see Tuberculosis, Pulmonary
Phycomycetes   QW 180.5.P4
Phyllodes Tumor   WP 870
Phylloquinone see Phytonadione
Phylogeny   QH 367.5
Physarum   QW 180.5.M9
Physcomitrella see Mosses
Physiatry see Physical Medicine
Physical Agents see Meteorological Factors; names
  of specific agents, e.g., Heat
Physical Conditioning, Human see Exercise Therapy
Physical Disability see Disabled
Physical Education and Training   QT 255
Physical Effort see Exertion
Physical Endurance   QT 255
  Special topics, by subject
Physical Examination   WB 200–288
  For legal establishment of life   W 789
  Aged   WT 141
  Child   WS 141
  Infant   WS 141
Physical Examination, Preadmission see Diagnostic
  Tests, Routine
Physical Fitness   QT 255
  For automobile driving   WA 275
  In aviation medicine   WD 705
  In space medicine   WD 752
Physical Medicine   WB 460–545
Physical Optics see Optics
Physical Therapy   WB 460–545
  General works   WB 460
  Hospital departments   WX 223

  In psychiatry   WM 405–412
  Veterinary   SF 925
Physical Therapy Department, Hospital   WX 223
Physically Challenged see Disabled Persons
Physically Handicapped see Disabled Persons
Physician Assignment Acceptance see Medicare
  Assignment
Physician Assistants   W 21.5
Physician Impairment
  Medicine   W 21
  For general impairment of physicians in various
    specialties, class in the number for the
    profession where applicable
Physician–Nurse Relations
  From the physician's perspective   W 62
  From the nurse's perspective   WY 87
Physician–Patient Relations   W 62
  Adolescence   WS 462
  Child   WS 105.5.I5
  Infant   WS 105.5.I5
  In psychiatry   WM 62
  In surgery   WO 62
Physician Shortage Area see Medically Underserved
  Area
Physicians
  Arabic   WZ 80.5.A8
  Biography
    Collective   WZ 112–150
    Individual   WZ 100
  Directories   W 22
  Islamic   WZ 80.5.A8
  Liability   W 44
    See also Insurance, Liability   W 44, etc.
  Literary & artistic works   WZ 350
  Military   WZ 112.5.M4
  Social relations   W 62
  See also names of ethnic groups, e.g., Blacks
    WZ 80.5.B5, etc.; other special topics
Physicians' Assistants see Physician Assistants
Physicians' Extenders see Physician Assistants
Physicians, Family   W 89
  See also Family Practice   WB 110, etc.
Physicians' Offices
  Management   W 80
  Planning and construction   WX 140
Physician's Practice Patterns   W 87
Physician's Role   W 62
Physicians, Women   W 21
  Biography
    Collective   WZ 150
    Individual   WZ 100
  History of their place in medicine   WZ 80.5.W5
  See also special topics under Physicians
Physics   QC
  Biological see Biophysics   QT 34, etc.
  Radiologic see Health Physics   WN 110
Physiognomy   BF 840–861
  See also Facial Expression   WB 275, etc.
Physiologic Availability see Biological Availability
Physiological Adaptation see Adaptation,
  Physiological
Physiological Chemistry see Biochemistry
Physiological Optics see Optometry; Vision

Physiological Processes
    Domestic animals   SF 768–768.2
    General   QT 4
    Human (General)   QT 104
    Plants see Plant Physiology   QK 710–899
    Wild animals   QP, etc.
    Special topics, by subject
    See also Adaptation, Physiological   QT 140,
      etc.; Physiology   QT, etc.; specific physiology
      terms, and indentions for physiology under
      various topics
Physiological Psychology see Psychophysiology
Physiologists see Biography   WZ 112.5.P5, etc.,
    and Directories   QT 22 under Physiology
Physiology   QT
    Bacterial see Bacterial Physiology   QW 52
    Biography
      Collective   WZ 112.5.P5
      Individual   WZ 100
    Blood see Blood Physiology   WH 100
    Cardiovascular see Cardiovascular Physiology
      WG 102
    Cell see Cell Physiology   QH 631
    Cold climate   QT 160
    Dental see Dental Physiology   WU 102
    Digestive see Digestive Physiology   WI 102
    Desert climate   QT 150
    Directories   QT 22
    Domestic animals   SF 768–768.2
    Experimental   QT 25
    Fetus   WQ 210.5
    Hot climate   QT 150
    Human (General)   QT 104
    Labor   WQ 305
    Musculoskeletal see Musculoskeletal Physiology
      WE 102
    Neurological see Neurophysiology   WL 102;
      Nervous System Physiology   WL 102
    Nursing texts   QT 104
    Ocular see Ocular Physiology   WW 103
    Plant see Plant Physiology   QK 710–899
    Psychological see Psychophysiology   WL 103
    Respiratory see Respiratory Physiology   WF
      102
    Skin see Skin Physiology   WR 102
    Surgical   WO 102
    Urinary tract see Urinary Tract Physiology   WJ
      102
    Viral see Viral Physiology   QW 160
    Wild animals   QP, etc.
    Particular systems, organism or parts, by subject
    See also Anthropology, Physical   GN 50.2–298;
      Physiological Processes   QT 4, etc.; and
      Physiology under organs and organ systems
Physiology, Comparative   QT 4
    Domestic animals only   SF 768–768.2
    Wild animals only   QP 33
Physiopathology see Pathology
Physiotherapy see Physical Therapy
Physostigmine   QV 124
Phytagglutinins see Lectins
Phytic Acid   QU 75
Phytin see Phytic Acid

Phytochrome   QK 898.P67
Phytohaemagglutinins see Plant Agglutinins
Phytohemagglutinins   QK 898.P8
    Hemagglutination   QW 640
Phytohormones see Plant Growth Regulators
Phytomenadione see Phytonadione
Phytomitogens see Lectins
Phytonadione   QV 195
Phytophagineae see Plant Viruses
Pia Mater   WL 200
Pial Vein see Cerebral Veins
Pica   WM 175
Picibanil
    As antineoplastic agents   QV 269
Pick's Disease of Brain see Dementia
Pick's Disease of Heart see Pericarditis, Constrictive
Picloram
    Public health   WA 240
Picodnaviruses see Parvoviridae
Picornaviridae   QW 168.5.P4
Picornaviridae Infections   WC 501
Picornavirus Infections see Picornaviridae Infections
Picrates   QV 223
Picric Acid see Picrates
Picrotoxin   QV 103
Pictorial Works see Form number 17 in any NLM
    schedule where applicable or appropriate LC
    number
Picture Archiving and Communication Systems see
    Radiology Information Systems
Picture Archiving, Radiologic see Radiology
    Information Systems
Picture Frustration Study see Rosenzweig
    Picture–Frustration Study
Piebald Skin see Albinism; Pigmentation Disorders;
    Vitiligo
Pig Skin Dressings see Biological Dressings
Pig-Tailed Monkey see Macaca nemestrina
Pigeon Breeder's Lung see Bird Fancier's Lung
Pigeons   QL 696.C63
    Diseases   SF 994.6
Pigment Epithelium of Eye   WW 103
    Of particular parts of the eye, with the part, e.g.,
      Retinal Pigment Epithelium   WW 270
Pigmentary Retinopathy see Retinitis Pigmentosa
Pigmentation
    Anthropology   GN 197
    Manifestations of disease   WR 143
    Physiology   WR 102
Pigmentation Disorders   WR 265–267
    Manifestations of disease   WR 143
Pigments   QU 110
    Animals
      Domestic   SF 768–768.2
      Wild   QP 670–671
    Plants
      Biochemistry   QD 441
      Botany   QK 898.P7
    See also Porphyrins   QU 110, etc.; names of
      other specific pigments
Pigs see Swine
Pike see Salmonidae
Pilar Cyst see Epidermal Cyst

Piles see Hemorrhoids
Pili, Bacterial see Pili, Sex
Pili, Sex   QW 51
Pills see Nostrums; Tablets
Pilocarpine   QV 122
Pilonidal Cyst see Pilonidal Sinus
Pilonidal Sinus   WE 750
Pineal Body   WK 350
Pinealoma   WK 350
Pinna see Ear, External
Pinnipedia   QL 737.P64
Pinta   WC 422
Pinworm see Oxyuroidea
Piperacillin   QV 354
Pipradol see Pipradrol
Pirenzepine
    As an anti-ulcer agent   QV 69
Piroplasmosis see Babesiosis
Piroxicam   QV 95
Pit and Fissure Sealants   WU 190
Pit Viper Venoms see Crotalid Venoms
Pitch Discrimination   WV 272
Pitch Perception   WV 272
Pithecinae see Cebidae
Pituitary Adenoma, Prolactin-Secreting see
    Prolactinoma
Pituitary-Adrenal Function Tests   WK 510
Pituitary-Adrenal System   WK 510
Pituitary Diseases   WK 500-590
Pituitary Dwarfism see Dwarfism, Pituitary
Pituitary Function Tests   WK 502
    See also Pituitary-Adrenal Function Tests   WK
    510
Pituitary Gland   WK 500-590
Pituitary Gland, Anterior   WK 510
Pituitary Gland, Posterior   WK 520
Pituitary Growth Hormone see Somatotropin
Pituitary Hormone Release Inhibiting Hormones
    WK 515
Pituitary Hormone-Releasing Hormones   WK 515
Pituitary Hormones   WK 502
Pituitary Hormones, Anterior   WK 515
Pituitary Hormones, Posterior   WK 520
Pituitary Neoplasms   WK 585
Pityriasis   WR 204
    Linguae see Glossitis, Benign Migratory   WI
    210
Pivampicillin   QV 354
PIXE see Spectrometry, X-Ray Emission
Pizotifen see Pizotyline
Pizotyline
    As a serotonin antagonist   QV 126
Placebos   WB 330
Placement Agencies, Nursing see Employment
Placenta   WQ 212
    Growth and Development see Placentation   QS
    645
Placenta Diseases   WQ 212
Placental Extracts
    Pharmacology   QV 370
    Therapeutic use (General)   WB 391
    Used for treatment of particular disorders, with
    the disorder or system

Placental Function Tests   WQ 212
Placental Hormones   WK 920
Placental Insufficiency   WQ 212
Placental Lactogen   WK 920
Placental Proteins see Pregnancy Proteins
Placental Villi see Chorionic Villi
Placentation   QS 645
Placentoma, Normal see Placenta
Placentome see Placenta
Plague   WC 350-355
    Cattle see Rinderpest   SF 966
    Fowl see Fowl Plague   SF 995.6.F59
Plague Vaccine   WC 350
Planigraphy, X-Ray see Tomography, X-Ray
Plankton
    Aquatic biology (General)   QH 90.8.P5
    Freshwater biology   QH 96.8.P5
    Marine biology   QH 91.8.P5
    Plant ecology   QK 933-935
    Zoology
        Freshwater   QL 143
        Ocean   QL 123
Planned Parenthood see Family Planning
Planning, Health and Welfare see Health Planning
Planning, Health Facility see Health Facility
    Planning
Planning Techniques
    Health administration   WA 525-546
    Health services   W 84-84.8
    Hospital administration   WX 150
    Hospital facility   WX 140
    In other particular areas, by subject
Planning Theories see Planning Techniques
Plant Agglutinins see Lectins
Plant Diseases   SB 599-795
    Biological control   SB 975-978
    General works   SB 731
    Trees   SB 761-767
Plant Extracts   QV 766
Plant Extracts, Chinese see Drugs, Chinese Herbal
Plant Growth Regulators   QK 745
Plant Hormones see Plant Growth Regulators
Plant Lice see Aphids
Plant Microbiology see Microbiology; Plant Viruses
Plant Oils
    Biochemistry   QU 86
    Chemical technology   TP 680 684
    Public health aspects   WA 722
Plant Physiology   QK 710-899
Plant Poisoning   WD 500-530
    Veterinary   SF 757.5
    See also Milk Sickness   WD 530
Plant Proteins   QK 898.P8
    In nutrition   QU 55
Plant Tumors   SB 741.5
    Of specific plants with the plant, e.g., tree galls
    in   SB 767
Plant Viruses   QW 163
Plantar Prints see Dermatoglyphics
Plants   QK
    Chemistry   QK 861-899
    Cytology   QK 725
    Histology   QK 671

Lice see Aphids   QX 503, etc.
Microbiology   QW 60
Physiology see Plant Physiology   QK 710–899
Poisons see Plants, Toxic   WD 500–530
Plants, Edible   QK 98.5
    As a dietary supplement in health or disease
        WB 430–432
Plants, Medicinal   QV 766–770
    Atlases   QV 717
    Culture   SB 293–295
    See also specific names of medicinal plants
Plants, Toxic   WD 500–530
Plaque Therapy, Radioisotope see Brachytherapy
Plasma   WH 400
    Blood transfusion   WB 356
Plasma Cell Antigens PC–1 see Antigens,
    Differentiation, B–Lymphocyte
Plasma Cell Dyscrasias see Paraproteinemias
Plasma Cells   WH 400
Plasma Exchange   WB 356
Plasma Expanders see Plasma Substitutes
Plasma Membrane see Cell Membrane
Plasma Prokallikrein see Prekallikrein
Plasma Proteins see Blood Proteins
Plasma Substitutes   WH 450
Plasma Transglutaminase see Protein–Glutamine
    gamma–Glutamyltransferase
Plasma Volume   WG 106
Plasma Volume Expanders see Plasma Substitutes
Plasmacytes see Plasma Cells
Plasmalogens   QU 93
Plasmapheresis   WH 460
Plasmids   QW 51
Plasminogen
    Enzymology   QU 142
    Blood coagulation   WH 310
Plasminogen Activator Inhibitor 3 see Protein C
    Inhibitor
Plasminogen Activator Inhibitors see Plasminogen
    Inactivators
Plasminogen Activator, Tissue–Type see Tissue
    Plasminogen Activator
Plasminogen Activator, Urokinase–Type see
    Urokinase
Plasminogen Activators
    Biochemistry   QU 142
    Blood coagulation   WH 310
Plasminogen Inactivators   QU 136
Plasminokinase see Streptodornase and Streptokinase
Plasmodium   QX 135
Plasmodium Infections see Malaria
Plasmosome see Cell Nucleolus
Plaster, Adhesive see Bandages
Plaster Casts see Casts, Surgical
Plaster of Paris see Calcium Sulfate
Plasters see Dermatologic Agents; Irritants
Plastic Casts see Casts, Surgical
Plastic Surgery see Surgery, Plastic
Plasticity, Neuronal see Neuronal Plasticity
Plastics
    Chemical technology   TP 1101–1185
    Used for special purposes by subject, e.g., in
        plastic surgery   WO 640

Platelet Activating Factor   QU 93
    In blood coagulation   WH 310
Platelet Adhesiveness   WH 310
Platelet Aggregation   WH 310
Platelet Aggregation Inhibitors   QV 180
Platelet Antagonists see Platelet Aggregation
    Inhibitors
Platelet Antiaggregants see Platelet Aggregation
    Inhibitors
Platelet–Derived Growth Factor   QU 107
Platelet Function Tests   QY 410
Platelet Transforming Growth Factor see
    Transforming Growth Factor beta
Platelet Transfusion   WB 356
Plateletpheresis   WH 460
Platelets see Blood Platelets
Platelets, Blood see Blood Platelets
Platinum
    Inorganic chemistry   QD 181.P8
    Pharmacology   QV 290
Platinum Black see Platinum
Platinum Diamminodichloride see Cisplatin
Platybasia   WE 730
Platyhelminths   QX 350–422
Platyrrhina see Cebidae
Play and Playthings
    Child psychology   WS 105.5.P5
    Physical education   QT 255
    Projective techniques   WM 145.5.P8
    Preschool children   LB 1140.35.P55
    Psychology (General)   BF 717
    Recreation   QT 250
    School children   LB 1177; LB 3031
Play Therapy   WS 350.2
    Activity therapy   WM 450
    Special topics by subject, e.g., Hospitalized Child
        WS 105.5.H7
Pleasure–Pain Principle
    Psychoanalysis   WM 460.5.P5
    Psychology   BF 515
Plethysmography   WG 141.5.P7
    Special topics, by subject, e.g., in the diagnosis
        of Thrombosis   WG 610
Plethysmography, Impedance   WG 141.5.P7
    Special topics, by subject, e.g., diagnosis of
        Arteriosclerosis   WG 550
Plethysmography, Impedance, Transthoracic see
    Cardiography, Impedance
Plethysmography, Whole Body   WF 141.5.P7
    Special topics, by subject, e.g., in Tracheal
        Stenosis   WF 490
Pleura   WF 700–746
    Secretion   QY 210
    Tuberculosis see Tuberculosis, Pleural   WF 390
    See also Pleuropneumonia   WC 202
Pleural Cavity see Pleura
Pleural Effusion   WF 700
    Clinical analysis   QY 210
Pleural Fluid see Secretion   QY 210 under Pleura
Pleural Neoplasms   WF 700
Pleural Rub see Respiratory Sounds
Pleurisy   WF 744
Pleurisy, Tuberculous see Tuberculosis, Pleural

ALWAYS CONSULT MAIN SCHEDULES. USE NUMBER ASSIGNED ONLY WHEN
SUBJECT REPRESENTS MAJOR EMPHASIS OF WORK BEING CLASSIFIED

Pleuritis see Pleurisy

Pleurodynia, Epidemic   WC 500

Pleuropneumonia   WC 202
    Veterinary   SF 831
    In cattle   SF 964

Pleuropneumonia–Like Organisms see Mycoplasma

Plicamycin   QV 269

Plumbing see Sanitary Engineering

Plumbism see Lead Poisoning

Plummer–Vinson Syndrome   WI 250

Pluralism see Cultural Diversity

Plutonium   WN 420
    Nuclear physics   QC 796.P9
    See also special topics under Radioisotopes

Pneumatosis Cystoides Intestinalis   WI 400

Pneumococcal Infections   WC 217
    See also Pneumonia, Pneumococcal   WC 204

Pneumoconiosis   WF 654

Pneumoencephalography   WL 141

Pneumogastric Nerve see Vagus Nerve

Pneumology see Pulmonary Disease (Specialty)

Pneumomediastinum see Mediastinal Emphysema

Pneumomediastinum, Diagnostic   WF 975

Pneumonectomy   WF 668

Pneumonia   WC 202–209
    Friedlaender's pneumonia   WC 209
    Veterinary   SF 831

Pneumonia, Aspiration   WC 209

Pneumonia, Interstitial see Lung Diseases, Interstitial

Pneumonia, Lipid   WC 209

Pneumonia, Lobar see Pneumonia, Pneumococcal

Pneumonia, Mycoplasma   WC 209

Pneumonia, Pneumococcal   WC 204

Pneumonia, Staphylococcal   WC 204

Pneumonia, Viral   WC 207
    Veterinary   SF 831

Pneumonitis, Hypersensitivity, Avian see Bird
Fancier's Lung

Pneumonitis, Interstitial see Lung Diseases,
Interstitial

Pneumonology see Pulmonary Disease (Specialty)

Pneumonolysis   WF 668

Pneumoperitoneum   WI 575

Pneumoperitoneum, Artificial   WI 141
    Used for diagnosis of particular disorders, with
    the disorder or system

Pneumoradiography   WN 200

Pneumoretroperitoneum see
Retropneumoperitoneum

Pneumothorax   WF 746

Pneumothorax, Artificial   WF 768

Pocket, Periodontal see Periodontal Pocket

Podiatry   WE 890

Podophyllum
    As an antineoplastic agent   QV 269
    As a cathartic   QV 75
    As a medicinal plant   QV 767
    Poisoning   WD 500

Poetry   PN 6099–6110
    About medicine   WZ 330
    By physicians   WZ 350
    Light verse in medicine and related fields   WZ
    305–305.5

Point–of–Care Systems
    In hospitals (General)   WX 162
    Special topics, by subject

Point of Care Technology see Point–of–Care
Systems

Poison Control Centers   QV 600
    Directories   QV 605
    In hospitals   WX 215

Poison Ivy see Toxicodendron

Poison Ivy Dermatitis see Dermatitis,
Toxicodendron

Poisoning   QV 600–667
    Animal see Animals, Poisonous   WD 400–430;
      Fishes, Poisonous   WD 405; Bites and Stings
      WD 400–430
    Carbon monoxide see Carbon Monoxide
      Poisoning   QV 662
    Fluoride see Fluoride Poisoning   QV 282, etc.
    Food see Food Poisoning   WC 268
    Gas see Gas Poisoning   QV 662, etc.
    Industrial   WA 465
      Medicolegal Aspects   W 925
    Lead see Lead Poisoning   QV 292
    Mercury see Mercury Poisoning   QV 293
    Mushroom see Mushroom Poisoning   WD 520
    Plant see Plant Poisoning   WD 500–530
    Salmonella food see Salmonella Food Poisoning
      WC 268
    Staphylococcal food see Staphylococcal Food
      Poisoning   WC 268
    Veterinary   SF 757.5
    See also names of particular poisonous animals,
      bacteria, chemicals, insects, plants, viruses, etc.,
      and the field Toxicology

Poisonous Animals see Animals, Poisonous

Poisonous Fishes see Fishes, Poisonous

Poisonous Gases see Gases

Poisonous Plants see Plants, Toxic

Poisons   QV 600–667
    Corrosive   QV 612
    Detection see Laboratory manuals   QV 602 and
      Methods   QV 602 under Toxicology
    Industrial protection   WA 465
    Inorganic   QV 610–618
    Organic   QV 627–633
    Public health aspects   WA 730
    Volatile   QV 633
    See also names of specific poisons

Polar Regions see Cold Climate

Polarization Microscopy see Microscopy,
Polarization

Polarography
    Organic analysis   QD 272.E4
    Quantitative analysis   QD 116.P64

Policy Making
    General   H 97
    In special topics, by subject

Poliodystrophia Cerebri see Cerebral Sclerosis,
Diffuse

Poliomyelitis   WC 555
    Prevention & control   WC 556

Poliomyelitis Immunization see Prevention & control
WC 556 under Poliomyelitis

Poliosis see Hair Color
Poliovirus Vaccine   WC 556
Poliovirus Vaccine, Oral   WC 556
Polioviruses   QW 168.5.P4
Polioviruses, Human 1–3   QW 168.5.P4
Polishes see Industrial Oils
Polishes, Dental see Dentifrices
Political Activity see Politics
Political Systems   JC
   In psychoanalysis, psychoanalytic therapy, or
     psychoanalytic interpretation   WM 460.5.P7
   Related to special topics, by subject
   See also names of specific systems, e.g.,
     Communism   HX 72–73; 626–780.7, etc.
Politics   J (rarely used)
   Special topics, by subject
Pollen   QK 658
   As an allergen   QW 900
   As a food preparation   WB 447
Pollinosis see Hay Fever
Pollution see Names of specific kinds of pollution,
   e.g., Air Pollution
Polonium   WN 420
   Nuclear physics   QC 796.P6
   See also special topics under Radioisotopes
Poly Adenosine Diphosphate Ribose   QU 57
Poly ADP Ribose see Poly Adenosine Diphosphate
   Ribose
Poly ADP Ribose Polymerase see NAD+
   ADP–Ribosyltransferase
Poly ADP Ribose Synthetase see NAD+
   ADP–Ribosyltransferase
Poly I–C
   Immunology   QW 800
   Pharmacology   QV 268.5
Polyacrylamide Gel Electrophoresis,
   Two–Dimensional see Electrophoresis, Gel,
   Two–Dimensional
Polyamides see Nylons
Polyamines   QU 61
   Organic chemistry
     Aliphatic   QD 305.A8
     Aromatic   QD 341.A8
Polyangiaceae see Myxococcales
Polyangium see Myxococcales
Polyarteritis Nodosa   WG 518
Polyarthritis see Arthritis
Polyarthritis Rheumatica see Rheumatic Fever
Polybrominated Biphenyls
   As carcinogens   QZ 202
   Toxicology   QV 633
Polybromobiphenyl Compounds see Polybrominated
   Biphenyls
Polychemotherapy see Drug Therapy, Combination
Polychlorinated Biphenyls
   As air pollutants   WA 754, etc.
   As water pollutants   WA 689
   Organic chemistry   QD 341.H9
   Toxicology (General)   QV 633
Polychlorobiphenyl Compounds see Polychlorinated
   Biphenyls
Polychloroethylene see Polyvinyl Chloride
Polycyclic Compounds see Polycyclic

Hydrocarbons
Polycyclic Hydrocarbons
   Organic chemistry
     Aliphatic QD 305.H9
     Aromatic   QD 341.H9
   Toxicology   QV 633
Polycystic Kidney see Kidney, Polycystic
Polycystic Ovary Syndrome   WP 320
Polycythemia   WH 180
Polycythemia Vera   WH 180
Polydeoxyribonucleotide Ligases see DNA Ligases
Polydeoxyribonucleotide Synthetases see DNA
   Ligases
Polyergin see Transforming Growth Factor beta
Polyethylene Terephthalates
   Inguinal hernia repair   WI 960
   Production   TP 1180.P65
   Used for other special purposes, by subject
Polyethylenes
   Chemical technology   TP 1180.P65
   Used for special purposes, by subject, e.g., in
     drainage for middle ear surgery   WV 230
Polygenic Inheritance
   Medical genetics (General)   QZ 50
   Of a particular disease, with the disease
Polyglucoses see Glucans
Polyglutamate Folates see Pteroylpolyglutamic
   Acids
Polygonum see Plants, Medicinal
Polyhedrosis Viruses   QW 162
Polyisocyanates see Polyurethanes
Polyisoprenyl Phosphate Sugars   QU 75
   As glycolipids   QU 85
Polyisoprenyl Phosphates
   Biochemistry   QU 85
   Toxicology   QV 633
Polymenorrhea see Menstruation Disorders
Polymerase Chain Reaction   QH 450.3
Polymers   QD 380–388
   Classify by use where possible, e.g., in dentistry
     WU 190; in medicine   QT 37.5.P7
Polymorphism (Genetics)   QH 455
Polymorphonuclear Leukocytes see Neutrophils
Polymyalgia Rheumatica   WE 550
Polymyxin E see Colistin
Polyneuritis   WL 544
Polyneuritis Endemica see Beriberi
Polynuclear Aromatic Hydrocarbons see Polycyclic
   Hydrocarbons
Polynucleotide Vaccines see Vaccines, DNA
Polynucleotides   QU 57
Polyomavirus   QW 165.5.P2
Polyomavirus hominis 1   QW 165.5.P2
Polyomavirus macacae   QW 165.5.P2
Polypeptides see Peptides
Polyphosphates   QV 285
Polyploidy   QH 461
   Plant breeding   SB 123
Polyposis see Polyps
Polyposis Coli, Familial see Adenomatous Polyposis
   Coli
Polyposis Syndrome, Familial see Adenomatous
   Polyposis Coli

**ALWAYS CONSULT MAIN SCHEDULES. USE NUMBER ASSIGNED ONLY WHEN
SUBJECT REPRESENTS MAJOR EMPHASIS OF WORK BEING CLASSIFIED**

Polyproteins see Proteins
Polyps   QZ 200
    Localized, by site
    See also Colonic Polyps   WI 529; Intestinal
        Polyps   WI 430; Nasal Polyps   WV 300
Polyradiculitis   WL 400
Polyradiculoneuritis   WL 544
Polysaccharides   QU 83
Polysaccharides, Bacterial   QW 52
Polyurethanes
    Chemical technology   TP 1180.P8
    Used for special purposes, by subject, e.g., in
        tubing for tracheal prosthesis   WF 490
Polyvidon see Povidone
Polyvinyl Chloride
    Chemical technology   TP 1180.V48
Polyvinylpyrrolidone see Povidone
Polyvinylpyrrolidone Iodine see Povidone–Iodine
Polyvinyls
    Chemical technology   TP 1180.V48
    Used for particular purposes, by subject, e.g., in
        Blood Bags   WH 460
Pompholyx see Eczema, Dyshidrotic
Pongidae   QL 737.P96
    As laboratory animals   QY 60.P7
    Diseases   SF 997.5.P7
Pongo pygmaeus   QL 737.P96
    Diseases   SF 997.5.P7
    As laboratory animals   QY 60.P7
Pons   WL 310
Pontocaine see Tetracaine
Poor, Medical Care see Medical Indigency
Popliteal Artery   WG 595.P6
    See also Blood Supply   WE 870 under Knee
Popliteal Space see Knee
Popliteal Vein   WG 625.P6
    See also Blood Supply   WE 870 under Knee
Poppy see Papaver
Popular works
    Cardiovascular system   WG 113
    Dentistry   WU 80
    Digestive system   WI 113
    Geriatrics   WT 120
    Gynecology   WP 120
    Medicine (General)   WB 120–130
    Neoplasms   QZ 201
    Obesity   WD 212
    Obstetrics   WQ 150
    Ophthalmology   WW 80
    Psychiatry   WM 75
    Surgery   WO 75
    Special topics, by subject
Population   HB 848–3697
    Genetics see Genetics, Population   QH 455, etc.
    Health problems of special population groups
        WA 300–395
        Movement   HB 1951–2577
        See also Demography   HB 848–3697
Population Characteristics   HB 848–3697
    Health problems of special population groups
        WA 300–395
Population Control   HB 848–871
    Population policy   HB 883.5

    See also Family Planning   HQ 763.5–767.7
Population Density   HB 1953
Population Distribution see Demography
Population Dynamics   QH 352
    Special topics, by subject
Population Explosion see Population Growth
Population Growth   HB 848–871
Population Size see Population Density
Population Surveillance
    Epidemilological studies   WA 105
    See also names of specific types of surveys, e.g.,
        Health Surveys   WA 900, etc.
Poradenitis Nostras see Lymphogranuloma
Venereum
Porcelain see Dental Porcelain
Porcine Influenza Virus Type A see Influenza A
Virus, Porcine
Porcine Xenograft Bioprosthesis see Bioprosthesis
Porcine Xenograft Dressings see Biological
Dressings
Porcupines see Rodentia
Porifera   QL 370.7–374.2
Pornography see Erotica
Porphyria   WD 205.5.P6
    Special types, by system in which produced
Porphyrins   QU 110
    Special types, by system in which produced, e.g.,
        those related to hemorlobin   WH 190
Porpoises   QL 737.C434
Port Quarantine see Quarantine
Portacaval Shunt, Surgical   WI 720
Portal Hypertension see Hypertension, Portal
Portal System   WI 720
Portal Vein   WI 720
Portasystemic Shunt, Surgical   WI 720
Portasystemic Shunt, Transjugular Intrahepatic
WI 720
Portography   WI 720
Portosystemic Encephalopathy see Hepatic
Encephalopathy
Portosystemic Shunt, Surgical see Portasystemic
Shunt, Surgical
Portosystemic Shunt, Transjugular Intrahepatic see
    Portasystemic Shunt, Transjugular Intrahepatic
Portraits   N 7575–7624.5
    Of physicians and other specialists in medically
    related fields in the appropriate biography
    number in   WZ
Position Description see Job Description
Position, Sense of see Orientation
Positioning, Radiography see Technology,
Radiologic
Positive End–Expiratory Pressure see
Positive–Pressure Respiration
Positive–Pressure Respiration   WF 145
    In first aid   WA 292
Positive Reinforcement see Reinforcement
(Psychology)
Positron–Emission Tomography see Tomography,
Emission–Computed
Positrons see Electrons
Posology see Administration & dosage   QV 748
    under Drugs; Prescriptions, Drug

**ALWAYS CONSULT MAIN SCHEDULES. USE NUMBER ASSIGNED ONLY WHEN
SUBJECT REPRESENTS MAJOR EMPHASIS OF WORK BEING CLASSIFIED**

Post and Core Technique   WU 515
Post–Surgical Nursing see Postanesthesia Nursing
Post–Transcriptional RNA Modification see RNA
    Processing, Post–Transcriptional
Post–Translational Protein Modification see Protein
    Processing, Post–Translational
Post–Traumatic Stress Disorders see Stress
    Disorders, Post–Traumatic
Postage Stamps see Philately
Postanesthesia Nursing   WY 154
Postcoital Contraceptives see Contraceptives,
    Postcoital
Posterior Chamber see Eye
Posterior Lobe Hormones see Pituitary Hormones,
    Posterior
Posterior Vitreous Detachment see Vitreous
    Detachment
Postgastrectomy Syndromes   WI 380
Postgraduate Education see Education, Graduate;
    names of specific types of graduate education, e.g.,
    Education, Pharmacy, Graduate
Postimplantation Phase   WQ 205
Postmarketing Product Surveillance see Product
    Surveillance, Postmarketing
Postmenopausal Bone Loss see Osteoporosis,
    Postmenopausal
Postmenopausal Hormone Replacement Therapy see
    Estrogen Replacement Therapy
Postmenopausal Osteoporosis see Osteoporosis,
    Postmenopausal
Postmortem Changes   QZ 35
Postmortem Examination see Autopsy
Postnatal Care   WQ 500
    See also Postnatal Nursing   WY 157.3 under
        Obstetrical Nursing
Postnatal Depression see Depression, Postpartum
Postnidation Phase see Postimplantation Phase
Postoperative Care   WO 183
    Geriatric surgery   WO 950
    Pediatric surgery   WO 925
    See also Perioperative Nursing   WY 161
Postoperative Complications   WO 184–185
    Specific complications, by site
Postoperative Hemorrhage   WO 184
Postoperative Period   WO 183
Postoperative Wound Infection see Surgical Wound
    Infection
Postpartum Depression see Depression, Postpartum
Postpartum Hemorrhage   WQ 330
Postpartum Period see Puerperium
Postphlebitic Disease see Postphlebitic Syndrome
Postphlebitic Syndrome   WG 610
Postphlebitic Ulcer see Postphlebitic Syndrome
Posture   WE 103
Postviral Fatigue Syndrome see Fatigue Syndrome,
    Chronic
Potassium   QV 277
    Inorganic chemistry   QD 181.K1
    Metabolism   QU 130
    Toxicology   QV 277
Potassium Antimonyltartrate see Antimony
    Potassium Tartrate
Potassium Canrenoate see Canrenoate Potassium

Potassium Channels   QH 603.I54
Potassium Chloride
    Inorganic chemistry   QD 181.K1
    Pharmacology   QV 280
Potassium Deficiency   WD 105
    Veterinary   SF 855.P67
Potassium Isotopes
    Inorganic chemistry   QD 181.K1
    Pharmacology   QV 277
Potassium Permanganate   QV 229
Potassium Pump see Na(+)-K(+)-Exchanging
    ATPase
Pottos see Lorisidae
Pott's Disease see Tuberculosis, Spinal
Poultry
    Anatomy   SF 767.P6
    Culture   SF 481–507
    Physiology   SF 768.2.P6
Poultry Diseases   SF 995–995.6
Poultry Products
    As a dietary supplement in health or disease
        WB 426
    Public health aspects   WA 707
    See also Eggs   WA 703, etc.
Poverty
    Economic conditions   HC 79.P6
        By country   HC 94–1085
    Welfare   HV 40–4630
Poverty Areas
    Health problems (General)   WA 30
    Special topics, by subject
Povidone   WH 450
Povidone–Iodine
    As an anti–infective agent   QV 231
Powders   QV 785
    As adsorbent dermatological agents   QV 63
    As adsorbent gastrointestinal agents   QV 66
Power, Personal see Power (Psychology)
Power Plants   TJ 164
    Prevention and control of accidents and diseases
        WA 440–495
Power, Professional see Power (Psychology)
Power (Psychology)
    As an expression of will   BF 608–618, etc.
        Manipulation or control by others   BF 632.5
        Self control, willpower, etc   BF 632
    Other aspects, by subject
Power, Social see Power (Psychology)
Power Sources, Bioelectric see Bioelectric Energy
    Sources
Poxviridae   QW 165.5.P6
Poxviridae Infections   WC 584–590
Poxvirus Infections see Poxviridae Infections
Poxvirus myxomatis see Myxoma Virus
Poxvirus officinale see Vaccinia Virus
Poxvirus variolae see Variola Virus
PPLO see Mycoplasma
Practical Nurses see Nurses; Nursing, Practical
Practice see Family Practice; General Practice,
    Dental; Group Practice; Group Practice, Dental;
    Group Practice, Prepaid; Institutional Practice;
    Mortuary Practice; Partnership Practice; Private
    Practice; Professional Practice; See also Medicine

ALWAYS CONSULT MAIN SCHEDULES. USE NUMBER ASSIGNED ONLY WHEN
SUBJECT REPRESENTS MAJOR EMPHASIS OF WORK BEING CLASSIFIED

Premenstrual Tension see Premenstrual Syndrome
Prenatal Care   WQ 175
Prenatal Diagnosis   WQ 209
   For hereditary diseases specifically   QZ 50
Prenatal Diagnosis, Ultrasonic see Ultrasonography,
   Prenatal
Prenatal Exposure Delayed Effects   WQ 210
Prenatal Structures see Embryonic Structures
Prenidation Phase see Preimplantation Phase
Preoperative Care   WO 179
   Geriatric surgery   WO 950
   Pediatric surgery   WO 925
   Preparation of patient for anesthesia   WO 234
Prepaid Dental Care see Insurance, Dental
Prepaid Group Health Organizations see Health
   Maintenance Organizations
Prepaid Group Practice see Group Practice, Prepaid
Preparatory Manipulation, Obstetric see Methods
   WQ 415–430 under Delivery
Prepayment Medical Plans see Insurance, Health
Preprosthetic Oral Surgery see Surgery, Oral,
   Preprosthetic
Preprosthetic Oral Surgical Procedures see Oral
   Surgical Procedures, Preprosthetic
Prepuce see Penis
Presbyopia   WW 300
Presbytis see Cercopithecidae
Prescription Fees   QV 736
Prescription Insurance see Insurance, Pharmaceutical
   Services
Prescriptions, Drug
   Dental   WU 166
   Formularies   QV 740
   Pharmacopoeias   QV 738
   Veterinary   SF 916.5
   Writing   QV 748
Prescriptions, Non-Drug
   For specific subjects, with the subject, e.g.,
      Hearing aids   WV 274
Presentation, Breech see Breech Presentation
Presentation, Fetal see Labor Presentation
Presentation (Obstetrics) see Labor Presentation
Preservation, Biological   QH 324
   Blood see Blood Preservation   WH 460, etc.
   Dead bodies see Embalming   WA 844
   Drugs see Drug Storage   QV 754, etc.
   Food see Food Preservation   WA 710
   Organs see Tissue Preservation   WO 665, etc.
Preservation, Food see Food Preservation
Preservatives, Pharmaceutical   QV 820
Pressoreceptors   WL 102.9
Pressure
   Therapeutic use   WB 890
      See also Atmospheric pressure   WD 710, etc.;
      Blood Pressure   WG 106, etc.; Intracranial
      Pressure   WL 102, etc.; Intraocular
      Pressure   WW 103, etc.
Pressure Sore see Decubitus Ulcer
Pressure Ulcer see Decubitus Ulcer
Prevalence Studies see Cross–Sectional Studies
Prevention of accidents see Accident Prevention
Prevention of Infectious Diseases see Communicable
   Disease Control; names of specific diseases

Prevention, Primary see Primary Prevention
Preventive Dentistry   WU 113–113.7
Preventive Health Services   WA 108
   See also Immunization   QW 800–815, etc.
Preventive Inoculation see Immunization
Preventive Medicine   WA 108–245
Preventive Psychiatry   WM 31.5
Priapism   WJ 790
Primaquine   QV 258
Primary Care Physicians see Physicians, Family
Primary Health Care   W 84.6
Primary Nursing Care   WY 101
Primary Prevention   WA 108–245
   Of particular conditions, by subject
Primates   QL 737.P9–737.P968
   As laboratory animals   QY 60.P7
   As pets   SF 459.P3
   Diseases   SF 997.5.P7
   Human emphasis, in NLM schedules, by subject
   Zoo and captive wild animal culture   SF
      408.6.P75
Printers' Marks   Z 235–236
Printing   Z 116–264.5
Prinzmetal's Angina see Angina Pectoris, Variant
Prion Diseases   WL 300
Prion Proteins see Prions
Prions   QU 55
Priorities, Health see Health Priorities
Prisoners
   Human experimentation   QV 20.5
      In special areas, by subject
   Psychology of prisoners of war   BF 727.P7
   Reform of   HV 9261–9430.7
   Special topics, by subject, e.g., Psychotherapy
      of Prisoners   WM 420
Prisoner's Dilemma see Game Theory
Prisons   HV 8301–9025
   Hygiene and medical service   HV 8833–8844
   Psychiatric services   HV 8841
   Sex in prisons   HV 8836
Privacy
   Applied psychology   BF 637.P74
   Medical records confidentiality   WX 173
   Special topics, by subject
   See also Civil Rights
Privacy Act see Privacy
Privacy Act see Privacy
Privacy of Space see Personal Space
Private Nursing see Nursing, Private Duty
Private Practice   W 89
   By country   WB 50
   Nursing see Nursing, Private Duty   WY 127
   Textbooks for   WB 100
Privatization
   In special fields, by subject, e.g. Mental Health
      Services   WM 30, etc.
Privileged Communication see Confidentiality
PRL–Secreting Pituitary Adenoma see Prolactinoma
PRO Professional Review Organizations see
   Professional Review Organizations
Probabilistic Models see Models, Statistical
Probability   QA 273–274.8
Probability Learning   QA 273.2

Educational psychology   LB 1051
Probability Theory   QA 273–274.8
  Special topics, by subject
Problem–Oriented Medical Records see Medical
  Records, Problem–Oriented
Problem Solving   BF 449
  Child   WS 105.5.D2
  Infant   WS 105.D2
Problems
  (Form number 18.2 in any NLM schedule where
  applicable)
Probucol   QU 95
  Organic chemistry   QD 341.P5
Procaine   QV 115
  In veterinary pharmacology   SF 918.P75
  In veterinary anesthesiology   SF 914
Procarbazine
  Antineoplastic agent   QV 269
    Therapeutic use   QZ 267
  Other special topics, by subject
Procolobus see Colobus
Proconvertin see Factor VII
Proctitis   WI 600
Proctocolitis, Hemorrhagic see Colitis, Ulcerative
Proctocolitis, Ulcerative see Colitis, Ulcerative
Proctological Surgery see Surgery   WI 650 under
  Rectum
Proctology see Colorectal Surgery
Proctoscopy   WI 620
Proctosigmoidoscopy see Sigmoidoscopy
Prodrugs   QV 785
Product Labeling   WA 250
  Of specific products, by subject
  See also Drug Labeling   QV 835
Product Labeling, Drug see Drug Labeling
Product Surveillance, Postmarketing
  Of specific product, with the product
Productivity see Efficiency
Proenzymes see Enzyme Precursors
Proerythroblasts see Erythroblasts
Professional Competence   W 21
  Dentists   WU 21
  Nurses   WY 16
  Pharmacists   QV 21
  As an educational measurement
    Works about (Form number 18 in any NLM
      schedule where applicable)
    Actual tests (Form number 18.2 in any NLM
      schedule where applicable)
Professional Corporations   W 87
Professional Impairment
  Medicine   W 21
  For general impairment in other specialties, class
    in the number for the profession where
    applicable
Professional Liability see Liability, Legal
Professional–Patient Relations
  Allied health personnel   W 21.5
  Hospital personnel   WX 159
  Particular specialty, with the specialty
  See also specific professional relationships with
    the patient, e.g., Physician–Patient Relations
    W 62, etc.

Professional Practice
  Medicine as a career   W 21
  Types of professional practice   W 87
  See also names of specialties in medicine and
    allied fields, e.g., Nursing   WY 16; form
    number 21 in any other NLM schedule where
    applicable
Professional Review Organizations   W 84
  By specialty, in the number for the profession,
    e.g.,   QV 21
Professional Staff Committees
  In schools
    (Form number 19–20 in any NLM schedule
      where applicable)
  In hospitals   WX 159
Professional Standards Review Organizations see
  Professional Review Organizations
Professions see Names of professions, e.g., Nursing
Profibrinolysin see Plasminogen
Proflavine
  As a local anti–infective agent   QV 220
Progenitor Cells see Stem Cells
Progenitor Cells, Hematopoietic see Hematopoietic
  Stem Cells
Progeria   WS 104
  In adults see Werner Syndrome   QZ 45
Progestational Hormones   WP 530
Progesterone   WP 530
Progesterone Receptors see Receptors, Progesterone
Progestin Receptors see Receptors, Progesterone
Progestins see Progestational Hormones
Progestogens see Progestational Hormones
Proglumide Receptors see Receptors,
  Cholecystokinin
Prognathism   WU 440
Prognosis   WB 142
  See also names of particular diseases
Prognostic Nutritional Index (PNI) see Nutrition
  Assessment
Program Evaluation
  Health Services   W 84
  Other special topics, by subject being evaluated
Program Evaluation, Nursing see Nursing
  Evaluation Research
Programmable Implantable Insulin Pump see Insulin
  Infusion Systems
Programmable Implantable Medication Systems see
  Infusion Pumps, Implantable
Programmed Instruction   LB 1028.5–1028.7
  (Form number 18.2 in any NLM schedule where
  applicable)
Programmed Instruction, Computerized see
  Computer–Assisted Instruction
Programmed Learning see Programmed Instruction
Programming, Linear   T 57.74–57.79
  Special topics, by subject
Progressive Lenticular Degeneration see
  Hepatolenticular Degeneration
Progressive Lipodystrophy see Lipodystrophy
Progressive Muscular Atrophy see Muscular
  Atrophy, Spinal
Progressive Muscular Dystrophy see Muscular
  Dystrophy

Progressive Patient Care   W 84.7–84.8
   Of hospital patients   WX 162–162.5
Proinsulin   WK 820
Projection   WM 193.5.P7
   Adolescence   WS 463
   Child   WS 350.8.D3
   Infant   WS 350.8.D3
Projections and Predictions see Forecasting
Projective Techniques   WM 145.5.P8
   Adolescence   WS 462
   Child   WS 105.5.E8
   See also Psychological Tests   BF 176
Prokaryotic Cells   QW 51
Prolactin   WK 515
   Veterinary medicine   SF 768.3
Prolactin–Producing Pituitary Adenoma see
   Prolactinoma
Prolactinoma   WK 585
Prolapsed Disk see Intervertebral Disk Displacement
Proliferative Phase see Menstrual Cycle
Proline   QU 60
Prolongation of life see Longevity; Rejuvenation
Prolonged–Action Preparations see Delayed–Action
   Preparations
Promethium   WN 420
   Nuclear physics   QC 796.P5
   See also special topics under Radioisotopes
Promoter (Genetics) see Promoter Regions
   (Genetics)
Promoter Regions (Genetics)   QH 450.2
Promotion of Health see Health Promotion
Promyelocytes see Granulocytes
Pronormoblasts see Erythroblasts
PROPAC see Prospective Payment Assessment
   Commission
Propafenone   QV 150
Propaganda   HM
Propamidine see Antiprotozoal Agents
Propanidid   QV 81
Propanol see 1–Propanol
Propanolamines
   Organic chemistry   QD 305.A4
   Pharmacology   QV 82
   Used for specific purposes, by subject, e.g., as
   a betablocker   QV 132
Properdin   WH 400
   Clinical analysis   QY 455
   Complement action   QW 680
   In other biological processes, by subject
Prophage Integration see Lysogeny
Propheniramine see Pheniramine
Prophenpyridamine see Pheniramine
Prophylactic Immunization see Vaccination
Prophylaxis see Dental Prophylaxis; diseases for
   which prevention and control measures are
   prescribed
Propionates   QU 98
Propionibacteriaceae   QW 120
Propionibacterium   QW 120
Propionic Acids   QU 98
Propiophenones
   Organic chemistry   QD 341.K2
   Pharmacology   QV 150

Propolis
   Used for special purposes, by subject
Propranolol   QV 132
Proprioception   WE 103
Proptosis see Exophthalmos
Propyl Gallate
   As a carcinogen   QZ 202
Prosencephalon see Embryology   WL 300 under
   Brain
Prosimii see Strepsirhini
Prospective Payment Assessment Commission
Prospective Payment System
   Hospitals   WX 157
Prospective Pricing see Prospective Payment System
Prospective Reimbursement see Prospective
   Payment System
Prospective Studies
   In epidemiology   WA 105
   Special topics, by subject
Prostacyclins see Epoprostenol
Prostaglandin Antagonists   QU 90
Prostaglandin–Endoperoxide Synthase   QU 140
Prostaglandin Endoperoxides   QU 90
Prostaglandin E1 see Alprostadil
Prostaglandin F2 see Dinoprost
Prostaglandin F2alpha see Dinoprost
Prostaglandin Inhibitors see Prostaglandin
   Antagonists
Prostaglandin Receptors see Receptors,
   Prostaglandin
Prostaglandin Synthesis Antagonists see
   Anti–Inflammatory Agents, Non–Steroidal
Prostaglandins   QU 90
Prostaglandins A   QU 90
Prostaglandins E   QU 90
Prostaglandins F   QU 90
Prostaglandins I see Epoprostenol
Prostaglandins I2 see Epoprostenol
Prostaglandins X see Epoprostenol
Prostanoic Acids   QU 90
Prostate   WJ 750
Prostatectomy   WJ 768
Prostatectomy, Transurethral see Prostatectomy
Prostatic Diseases   WJ 752
Prostatic Hyperplasia   WJ 752
Prostatic Hypertrophy see Prostatic Hyperplasia
Prostatic Hypertrophy, Benign see Prostatic
   Hyperplacia
Prostatic Neoplasms   WJ 752
Prostatitis   WJ 752
Prostheses and Implants   WE 172
   See also Prosthesis; Prosthesis Implantation;
   names of specific implants or prostheses
Prosthesis   WE 172
   Blood vessels see Blood Vessel Prosthesis   WG
   170
   Cleft palate see Palatal Obturators   WV 440
   Dental see Dental Prosthesis   WU 500–530
   Heart valve see Heart Valve Prosthesis   WG
   169
   Joint see Joint Prosthesis   WE 312
   Mandibular see Mandibular Prosthesis   WU 600
   Maxillofacial see Maxillofacial Prosthesis
   WU 600

Ocular see Eye, Artificial   WW 358; Lenses,
   Intraocular   WW 358
Periodontal see Periodontal Prosthesis   WU 240
Plastic surgery   WO 640
Veterinary   SF 901
See also Prosthesis Implantation   WE 172
Prosthesis, Dental see Dental Prosthesis
Prosthesis Design   WE 172
   Localized, by site
Prosthesis Failure
   Equipment failure (General)   W 26
   Of particular prosthesis, with the prosthesis
Prosthesis Fitting   WE 172
   For particular prosthesis, with the prosthesis
Prosthesis Implantation   WE 172
   Of specific prosthesis, with the prosthesis
   See also Prosthesis   WE 172; names of specific
      implants, prostheses, or prosthesis implantation
Prosthesis Loosening see Prosthesis Failure
Prosthodontics   WU 500
   See also Dental Prosthesis   WU 500–530
Prostitution   HQ 101–440.7
Protactinium   WN 420
   Nuclear physics   QC 796.P2
   See also special topics under Radioisotopes
Protease Antagonists see Protease Inhibitors
Protease Inhibitors   QU 136
Proteases see Peptide Hydrolases
Protective Clothing   WA 260
   In industry   WA 485
Protective Devices   WA 260
   In hospitals   WX 185
   In industry   WA 485
      Aviation   WD 740
      Ophthalmology   WW 505
      Professions   WA 487
   In ophthalmology (General)   WW 113
   Respiratory   WF 26
   For particular parts of the body (when not
      covered by above) use form number 26 in any
      schedule where applicable
Protein A see Staphylococcal Protein A
Protein Binding   QU 55
Protein–Bound Iodine Test see Thyroid Function
Tests
Protein C
   As an anticoagulant   QV 193
Protein C Inhibitor   QU 136
Protein–Calorie Malnutrition see Protein–Energy
   Malnutrition
Protein Conformation   QU 55
Protein Deficiency   WD 105
   Veterinary   SF 855.P76
Protein Denaturation   QU 55
Protein–Energy Malnutrition   WD 105
Protein Engineering   TP 248.65.P76
Protein–Glutamine gamma–Glutamyltransferase
   WH 310
   Clinical examination   QY 410
   Pharmacology   QV 195
Protein Hydrolysates   QU 55
Protein–Losing Enteropathies   WI 400

Protein Methylases see Protein Methyltransferases
Protein Methyltransferases   QU 141
Protein Phosphatase see Phosphoprotein
   Phosphatase
Protein Processing, Post–Translational   QH 450.6
Protein Sensitization see Hypersensitivity
Protein Structure, Primary see Amino Acid
   Sequence
Protein Structure, Quaternary see Protein
   Conformation
Proteinase Inhibitors see Protease Inhibitors
Proteins   QU 55
   Antigens and antibodies   QW 570–680
   Bacterial see Bacterial Proteins   QW 52
   Blood see Blood Proteins   QY 455, etc.
   Carrier see Carrier Proteins   QU 55
   Cerebrospinal fluid see Cerebrospinal Fluid
      Proteins   WL 203, etc.
   Dietary see Dietary Proteins   QU 55, etc.
   Eye see Eye Proteins   WW 101
   Milk see Milk Proteins   WA 716, etc.
   Muscle see Muscle Proteins   WE 500
   Myeloma see Myeloma Proteins   WH 540
   Neoplasm see Neoplasm Proteins   QZ 200
   Nerve tissue see Nerve Tissue Proteins   WL
      104
   Plant see Plant Proteins   QK 898.P8
   Viral see Viral Proteins   QW 160
   With drug action on a particular system in   QV
   Localized elsewhere, by site
   See also names of other specific proteins
Proteins, Acute Phase see Acute Phase Proteins
Proteinuria   WJ 343
Proteinuria–Edema–Hypertension Gestosis see
   Gestosis, EPH
Proteoglycans   QU 55
Proteolytic Enzymes see Peptide Hydrolases
Protestantism see Christianity
Proteus   QW 138.5.P7
Prothrombin   WH 310
   Clinical analysis   QY 410
Prothrombin Time   QY 410
Protirelin   WK 515
Proto–Oncogenes   QZ 202
Protocol–Directed Therapy, Computer–Assisted see
   Therapy, Computer–Assisted
Protocols, Clinical see Clinical Protocols
Protoheme see Heme
Proton–Induced X–Ray Emission Spectrometry see
   Spectrometry, X–Ray Emission
Proton–Translocating ATPase Complex see
   H(+)–Transporting ATP Synthase
Protons   WN 415–420
   In health physics   WN 110
   In nuclear physics (General)   QC
      793.5.P72–793.5.P729
Protoplasts
   Bacteria   QW 51
   Plants   QK 725
Protoporphyrins
   General   QU 110
   Special types, by system in which produced
Protosteliomycetes see Myxomycetes

Protozoa   QX 50-151
Protozoan Infections   WC 700-770
   Veterinary see Protozoan Infections, Animal
      SF 780.6
Protozoan Infections, Animal   SF 780.6
Protracted Pregnancy see Pregnancy, Prolonged
Proverbs see Aphorisms and Proverbs
Proverbs, Medical see Aphorisms and Proverbs
Provocation Tests, Bronchial see Bronchial
   Provocation Tests
Provocation Tests, Nasal see Nasal Provocation
   Tests
Proxemics see Spatial Behavior
Proxy
   Special topics, by subject
Prurigo   WR 282
Pruritus   WR 282
Pruritus Ani   WI 600
Pruritus Vulvae   WP 200
Psammomys see Gerbillinae
Pseudarthrosis   WE 180
Pseudobulbar Paralysis see Paralysis
Pseudoephedrine see Ephedrine
Pseudoglobulins see Serum Globulins
Pseudohypoparathyroidism   WD 200.5.C2
   Inborn error   WD 205.5.M3
Pseudomonadaceae   QW 131
Pseudomonas   QW 131
Pseudomonas aeruginosa   QW 131
Pseudomonas fluorescens   QW 131
Pseudomonas Infections   WC 330
Pseudoneurotic Schizophrenia see Schizotypal
   Personality Disorder
Pseudonyms see Anonyms and Pseudonyms
Pseudopelade see Alopecia
Pseudopolyarthritis, Rhizomelic see Polymyalgia
   Rheumatica
Pseudopsychopathic Schizophrenia see Schizotypal
   Personality Disorder
Pseudorabies   SF 809.A94
Pseudorabies Virus see Herpesvirus 1, Suid
Pseudosclerosis see Hepatolenticular Degeneration
Pseudotuberculosis Infections, Yersinia see Yersinia
   pseudotuberculosis Infections
Pseudotuberculosis, Pasteurella see Yersinia
   pseudotuberculosis Infections
Pseudotumor Cerebri   WL 348
Psilocybine   QV 77.7
   Indian ritual use   E 98.R3
Psilosis see Celiac Disease
Psittacosis see Ornithosis
Psittacosis-Lymphogranuloma Group see Chlamydia
Psoralen Ultraviolet A Therapy see PUVA Therapy
Psoralens   QV 60
   As sunscreens   QV 63
Psoriasis   WR 205
PSRO see Professional Review Organizations
Psychasthenia see Neurasthenia
Psychedelic Agents see Hallucinogens
Psychiatric Aides   WY 160
Psychiatric Aspects of Aerospace Medicine see
   Aerospace Medicine
Psychiatric Department, Hospital   WM 27-28

   In a children's hospital   WS 27-28
Psychiatric Nursing   WY 160
   Education   WY 18-18.5
Psychiatric Social Work see Social Work,
   Psychiatric
Psychiatric Status Rating Scales   WM 141
Psychiatrist-Patient Relations see Physician-Patient
   Relations
Psychiatrists see Biography   WZ 112.5.P6, etc., and
   Directories   WM 22 under Psychiatry
Psychiatry   WM
   Adolescents see Adolescent Psychiatry   WS 463
   Biography
      Collective   WZ 112.5.P6
      Individual   WZ 100
   Case studies   WM 40-49
      In mental retardation   WM 302
   Child see Child Psychiatry   WS 350-350.8
   Counseling   WM 55, etc.
   Directories   WM 22
   Experimental   WM 20
      Techniques   WM 25
   Geriatric see Geriatric Psychiatry   WT 150
   Insurance see Insurance, Psychiatric   W 270,
      etc.
   Legislation & jurisprudence   WM 32-33
   Medicolegal see Forensic Psychiatry   W 740
   Nursing see Psychiatric Nursing   WY 160
   Office management   WM 30
   Aged   WT 150
   Preventive see Community Psychiatry   WM
      31.5, etc.
   Social see Psychiatry, Community   WM
      30.6-31.5; Socioenvironmental Therapy   WM
      428
   See also Forensic Psychiatry   W 740
Psychiatry, Biological see Biological Psychiatry
Psychiatry, Community see Community Psychiatry
Psychiatry, Geriatric see Geriatric Psychiatry
Psychiatry, Military see Military Psychiatry
Psychic Energizers see Antidepressive Agents
Psychic Maladjustment see Personality Disorders
Psychical Research see Parapsychology
Psychoacoustics   WV 270
Psychoactive Agents see Psychotropic Drugs
Psychoanalysis   WM 460-460.5
   Adolescence   WS 463
   Aged   WT 150
   Child   WS 350.5
Psychoanalytic Interpretation   WM 460.7
   Adolescence   WS 463
   Aged   WT 150
   Child   WS 350.5
   Of art and literature   WM 49
   Of famous people from their works   WZ 313
Psychoanalytic Theory   WM 460
Psychoanalytic Therapy   WM 460.6
   Adolescence   WS 463
   Child   WS 350.2
Psychodrama   WM 430.5.P8
   Child   WS 350.2
Psychogenetics see Genetics, Behavioral
Psychogeriatrics see Geriatric Psychiatry

Psychoimmunology see Psychoneuroimmunology
Psycholinguistics   BF 455-463
  Child   WS 105.5.C8
  Infant   WS 105.5.C8
  Language development   LB 1139.L3
Psychological aspects of Aerospace Medicine see
  Aerospace Medicine
Psychological Tests   BF 176
  Child   WS 105.5.E8
  In psychiatry   WM 145
  Infant   WS 1015.5.E8
  See also Projective Techniques   WM 145.5.P8;
    Intelligence Tests   BF 431-433; Personality
    Tests   BF 698.5-698.8; and names of specific
    tests in the LC subject authority file
Psychological Theory   BF 38-64
Psychological Warfare   UB 275-277
Psychology   BF
  Abnormal   WM
  Adolescent see Adolescent Psychology   WS 462
  As a career   BF 75-76
  Biography   WZ 100
  Biography, Collective   BF 109
  Child see Child Psychology   WS 105
  Counseling   WM 55
  Criminal see Criminal Psychology   HV
    6080-6113
  Crowd   HM
  Directories   BF 30
  Geriatric   WT 145
  In aviation medicine   WD 730
  In space medicine   WD 754
  Mass   HM
  Nursing   WY 87
  Pathological see Psychopathology   WM, etc.
  Phenomenological   BF 204.5
  Physiological see Psychophysiology   WL 103
  Sex   BF 692
  War see Psychology, Military   U 22.3;
    Psychological Warfare   UB 275-277
Psychology, Applied   BF 636-637
Psychology, Clinical   WM 105
  Child   WS 105
  Infant   WS 105
Psychology, Comparative
  Animals (primarily)   QL 751
  Human   BF 660-685
Psychology, Criminal see Criminal Psychology
Psychology, Educational   LB 1051-1091
Psychology, Experimental   BF 181-198.7
  Child   WS 105
  Infant   WS 105
  Laboratory manuals   BF 79
  Works about research   BF 76.5
Psychology, Industrial   HF 5548.8
  Mental health of working people   WA 495
Psychology, Medical   WB 104
  Special topics, by subject
Psychology, Military   U 22.3
Psychology, Pastoral see Pastoral Care
Psychology, Physiological see Psychophysiology
Psychology, Schizophrenic see Schizophrenic
  Psychology

Psychology, Self see Self Psychology
Psychology, Social   HM
  Adolescence   WS 462
  Child   WS 105
  Infant   WS 105
Psychometrics   BF 39
Psychomotor Disorders   WM 197
  Of the retarded child   WS 107.5.P7
  See also names of specific disorders
Psychomotor Performance   WE 104
Psychoneuroimmunology   WL 103.7
Psychoneuroses see Neuroses
Psychopathic Personality see Antisocial Personality
  Disorder
Psychopathology   WM
  Child   WS 350
  Infant   WS 350
Psychopharmaceuticals see Psychotropic Drugs
Psychopharmacology   QV 77
  Drug therapy of mental disorders   WM 402
Psychophysics   WL 702
Psychophysiologic Disorders   WM 90
  Child   WM 90
  Infant   WM 90
  Sex disorders   WM 611
Psychophysiology   WL 103
Psychoses see Psychotic Disorders
Psychoses, Alcoholic   WM 274
Psychoses, Drug see Psychoses, Substance-Induced
Psychoses, Organic see Delirium, Dementia,
  Amnestic, Cognitive Disorders
Psychoses, Paranoid see Paranoid Disorders
Psychoses, Senile see Dementia, Senile
Psychoses, Substance-Induced   WM 220
Psychoses, Toxic see Psychoses, Substance-Induced
Psychoses, Traumatic see Delirium, Dementia,
  Amnestic, Cognitive Disorders
Psychosexual Development   BF 692
  Adolescence   WS 462
  Child   WS 105.5.P3
  Infant   WS 105.5.P3
Psychosexual Disorders see Sexual Dysfunctions,
  Psychological
Psychosexual Dysfunctions see Sexual Dysfunctions,
  Psychological
Psychosis, Brief Reactive see Psychotic Disorders
Psychosis, Involutional see Depression, Involutional
Psychosis, Manic-Depressive see Bipolar Disorder
Psychosocial Deprivation   HM
  Adolescents   WS 462
  In infants and children
    Psychological aspects   WS 105.5.D3
    Welfare   WA 320
Psychosocial Support Systems see Social Support
Psychosomatic Disorders see Psychophysiologic
  Disorders
Psychosomatic Medicine   WM 90
  Diseases see Psychophysiologic Disorders   WM
  90, etc.
Psychosurgery   WL 370
Psychotherapeutic Processes   WM 420
  Adolescence   WS 463
  Aged   WT 150

Child   WS 350.2
Infant   WS 350.2
Psychotherapy   WM 420
Adolescence   WS 463
Aged   WT 150
Child   WS 350.2
Infant   WS 350.2
Psychotherapy, Brief   WM 420.5.P5
Psychotherapy, Cognitive see Cognitive Therapy
Psychotherapy, Group   WM 430–430.5
Child   WS 350.2
See also names of specific types of group therapy,
e.g., Sensitivity Training Groups   WM
430.5.S3, etc.
Psychotherapy, Multiple   WM 420.5.P7
Psychotherapy, Rational see Psychotherapy,
Rational–Emotive
Psychotherapy, Rational–Emotive   WM 420.5.P8
Psychotic Disorders   WM 200–220
Functional   WM 202
Adolescence   WS 463
Child   WS 350–350.8
Infant   WS 350–350.8
Psychotomimetic Agents see Hallucinogens
Psychotomimetic Drugs see Hallucinogens
Psychotropic Drugs   QV 77.2–77.9
PTCA see Angioplasty, Transluminal, Percutaneous
Coronary
PtdIns see Phosphatidylinositols
Pteridines
In folic acid   QU 188
Organic chemistry   QD 401
Pterins   QU 110
Pteroylglutamic Acid see Folic Acid
Pteroylpolyglutamic Acids   QU 188
Pterygium   WW 212
Ptomaine Poisoning see Food Poisoining
Ptosis, Eyelid see Blepharoptosis
PTSD see Stress Disorders, Post–Traumatic
Puberty   WS 450
Puberty, Delayed   WS 450
Puberty, Precocious   WS 450
Pubic Bone   WE 750
Surgery to facilitate delivery   WQ 430
Pubic Symphysis   WE 750
Surgery   WE 750
To facilitate delivery   WQ 430
See also Symphysiotomy   WQ 430
Pubiotomy see Surgery   WQ 430 under Pubic Bone
Public Advocacy see Consumer Advocacy
Public Assistance   HV 687–4630
For maternal and child welfare (Public health
aspects)   WA 310–320
For medicosocial problems of the aged   WT
30
See also more specific headings, e.g., Medicaid
W 250
Public Baths see Baths
Public Carriers see Transportation
Public Health   WA
As a profession   WA 21
Impact of environment on public health see
Environmental Health   WA 30, etc.

Statistics   WA 900
See also Morbidity   WA 900; Vital statistics
HB, etc.
Workers see Allied Health Personnel   W 21.5,
etc.; Health Manpower   W 76
Public Health Administration   WA 525–590
Public Health Dentistry   WU 113
Public Health Nursing   WY 108
Education   WY 18
Government (General)   WY 130
Indian services   WY 130
See also Military Nursing   WY 130
Public Health Schools see Schools, Public Health
Public Health Surveillance see Population
Surveillance
Public Housing
Hotels   WA 799, etc.
Low cost housing   HD 7288.77–7288.78
Rural   HD 7289
Sanitary control   WA 795–799
Public Opinion   HM
Specific topics, by subject
Public Policy
Abortion   HQ 767
Laetrile   QZ 267
Other areas, by subject
Public Relations   HM
Specific relations by subject, professions, or
named group of persons involved
Publishers' Catalogs see Catalogs, Publishers'
Publishing   Z 278–544
Medical   WZ 345
Puericulture see Child Care
Puerperal Disorders   WQ 500–505
Puerperal Infection   WQ 505
Puerperium   WQ 500–505
Puerto Ricans see Hispanic Americans
Pulex see Fleas
Pulmonary Alveolar Proteinosis   WF 600
Pulmonary Alveoli   WF 600
Pulmonary Artery   WG 595.P8
See also Blood Supply   WF 600 under Lungs;
Pulmonary Circulation   WF 600
Pulmonary Circulation   WF 600
Pulmonary Coin Lesion see Coin Lesion, Pulmonary
Pulmonary Diffusing Capacity   WF 141
Pulmonary Disease, Chronic Obstructive see Lung
Diseases, Obstructive
Pulmonary Disease (Specialty)   WF 100
Pulmonary Diseases see Lung Diseases
Pulmonary Edema   WF 600
Pulmonary Embolism   WG 420
Pulmonary Emphysema   WF 648
Pulmonary Fibrosis   WF 600
Pulmonary Function Tests see Respiratory Function
Tests
Pulmonary Gas Exchange   WF 102
Used for diagnostic aspects   WF 141
Pulmonary Heart Disease   WG 420
Pulmonary Incompetence see Pulmonary Valve
Insufficiency
Pulmonary Medicine see Pulmonary Disease
(Specialty)

Pulmonary Neoplasms see Lung Neoplasms
Pulmonary Nodule, Solitary see Coin Lesion,
  Pulmonary
Pulmonary Regurgitation see Pulmonary Valve
  Insufficiency
Pulmonary Stenosis see Pulmonary Valve Stenosis
Pulmonary Surfactants   WF 600
Pulmonary Surgical Procedures   WF 668
Pulmonary Tuberculosis see Tuberculosis,
  Pulmonary
Pulmonary Valve   WG 269
Pulmonary Valve Incompetence see Pulmonary
  Valve Insufficiency
Pulmonary Valve Insufficiency   WG 269
Pulmonary Valve Stenosis   WG 269
Pulmonary Veins   WG 625 P8
    See also Blood Supply   WF 600 under Lungs;
      Pulmonary Circulation   WF 600
Pulmonary Ventilation   WF 102
Pulmonology see Pulmonary Disease (Specialty)
Pulp see Dental Pulp
Pulp Canal see Dental Pulp Cavity
Pulp Capping see Dental Pulp Capping
Pulp Chamber see Dental Pulp Cavity
Pulpitis   WU 230
Pulpotomy   WU 230
Pulsatile Flow   WG 106
Pulse
    Cardiovascular diagnosis   WG 141
    General diagnosis   WB 282
    Hemodynamics   WG 106
Pulse Oximetry see Oximetry
Pulse Radiolysis   QD 643.P84
Pulsus Alternans see Arrhythmia
Pulverization see Drug Compounding; Powders
Pumping, Intra-Aortic Balloon see Intra-Aortic
  Balloon Pumping
Pumps, Heart-Assist see Heart-Assist Devices
Pumps, Infusion see Infusion Pumps
Punched-Card Systems   Z 695.92
    Special topics, by subject
Puncture Biopsy see Biopsy, Needle
Puncture Fluids see Body Fluids; Laboratory
  Techniques and Procedures; Exudates and
  Transudates
Punctures   WB 373-377
    Cisternal   WB 377
    Sternal   WH 380
    Ventricular   WB 377
    See also Amniocentesis   WQ 209; Biopsy,
      Needle   WB 379, etc.; Spinal Puncture   WB
      377, etc.
Punishment
    Adolescence   WS 462-463
    Child   WS 105.5.C3
    Infant   WS 105.5.C3
    Conditioned response   BF 319.5.P8
    Theory of (Penology)   K 5103
Pupil   WW 240
    Dilatation   WW 240
      See also Dilatation, Pathologic   WW 240, etc.
    Dilators   QV 134
Pupillary Reflex see Reflex, Pupillary

Puppets see Play and Playthings
Purchasing, Hospital   WX 157
Pure Food Laws see Food and drug laws   WA
  697 under Legislation, Drug
Pure Red-Cell Aplasia see Red-Cell Aplasia, Pure
Purgatives see Cathartics
Purification see Environment, Controlled;
  Sterilization
Purine-Nucleoside Phosphorylase   QU 141
Purine Nucleosides   QU 57
    Pharmacology   QV 185
Purine-Pyrimidine Metabolism, Inborn Errors
  WD 205.5.P8
    See also Gout   WE 350
Purine Receptors see Receptors, Purinergic
Purinergic Receptors see Receptors, Purinergic
Purines
    Constituents of nucleic acids   QU 58
    Organic chemistry   QD 401
    Stimulants   QV 107
Purkinje Cells   WL 320
Purple Membrane see Bacteriorhodopsin
Purpura   WH 314-320
Purpura, Thrombocytopenic   WH 315
Purpura, Thrombopenic see Purpura,
  Thrombocytopenic
Pursuit, Saccadic see Saccades
Pus see Suppuration
Pustulants see Irritants
Pustular Dermatosis, Subcorneal see Skin Diseases,
  Vesiculobullous
Pustular Psoriasis of Palms and Soles see Psoriasis
Pustulosis of Palms and Soles see Psoriasis
Pustulosis Palmaris et Plantaris see Psoriasis
PUVA Therapy   WB 480
PVP-Iodine see Povidone-Iodine
Pyelitis   WJ 351
Pyelocystitis see Pyelitis
Pyelography see Urography
Pyelonephritis   WJ 351
Pyelonephritis, Acute Necrotizing see Kidney
  Papillary Necrosis
Pyelophlebitis see Phlebitis
Pyemia see Septicemia
Pygathrix see Cercopithecidae
Pygmy Chimpanzee see Pan paniscus
Pyknolepsy see Epilepsy, Absence
Pyloric Antrum   WI 387
Pyloric Stenosis   WI 387
Pylorospasm see Spasm
Pylorus   WI 387
Pyoctanium aureum see Benzophenoneidum
Pyoderma   WR 220
Pyonephrosis see Pyelonephritis
Pyopneumothorax see Pneumothorax
Pyorrhea Alveolaris see Periodontal Diseases
Pyothorax see Empyema
Pyramidal Tracts   WL 400
Pyrans   QV 138.C1
    Organic chemistry   QD 405
Pyrazinopyrimidines see Pteridines
Pyrazoles
    Organic chemistry   QD 401

ALWAYS CONSULT MAIN SCHEDULES. USE NUMBER ASSIGNED ONLY WHEN
SUBJECT REPRESENTS MAJOR EMPHASIS OF WORK BEING CLASSIFIED

Pharmacology   QV 95
Pyrethrum
   As an insecticidal plant   SB 292.P8
   Public health aspects   WA 240
Pyretotherapy see Hyperthermia, Induced
Pyrexia see Fever
Pyridazines   QV 150
   As antirheumatoid agents   QV 95
   Organic chemistry   QD 401
Pyridines
   Enzyme inhibitors   QU 143
   Organic chemistry   QD 401
Pyridinium Compounds
   Enzymology   QU 135
   Organic chemistry   QD 401
Pyridinones see Pyridones
Pyridones
   As anti-arteriosclerosis agents   QV 150
   Organic chemistry   QD 401
Pyridoxal   QU 195
Pyridoxine   QU 195
Pyridoxine Deficiency   WD 120
Pyrimethamine   QV 256
Pyrimidines
   Constituents of nucleic acids   QU 58
   Organic chemistry   QD 401
Pyrocatechols see Catechols
Pyrogallol   QV 223
Pyrogens
   As substances causing fever   WB 152
   Special topics, by subject
Pyromania see Firesetting Behavior
Pyrophosphatases   QU 136
Pyrophosphates see Diphosphates
Pyrosis see Heartburn
Pyrroles
   As antirheumatoid agents   QV 95
   In heme and porphyrin chemistry   WH 190
   Organic chemistry   QD 401
Pyrrolidines
   As antineoplastic agents   QV 269
   Organic chemistry   QD 401
Pyruvaldehyde   QU 98
Pyruvate Oxidase   QU 140
Pyruvates   QU 98
   Organic chemistry
     Aliphatic compounds   QD 305.A2
Pyuria   WJ 151
   In urine analysis   QY 185

Q

Q Fever   WC 625
QALY see Quality-Adjusted Life Years
Qi see Ch'i
Quackery   WZ 310
   Supposed antineoplastic agents   QV 269
Quadrigeminal Plate see Corpora Quadrigemina
Quadriplegia   WL 346
   Veterinary   SF 895
Quality-Adjusted Life Years
   Demography   HB 1322
   Special topics, by subject

   See also Quality of Life   WA 30
Quality Assessment, Health Care see Quality
   Assurance, Health Care
Quality Assurance, Health Care   W 84
   Special topics, by subject
Quality Circles see Management Quality Circles
Quality Control
   Drugs   QV 771
     Public health aspects   WA 730
   Food (Flavor, texture, appearance)   TP 372.5
     Public health aspects   WA 695-722
   Health services   W 84
   Hospitals   WX 153
     See also Facility Regulation and Control   WX
     153
   Nursing   WY 16
   Psychiatry   WM 30
   Sanitation   WA 672
   Other particular products or procedures, by
     subject
   Of other specialty fields, in the number for the
     profession, e.g. Dentistry   WU 21
Quality Indicators see Quality Indicators, Health
   Care
Quality Indicators, Health Care
   General   W 84
   Special topics, by subject
Quality of Health Care
   General   W 84
   Hospitals   WX 153
   Private practice   WB 50
   Public health   WA 525-546
Quality of Life   WA 30
   Specific topics, by subject
Quantum Theory   QC 173.96-174.52
Quarantine   WA 230
   Law   WA 32-33
   Port and maritime   WA 234
   Veterinary medicine   SF 740
     By locality   SF 621-723
Quarantine Hospitals see Hospitals, Special
Quartz
   Toxicology   QV 610
Questionnaires
   Research (Form number 20 or 20.5 in any NLM
     schedule where applicable)
   Statistical methods in psychology   BF 39
   Surveys
     Health   WA 900
     Nutrition   QU 146
   Special topics, by subject
Queuing Theory see Systems Theory
Quick Test see Prothrombin Time
Quinacrine   QV 258
Quinalbarbitone see Secobarbital
Quinazolines
   As antihypertensive agents   QV 150
   Organic chemistry   QD 401
Quincke's Edema see Angioneurotic Edema
Quinidine   QV 155
Quinine   QV 257
Quinolines
   As anti-infective agents   QV 250

**ALWAYS CONSULT MAIN SCHEDULES. USE NUMBER ASSIGNED ONLY WHEN
SUBJECT REPRESENTS MAJOR EMPHASIS OF WORK BEING CLASSIFIED**

Organic chemistry   QD 401
Quinolinic Acids
    Biochemistry   QU 65
    Organic chemistry   QD 401
Quinolinium Compounds
    As anti–infective agents   QV 250
    Organic chemitry   QD 401
Quinolinols see Hydroxyquinolines
Quinolinones see Quinolones
Quinolone Anti–Infective Agents see Anti–Infective
    Agents, Quinolone
Quinolones   QV 250
Quinones
    Organic chemitry   QD 341.Q4
Quinoxalines
    As anti infective agents   QV 250
    Organic chemistry   QD 401
Quintan Fever see Trench Fever
Quinuclidines
    As autonomic drugs (general)   QV 120
    Organic chemistry   QD 401
Quokkas see Kangaroos

R

R Factors   QW 51
R Plasmids see R Factors
Rabbit Aorta Contracting Substance see
    Thromboxane A2
Rabbit Fever see Tularemia
Rabbits
    As laboratory animals   QY 60.L3
    Culture   SF 451–455
    Diseases (Domestic and Wild)   SF 997.5.R2
    Wild   QL 737.L32
Rabies   WC 550
    Veterinary   SF 797
Rabies Vaccine   WC 550
Rabies Virus   QW 168.5.R2
Raccoon Dogs see Carnivora
Race see Racial Stocks
Race Psychology see Ethnopsychology
Race Relations   HT 1503–1595
    Adolescent   WS 462
    Child   WS 105.5.S6
    Discrimination (non–MeSH usage)
        In education   LC 212–212.73
        In employment   HD 4903–4903.5
        In housing   HD 7288.75–7288.76
        In particular countries (General) by country
            D, E, or F schedules
Races, Diseases of see Diseases   WB 720 under
    Ethnic Groups
Rachitis see Rickets
Racial Stocks   GN 537–673
    Miscegenation   GN 254
    See also special topics under Ethnic Groups
Racquet Sports   QT 260.5.R2
Radar   TK 6573–6595
    Special topics, by subject
Rademacherism see Alternative Medicine
Radial Keratotomy see Keratotomy, Radial
Radiant Warmers, Infant see Incubators, Infant

Radiation   WN
    As a cause of disease (Pathology)   QZ 57
    Physics (General)   QC 474–496.9
Radiation Biology see Radiobiology
Radiation Counters see Instrumentation   WN 150
    under Technology, Radiologic; Scintillation
    Counting; Whole–Body Counting
Radiation Dosage
    Measurement, tolerance, safety measures   WN
    665
    See also Radiotherapy Dosage   WN 250.5.X7,
    etc.
Radiation Effects   WN 600–630
    See also names of organs, organisms, chemicals,
    drugs, or processes affected
Radiation Genetics   WN
    Animal   WN 620
    General works   WN 610
    Human   WN 620
    Plant   WN 630
Radiation–Induced Dermatitis see Radiodermatitis
Radiation Injuries   WN 610–650
    In industry   WA 470
    Prevention & control   WN 650
    Veterinary   SF 757.8
    See also Adverse effects   WN 200 under
        Radiography; Adverse effects   WN 250 under
        Radiotherapy; Adverse Effects   WN 300
        under Radium
Radiation Injuries, Experimental   WN 620
Radiation, Ionizing
    General works   WN 105
Radiation Monitoring   WN 650
Radiation, Nonionizing
    Diseases caused by   WD 605
    Diagnostic use   WB 288
    General medical use   WB 117
    General physiological effects   QT 162.U4
    Therapeutic use   WB 480
    Used for special purposes, by subject
    See also names of specific forms of nonionizing
        radiation, e.g., Light   WB 117, etc.
Radiation Protection   WN 650
    In industry   WA 470
    See also Radioactive Waste   WA 788
Radiation–Protective Agents   WN 650
Radiation Sensitivity see Radiation Tolerance
Radiation–Sensitizing Agents   WN 610
Radiation Sickness see Radiation Injuries
Radiation Syndrome see Radiation Injuries
Radiation Therapy, Computer–Assisted see
    Radiotherapy, Computer–Assisted
Radiation Tolerance   WN 650
    In treating particular conditions, with the
        condition, e.g., in the radiotherapy of neoplasms
        QZ 269
Radiation, Visible see Light
Radiation, Whole–Body see Whole–Body Irradiation
Radicular Cyst   WU 240
Radiculitis   WL 400
Radiesthesia   WB 960
Radio
    In general education   LB 1044.5–1044.6

Radionuclide Tomography, Single–Photon Emission–Computed see Tomography, Emission–Computed, Single–Photon
Radionuclides see Radioisotopes
Radiopaque Media see Contrast Media
Radiopharmaceuticals   WN 415–450
    Adverse effects   WN 610–630
    Diagnostic Use   WN 445
    Therapeutic Use   WN 450
    Used for special purposes, by subject
Radioscopy see Fluoroscopy
Radiosensitivity see Radiation Tolerance
Radiosurgery   WL 368
Radiotherapy
    Adverse effects   WN 250
    Anti–neoplastic see Radiotherapy   QZ 269
      under Neoplasms
    Dermatology   WR 660
    General works   WN 250
    Radioisotopes see Therapeutic use   WN 450
      under Radioisotopes
    Radium see Therapeutic use   WN 340 under
      Radium
    Veterinary   SF 757.8
    X–ray therapy   WN 250.5.X7
    See also names of diseases for which therapy is used
Radiotherapy, Computer–Assisted   WN 250.5.R2
Radiotherapy, Conformal   WN 250.5.R2
Radiotherapy Dosage
    Radioisotopes   WN 450
    Radium   WN 340
    X–rays   WN 250.5.X7
    See also Radiation Dosage   WN 665
Radiotherapy Dose Fractionation see Dose Fractionation
Radiotherapy, High–Energy   WN 250.5.R3
    See also special topics under Radiotherapy
Radiotherapy, Interstitial see Brachytherapy
Radiotherapy, Intracavity see Brachytherapy
Radiotherapy Planning, Computer–Assisted   WN 250.5.R2
Radiotherapy, Surface see Brachytherapy
Radiovisiography, Dental see Radiography, Dental, Digital
Radium   WN 300–340
    Adverse effects   WN 300
    Inorganic chemistry   QD 181.R1
    Therapeutic use   WN 340
Radius   WE 820
Radius Fractures   WE 820
Radon   WN 300–340
    General works   WN 300
    Therapeutic use   WN 340
Rage   BF 575.A5
    Adolescence   WS 462
    Child   WS 105.5.E5
    Infant   WS 105.5.E5
Raillietina see Cestoda
Raillietiniasis see Cestode Infections
Railroads
    Accidents   WA 275
    Occupational medicine   WA 400–495

    Nursing service   WY 143
    Sanitary control of public carriers   WA 810
Rain
    Meteorology   QC 924.5–926.2
    Special topics, by subject, e.g., Air Pollution   WA 754
Rales see Respiratory Sounds
Raman Spectroscopy see Spectrum Analysis, Raman
Ramps see Architectural Accessibility
Ramsay Hunt Paralysis Syndrome see Parkinson Disease
Random Allocation
    (Form number 20 or 20.5 in any NLM schedule where applicable)
Randomization see Random Allocation
Randomized Controlled Trials
    Special topics, by subject
    See also Clinical Trials
Ranitidine
    As an anti–ulcer agent   QV 69
Rape
    Criminology   HV 6558–6569
    Medicolegal aspects   W 795
    Therapy for victims   WM 401
Rapeseed see Brassica
Raphe Nuclei   WL 310
Rapid Eye Movements see Sleep, REM
Raptors
    Diseases   SF 994.5
Rare Books
    Works about   Z 688.R3
    Medical books by period (if old)   WZ 220–270
    By subject, if post 1801 or post–Americana
ras Genes see Genes, ras
Rat–Bite Fever   WC 390
Rat Virus see Parvovirus
Rate Setting and Review
    General   W 74
    Hospitals   WX 157
Rational–Emotive Psychotherapy see Psychotherapy, Rational–Emotive
Rationalization   WM 193.5.R1
Rationing, Health Care see Health Care Rationing
Rats
    Diseases   SF 997.5.R3
    As laboratory animals   QY 60.R6
    Public health aspects see Rodent Control   WA 240
Rats, Bandicoot see Muridae
Rats, Brattleboro
    As laboratory animals   QY 60.R6
Rats, Inbred CDF see Rats, Inbred F344
Rats, Inbred Fischer 344 see Rats, Inbred F344
Rats, Inbred F344
    As laboratory animals   QY 60.R6
Rats, Inbred SHR
    As laboratory animals   QY 60.R6
Rats, Inbred Strains
    As laboratory animals   QY 60.R6
Rats, Laboratory see Rats
Rats, Long–Evans
    As laboratory animals   QY 60.R6

Rats, Mutant Strains
    As laboratory animals   QY 60.R6
Rats, Norway see Rats
Rats, Sand see Gerbillinae
Rats, Spontaneously Hypertensive see Rats, Inbred
    SHR
Rattlesnake Venoms see Crotalid Venoms
Rattus see Muridae
Rattus norvegicus see Rats
Rauwolfia   QV 150
Rauwolfia Alkaloids   QV 150
Rauwolscine see Yohimbine
Raw Food Diet see Diet
Raynaud's Disease   WG 570
Reactants, Acute Phase see Acute Phase Proteins
Reaction, Acute-Phase see Acute-Phase Reaction
Reaction Time   BF 317
Reactive Disorders see Adjustment Disorders
Reactive Site see Binding Sites
Readiness Potential see Contingent Negative
    Variation
Reading
    Education (General)   LB 1050–1050.75
    Children with learning disabilities   LC
        4704–4803
    Mentally disabled children   LC 4620
    Medical aspects of problems associated with poor
        vision   WW 480
    Psychology   BF 456.R2
    See also Dyslexia   WL 340.6; Dyslexia,
        Acquired   WL 340.6
Reading Disability, Acquired see Dyslexia, Acquired
Reading Disability, Developmental see Dyslexia
Reading, Therapeutic see Bibliotherapy
Reagent Kits, Diagnostic   QY 26
    Used for particular tests, by subject, e.g., for
        hemoglobin examination   QY 455
Reagents see Indicators and Reagents
Reagins   QW 575
    Associated with hypersensitivity   QW 900
Real-Time Systems see Computer Systems
Reality Testing
    Child psychology   WS 105.5.S3
    Psychoanalysis   WM 460.5.E3
Recall   BF 370–385
    Child   WS 105.5.M2
    Infant   WS 105.5.M2
Receptor-Mediated Signal Transduction see Signal
    Transduction
Receptors, Acetylcholine see Receptors, Cholinergic
Receptors, Adenosine see Receptors, Purinergic P1
Receptors, ADP see Receptors, Purinergic P2
Receptors, Adrenergic   WL 102.8
Receptors, Adrenergic, alpha   WL 102.8
Receptors, Adrenergic, beta   WL 102.8
Receptors, alpha-Adrenergic see Receptors,
    Adrenergic, alpha
Receptors, Angiotensin   QU 68
Receptors, Antigen   QW 573
Receptors, Antigen, T-Cell   QW 573
Receptors, ATP see Receptors, Purinergic P2
Receptors, Benzodiazepine see Receptors, GABA-A
Receptors, Benzodiazepine-GABA see Receptors,

GABA-A
Receptors, beta-Adrenergic see Receptors,
    Adrenergic, beta
Receptors, Caerulein see Receptors, Cholecystokinin
Receptors, Caffeine see Receptors, Purinergic
Receptors, Cell Surface
    Biochemistry   QU 55
    Immunochemistry   QW 504.5
    Pharmacology   QV 38
Receptors, Cholecystokinin   WK 170
Receptors, Cholinergic   WL 102.8
Receptors, Complement   QW 680
Receptors, Corticosteroid see Receptors,
    Glucocorticoid
Receptors, Diazepam see Receptors, GABA-A
Receptors, Diiodotyrosine see Receptors, Thyroid
    Hormone
Receptors, Dopamine   WL 102.8
Receptors, Drug   QV 38
Receptors, Endogenous Substances see Receptors,
    Cell Surface
Receptors, Epidermal Growth Factor-Urogastrone
    WK 170
Receptors, Estrogen   WP 522
Receptors, Fc   QW 601
Receptors, GABA-A   QU 60
Receptors, GABA-Benzodiazepine see Receptors,
    GABA-A
Receptors, gamma-Aminobutyric Acid see
    Receptors, GABA
Receptors, Gastrin see Receptors, Cholecystokinin
Receptors, Gastrointestinal Hormone   WK 170
Receptors, Glucocorticoid   WK 150
Receptors, Growth Hormone see Receptors,
    Somatotropin
Receptors, Histamine   QV 157
    See also Histamine H1 Receptor Blockaders
        QV 157
Receptors, Histamine H2   QV 157
Receptors, Hormone   WK 102
    Localized, by site
    See also names of specific hormone receptors
Receptors, IL-2 see Receptors, Interleukin-2
Receptors, Immunologic   QW 570
    Immunochemistry   QW 504.5
Receptors, Interleukin-2   QW 568
Receptors, LDL   QU 95
Receptors, Low Density Lipoprotein see Receptors,
    LDL
Receptors, Muscarinic   WL 102.8
Receptors, Muscimol see Receptors, GABA-A
Receptors, N-Methyl-D-Aspartate   QU 60
    As neurotransmitter   QV 126
    In synaptic transmission   WL 102.8
Receptors, Neural see Receptors, Sensory
Receptors, Neurohumor see Receptors,
    Neurotransmitter
Receptors, Neurotransmitter   WL 102.8
Receptors, Nicotinic   WL 102.8
Receptors, Pancreozymin see Receptors,
    Cholecystokinin
Receptors, Pheromone see Chemoreceptors
Receptors, Progesterone   WP 530

Receptors, Progestin see Receptors, Progesterone

Receptors, Proglumide see Receptors, Cholecystokinin

Receptors, Prostaglandin   QU 90

Receptors, Purinergic   QU 58

Receptors, Purinergic P1   QU 58

Receptors, Purinergic P2   QU 58

Receptors, Sensory   WL 102.9

Receptors, Sincalide see Receptors, Cholecystokinin

Receptors, Somatotropin   WK 515

Receptors, Steroid   WK 150

Receptors, Stretch see Mechanoreceptors

Receptors, Synaptic see Receptors, Neurotransmitter

Receptors, T–Cell Growth Factor see Receptors, Interleukin-2

Receptors, Tetragastrin see Receptors, Cholecystokinin

Receptors, Theophylline see Receptors, Purinergic

Receptors, Thyroid Hormone   WK 202

Receptors, Thyroxine see Receptors, Thyroid Hormone

Receptors, Transforming Growth Factor Alpha see Receptors, Epidermal Growth Factor–Urogastrone

Receptors, Triiodothyronine see Receptors, Thyroid Hormone

Receptors, Urogastrone see Receptors, Epidermal Growth Factor–Urogastrone

Receptors, Virus   QW 160

Receptosomes see Endosomes

Recklinghausen's Disease of Bone see Osteitis Fibrosa Cystica

Recklinghausen's Disease of Nerve see Neurofibromatosis

Recombinant DNA see DNA, Recombinant

Recombinant DNA Vaccines see Vaccines, DNA

Recombinant Interferon Alfa–2c see Interferon Alfa, Recombinant

Recombinant Proteins   QU 55
   Biotechnology   TP 248.65.P76

Recombination, Genetic   QH 443–450.6

Reconstructive Surgical Procedures   WO 600–640
   Specific locations, by site
   See also Cosmetic Techniques; Surgery, Plastic; specific reconstructive surgical procedures, e.g., Blepharoplasty   WW 205; Mammaplasty WP 910; Rhinoplasty   WV 312

Record Linkage, Medical see Medical Record Linkage

Records
   Bibliographical on magnetic tape   Z 699–699.5
   Government administration   JF 1521
   Hospital see Hospital Records   WX 173
   Public records and privacy   JC 596–596.2
   Statistical   HA 38–39
   See also Dental Records   WU 95; Medical Records   WX 173, etc.; Nursing Records WY 100.5

Records Control see Forms and Records Control

Recovery of Function
   In brain injuries   WL 354, etc.
   Special topics, by subject

Recovery Period, Anesthesia see Anesthesia

Recovery Period

Recovery Room   WX 218

Recovery Room Nursing see Postanesthesia Nursing

Recreation   QT 250
   Centers (General works)   GV 182
      For leisure activities and outdoor games   QT 250
      See also Fitness Centers   QT 255

Recrudescence see Recurrence

Rectal Diseases   WI 600
   Surgery   WI 650

Rectal Drug Administration see Administration, Rectal

Rectal Fistula   WI 605
   See also Rectovaginal Fistula   WP 180

Rectal Neoplasms   WI 610

Rectal Prolapse   WI 600

Rectal Surgery (Specialty) see Colorectal Surgery

Rectocolitis, Hemorrhagic see Colitis, Ulcerative

Rectocolitis, Ulcerative see Colitis, Ulcerative

Rectovaginal Fistula   WP 180

Rectum   WI 600–650
   Anesthesia by see Anesthesia, Rectal   WO 290
   Feeding by see Tube feeding   WB 410
   Medication by see Enema   WB 344;
      Suppositories   QV 785
   Surgery (General)   WI 650

Recurrence   QZ 140
   Of specific diseases, with the disease

Red Blood Cell Count see Erythrocyte Count

Red Blood Cell Membrane Sialoglycoprotein see Glycophorin

Red Blood Cell Transfusion see Erythrocyte Transfusion

Red Blood Cells see Erythrocytes

Red Bugs see Trombiculid Mites

Red–Cell Aplasia, Pure   WH 155

Red Cell Ghost see Erythrocyte Membrane

Red Cell Mass see Erythrocyte Volume

Red Cell Substitutes see Blood Substitutes

Red Cross
   Army services   UH 535–537
   Disasters   HV 560–583
   Navy services   VG 457
   Nursing   WY 137

Red Marrow see Bone Marrow

Red Mites see Trombiculid Mites

Red Monkey see Erythrocebus patas

Red Nucleus   WL 310

Red Tide see Dinoflagellida

Redox see Oxidation–Reduction

Reductases see Oxidoreductases

Reductive Enzymes see Oxidoreductases

Reduviidae   QX 503

Reeler Mice see Mice, Neurologic Mutants

Reference Books
   General   Z 711
   On special topics, by subject

Reference Books, Medical
   Bibliography   ZWB 100
   On special topics, by subject, e.g., Dictionary of Nutrition   QU 13

Reference Ranges see Reference Values

Reference Standards
  Drugs   QV 771
  Of other products, by subject
Reference Values
  (Form number 16 in any NLM schedule where applicable)
Referral and Consultation
  Initiated by the nurse practitioner   WY 90
  Initiated by the physician   W 64
  Initiated by the psychiatrist   WM 64
  Initiated by the surgeon   WO 64
  In other specific specialties, in the number for interpersonal relationships or lacking that, in the general works number
  Specific conditions discussed, by subject
Reflex   WL 106
  Psychogalvanic see Galvanic Skin Response   WM 145, etc.
  See also Conditioning, Classical   BF 319 and other types of conditioning
Reflex, Abnormal   WL 340
Reflex, Acoustic
  In hearing assessment   WV 274
Reflex, Conditioned see Conditioning, Classical
Reflex Epilepsy see Epilepsy
Reflex, Pharyngeal see Gagging
Reflex, Psychogalvanic see Galvanic Skin Response
Reflex, Pupillary   WW 240
Reflex, Stretch   WL 106
Reflex Sympathetic Dystrophy   WL 600
Reflex, Tendon see Reflex, Stretch
Reflex, Vestibulo–Ocular   WV 255
Reflexology see Massage
Reflexotherapy   WB 962
Refraction, Ocular   WW 300–320
Refractive Disorders see Refractive Errors
Refractive Errors   WW 300–320
  Diagnosis   WW 300
Refractive Index see Refractometry
Refractometry   QC 387
Refrigeration
  Biological products   WA 730
  Blood   WH 460
  Chemical technology   TP 490–497
  Drugs   WA 730;   QV 754
  Food   WA 710
  Organs   WO 665
  Specimen handling   QY 25, etc.
Refrigeration Anesthesia see Anesthesia, Refrigeration
Refsum Disease, Infantile see Peroxisomal Disorders
Refugees
  Health problems   WA 300
  Mental health problems   WA 305
  Relief   HV 640–640.5
Refuse Disposal
  Industrial bacteriology   QW 75
  Public health aspects
    General   WA 780
    Industrial   WA 788
    Solid and fluid waste combined (General)   WA 778
  See also names of specific types of waste and waste disposal, e.g., Industrial Waste, Radioactive Waste, Medical Waste, Medical Waste Disposal, etc.
Regeneration
  Biology   QH 499
  Bone see Bone Regeneration   WE 200
  Liver see Liver Regeneration   WI 702
  Local reaction to injury (Pathology)   QZ 150
  Nerve see Nerve Regeneration   WL 102
  Other specific areas, with the area affected
  See also Wound Healing   WO 185, etc.
Regional Anatomy see Anatomy, Regional
Regional Anesthesia see Anesthesia, Conduction
Regional Blood Flow   WG 106
Regional Health Planning   WA 541
Regional Hospital Planning see Hospital Planning
Regional Medical Programs   WA 541
Regional Perfusion see Perfusion, Regional
Regional Surgery see Surgery; names of organs or regions treated
Registration see Birth Certificates; Death Certificates; Licensure; Notifiable disease registration   WA 55 under Communicable Disease Control
Registries
  Of mental diseases
    Administration of registries   WM 30
    Statistics themselves   WM 16
  Of neoplastic diseases   QZ 200
  Of notifiable diseases   WA 55, etc.
  Of other diseases or types of data
    (Form number 16 in any NLM schedule where applicable)
Regression Analysis   QA 278.2
  Special topics, by subject
Regression Diagnostics see Regression Analysis
Regression (Psychology)   WM 193.5.R2
  Adolescence   WS 463
  Child   WS 350.8.D3
  Infant   WS 350.8.D3
Regulation of Gene Expression see Gene Expression Regulation
Regulation of Gene Expression, Bacterial see Gene Expression Regulation, Bacterial
Regulation of Gene Expression, Enzymologic see Gene Expression Regulation, Enzymologic
Regulation of Gene Expression, Neoplastic see Gene Expression Regulation, Neoplastic
Regulation of Gene Expression, Viral see Gene Expression Regulation, Viral
Regurgitation, Gastric see Gastroesophageal Reflux
Rehabilitation   WB 320
  Disabled veterans   UB 360–366
  Educational   LC 4001–4824
  General works on physically disabled   WB 320
  Of the blind   HV 1573–2349
    Medical   WW 276
    See also Rehabilitation under Visually Impaired Persons   WW 276, etc.
  Of the deaf, etc.   HV 2353–2990.5, etc.
    Medical rehabilitation   WV 270–280
    See also Rehabilitation of Hearing Impaired   WV 270–280, etc.

Of the mentally ill   WM 400–460.6
Orthopedic devices for see Orthopedic
  Equipment   WE 172
Physical therapy   WB 460
Physically disabled child   WS 368
  Psychological problems   WS 105.5.H2
Retarded child see Mental Retardation   WS
  107.5.R3
Sociological aspects   HD 7255–7256
Videotherapy in psychiatry   WM 450.5.V5
See also names of particular disabilities or diseases
  being treated
Rehabilitation Centers
  For the mentally ill or disabled; alcoholics and
    drug addicts   WM 29
  For the physically disabled   WB 29
  See also Halfway houses   WM 29, etc.; Sheltered
    workshops   WB 29, etc.
Rehabilitation Nursing   WY 150.5
  Of particular diseases, with the nursing number
    for the disease
Rehabilitation of Hearing Impaired
  Physical & medical   WV 270–280
  Social   HV 2353–2990.5
  See also specific rehabilitation devices and
    procedures, e.g., Hearing Aids   WV 274; Sign
    Language   HV 2474–2476
Rehabilitation, Vocational   HD 7255–7256
  See also Occupational Therapy   WB 555, etc.
Rehydration see Fluid Therapy
Rehydration, Oral see Fluid Therapy
Rehydration Solutions   QV 786
  Used for special purposes, by subject
Reimbursement, Health Insurance see Insurance,
  Health, Reimbursement
Reimbursement, Incentive
  Hospitals   WX 157
Reimbursement Mechanisms
  Dentistry   WU 77
  Hospitals   WX 157
  Medicine   W 80
  Nursing   WY 77
  Pharmacy   QV 736
  In other specific fields, by subject
Reimbursement, Prospective see Prospective
  Payment System
Reimplantation see Replantation
Reimplantation, Tooth see Tooth Replantation
Reindeer   QL 737.U55
  Diseases   SF 997.5.D4
Reinforcement (Psychology)   BF 319.5.R4
  Associated with psychoanalysis   WM 460.5.R2
Reinforcement Schedule   BF 319.5.R4
Reinforcement, Social   HM
Reinforcement, Verbal   LB 1065
Rejuvenation   WJ 875
rel Genes see Oncogenes
Relapse see Recurrence
Relapsing Fever   WC 410
Relationship, Blood see Consanguinity; Family;
  Paternity; Twins
Relative Risk see Risk

Relative Value Scales
  Dental   WU 77
  Hospital   WX 157
  Medical   W 74
  Nursing   WY 77
  Pharmaceutical   QV 736
  For other services, by subject
Relative–Value Schedules see Relative Value Scales
Relaxation
  Hygiene   QT 265
  Mental health   WM 75, etc.
  Physical therapy   WB 545
Relaxation Techniques
  Behavior therapy   WM 425.5.R3
  Hygiene   QT 265
  Mental health   WM 75
  Physical therapy   WB 545
Relaxation Therapy see Relaxation Techniques
Relaxin   WP 530
Reliability and Validity see Reproducibility of
  Results
Relief Work   HV 553–555
  Hospital emergency service   WX 215
  See also special topics under Disasters
Religion   BL–BX
  In psychoanalysis   WM 460.5.R3
    See also Religion and Psychology   BL 53,
      etc.
Religion and Medicine
  Ethical considerations
    Church's   BL 65.M4
    Doctor's   W 50
  In literature   WZ 330
  Mental healing aspects   WB 885
  Mental health aspects   WM 61
  Other aspects, by subject
  See also specific religions, e.g., Christian Science
    BX 6903–6997, etc.
Religion and Psychology
  Psychology of religion   BL 53
  Therapeutic aspects   WM 61
  See also Mental Healing   WB 880–885; Pastoral
    Care   WM 61
Religion and Science   BL 239–265
Religion and Sex   HQ 63
  In psychoanalysis   WM 460.5.R3
Religious Beliefs see Religion
REM   WL 108
Remedial Teaching   LB 1029.R4
  Special students, by type, e.g., the deaf   HV
    2417–2990.5
Remedies see Therapeutics
Remission Induction   WB 300
  Special topics, by subject
Remission, Spontaneous   QZ 140
  In specific diseases, with the disease
Remission, Spontaneous Neoplasm see Neoplasm
  Regression, Spontaneous
Renal Agents
  Therapeutic use   WJ 166
  See also Anti-Infective Agents, Urinary   QV
    243; Diuretics   QV 160; Uricosuric Agents
    QV 98

ALWAYS CONSULT MAIN SCHEDULES. USE NUMBER ASSIGNED ONLY WHEN
SUBJECT REPRESENTS MAJOR EMPHASIS OF WORK BEING CLASSIFIED

Renal Aminoaciduria see Aminoaciduria, Renal
Renal Artery   WG 595.R3
 See also Blood supply   WJ 301 under Kidney
Renal Artery Obstruction   WJ 300
Renal Artery Stenosis see Renal Artery Obstruction
Renal Calculi see Kidney Calculi
Renal Circulation   WJ 301
Renal Dialysis, Home see Hemodialysis, Home
Renal Disease, End–Stage see Kidney Failure,
 Chronic
Renal Failure, Acute see Kidney Failure, Acute
Renal Failure, Chronic see Kidney Failure, Chronic
Renal Failure, End–Stage see Kidney Failure,
 Chronic
Renal Function Tests see Kidney Function Tests
Renal Hormones see Hormones
Renal Hypertension see Hypertension, Renal
Renal Insufficiency see Kidney Failure, Acute;
 Kidney Failure, Chronic
Renal Insufficiency, Acute see Kidney Failure,
 Acute
Renal Insufficiency, Chronic see Kidney Failure,
 Chronic
Renal Osteodystrophy   WD 200.5.C2
Renal Papillitis, Necrotizing see Kidney Papillary
 Necrosis
Renal Transplantation see Kidney Transplantation
Renal Tubular Transport   WJ 301
Renal Tubular Transport, Inborn Errors   WJ 301
Renal Veins   WG 625.R3
 See also Blood supply   WJ 301 under Kidney
Renin   WK 180
 Enzymology   QU 136
Renin–Angiotensin–Aldosterone System see
 Renin–Angiotensin System
Renin–Angiotensin System
 Enzymology   QU 136
 In hemodynamics   WG 106
Renin–Substrate see Angiotensinogen
Rennin see Chymosin
Renography see Radioisotope Renography
Reoperation   WO 500
 For specific condition, with the condition
Reoviridae   QW 168.5.R15
Reoviruses see Reoviridae
Reperfusion Injury   QZ 170
 Localized, by site
  As a postoperative complication   WO 184
Reperfusion Injury, Myocardial see Myocardial
 Reperfusion Injury
Reperfusion, Myocardial see Myocardial
 Reperfusion
Repetition Strain Injury see Cumulative Trauma
 Disorders
Replacement Therapy, Estrogen see Estrogen
 Replacement Therapy
Replacement Therapy, Hormone see Hormone
 Replacement Therapy
Replantation   WO 700
 Localized, by specific organ or tissue
Replantation, Tooth see Tooth Replantation
Repression   WM 193.5.R4
 Adolescence   WS 463

 Child   WS 350.8.D3
 Infant   WS 350.8.D3
Reproducibility of Results
 Used for special purposes, by subject
Reproduction
 Animals, Domestic
  General   SF 887
  Specific   SF 768.2.A–Z
 Animals, Wild
  General   QP 251–285
  Specific   QL 364–739.2
 Bacteria   QW 52
 Drugs affecting   QV 170–177
 Fishes   SH 165
 General biology   QH 471–489
 Human   WQ 205–208
 Plant ecology   QK 925–929
 Plant physiology   QK 825–830
 See also Genitalia   WJ 100, etc.; Reproduction
  Techniques   WQ 208; Urogenital System
  WJ, etc.
Reproduction Techniques   WQ 208
Reproductive Control Agents   QV 170
Reproductive History   WQ 205
Reproductive System see Genitalia; Reproduction;
 Urogenital System
Reptile Poisons see Snake Venoms
Reptiles   QL 665–666
 As poisonous animals   WD 410
 Diseases   SF 997.5.R4
Rescue Work
 First aid   WA 292
 Medical emergencies   WB 105
 For specific conditions, by subject
Research
 (Form number 20 or 20.5 in any NLM schedule
  where applicable)
 Anesthesia   WO 220
 Genetics   QH 440
  For the biochemist   QU 20
 Internal medicine   WB 25
 Neoplasms   QZ 206
 Radiology   WN 20
 Scientific   Q 179.9–180.6
 Space medicine   WD 751
 Other fields outside the NLM area, in appropriate
  LC number
Research, Clinical Nursing see Clinical Nursing
 Research
Research, Dental see Dental Research
Research Design
 (Form number 20–20.5 in any NLM schedule
  where applicable)
 Science   Q 180.A1, etc.
 See also Epidemiologic Research Design   WA
  105, etc.
Research, Health Services see Health Services
 Research
Research Institutes see Academies and Institutes
Research, Nursing see Nursing Research
Research, Nursing Administration see Nursing
 Administration Research
Research, Nursing Education see Nursing Education

Research
Research, Nursing Evaluation see Nursing
    Evaluation Research
Research, Nursing Methodology see Nursing
    Methodology Research
Research Personnel
    Medical   W 20.5
    Scientific (General)   Q 180.A5–Z [by country]
    Directories   Q 145
    See also names of fields in which research is done
Research Protocols, Clinical see Clinical Protocols
Research Support
    (Form number 20–20.5 in any NLM schedule
    where applicable)
    Science   Q 180–180.5
Reserpine   QV 150
Residence Characteristics
    Demography   HB 1951–2577
    Housing   HD 7285–7391
        Public health aspects   WA 795
        Public housing   HD 7288.77–7288.78
Residencies see Internship and Residency
Residency, Dental see Internship and Residency
Residency, Medical see Internship and Residency
Residency, Nonmedical see Internship, Nonmedical
Residential Facilities
    For children   WS 27–28
    For the mentally ill   WM 29
    For the physically ill   WB 29
    See also Foster home care   HV 875, etc.
Residential Mobility   HB 1954
    Of health manpower   W 76
    Of other special groups, by subject
Residential Treatment
    Institutions
        General   WM 29
        Adolescence   WS 27–28
        Child   WS 27–28
        Infant   WS 27–28
    Programs
        General   WM 445
        Adolescence   WS 463
        Child   WS 350.2
        Infant   WS 350.2
Resin Cements   WU 190
Resins
    Chemical technology   TP 978–979.5
    In dentistry   WU 190
    Pharmaceutical preparation   QV 785
    Used for special purposes, by subject, e.g., in the
        treatment of mandibular fractures   WU 610
Resins, Synthetic
    Chemical technology   TP 978–979.5
    Dentistry   WU 190
    Pharmaceutic preparation   QV 785
    Used for special purposes, by subject
    See also Acrylic Resins   WU 190, etc;
        Composite Resins   WU 190; Epoxy Resins
        WU 190, etc.
Resistance Factors see R Factors
Resistance, Natural see Immunity, Natural
Resistance to Infection see Infection
Resistance Transfer Factor see F Factor

Resorcinols   QV 223
Resorts see Health Resorts
Resorts, Health see Health Resorts
Resource Allocation see Health Care Rationing
Resource–Based Relative Value Scale see Relative
    Value Scales
Resource Guides
    (Form number 39 in any NLM schedule where
    applicable)
    Anesthesiology   WO 231
    Animal poisoning   WD 401
    Aviation and space medicine   WD 701
    Dentistry   WU 49
    Diseases and injuries caused by physical agents
        WD 601
    Embryology   QS 629
    Forensic medicine and dentistry   W 639
    Histology   QS 529
    Immunologic diseases. Hypersensitivity.
        Collagen diseases   WD 301
    Immunology   QW 539
    Medicine   W 49
    Metabolic diseases   WD 200.1
    Nursing   WY 49
    Nutrition disorders   WD 101
    Pharmacy   QV 735
    Physiology   QT 29
    Plant poisoning   WD 501
    Psychiatry   WM 34
    Toxicology   QV 607
    See also Abstracts; Bibliography; Directories;
        Handbooks; Indexes
Respiration   WF 102
    Anesthesia see Anesthesia, Inhalation   WO 277
    Biochemistry   WF 110
    In physical examination   WB 284
    Skin   WR 102
Respiration, Artificial
    Anesthesia complications   WO 250
    First Aid   WA 292
Respiration, Cell see Cell Respiration
Respirators see Ventilators, Mechanical
Respirators, Air–Purifying see Respiratory
    Protective Devices
Respirators, Industrial see Respiratory Protective
    Devices
Respiratory Acidosis see Acidosis, Respiratory
Respiratory Airflow see Pulmonary Ventilation
Respiratory Alkalosis see Alkalosis, Respiratory
Respiratory Care Units   WF 27–28
Respiratory Center   WL 310
Respiratory Chain see Electron Transport
Respiratory Diseases see Respiratory Tract Diseases
Respiratory Distress Syndrome   WS 410
Respiratory Distress Syndrome, Adult   WF 140
Respiratory Drug Administration see
    Administration, Inhalation
Respiratory Exchange see Respiration
Respiratory Failure see Respiratory Insufficiency
Respiratory Function Tests
    General physical examination   WB 284
    Respiratory diagnosis   WF 141
Respiratory Hypersensitivity   WF 150

ALWAYS CONSULT MAIN SCHEDULES. USE NUMBER ASSIGNED ONLY WHEN
SUBJECT REPRESENTS MAJOR EMPHASIS OF WORK BEING CLASSIFIED

See also Asthma   WF 553; Farmer's Lung
    WF 652; Hay Fever   WV 335
Respiratory Insufficiency   WF 140
Respiratory Mechanics   WF 102
Respiratory Muscles   WF 101–102
Respiratory Paralysis   WF 140
Respiratory Physiology   WF 102
Respiratory Protective Devices   WF 26
Respiratory Sounds   WF 102
Respiratory Stimulants see Respiratory System
    Agents
Respiratory Syncytial Viruses   QW 168.5.P2
Respiratory System   WF
    Abnormalities see Respiratory System
      Abnormalities   WF 101
    Child   WS 280
    Drugs affecting see names of particular agents
      or groups of agents, e.g., Antibiotics   QV 350
    Infant   WS 280
    Physiology see Respiratory System Physiology
      WF 102
Respiratory System Abnormalities   WF 101
    Child   WS 280
    Infant   WS 280
Respiratory System Agents   QV 120
    See also specific kinds of agents, e.g., Antitussive
      Agents   QV 76, etc.
Respiratory Therapy   WB 342
    For disease of the respiratory system   WF 145
    For disease of the respiratory system in animals
      SF 831
Respiratory Therapy Department, Hospital   WF
    27–28
Respiratory Tract Diseases   WF 140–900
    Child   WS 280
    Infant   WS 280
    Nursing   WY 163
    Signs and symptoms see Signs and Symptoms,
      Respiratory   WF 143
    Veterinary   SF 831
    See also names of specific diseases
Respiratory Tract Fistula   WF 140
Respiratory Tract Infections
    General   WF 140
    Child   WS 280
    Infant   WS 280
    Veterinary   SF 831
    Viral   WC 505–510
      General works   WC 505
    See also name of specific infections
Respiratory Tract Neoplasms   WF 450
Response, Acute–Phase see Acute–Phase Reaction
Response Latency see Reaction Time
Response Time see Reaction Time
Responsibility for Injuries see Forensic Medicine
Responsibility, Social see Social Responsibility
Rest
    Hygienic   QT 265
    Therapeutic   WB 545
Restaurants   WA 799
Resting Phase see Interphase
Resting Potentials see Membrane Potentials

Restraint, Physical
    Of mental patients   WM 35
    Veterinary (Surgery)   SF 911
    See also Immobilization   WE 168; Protective
      Devices   WX 185, etc.
Restriction Endonucleases see DNA Restriction
  Enzymes
Resume, Job see Job Application
Resurrectionists see Cadaver
Resuscitation
    Accidents in anesthesia   WO 250
    First aid   WA 292
    Child   WS 100
    Infant   WS 100
    Of the newborn   WQ 450
Resuscitation Decisions see Resuscitation Orders
Resuscitation Orders
    General works   W 84.7
    In hospitals   WX 162
    Ethical aspects   W 50
    See also Right to Die
Retarded Child see Mental Retardation
Retention (Psychology)   BF 370–385
    Child   WS 105.5.M2
    Infant   WS 105.5.M2
    Physiology   WL 102
Reticular Formation   WL 310
Reticulocytes   WH 150
Reticuloendothelial Cytomycosis see Histoplasmosis
Reticuloendothelial System   WH 650
Reticuloendotheliosis   WH 650
Reticuloendotheliosis, Leukemic see Leukemia,
  Hairy Cell
Reticulolymphosarcoma see Lymphoma
Reticulosis see Reticuloendotheliosis
Reticulum–Cell Sarcoma see Lymphoma,
  Large–Cell
Retina   WW 270
Retinal Artery   WG 595.R38
Retinal Degeneration   WW 270
Retinal Detachment   WW 270
Retinal Diseases   WW 270
Retinal Ganglion Cells   WW 270
Retinal Hemorrhage   WW 270
Retinal Neoplasms   WW 270
Retinal Perforations   WW 270
Retinal Pigment Epithelium see Pigment Epithelium
  of Eye
Retinal Pigments   WW 270
Retinal Vein   WG 625.R38
Retinal Vessels   WW 270
    See also Retinal Artery   WG 595.R38; Retinal
      Vein   WG 625.R38
Retinitis   WW 270
Retinitis Pigmentosa   WW 270
Retinoblastoma   WW 270
Retinoic Acid see Tretinoin
Retinoids   QU 167
Retinol see Vitamin A
Retinopathy of Prematurity   WW 270
Retinoscopy see Diagnosis   WW 300 under
  Refractive Errors
Retirement   HQ 1062–1063.2

As a problem of aging   WT 30
Housing for   HD 7287.9–7287.92
Pensions, etc.   HD 7105–7105.45
Retirement Benefits see Pensions
Retreatment
      Of a particular disease, with the disease
Retrocochlear Diseases   WL 330
      See also Hearing Loss, Sensorineural   WV
      270–276
Retrognathism   WU 440
Retrolental Fibroplasia see Retinopathy of
   Prematurity
Retroperitoneal Fibrosis   WI 575
Retroperitoneal Neoplasms   WI 575
Retroperitoneal Space   WI 575
Retropneumoperitoneum   WI 575
Retrospective Studies
      Epidemiology   WA 105
      Other special topics, by subject
Retroviridae   QW 168.5.R18
Retroviridae Infections   WC 502
Retrovirus Infections see Retroviridae Infections
Retroviruses see Retroviridae
Reuptake Inhibitors, Neurotransmitter see
   Neurotransmitter Uptake Inhibitors
Reverse Immunoblotting see Immunoblotting
Reverse Transcription see Transcription, Genetic
Review Literature
      On special topics, by subject
Revision, Joint see Reoperation
Revision, Surgical see Reoperation
Reward
      Conditioned response   BF 319
      School management   LB 3025
Reye Syndrome   WS 340
Rh Factors see Rh–Hr Blood–Group System
Rh–Hr Blood–Group System   WH 425
Rh Isoimmunization   WH 425
Rhabdomyolysis   WE 550
Rhabdomyosarcoma   QZ 345
      Localized, by site
Rhabdoviridae   QW 168.5.R2
Rhamnus
      As a medicinal plant   QV 766
      Poisoning   WD 500
Rhenium
      Inorganic chemistry   QD 181.R4
      Pharmacology   QV 290
Rheography see Plethysmography, Impedance
Rheology   QC 189.5
      Blood   WG 106
Rhesus Blood–Group System see Rh–Hr
   Blood–Group System
Rhesus Monkey see Macaca mulatta
Rhetinic Acid see Glycyrrhetinic Acid
Rheum see Rhubarb
Rheumatic Diseases   WE 544
      Acute articular see Rheumatic Fever   WC 220
Rheumatic Fever   WC 220
Rheumatic Heart Disease   WG 240
Rheumatism see Rheumatic Diseases
Rheumatism, Articular, Acute see Rheumatic Fever
Rheumatism, Muscular see Fibromyalgia

Rheumatism, Peri–Extra–Articular see Polymyalgia
   Rheumatica
Rheumatoid Arthritis see Arthritis, Rheumatoid
Rheumatoid Factor   WE 346
Rheumatoid Spondylitis see Spondylitis, Ankylosing
Rheumatology   WE 140
      See also names of specific musculoskeletal
      diseases
Rhinencephalon see Limbic System
Rhinitis   WV 335
      Veterinary   SF 891
Rhinitis, Allergic, Nonseasonal see Rhinitis, Allergic,
   Perennial
Rhinitis, Allergic, Perennial   WV 335
Rhinitis, Allergic, Seasonal see Hay Fever
Rhinitis, Atrophic   WV 335
      Veterinary   SF 891
Rhinitis, Vasomotor   WV 335
Rhinology see Otolaryngology
Rhinopharynx see Nasopharynx
Rhinoplasty   WV 312
Rhinoscleroma   WV 300
Rhinosporidiosis   WC 450
Rhinovirus   QW 168.5.P4
Rhizanesthesia see Anesthesia, Conduction
Rhizobium   QW 131
Rhizotomy   WL 368
Rhodanates see Thiocyanates
Rhodopsin   WW 270
Rhombencephalic Sleep see Sleep, REM
Rhonchi see Respiratory Sounds
Rhubarb
      As a medicinal plant   QV 766
      As a cathartic   QV 75
Rhus see Toxicodendron
Rhus Dermatitis see Dermatitis, Toxicodendron
Rhythm Method   WP 630
Rhythmicity see Periodicity
Rhytidoplasty   WE 705
Ribavirin
      As an antiviral agent   QV 268.5
Riboflavin   QU 191
Riboflavin Deficiency   WD 124
Ribonucleases   QU 136
Ribonucleic Acid see RNA
Ribonucleoproteins   QU 56
Ribonucleoside Diphosphate Reductase   QU 140
Ribosomal RNA see RNA, Ribosomal
Ribosomes   QH 603.R5
Ribovirin see Ribavirin
Ribozymes see RNA, Catalytic
Ribs   WE 715
Rice
      As a dietary supplement in health or disease
      WB 431
      Cultivation   SB 191.R5
Ricin
      As a toxin   QW 630.5.R5
Ricinus   QV 75
Rickets   WD 145
Rickets, Renal see Renal Osteodystrophy
Rickettsia   QW 150
      As a cause of disease   QZ 65

**ALWAYS CONSULT MAIN SCHEDULES. USE NUMBER ASSIGNED ONLY WHEN
SUBJECT REPRESENTS MAJOR EMPHASIS OF WORK BEING CLASSIFIED**

Rickettsia Infections   WC 600–660
  General works   WC 600
    Mite–borne   WC 630–635
    Tick–borne   WC 620–625
    Veterinary   SF 809.R52
Rickettsiaceae   QW 150
Rickettsiaceae Infections   WC 600–635
Rickettsial Vaccines   WC 600
Rickettsiales   QW 150
Rickettsialpox   WC 635
Rickettsias see QW 149 for works including
  Rickettsias and Chlamydias treated together
Rifampicin see Rifampin
Rifampin   QV 268
Rifamycins   QV 350
Rifomycins see Rifamycins
Rift Valley Fever   WC 524
Rift Valley Fever Virus   QW 168.5.B9
Right to Die   W 85.5
Right to Treatment see Patient Advocacy
Right Ventricular Dysplasia, Arrhythmogenic see
  Arrhythmogenic Right Ventricular Dysplasia
Rightsizing see Personnel Downsizing
Rigidity, Decerebrate see Decerebrate State
Riley–Day Syndrome see Dysautonomia, Familial
Rinderpest   SF 966
Ringworm see Tinea
Risk
  In specific topics, by subject
Risk Adjustment
  Used in evaluation of quality of health care
    General   W 84
    Hospitals   WX 153
  Special topics, by subject
Risk Behavior see Risk–Taking
Risk Factors
  In a particular subject, with the subject
Risk Management
  Hospitals   WX 157
  For other topics, class by subject if specific; if
    general, in economics number where available
Risk Sharing, Financial
  General   W 74
  Other topics, class by subject if specific; if general,
    in economics number where available
Risk–Taking
  Psychology   BF 637.R57
Ritodrine
  Used in controlling premature labor   WQ 330
RNA   QU 58.7
RNA, Antisense   QU 58.7
RNA, Bacterial   QW 52
RNA Caps   QU 58.7
RNA, Catalytic   QU 58.7
RNA–Dependent RNA Polymerase see RNA
  Replicase
RNA, Double–Stranded   QU 58.7
RNA, Messenger   QU 58.7
RNA, Messenger, Splicing see RNA Splicing
RNA, Neoplasm
  In cancer research   QZ 206
RNA Nucleotidyltransferases   QU 141
RNA Polymerases see DNA–Directed RNA

Polymerase
RNA Processing, Post–Transcriptional   QH 450.2
RNA Replicase   QU 141
RNA, Ribosomal   QU 58.7
RNA, Ribosomal, Self–Splicing see RNA, Catalytic
RNA Rodent Viruses see RNA Viruses
RNA, Satellite   QU 58.7
RNA Sequence see Base Sequence
RNA Sequence Analysis see Sequence Analysis,
  RNA
RNA, Small Nuclear   QU 58.7
RNA Splicing   QH 450.2
RNA Synthesis Inhibitors see Nucleic Acid
  Synthesis Inhibitors
RNA, Transfer   QU 58.7
RNA, Transfer, Amino Acyl   QU 58.7
RNA, Viral   QW 168
RNA Virus Infections   WC 501
RNA Viruses
  General works   QW 168
  Specific viruses   QW 168.5.A–Z
RNase see Ribonucleases
Ro 10–9359 see Etretinate
Ro 15–1788 see Flumazenil
Robotics   TJ 210.2–211.47
  Biomedical engineering   QT 36
  Used for special purposes, by subject, e.g., in
    clinical laboratory procedures   QY 23
Rock Fever see Brucellosis
Rocky Mountain Spotted Fever   WC 620
Rod–Cone Dystrophy see Retinitis Pigmentosa
Rodent Control   WA 240
Rodent Diseases   SF 997.5.R64
Rodentia   QL 737.R6–737.R688
  As laboratory animals   QY 60.R6
Rodenticides
  Agriculture   SB 951.8
  Public health aspects   WA 240
Rods and Cones   WW 270
Roentgen Radiation see Radiation, Ionizing
Roentgen Rays see X–Rays
Roentgenkymography see Electrokymography
Roentgenograms see Radiography
Roentgenography see Radiography
Roentgenography, Dental see Radiography, Dental
Roentgenology see Radiation, Ionizing
Roentgenotherapy see X–Ray Therapy
Roeteln see Rubella
Rogerian Therapy see Nondirective Therapy
Role
  Parents   WS 105.5.F2
  Physician   W 62
  Sexual psychology   BF 692–692.5
  Social   HM
  See also Self Concept   BF 697, etc.
Role Concept see Role
Role Playing   WM 430.5.P8
  Adolescence   WS 463
  Child   WS 350.2
Romano–Ward Syndrome see Long QT Syndrome
Root Canal see Dental Pulp Cavity
Root Canal Filling Materials   WU 190
Root Canal Therapy   WU 230

Root Resection see Apicoectomy
Root Resorption   WU 230
Root Scaling see Dental Scaling
Rorschach Test   WM 145.5.R7
Rosa see Rosales
Rosacea see Acne Rosacea
Rosales
    As a dietary supplement in health or disease
        WB 430
    As a medicinal plant   QV 766
    See also names of specific plants and processed
        foods, e.g., Wine   WB 444, etc.
Rosaniline Dyes   QV 240
Rose Bengal   QV 240
Rosemary see Lamiaceae
Rosenzweig Picture–Frustration Study   WM
    145.5.R8
    Adolescence   WS 462
    Child   WS 105.5.E8
    In psychology   BF 698.8.R6
    Infant   WS 105.5.E8
Roseola, Epidemic see Measles
Roseola Infantum see Exanthema Subitum
Rosidae see Rosales
Rotation
    Aviation medicine   WD 720
    Motion sickness   WD 630
    Of the eye   WW 103
    Special topics, by subject
Rotavirus   QW 168.5.R15
Rotavirus Infections   WC 501
Rouget Cells see Pericytes
Roughage see Dietary Fiber
Round Window   WV 250
Roundworms see Nematoda
Rous–Associated Virus see Leukosis Virus, Avian
Rous Sarcoma see Sarcoma, Avian
Rous Sarcoma Virus see Sarcoma Viruses, Avian
Roussy–Levy Syndrome see Charcot–Marie Disease
Routine Diagnostic Tests see Diagnostic Tests,
    Routine
Roxithromycin   QV 350.5.E7
Royal Free Disease see Fatigue Syndrome, Chronic
RU–486 see Mifepristone
Rubber
    Agriculture   SB 289–291
    Industry   TS 1870–1935
    Used in artificial parts, with specific part
Rubber Allergy see Latex Allergy
Rubber Silicone see Silicone Elastomers
Rubefacients see Irritants
Rubella   WC 582
Rubella Vaccine   WC 582
Rubella Virus   QW 168.5.R8
Rubeola see Measles
Rubidium
    Inorganic chemistry   QD 181.R3
    Metabolism   QU 130
    Pharmacology   QV 275
Rubinstein–Taybi Syndrome   QS 675
Rubivirus   QW 168.5.R8
Ruffini's Corpuscles see Thermoreceptors
Rumen   QL 862

Domestic animals   SF 851
Ruminantia see Ruminants
Ruminants   QL 737.U5
    Diseases   SF 997.5.U5
    Physiology   SF 768.2.R8
Rumination, Obsessive see Compulsive Behavior
Runaway Behavior
    Adolescents   WS 463
    Child   WS 350.8.R9
Running   QT 260.5.R9
Runt Disease see Graft vs Host Disease
Rupture   QZ 55
    Localized, by site
Rural Health   WA 390
Rural Health Services   WA 390
Rural Population
    Demography   HB 2371–2577
    Health problems see Rural Health   WA 390
    Other aspects, by subject
    See also Housing   HD 7289, etc.; Public Housing
        HD 7288.77–7288.78
Russell's Viper Venom Time see Prothrombin Time
Russian Baths see Baths
Ruthenium
    Inorganic chemistry   QD 181.R9
    Pharmacology   QV 290
Rutin   QU 220

S

S–Adenosylhomocysteine   QU 60
S–Adenosylmethionine   QU 57
S Cells (Intestine) see Endocrine Cells of Gut
Sabin Vaccine see Poliovirus Vaccine, Oral
Saccades   WW 400
Saccadic Eye Movements see Saccades
Saccharide–Mediated Cell Adhesion Molecules see
    Cell Adhesion Molecules
Saccharides see Carbohydrates; Disaccharides;
    Monosaccharides; Oligosaccharides;
    Polysaccharides
Saccharin   WA 712
Saccharomyces   QW 180.5.A8
Saccharomycetales   QW 180.5.A8
Sacral Plexus see Lumbosacral Plexus
Sacral Region see Sacrococcygeal Region
Sacrococcygeal Region   WE 750
Sacroiliac Joint   WE 750
Sadism   WM 610
Sadomasochism see Sadism; Masochism
Safety   WA 250–288
Safety, Consumer Product see Consumer Product
    Safety
Safety Devices see Protective Devices
Safety Equipment see Protective Devices
Safety, Equipment see Equipment Safety
Safety Glasses see Eye Protective Devices
Safety Lenses see Eye Protective Devices
Safety Management
    General   WA 250–288
    In hospitals   WX 185
    In occupational settings   WA 485–491
    Radiation   WN 650

ALWAYS CONSULT MAIN SCHEDULES. USE NUMBER ASSIGNED ONLY WHEN
SUBJECT REPRESENTS MAJOR EMPHASIS OF WORK BEING CLASSIFIED

In specific types of facilities, class with type of facility in the number for administration if number for safety or accident prevention is unavailable; in the general works number if both are lacking

Sage see Lamiaceae

Saimiri   QL 737.P925
    Diseases   SF 997.5.P7
    As laboratory animals   QY 60.P7

Saimirine Herpesvirus 2 see Herpesvirus 2, Saimirine

Salaam Seizures see Spasms, Infantile

Salamanders see Urodela

Salaries and Fringe Benefits
    Economic theory   HD 4909–4912
    Fringe benefits (General)   HD 4928.N6
    In hospitals   WX 157
    Of dentists   WU 77
    Of nurses   WY 77
    Of physicians   W 79
    Of other specialties, by type, e.g., of psychiatric nurses   WY 160

Salicylates   QV 95

Salicylic Acids   QV 60

Salientia see Anura

Saline see Sodium Chloride

Saline Infusion see Infusions, Parenteral; Sodium Chloride

Saline Solution, Hypertonic   WB 354

Saliva   QY 125

Salivary Duct Calculi   WI 230

Salivary Duct Stones see Salivary Duct Calculi

Salivary Ducts   WI 230

Salivary Gland Diseases   WI 230

Salivary Gland Fistula   WI 230

Salivary Gland Neoplasms   WI 230

Salivary Gland Virus Disease see Cytomegalovirus Infections

Salivary Gland Viruses see Cytomegalovirus

Salivary Glands   WI 230

Salk Vaccine see Poliovirus Vaccine

Salmonella   QW 138.5.S2

Salmonella arizonae   QW 138.5.S2

Salmonella Food Poisoning   WC 268

Salmonella Infections   WC 269

Salmonella Infections, Animal   SF 809.S24

Salmonella paratyphi B see Salmonella schottmuelleri

Salmonella schottmuelleri   QW 138.5.S2

Salmonella typhi   QW 138.5.S2

Salmonella typhosa see Salmonella typhi

Salmonellosis see Salmonella Infections

Salmonidae
    Anatomy and physiology   QL 638.S2
    Diseases   SH 179.S3

Salpingography see Hysterosalpingography

Salt-Free Diet see Diet, Sodium-Restricted

Salts
    Inorganic chemistry   QD 189–193
    Microorganism metabolism   QW 52
    See also names of specific salts, e.g. Sodium Chloride   QV 273, etc.

Sampling Studies
    Epidemiology   WA 105–106, etc.

Psychology   BF 39

Research
    (Form number 20 or 20.5 in any NLM schedule where applicable)

Surveys
    Health   WA 900
    Nutrition   QU 146
    Special topics, by subject

Sanatorium Regimen in Tuberculosis see Rehabilitation   WF 330, etc. under Tuberculosis, Pulmonary

Sand Baths see Ammotherapy

Sand-Dollar see Sea Urchins

Sandfly Fever see Pappataci Fever

Sanitary Codes see Legislation   WA 32 under Sanitation

Sanitary Conditions, Epidemic Factor see Communicable Disease Control; Public health   WA 30 under Socioeconomic Factors

Sanitary Control see Environment, Controlled

Sanitary Engineering   WA 671
    See also specific topics, e.g. Refuse Disposal   WA 780, etc.

Sanitation   WA 670–847
    Housing   WA 795
    Occupational   WA 440
    Inspection   WA 672
        See also Food Inspection   WA 695; Quality Control   WA 672, etc.
    Legislation   WA 32–33
    Rural   WA 390
    School   WA 350–351
    Surveys   WA 672

Santonin   QV 253

Sao Paulo Typhus see Rocky Mountain Spotted Fever

Saphenous Vein   WG 625.S2

Sapogenins
    Biochemistry   QU 85

Saponins   QU 75

Saralasin   QU 68

Sarcodina   QX 55

Sarcoidosis   QZ 140
    Localized, by site

Sarcolemma   WE 500

Sarcoma   QZ 345
    Localized, by site

Sarcoma, Avian
    Experimental in the interest of humans   QZ 345

Sarcoma, Ewing's   WE 258
    Localized, by site

Sarcoma, Germinoblastic see Lymphoma

Sarcoma, Kaposi   QZ 345
    Localized, by site

Sarcoma, Lymphatic see Lymphoma, Diffuse

Sarcoma, Osteogenic see Osteosarcoma

Sarcoma, Reticulum-Cell see Lymphoma, Large-Cell

Sarcoma, Rous see Sarcoma, Avian

Sarcoma, Synovial   WE 300
    Localized, by site

Sarcoma Virus, Feline   QW 166

Sarcoma Viruses, Avian   QW 166

Sarcoptes scabiei   QX 475
Sarcoptidae see Mites; Sarcoptes scabiei
Sarcosomes see Mitochondria, Muscle
Satellite DNA see DNA, Satellite
Satellite RNA see RNA, Satellite
Satire see Wit and Humor
Sauna see Baths, Finnish
Savanna Baboons see Papio
Savings Accounts, Medical see Medical Savings
  Accounts
Scabies   WR 365
    Veterinary   SF 810.S26
Scalded Skin Syndrome, Nonstaphylococcal see
  Epidermal Necrolysis, Toxic
Scalds see Burns
Scalenus Anticus Syndrome see Thoracic Outlet
  Syndrome
Scaling, Dental see Dental Scaling
Scaling, Root see Dental Scaling
Scaling, Subgingival see Dental Scaling
Scaling, Supragingival see Dental Scaling
Scalp   WR 450
Scalp Dermatoses   WR 450
Scanning Electron Microscopy see Microscopy,
  Electron, Scanning
Scanning, Radioisotope see Radionuclide Imaging
Scapula   WE 810
Scarlatina see Scarlet Fever
Scarlet Fever   WC 214
Scarpa's Ganglion see Vestibular Nerve
Scars see Cicatrix
Scattering, Radiation
    Biomedical uses   WB 117
    Physical optics   QC 427.4
Schamberg's Disease see Pigmentation Disorders
Schaumann's Disease see Sarcoidosis
Schedules, Patient see Appointments and Schedules
Scheie's Syndrome see Mucopolysaccharidosis I
Scheuermann's Disease   WE 725
Schistosoma   QX 355
Schistosomiasis   WC 810
Schistosomiasis, Intestinal see Schistosomiasis
  mansoni
Schistosomiasis japonica   WC 810
Schistosomiasis mansoni   WC 810
Schizoaffective Disorder see Psychotic Disorders
Schizoid Personality Disorder   WM 203
Schizomycetes see Bacteria
Schizophrenia   WM 203
Schizophrenia, Borderline see Schizotypal
  Personality Disorder
Schizophrenia, Catatonic   WM 203
Schizophrenia, Childhood   WM 203
Schizophrenia, Disorganized   WM 203
Schizophrenia, Hebephrenic see Schizophrenia,
  Disorganized
Schizophrenia, Latent see Schizotypal Personality
  Disorder
Schizophrenia, Paranoid   WM 203
Schizophrenia, Pseudoneurotic see Schizotypal
  Personality Disorder
Schizophrenic Disorders see Schizophrenia
Schizophrenic Language   WM 203

Schizophrenic Psychology   WM 203
Schizophreniform Disorders see Psychotic Disorders
Schizosaccharomyces   QW 180.5.A8
Schizotypal Personality Disorder   WM 203
Scholarships see Fellowships and Scholarships
School Admission Criteria   LB 2351-2351.6
    (Form number 18 in any NLM schedule where
    applicable)
School Dentistry
    Services offered   WA 350-351
    Specific dental problems   WU
School Dropouts see Student Dropouts
School Health Services   WA 350
    Mental health   WA 352
    See also Student Health Services   WA 350-353
School Nursing   WY 113
    Education   WY 18-18.5
Schools   L
    (Form number 19 in any NLM schedule where
    applicable)
    For exceptional children   LC 3951-4801
    For the blind   HV 1618-2349
    For the deaf   HV 2417-2990.5
    For the deaf-mute   HV 2417-2990.5
Schools, Dental   WU 19
Schools, Health Occupations   W 19
Schools, Library see Library Schools
Schools, Medical   W 19
Schools, Nursery   LB 1140-1140.5
    Public health aspects   WA 350-352
Schools, Nursing   WY 19
Schools, Pharmacy   QV 19
Schools, Public Health   WA 19
Schools, Veterinary   SF 756.3-756.37
Schueller-Christian Disease see
  Hand-Schueller-Christian Syndrome
Schwalbe's Nucleus see Vestibular Nuclei
Schwannoma see Neurilemmoma
Schwannoma, Acoustic see Neuroma, Acoustic
Schwartz-Jampel Syndrome see
  Osteochondrodysplasias
Sciatic Nerve   WL 400
Sciatica   WE 755
Science   Q
    Biography
        Collective   Q 141
        Individual   WZ 100
    Directories   Q 145
    General works   Q 158-158.5
    History (General)   Q 125
Scientific Misconduct   Q175.37
    Special topics, by subject
Scientific Societies see Societies, Scientific
Scientology see Alternative Medicine; Philosophy
Scintigraphy see Radionuclide Imaging
Scintigraphy, Computed Tomographic see
  Tomography, Emission-Computed
Scintillation Counting   WN 660
Scintiphotography see Radionuclide Imaging
Sciuridae   QL 737.R68
    As laboratory animals   QY 60.R6
Sclera   WW 230
    Abnormalities   WW 230

**ALWAYS CONSULT MAIN SCHEDULES. USE NUMBER ASSIGNED ONLY WHEN
SUBJECT REPRESENTS MAJOR EMPHASIS OF WORK BEING CLASSIFIED**

Scleritis   WW 230
Scleral Buckling   WW 230
Scleroderma, Circumscribed   WR 260
Scleroderma, Diffuse see Scleroderma, Systemic
Scleroderma, Localized see Scleroderma,
   Circumscribed
Scleroderma, Systemic   WR 260
Scleroma, Nasal see Rhinoscleroma
Scleroproteins (Non MeSH)   QU 55
Sclerosing Solutions   QV 786
Sclerosis   QZ 190
   Disseminated see Multiple Sclerosis   WL 360
   Hereditary spinal see Friedreich's Ataxia   WL
      390
   Progressive systemic see Scleroderma, Systemic
      WR 260
Sclerosis, Disseminated see Multiple Sclerosis
Sclerosis, Hereditary Spinal see Friedreich's Ataxia
Sclerosis, Progressive Systemic see Scleroderma,
   Systemic
Sclerostomy
   For glaucoma   WW 290
Sclerotherapy   WB 354
   Special topics, by subject
Sclerotinia see Ascomycota
Scoliosis   WE 735
Scopolamine   QV 134
Scopolamine Derivatives   QV 134
Scopolamine-Morphine Anesthesia see Anesthesia,
   Obstetrical; Preanesthetic Medication
Scorbutus see Scurvy
Scorpion Venoms   WD 420
Scorpions   QX 469
   Sting see Arachnidism   WD 420
Scrapie Agent see Prions
Scrapie-Associated Fibrils see Prions
Scrapie Virus see Prions
Screen-Film Systems, X-Ray see X-Ray
   Intensifying Screens
Screens, Radiographic see Instrumentation   WN
   150 under Radiography
Scrofula see Tuberculosis, Lymph Node
Scrofuloderma see Tuberculosis, Cutaneous
Scrotum   WJ 800
Scrub Typhus   WC 630
Sculpture
   Related to medicine   WZ 330
   Related to psychiatry   WM 49
Scurvy   WD 140
Sea Anemone Venoms see Coelenterate Venoms
Sea Bathing see Balneology; Swimming;
   Thalassotherapy
Sea Pollution see Seawater; Water Pollution
Sea Urchins   QL 384.E2
Seafood
   As a dietary supplement in health or disease
      WB 426
   Inspection   WA 707
   Preservation   WA 710
   Sanitation   WA 703
   Supply   WA 703
Sealants, Tooth see Pit and Fissure Sealants
Sealed Cabin Ecology see Ecological Systems,

Closed
Seasickness see Motion Sickness
Seasons
   Astronomical geography   QB 637.2–637.8
   Atmospheric temperature   QC 903–906
   Folklore   GR 930
   Medical climatology   WB 700
Seawater
   Balneology   WB 525
   Ecology   QH 541.5.S3
   Marine biology   QH 91–95.9
   Microbiology see Plankton   QH 90.8.P5, etc.;
      Water Microbiology   QW 80
   Oceanography   GC 100–181
   Pollution
      Bathing beaches   WA 820
      Industrial waste   WA 788
      See also Water Pollution   WA 689
Seaweed   QK 564–580
Sebaceous Cyst see Epidermal Cyst
Sebaceous Gland Diseases   WR 410
Sebaceous Gland Neoplasms   WR 410
Sebaceous Glands   WR 410
Seborrhea see Dermatitis, Seborrheic
Secobarbital   QV 88
Second-Look Surgery see Reoperation
Second Messenger Systems   QU 120
Second Opinion see Referral and Consultation
Secretaries, Medical see Medical Secretaries
Secretin   WK 170
Secretin Cells see Endocrine Cells of Gut
Secretory Granules see Cytoplasmic Granules
Secretory Phase see Menstrual Cycle
Secretory Rate   QU 120
Security Measures
   Hospitals   WX 185
   Libraries   Z 679.6
Sedation, Conscious see Conscious Sedation
Sedatives see Hypnotics and Sedatives
Sedimentation of Blood see Blood Sedimentation
Seeds
   As a dietary supplement in health and disease
      WB 431
   Botany   QK 661
   Plant culture   SB 113.2–118.46
   Toxic   WD 500
Seizures   WL 340
Seizures, Febrile see Convulsions, Febrile
Selection (Genetics)   QH 455
   See also Natural Selection   QH 375
Selegiline
   As an antiparkinson agent   QV 80
Selenium
   Inorganic chemistry   QD 181.S5
   Metabolism   QU 130.5
   Pharmacology   QV 138.S5
Self see Ego
Self Assessment (Psychology)   BF 697
   Child   WS 105.5.S3
Self Care   WB 327
   For particular conditions, with the condition
Self Care (Rehabilitation) see Activities of Daily
   Living

Self-Care Units   WX 200
Self Concept   BF 697
    Child   WS 105.5.S3
    Infant   WS 105.5.S3
Self Determination see Freedom
Self Disclosure   BF 697.5.S427
    Child   WS 105.5.S3
Self Efficacy   BF 637.S38
Self Esteem see Self Concept
Self-Evaluation Programs
    In a particular field (Form number 18–18.2 in
      any NLM schedule where applicable)
    Other special topics, by subject
Self-Examination   WB 120
    For specific conditions, with the condition
Self-Help Devices   WB 320
    Catalogs   W 26
    For particular disability, by the disability
    See also specific types of devices
Self-Help Groups
    In mental disorders   WM 426
    In other areas, by subject
Self-Instruction Programs see Programmed
  Instruction
Self-Instruction Programs, Computerized see
  Computer-Assisted Instruction
Self Medication   WB 120
    Popular works   WB 120
Self-Monitoring, Blood Glucose see Blood Glucose
  Self-Monitoring
Self Mutilation   WM 100
    Special topics, by subject
Self Perception see Self Concept
Self Psychology   WM 460.5.E3
    See also Self Concept   BF 697, etc.
Self Realization see Achievement
Sella Turcica   WE 705
Selye Syndrome see General systemic reaction   QZ
  160 under Wounds and Injuries; Stress
Semantic Differential
    Used in psycholinguistics   BF 463
    As a personality test   BF 698.5
Semantics   P 325
Semen
    Analysis   QY 190
      Medicolegal   W 750
    Secretion
      Genital physiology   WJ 702
      Spermatozoa   WJ 834
Semen Preservation   WJ 834
    Artificial insemination   WQ 208
Semicircular Canals   WV 255
Semiconductors
    Electronics   TK 7871.85–7871.99
    Medical engineering   QT 36
    Photoelectronics   TK 8320–8334
    Physics   QC 610.9–611.8
Semilunar Bone   WE 830
Semilunar Cartilages see Menisci, Tibial
Seminal Vesicles   WJ 750
Seminiferous Tubules   WJ 830
Seminoma see Dysgerminoma
Semiochemicals see Pheromones

Semiology see Signs and Symptoms
Semisynthetic Vaccines see Vaccines, Synthetic
Semliki Forest Virus   QW 168.5.A7
Sendai Virus see Paramyxovirus
Senescence see Aging
Senile Osteoporosis see Osteoporosis
Senility see Aged
Sensation   WL 702
    Disorders
      Dermatological   WR 280
      General   WL 710
    See also Touch   WR 102; Smell   WV 301 and
      other sensations
Sense see Hearing; Orientation; Pain; Proprioception;
  Smell; Taste; Temperature Sense; Touch; Vision
Sense Organs   WL 700–710
Sensibilisinogens see Anaphylaxis
Sensitinogens see Allergens; Anaphylaxis
Sensitivity, Contact see Dermatitis, Contact
Sensitivity Training Groups
    Psychiatry   WM 430.5.S3
    Social psychology   HM
Sensitization see Anaphylaxis; Hypersensitivity
Sensitization, Immunologic see Immunization
Sensitizer see Antibodies
Sensory Aids
    Catalogs   W 26
    General   WL 26
    See also Eyeglasses   WW 350–354; Hearing Aids
      WV 274; other specific types in the
      equipment number, usually 26, for the field
Sensory Deprivation   WL 710
Sensory Motor Performance see Psychomotor
  Performance
Sensory System Agents   QV 76.5
    See also specific kinds of agents, e.g., Analgesics
      QV 95; Anesthetics, Local   QV 110–115
Sensory Thresholds   WL 705
    See also names of specific thresholds, e.g.,
      Auditory Threshold   WV 272, etc.
Seoul Virus see Hantavirus
Separation, Drugs see Drug Compounding
Sepsis   WC 240
Septal Nuclei   WL 314
Septic Sore Throat see Streptococcal Infections
Septicemia   WC 240
    Puerperal see Puerperal Infection   WQ 505
    Veterinary   SF 802
Septum, Nasal see Nasal Septum
Septum Pellucidum   WL 314
Sequence Analysis
    As a genetic technique (General)   QH 441
    Special topics, by subject
Sequence Analysis, DNA
    As a genetic technique (General)   QH 441
    Special topics, by subject
Sequence Analysis, RNA
    As a genetic technique (General)   QH 441
    Special topics, by subject
Sequence Data, Molecular see Molecular Sequence
  Data
Sequence Homology, Nucleic Acid   QU 58
Serial Learning   LB 1059

Serial Publications W1
  Bibliography
    General Z 6940–6967
    Medical and medically related ZW 1
      On specific subjects, NLM classification
      number for the subject preceded by letter
      Z
  Directories, handbooks, etc. (Asterisked form
    numbers in any NLM schedule where
    applicable)
  Government administrative reports and statistics
    W2
  Hospital administrative reports and statistics
    WX 2
  See also more specific terms, e.g., Newspapers
    Z 6940–6967, etc.; Periodicals W1, etc.
Serine QU 60
Serine Proteases see Serine Proteinases
Serine Proteinases QU 136
Serodiagnosis see Serologic Tests
Seroepidemiologic Studies
  Used for the detection of a specific disease, with
    the disease
Serologic Tests QY 265–275
Serology QW 570
Seromucoid see Orosomucoid
Seroprevalence see Seroepidemiologic Studies
Serotherapy see Immunization, Passive
Serotonin QV 126
Serotonin Antagonists QV 126
Serotonin Blockaders see Serotonin Antagonists
Serpin Superfamily see Serpins
Serpins QU 136
Serratia QW 138.5.S3
Sertoli Cell Tumor WJ 858
Sertraline
  As an antidepressive agent QV 77.5
Serum see Blood; Immune Sera; Serum Albumin;
  Serum Globulins
Serum Albumin WH 400
  Clinical analysis QY 455
Serum Globulins WH 400
  Immunoglobulins QW 601
Serum Markers see Biological Markers
Serum Proteins see Blood Proteins
Serum Sialomucin see Orosomucoid
Serum Sickness WD 330
Serum Thymic Factor see Thymic Factor,
  Circulating
Servicemen see Military Personnel
Services, Outsourced see Outsourced Services
Set (Psychology) BF 321
Sewage
  Bacteriology QW 80
  Disposal WA 785
    General waste disposal WA 778
  Water pollution WA 689
Sex
  Counseling WM 55
  General HQ 12–25
  Hygiene
    Female WP 120
    Male WJ 700

  In mental retardation WM 307.S3
  Medicolegal aspects W 795
  Organs see Genitalia WJ 700, etc.
  Psychoanalysis WM 460.5.S3
  Psychology BF 692
  Research HQ 60
Sex Behavior
  Human HQ 12–472
  Adolescence WS 462
  Child WS 105.5.S4
  Psychology BF 692
Sex Behavior, Animal QL 761
  Domestic animals SF 195–518
  Wild animals QL 364–739.3
Sex Characteristics
  Physical QS, QT
    Female WP 101
    Male WJ 101–102
  Psychological BF 692
Sex Chromatin QH 599
Sex Chromosome Abnormalities QS 677
Sex Chromosomes QH 600.5
Sex Counseling WM 55
Sex Determination (Analysis) WQ 206
  See also Sex Determination (Genetic) QS 638;
    Sex Differentiation QS 640
Sex Determination (Genetics) QS 638
  See also Sex Determination (Analysis) WQ 206;
    Sex Differentiation QS 640
Sex Determination Techniques see Sex
  Determination (Analysis)
Sex Deviations see Paraphilias
Sex Differences see Sex Characteristics
Sex Differentiation
  Embryogenic QS 640
Sex Differentiation Disorders WJ 712
  Veterinary SF 871
Sex Dimorphism see Sex Characteristics
Sex Disorders
  Female WP 610
  Male WJ 709
  Problems of mentally retarded WM 307.S3
  Psychophysiologic (General) WM 611
Sex Education HQ 34–59
  Of the mentally retarded LC 4601–4640.4 or
    HQ 54.3
    Sex problems WM 307.S3
  School texts QT 225
Sex Factor, Bacterial see F Factor
Sex Factor F see F Factor
Sex Factors
  As a cause of disease QZ 53
    See also Sex Ratio QH 455, etc.
  Demography HB 1741–1947
  Other special topics, by subject
Sex Hormones WK 900
  Female WP 520–530
  Male WJ 875
  See also names of specific hormones
Sex Manuals HQ 31
Sex Offenses
  Criminology HV 6556–6593
  Medicolegal aspects W 795

**ALWAYS CONSULT MAIN SCHEDULES. USE NUMBER ASSIGNED ONLY WHEN
SUBJECT REPRESENTS MAJOR EMPHASIS OF WORK BEING CLASSIFIED**

Sex Pili see Pili, Sex
Sex Predetermination see Sex Preselection
Sex Preselection   WQ 205
    Using genetic engineering techniques   QH 442
Sex Ratio
    Animals
        Domestic (Breeding)   SF 105
        Wild   QH 352
    Population genetics   QH 455
    Population statistics
        At birth by country   HB 911–1107
        General   HB 1741–1947
    Other special topics, by subject, e.g., Sex Ratio
        of children born with Huntington Chorea   WL
        390
Sex Reversal, Gonadal   WK 900
Sex Role see Gender Identity
Sex Selection see Sex Preselection
Sexology see Sex
Sexual Abuse, Child see Child Abuse, Sexual
Sexual Adjustment see Sex Disorders; Sex Manuals
Sexual and Gender Disorders   WM 611
Sexual Arousal Disorder see Sexual Dysfunctions,
    Psychological
Sexual Aversion Disorder see Sexual Dysfunctions,
    Psychological
Sexual Dysfunctions see Sexual Dysfunctions,
    Psychological
Sexual Dysfunctions, Psychological   WM 611
    Frigidity   WP 610
    See also Impotence   WJ 709; names of specific
        disorders, e.g., Paraphilias   WM 610
Sexual Harassment   HD 6060.3
Sexual Intercourse see Coitus
Sexual Partners
    Special topics, by subject
Sexuality
    Adolescence   WS 462
    Child   WS 105.5.S4
    Human   HQ 12–449
    Psychology   BF 692
Sexually Transmitted Diseases   WC 140–185
    General works   WC 140
    Gonorrhea   WC 150
        In the female   WP 157
SGOT see Aspartate Transaminase
SGPT see Alanine Transaminase
Shadow Test see Refraction, Ocular
Shamanism
    Alternative medicine   WB 885
    History   WZ 309
Shame   BF 575.S45
    Adolescence   WS 462
    Child   WS 105.5.E5
    Infant   WS 105.5.E5
Shared Paranoid Disorder   WM 205
Sharks   QL 638.9–638.95
Sharp Syndrome see Mixed Connective Tissue
    Disease
Sheathed Bacteria (Non Mesh) see Bacteria
Sheehan's Syndrome see Hypopituitarism
Sheep
    Domestic   SF 371–379

    Anatomy   SF 767.S5
    Physiology   SF 768.2.S5
    Wild   QL 737.U53
Sheep Diseases   SF 968–969
Shellfish
    As a dietary supplement in health or disease
        WB 426
    Culture   SH 365–380.92
    Diseases   SH 179.S5
    Poisoning   WD 405
    See also Crustacea   QX 463; Mollusca   QX
        675
Sheltered Workshops
    For the mentally disabled   WM 29
    For the physically disabled   WB 29
Sherman Antitrust Act see Antitrust Laws
Shiatsu see Acupressure
Shiatzu see Acupressure
Shigella   QW 138.5.S4
Shigella Infections see Dysentery, Bacillary
Shingles see Herpes Zoster
Shipping Fever Virus see Paramyxovirus
Ships
    Naval science   V
    Nursing service   WY 143
    Public health aspects   WA 810
    Quarantine   WA 234
Shivering   WB 152
Shock   QZ 140
    Anaphylactic see Anaphylaxis   QW 900
    Electric see Electric Injuries   WD 602, etc.
Shock, Anaphylactic see Anaphylaxis
Shock, Cardiogenic   WG 300
Shock, Endotoxic see Shock, Septic
Shock, Hemorrhagic
    Surgical complications   WO 149
    Injury   WO 700
Shock Lung see Respiratory Distress Syndrome,
    Adult
Shock, Septic   QZ 140
    In septicemia   WC 240
    Other special topics, by subject
    Pregnancy   WQ 240
Shock, Surgical   WO 149
Shock Therapy see Convulsive Therapy
Shock Therapy, Electric see Electroconvulsive
    Therapy
Shock Therapy, Insulin see Convulsive Therapy
Shock, Toxic see Shock, Septic
Shock, Traumatic   WO 700–820
Shock Waves, High-Energy see High-Energy Shock
    Waves
Shockwaves, Ultrasonic see Ultrasonics
Shoes   QT 245
    Orthopedic   WE 880–890
    Protective
        In sports   QT 260
        In industry   WA 485
Short-Term Psychotherapy see Psychotherapy,
    Brief
Short Waves see Radio Waves
Shorthand   Z 53–102
    Medical   W 80

**ALWAYS CONSULT MAIN SCHEDULES. USE NUMBER ASSIGNED ONLY WHEN
SUBJECT REPRESENTS MAJOR EMPHASIS OF WORK BEING CLASSIFIED**

Dictionaries   W 13
Shoulder   WE 810
Shoulder Dislocation   WE 810
Shoulder Fractures   WE 810
Shoulder-Girdle Neuropathy see Cervico-Brachial
  Neuralgia
Shoulder-Hand Syndrome   WE 810
Shoulder Impingement Syndrome   WE 810
Shoulder Joint   WE 810
Shoulder Pain   WE 810
Shrimp   QX 463
Shwartzman Phenomenon   QW 900
Shyness   BF 575.B3
SI Units see International System of Units
Sialadenitis   WI 230
Sialidase see Neuraminidase
Sialography   WI 230
Sialolithiasis, Ductal see Salivary Duct Calculi
Sialyltransferases   QU 141
Siamang see Hylobates
Siamese Twins see Twins, Conjoined
Sibling Relations   WS 105.5.F2
Sicca Syndrome see Sjogren's Syndrome
Sick Building Syndrome   WA 754
Sick Leave   HD 5115.5–5115.6
Sick Role   WM 178
    Special topics, by subject
Sick Sinus Syndrome   WG 330
Sickle Cell Anemia see Anemia, Sickle Cell
Sickle Cell Trait   WH 170
Sickness Insurance see Insurance, Health
SID see Sudden Infant Death
Siderophilin see Transferrin
Siderosis   WF 654
    Localized, by site, e.g., of the cornea,   WW 220
Sight see Vision
Sigma Element see Sigma Factor
Sigma Factor   QU 141
Sigma Initiation Factor see Sigma Factor
Sigma Subunit see Sigma Factor
Sigmoid   WI 560
Sigmoid Neoplasms   WI 560
Sigmoidoscopes see Endoscopes
Sigmoidoscopy   WI 620
Sign Language   HV 2474–2476
Signal Interpretation, Computer-Assisted see Signal
  Processing, Computer-Assisted
Signal Pathways see Signal Transduction
Signal Peptides   QU 68
Signal Processing, Computer-Assisted
    As equipment in special fields (Form number
    26.5 in any NLM schedule where applicable;
    e.g. Nursing WY 26.5)
Signal Processing, Digital see Signal Processing,
  Computer-Assisted
Signal Sequences, Peptides see Signal Peptides
Signal Transduction
    Cytology   QH 601
Signs and Location Directories see Location
  Directories and Signs
Signs and Symptoms
    Digestive system diseases see Signs and
    Symptoms, Digestive   WI 143

General   WB 143
Intestinal diseases   WI 405
Otorhinolaryngologic diseases   WV 150
Pain   WB 176
Respiratory tract diseases see Signs and
  Symptoms, Respiratory   WF 143
Specific diseases with disease, in diagnosis number
  if available
Thinness   WB 146
See also Eye Manifestations   WW 475, etc.;
  Neurologic Manifestations   WL 340, etc.; Oral
  Manifestations   WU 290; Skin Manifestations
  WR 143
Signs and Symptoms, Digestive   WI 143
Signs and Symptoms, Respiratory   WF 143
Silastics see Silicone Elastomers
Silica see Silicon Dioxide
Silicate Cement   WU 190
    Used for special purposes, by subject, e.g., in
    dental cavity treatment   WU 350
Silicate Fillings see Silicate Cement
Silicic Acid
    Toxicology   QV 610
Silicon
    Inorganic chemistry   QD 181.S6
    Metabolism   QU 130.5
    Toxicology   QV 618
Silicon Dioxide
    Inorganic chemistry   QD 181.S6
    Toxicology   QV 610
Silicone Elastomers
    Artificial organ construction (General)   WO 176
    Chemical technology   TP 248.S5
    Dental materials   WU 190
    Plastic surgery   WO 600–640
    Used in other particular procedures, with the
    procedure
Silicone Gels
    Used in breast implants   WP 910
Silicone Oils
    Chemical technology   TP 685
    Public health aspects   WA 722
    In the treatment of retinal detachment   WW 270
Silicones
    Analytical chemistry   QD 139.S5
    Chemical technology   TP 248.S5
    Plastic surgery   WO 600–640
    Used in other particular procedures, with the
    procedure
Silicopolyacrylate Cement see Glass Ionomer
  Cements
Silicosis   WF 654
Silicotuberculosis   WF 654
Silver   QV 297
    Metabolism   QU 130
Silver Nitrate
    Inorganic chemistry   QD 181.A3
    Pharmacology   QV 297
Simian Immunodeficiency Viruses see SIV
Simian T-Lymphotropic Virus Type III see SIV
Simian Virus 40 see Polyomavirus macacae
Simmonds' Disease see Hypopituitarism
Simplexvirus   QW 165.5.H3

**ALWAYS CONSULT MAIN SCHEDULES. USE NUMBER ASSIGNED ONLY WHEN
SUBJECT REPRESENTS MAJOR EMPHASIS OF WORK BEING CLASSIFIED**

Simuliidae   QX 505
Simulium see Simuliidae
Simvastatin
    As an anticholesteremic agent   QU 95
SIN-10 see Molsidomine
Sinapis see Mustard
Sincalide Receptors see Receptors, Cholecystokinin
Single Parent   HQ 759.915
    Special topics, by subject
Single-Parent Family see Single Parent
Single-Payer Plan see Single-Payer System
Single-Payer System   W 100-275
Single Person   HQ 800-800.4
    Widows and widowers   HQ 1058-1058.5
    Relations to adolescents   WS 462
    Relations to children   WS 105.5.F2
Single-Photon Emission-Computed Tomography
    see Tomography, Emission-Computed,
    Single-Photon
Single-Stranded DNA see DNA, Single-Stranded
Single-Stranded DNA Binding Proteins see
    DNA-Binding Proteins
Single-Tooth Implants see Dental Implants,
    Single-Tooth
Sinoatrial Node   WG 201-202
Sinus Arrhythmia see Arrhythmia, Sinus
Sinus Thrombosis   WL 355
Sinuses, Cranial see Cranial Sinuses
Sinuses, Paranasal see Paranasal Sinuses
Sinusitis   WV 340
Sinusitis, Maxillary see Maxillary Sinusitis
Siphonaptera see Fleas
Sipunculida see Nematoda
Sirenia   QL 737.S6-737.S63
sis Genes see Oncogenes
Sisomicin   QV 350.5.G3
Sisomycin see Sisomicin
Sissomicin see Sisomicin
Sister Chromatid Exchange   QH 445
Site-Directed Mutagenesis see Mutagenesis,
    Site-Directed
Site-Specific Mutagenesis see Mutagenesis,
    Site-Directed
Situational Ethics see Ethics
Situational Therapy see Milieu Therapy
Situs Inversus   QS 675
Situs Transversus see Situs Inversus
SIV   QW 166
SIV-1 see SIV
SIV-2 see SIV
Sixth Disease see Exanthema Subitum
Size Perception   WW 105
Sjogren's Syndrome   WE 346
Skeletal Age Measurement see Age Determination
    by Skeleton
Skeletal Fixation see Fracture Fixation
Skeletal Muscle Relaxants see Neuromuscular
    Agents
Skeletal Muscle Ventricle
    Used in cardiomyoplasty   WG 169
Skeletal System see Musculoskeletal System
Skeleton   WE 100-102
Skiascopy see Diagnosis   WW 300 under Refractive

Errors; Fluoroscopy
Skid Row Alcoholics
    Medical aspects   WM 274
    Sociological problems   HV 5050
Skiing   QT 260.5.S6
Skilled Nursing Facilities   WX 27-28
Skin   WR
    Drugs affecting see Dermatologic Agents   QV
    60-65
    Physiology see Skin Physiology   WR 102
    See also Dermis   WR 101; Epidermis   WR 101
Skin Abnormalities
    General   WR 218
Skin Absorption   WR 102
Skin Aging   WR 102
Skin Appendage Diseases   WR 390-475
Skin Diseases   WR
    General   WR 140
        Diagnosis   WR 141
    Child   WS 260
    Genetic see Skin Diseases, Genetic   WR 218
    Infant   WS 260
    Nursing   WY 154.5
    Papulosquamous   WR 204
    Radiotherapy   WR 660
    Surgery   WR 650
    Therapy   WR 650
    Veterinary   SF 901
Skin Diseases, Bullous see Skin Diseases,
    Vesiculobullous
Skin Diseases, Fungal see Dermatomycoses
Skin Diseases, Genetic   WR 218
Skin Diseases, Infectious   WR 220-245
    Bacterial   WR 220-245
    Fungal see Dermatomycosis   WR 300-340
    General works   WR 220
    Veterinary   SF 901
    Viral   WC 570-590, etc.
        General works   WC 570
Skin Diseases, Metabolic
    General   WR 140
    See also names of specific disorders, e.g., Adiposis
    Dolorosa   WD 214
Skin Diseases, Parasitic   WR 345
    Veterinary   SF 901
Skin Diseases, Vesicular see Skin Diseases,
    Vesiculobullous
Skin Diseases, Vesiculobullous   WR 200
Skin Drug Administration see Administration,
    Cutaneous
Skin Electric Conductance see Galvanic Skin
    Response
Skin Glands see Exocrine Glands
Skin Grafts see Skin Transplantation
Skin Manifestations   WR 143
Skin Neoplasms   WR 500
    Veterinary   SF 901
    See also Sebaceous Gland Neoplasms   WR 410;
        Sweat Gland Neoplasms   WR 400
Skin Physiology   WR 102
Skin Pigmentation   WR 102
    Disorders   WR 265
Skin Syphilis see Syphilis, Cutaneous

**ALWAYS CONSULT MAIN SCHEDULES. USE NUMBER ASSIGNED ONLY WHEN
SUBJECT REPRESENTS MAJOR EMPHASIS OF WORK BEING CLASSIFIED**

Skin Temperature   WR 102
Skin Tests   QY 260
Skin Transplantation   WO 610
Skin Tuberculosis see Tuberculosis, Cutaneous
Skin Ulcer   WR 598
Skin Wrinkling see Skin Aging
Skinfold Thickness
    Malnutrition   WD 105
    Obesity diagnosis   WD 210
Skull   WE 705
    Animal   QL
        Domestic   SF 901
        Wild   QL 822
        Anthropology   GN 71-131
Skull Base   WE 705
Skull Base Neoplasms   WE 707
Skull Fractures   WL 354
Skull Neoplasms   WE 707
Slang see Language; Philology; Vocabulary
Slaughter Houses see Abattoirs
Slaughterhouses see Abattoirs
Sleep   WL 108
    Drugs promoting   QV 85
    In personal hygiene   QT 265
    Physiology   WL 108
Sleep Apnea Syndromes   WF 143
Sleep Deprivation
    Experimental   WL 108
    In personal hygiene   QT 265
Sleep Disorders   WM 188
    See also names of specific disorders
Sleep, REM   WL 108
Sleep Stages   WL 108
Sleep Talking see Sleep Disorders
Sleep Terror Disorder see Sleep Disorders
Sleep Therapy see Rest; specific conditions for which
    therapy is used
Sleep Walking see Somnambulism
Sleeping Sickness see Encephalitis, Epidemic;
    Trypanosomiasis, African
Slim Disease see HIV Wasting Syndrome
Slime Bacteria see Myxococcales
Slime Molds, Plasmodial see Myxomycetes
Slime Molds, True see Myxomycetes
Slipped Disk see Intervertebral Disk Displacement
Slit-Lamp Microscopy see Microscopy
Slotted Attachment, Dental see Denture Precision
    Attachment
Slow Virus Diseases   WC 500
    See also names of specific diseases, e.g., Kuru
    WC 540
Slums see Poverty Areas
Small Nuclear RNA see RNA, Small Nuclear
Smallpox   WC 585-590
    Prevention & control   WC 588
Smallpox Vaccine   WC 588
    Used in the treatment of other diseases, with the
    disease
Smallpox Virus see Variola Virus
Smell   WV 301
Smith, Theobald, Phenomenon see Anaphylaxis
Smittia see Chironomidae

Smoke
    Air pollution   WA 754
    Tobacco   QV 137
        Public health aspects   WA 754
        Toxicology   QV 665
Smoke Inhalation Injury   WO 704
Smokeless Tobacco see Tobacco, Smokeless
Smokeless Tobacco Cessation see Tobacco Use
    Cessation
Smokers' Patches see Leukoplakia, Oral
Smoking
    Dependence   WM 290
    Effects   QV 137
    General   HV 5725-5770
Smoking Cessation   WM 290
Smoking, Passive see Tobacco Smoke Pollution
Snails   QX 675
Snake Bites   WD 410
Snake Poisons see Snake Venoms
Snake Venoms   WD 410
Snakeroot Poisoning see Milk Sickness
Snakes   QL 666.O6-666.O694
    Diseases   SF 997.5.R4
Sneddon-Wilkinson Disease see Skin Diseases,
    Vesiculobullous
Sneezing Gas see Toxicology   QV 665 under
    Smoke
Snoring   WF 143
Snuff see Tobacco, Smokeless
Soaps   QV 233
Soccer   QT 260.5.S7
Social Accountability see Social Responsibility
Social Adjustment   HM
    Adolescence   WS 462
    Child   WS 105.5.A8
    Infant   WS 105.5.A8
Social Alienation
    Adolescence   WS 463
    Child   WS 350.8.S6
    Infant   WS 350.8.S6
    Psychiatry   WM 600
    Sociology   HM
Social Behavior   HM
    Animals   QL 775
    Adolescence   WS 462
    Child   WS 105.5.S6
    Infant   WS 105.5.S6
Social Behavior Disorders
    Adolescence   WS 463
    Child   WS 350.8.S6
        See also Child Behavior Disorders   WS 350.6
    Infant   WS 350.8.S6
    Psychiatry (General)   WM 600
    Sociology   HM
    Television influence   HE 8700.6
Social Breakdown Syndrome see Social Alienation
Social Change
    Progress   HM
    Reform   HN
Social Class   HT 603-1445
    Adolescents   WS 462
    Child   WS 105.5.S6
Social Clubs, Therapeutic see Self-Help Groups

**ALWAYS CONSULT MAIN SCHEDULES.   USE NUMBER ASSIGNED ONLY WHEN
SUBJECT REPRESENTS MAJOR EMPHASIS OF WORK BEING CLASSIFIED**

Social Conditions   HN
Social Conformity   HM
Social Control, Formal
    Penology   HV 7240–9960
    Social elements, forces, laws   HM
    Special topics, by subject
Social Control, Informal   HM
    Primitive customs, e.g., Taboo   GN 493–495.2
    Special topics, by subject
Social Desirability   HM
Social Discrimination see Prejudice
Social Disorganization see Anomie
Social Distance   HM
    Adolescence   WM 462
    Child   WS 105.5.S6
    Infant   WS 105.5.S6
Social Dominance
    Anthropology
        Matriarchy   GN 479.5
        Patriarchy   GN 479.6
    In animals   QL 775
    Sociology   HM
    Leadership   BF 637.L4
Social Environment   HM
    Mental health   WM 31
Social Facilitation   BF 774
Social Identification
    Adolescence   WS 462
    Child   WS 105.5.S6
Social Insurance see Social Security
Social Interaction see Interpersonal Relations
Social Isolation
    Child   WS 105.5.D3
    Infant   WS 105.5.D3
    Psychology   BF 575.L7
    Social psychology   HM
Social Justice
    Special topics, by subject
Social Medicine   WA 31
Social Perception   HM
Social Planning   HN
Social Policy see Public Policy
Social Problems   HN
    Aged   WT 30
    Of the mentally retarded   WM 307.S6
        Of children   WS 107.5.P8
    Of the normal child   WS 105.5.S6
Social Psychiatry see Community Psychiatry
Social Psychology see Psychology, Social
Social Reinforcement see Reinforcement, Social
Social Responsibility
    Medical ethics   W 50
    Medical research   W 20.5
    Specific topics, by subject
Social Sciences   H
Social Security   HD 7090–7250.7
    Medical benefits   W 225–275
        See also Medicare   WT 31
Social Service see Social Work
Social Service, Psychiatric see Social Work,
    Psychiatric
Social Support
    Special topics, by subject

Social Values   HM
Social Welfare   HV 1–4959
    General works   HV 30–31
        By country   HV 85–525
Social Work
    General works   HV 6–696
    As a preventive health measure   WA 108
    Child   WA 310–320
    Hospitals   W 322
    Infant   WA 310–320
    Maternity   WA 310
    Medical   W 322
    Periodicals   W1
Social Work Department, Hospital   W 322
Social Work, Psychiatric   WM 30.5
Social Workers see Social Work
Socialization   HM
    Adolescents   WS 462
    Child   WS 105.5.S6
    Infant   WS 105.5.S6
Socialized Dentistry see State Dentistry
Socialized Medicine see State Medicine
Societies
    (Form number 1 in any NLM schedule where
        applicable. Include history)
    Fraternities in medicine and allied fields   W 20.9
    Other societies in appropriate LC number
Societies, Dental   WU 1
Societies, Hospital   WX 1
Societies, Medical   WB 1
    Fraternities   W 20.9
    Specialties (Form number 1 in any NLM schedule
        where applicable)
Societies, Nursing   WY 1
Societies, Pharmaceutical   QV 701
Societies, Scientific   Q 10–99
    See also types of societies above or subheading
        societies under specialty headings, e.g., Zoology
        QL 1
Sociocultural Change see Acculturation
Socioeconomic Factors
    Mental health   WM 31
    Public health   WA 30
    Other topics, by subject
Socioeconomic Status see Social Class
Socioenvironmental Therapy   WM 428–445
Sociology   HM–HX
    See also Social Medicine   WA 31; Social Work
        W 322, etc.; Social Work, Psychiatric   WM
        30.5
Sociology, Medical   WA 31
Sociometric Techniques   HM
Sociopathic Personality see Antisocial Personality
    Disorder
Sodium
    Inorganic chemistry   QD 181.N2
    Pharmacology   QV 275
Sodium Azide   QU 54
Sodium Bicarbonate see Bicarbonates
Sodium Cephalothin see Cephalothin
Sodium Channels   QH 603.I54
Sodium Chloride
    Metabolism   QU 130

**ALWAYS CONSULT MAIN SCHEDULES. USE NUMBER ASSIGNED ONLY WHEN
SUBJECT REPRESENTS MAJOR EMPHASIS OF WORK BEING CLASSIFIED**

Water–electrolyte balance   QU 105
Water–electrolyte imbalance   WD 220
   Pharmacology   QV 273
   Solution   QV 786
    Infusion   WB 354
Sodium Chloride Solution, Hypertonic see Saline Solution, Hypertonic
Sodium Cromoglycate see Cromolyn Sodium
Sodium, Dietary
   Metabolism   QU 130
   Pharmacology   QV 273
   Relation to a particular disorder, with the disorder
Sodium Glutamate
   Biochemistry   QU 60
   As a food additive   WA 712
Sodium Iodohippurate see Iodohippuric Acid
Sodium Isotopes
   Inorganic chemistry   QD 181.N2
   Pharmacology   QV 275
Sodium Nitroprusside see Nitroprusside
Sodium, Potassium Adenosinetriphosphatase see Na(+)-K(+)-Exchanging ATPase
Sodium, Potassium ATPase see Na(+)-K(+)-Exchanging ATPase
Sodium–Potassium Pump see Na(+)-K(+)-Exchanging ATPase
Sodium Pump see Na(+)-K(+)-Exchanging ATPase
Sodium Valproate see Valproic Acid
Sodoku see Rat–Bite Fever
Soft Contact Lenses see Contact Lenses, Hydrophilic
Soft Tissue Neoplasms   WD 375
   Localized, by site
Soft Tissue Radiography see Technology, Radiologic
Softball see Baseball
Softening, Brain see Encephalomalacia; Paresis
Software   QA 76.75–76.765
   In medicine (General)   W 26.55.S6
   In other special fields (Form number 26.5 in any NLM schedule where applicable)
Software Engineering see Software
Software Tools see Software
Soil   S 590–599.9
Soil Microbiology   QW 60
Soil Pollutants
   General public health aspects   WA 785
   Radioactive   WN 615
Soil Pollutants, Radioactive   WN 615
Solar Activity   QB 524–526
Solar Aging of Skin see Skin Aging
Solar Fever see Dengue
Solar Flares see Solar Activity
Solar Particle Events see Solar Activity
Solcoseryl see Actihaemyl
Soldiers see Military Personnel
Soldier's Heart see Neurocirculatory Asthenia
Sole, Foot see Foot
Solo Practice see Private Practice
Solubility   QD 543
   Pharmaceutical chemistry   QV 744
Solutions   QV 786
   Used for special purposes, by subject

See also specific solution terms, e.g., Contact Lens Solutions   WW 355; Ophthalmic Solutions   WW 166; Pharmaceutical Solutions   QV 786
Solvents
   Pharmaceutical chemistry   QV 744
   Solution chemistry   QD 544–544.5
   Toxicology   QV 633
Soman
   Biochemistry   QU 131
   Toxicology   QV 627
Somatic Cell Hybrids see Hybrid Cells
Somatic Gene Therapy see Gene Therapy
Somatization Disorder see Somatoform Disorders
Somatization Syndromes see Psychophysiologic Disorders
Somatoform Disorders   WM 170
Somatomammotropin, Chorionic see Placental Lactogen
Somatomammotropin Receptors see Receptors, Somatotropin
Somatomedin C see Insulin–Like Growth Factor I
Somatomedin MSA see Insulin–Like Growth Factor II
Somatosensory Cortex   WL 307
Somatosensory Evoked Potentials see Evoked Potentials, Somatosensory
Somatostatin   WK 515
Somatostatin–14 see Somatostatin
Somatotropin   WK 515
   Deficiency   WK 550
   As a cause of a particular disorder, with the disorder
Somatotropin (Human) see Somatropin
Somatotropin Receptors see Receptors, Somatotropin
Somatotropin Release Inhibiting Hormone see Somatostatin
Somatotypes   GN 66.5
Somatropin   WK 515
   Deficiency   WK 550
   As a cause of a particular disorder, with the disorder
Somnambulism   WM 188
Somniloquism see Sleep Disorders
Sonography, Speech see Sound Spectrography
Soporifics see Hypnotics and Sedatives; names of specific drugs
Sorbitol   QV 160
Sorbitol Dehydrogenase see Iditol Dehydrogenase
Sore Throat see Pharyngitis
Sore Throat, Septic see Streptococcal Infections
Sotalol   QV 132
Sound   QC 221–246
   Animal   QL 765
   Insect   QL 496.5
   See also Acoustics   WA 776, etc.; Hearing   WV 270; Noise   WA 776, etc.; Ultrasonics   WN 208, etc.; other particular topics associated with sound
Sound Localization   WV 272
Sound Spectrography   QC 246
   In a specific field, by subject
Southern Blotting see Blotting, Southern

Soy Beans see Soybeans
Soy Proteins   QU 55
    As a supplement in health or disease   WB 430
    Cookery for protein control   WB 430
Soybean Proteins see Soy Proteins
Soybeans
    As a dietary supplement in health or disease
    WB 430
    Cultivation   SB 205.S7
    Sanitary control   WA 703
Space Biology see Extraterrestrial Environment
Space Flight   WD 750-758
    Computers   WD 751.6
    Standards
        Physical   WD 752
    Psychological   WD 754
    Research   WD 751
Space Medicine see Space Flight
Space Perception   WW 105
    Concept formation in children   WS 105.5.D2
    Psychological aspects   BF 469
Space Suits   TL 1550
    In space medicine   WD 750-758
Spanish Americans see Hispanic Americans
Spasm   WL 340
    Bronchial see Bronchial Spasm   WF 500
    Drugs affecting   QV 85
    Pyloric   WI 150
    Affecting other parts of the body, with the part
Spasm, Hemifacial see Hemifacial Spasm
Spasmolytics see Parasympatholytics
Spasmophilia see Tetany
Spasms, Infantile   WS 340
Spasmus Nutans see Spasms, Infantile
Spastic Paralysis see Muscle Spasticity
Spastic Paraplegia see Paraplegia
Spasticity, Muscle see Muscle Spasticity
Spatial Behavior
    Anthropogeography   GF 51
    Psychology   BF 469
Spatial Orientation see Orientation
Spatial Vectorcardiography see Vectorcardiography
Specialism   W 90
Specialization see Specialism; Specialties, Dental;
    Specialties, Medical; Specialties, Nursing
Specialties, Dental   WU 21
Specialties, Medical   W 90
    See also names of particular specialties
Specialties, Nursing   WY 101-164
    Government   WY 130
    Indian service   WY 130
    Institutional   WY 125
    See also specific types of nursing, e.g.,
    Occupational Health Nursing   WY 141
Specialty Boards
    (Form number 21 in any NLM schedule where
    applicable)
Species Specificity
    Bacteriology   QW 700
    Special topics, with the affecting organism or the
    organism affected
Specimen Handling   QY 25
    In field other than clinical pathology, with the

field
SPECT see Tomography, Emission-Computed,
    Single-Photon
Spectacled Porpoises see Porpoises
Spectacles see Eyeglasses
Spectrin   WH 400
Spectrometry, Mass see Spectrum Analysis, Mass
Spectrometry, Near-Infrared see Spectroscopy,
    Near-Infrared
Spectrometry, Particle-Induced X-Ray Emission see
    Spectrometry, X-Ray Emission
Spectrometry, Proton-Induced X-Ray Emission see
    Spectrometry, X-Ray Emission
Spectrometry, X-Ray Emission
    Analysis of drinking water   WA 686
    Analytical chemistry   QD 96.X2
    Radiation physics   QC 482.S6
    Used for other purposes, by subject
Spectrometry, X-Ray Emission, Electron
    Microscopic see Electron Probe Microanalysis
Spectrometry, X-Ray Emission, Electron Probe see
    Electron Probe Microanalysis
Spectrometry, X-Ray Fluorescence see
    Spectrometry, X-Ray Emission
Spectrophotometry
    Analytical chemistry (General)   QD 95
    Quantitative analysis   QD 117.S64
    Used for special purposes, by subject, e.g.,
    Analysis of hormones   QY 330
Spectrophotometry, Atomic Absorption   QC
454.A2
    Used for special purposes, by subject, e.g., for
    blood chemical analysis   QY 450-490, etc.
Spectrophotometry, Infrared
    General qualitative and quantitative analysis
    QD 96.I5
    Organic chemistry   QD 272.S57
    Physics   QC 457
    Used for special purposes, by subject, e.g., for
    measuring impurities in the air   WA 754
Spectroscopy see Spectrum Analysis
Spectroscopy, Magnetic Resonance see Nuclear
    Magnetic Resonance
Spectroscopy, Mass see Spectrum Analysis, Mass
Spectroscopy, Near-Infrared
    General qualitative and quantitative analysis
    QD 96.I5
    Organic analysis   QD 272.S6
    Food analysis   TX 547.2.I53
    Used for special purposes, by subject
Spectroscopy, Nuclear Magnetic Resonance see
    Nuclear Magnetic Resonance
Spectrum Analysis
    Analytical chemistry   QD 95
    Organic analysis   QD 272.S6
Spectrum Analysis, Mass   QC 454.M3
Spectrum Analysis, Raman   QC 454.R36
Speech   WV 501
    Development see Language Development   WS
    105.5.C8, etc.
Speech Acoustics   WV 501
Speech, Alaryngeal   WV 540
Speech Articulation Tests   WV 501

In disorders of psychogenic origins   WM 475
In disorders of neurologic origins   WL 340.2
Speech Discrimination see Speech Perception
Speech Discrimination Tests   WV 272
Speech Disorders
   Associated with the larynx and other organs
     involved with speech   WV 500
   Neurologic   WL 340.2
   Psychogenic   WM 475
   Therapy   WL 340.2; WM 475; WV 500
     See also Speech Therapy   WM 475
   See also Deaf–Mutism   WV 280
Speech, Esophageal   WV 540
Speech Intelligibility
   Adolescence   WS 462
   Child   WS 105.5.C8
   Infant   WS 105.5.C8
   Physiological aspects   WV 501
   Speech disorders   WM 475, etc.
Speech–Language Pathology
   Neurologic   WL 340.2
   Psychogenic   WM 475
Speech Pathology see Speech–Language Pathology
Speech Perception   WV 272
Speech Production Measurement   WV 501
   In disorders of psychogenic origins   WM 475
   In disorders of neurologic origins   WL 340.2
Speech Reception Threshold Test   WV 272
Speech Sounds see Phonetics
Speech Synthesizers see Communication Aids for
  Disabled
Speech Therapy
   General   WL 340.2
   For disorders of neurologic origins   WL 340.2
   For disorders of psychogenic origins   WM 475
   See also Therapy   WL 340.2, etc., under Speech
     Disorders
Speechreading see Lipreading
Speed see Accidents, Traffic; Aircraft
Sperm see Spermatozoa
Sperm Immobilizing Agents   QV 177
Sperm–Ovum Interactions   WQ 205
Sperm Penetration see Sperm–Ovum Interactions
Spermatic Cord   WJ 780
Spermatic Cord Torsion   WJ 780
Spermatocidal Agents   QV 177
Spermatocytes   WJ 834
Spermatogenesis   WJ 834
Spermatogonia   WJ 834
Spermatophores see Spermatogonia
Spermatozoa   WJ 834
   Drugs destroying see Spermatocidal Agents
     QV 177
   Drugs immobilizing see Sperm–Immobilizing
     Agents   QV 177
Spermicidal Agents see Spermatocidal Agents
Spermiocytes see Spermatocytes
Spermophilus see Sciuridae
Sphaerophorus see Fusobacterium
Sphaerophorus Infections see Fusobacterium
  Infections
Sphagnum see Mosses
Sphagnum see Mosses

Sphenoid Bone   WE 705
Sphenoid Sinus   WV 358
Spherocytosis, Hereditary   WH 170
Spheroplasts   QW 51
Sphingolipidoses   WD 205.5.L5
   See also names of specific forms, e.g.,
     Niemann–Pick Disease   WD 205.5.L5
Sphingolipids   QU 85
Sphingomyelins   QU 93
Sphygmography see Blood Pressure Determination
Sphygmomanometers   WG 26
Sphygmomanometers, Continuous see Blood
  Pressure Monitors
Spider Bite see Arachnidism
Spider Monkey see Cebidae
Spider Venoms   WD 420
Spiders   QX 471
   Bites see Arachnidism   WD 420
Spin Labels
   Biological research   QH 324.9.S62
Spina Bifida see Spinal Dysraphism
Spina Bifida Aperta see Spina Bifida Cystica
Spina Bifida Cystica   WE 730
Spina Bifida Manifesta see Spina Bifida Cystica
Spina Bifida Occulta   WE 730
Spina Bifida, Open see Spina Bifida Cystica
Spinal Accessory Nerve see Accessory Nerve
Spinal Anesthesia see Anesthesia, Spinal
Spinal Bifida, Closed see Spina Bifida Occulta
Spinal Canal   WE 725
Spinal Cord   WL 400
Spinal Cord Compression   WL 400
Spinal Cord Diseases   WL 400
Spinal Cord Injuries   WL 400
Spinal Cord Neoplasms   WL 400
Spinal Cord Syphilis see Tabes Dorsalis
Spinal Curvatures   WE 735
   See also names of specific disorders, e.g.,
     Kyphosis, Lordosis, Scoliosis
Spinal Diseases   WE 725
   Veterinary   SF 901
Spinal Dysraphism   WE 730
Spinal Fluid Pressure see Cerebrospinal Fluid
  Pressure
Spinal Fractures   WE 725
Spinal Fusion   WE 725
Spinal Injuries   WE 725
Spinal Manipulation see Manipulation, Spinal
Spinal Muscular Atrophy see Muscular Atrophy,
  Spinal
Spinal Neoplasms   WE 725
Spinal Nerve Roots   WL 400
Spinal Nerves   WL 400
Spinal Osteophytosis   WE 725
   Veterinary   SF 901
Spinal Puncture
   Anesthesia see Anesthesia, Spinal   WO 305
   Clinical pathology
     Cerebrospinal fluid   QY 220, etc.
   General diagnosis   WB 377
   In neurology
     Cerebrospinal   WL 203, etc.
Spinal Stenosis   WE 725

Spine   WE 725–740
Spiral and Curved Bacteria   QW 154
Spiral Ganglion   WV 250
Spiral Organ see Organ of Corti
Spirillum   QW 154
Spiritual Healing see Mental Healing
Spiritualism   BF 1228–1389
Spiro Compounds
    As tranquilizing agents   QV 77.9
    Organic chemistry   QD 341.H9
Spirochaeta   QW 155
Spirochaetales   QW 155
Spirochaetales Infections   WC 400–425
    General works   WC 400
    Veterinary   SF 809.S6
Spirochete Infections see Spirochaetales Infections
Spirochetosis see Spirochaetales Infections
Spirolactone see Spironolactone
Spirometry
    General physical examination   WB 284
    Respiratory diagnosis   WF 141
Spironolactone   QV 160
Splanchnic Circulation   WI 900
Splanchnic Nerves   WL 610
Splanchnoptosis see Visceroptosis
Spleen   WH 600
    Blood supply   WH 600
Splenectomy   WH 600
Splenic Anemia see Hypersplenism
Splenic Artery   WG 595.S7
    See also Blood supply   WH 600 under Spleen
Splenic Diseases   WH 600
Splenic Neoplasms   WH 600
Splenic Rupture   WH 600
Splenic Vein   WI 720
Splenomegaly   WH 600
    Febrile tropical see Leishmaniasis, Visceral   WC 715
Splenoportography see Portography
Spliced Leader Peptides see Signal Peptides
Splicing, RNA see RNA Splicing
Splints   WE 26
Splints, Periodontal see Periodontal Splints
Split Genes see Genes
Spondylarthritis Ankylopoietica see Spondylitis, Ankylosing
Spondylitis   WE 725
Spondylitis, Ankylosing   WE 725
Spondyloepiphyseal Dysplasia see Osteochondrodysplasias
Spondylolisthesis   WE 730
Spondylosis see Spinal Osteophytosis
Spondylosis Deformans see Spinal Osteophytosis
Spontaneous Generation see Biogenesis
Spores   QW 190
    Of bacteria only in   QW 51
    Of cryptogams (other than fungi) in   QK 506
    Of fungi in   QW 180
Spores, Bacterial   QW 51
Spores, Fungal   QW 180
Sporotrichosis   WC 475
Sporozoa see Sporozoea
Sporozoea   QX 123–140

Sports   QT 260
Sports Equipment
    General   QT 26
    For a specific sport, with the sport
Sports Medicine   QT 261
    First aid   WA 292
Spotted Fever, Rocky Mountain see Rocky Mountain Spotted Fever
Spouse Abuse
    Counseling   WM 55
    Crime against the person   HV 6626–6626.23
Spouse Caregivers see Caregivers
Sprains and Strains   WE 175
Spreading Cortical Depression   WL 307
Sprue see Celiac Disease
Sprue, Tropical   WD 175
Sputum   QY 120
SQ 14225 see Captopril
Squalene   QU 85
    Organic chemistry   QD 416
Squint see Strabismus
Squirrel Monkey see Saimiri
Squirrels see Sciuridae
St. Anthony's Fire see Ergotism
St. Vitus' Dance see Chorea
STA–MCA Bypass see Cerebral Revascularization
Stabilizing Agents see Excipients
Stable Factor see Factor VII
Staff Development
    Job enrichment   HF 5549.5.J616
    Training of employees   HF 5549.5.T7
    In special fields, by subject
    See also Personnel Management
Staff Downsizing see Personnel Downsizing
Staffing and Scheduling see Personnel Staffing and Scheduling
Staggerer Mice see Mice, Neurologic Mutants
Staging, Neoplasm see Neoplasm Staging
Staining
    Bacteriology   QW 25
    Microscopy (General)   QH 237
    In medicolegal examination   W 750
Stammering see Stuttering
Standard Preparations see Reference Standards
Standardization, Drugs see Standards   QV 771 under Drugs
Standards see Name of specialties with subheading standards or, lacking that, the number for the specialty as a profession, e.g., in psychiatry; Hospitals; Professional standards review organizations; Quality control
Standards, Reference see Reference Standards
Stannum see Tin
Stapedectomy see Stapes Surgery
Stapedius   WV 230
Stapes   WV 230
Stapes Surgery   WV 230
    Treatment of otosclerosis   WV 265
Staphylocoagulase see Coagulase
Staphylococcal Clumping Factor see Coagulase
Staphylococcal Food Poisoning   WC 268
Staphylococcal Infections   WC 250
    Veterinary   SF 809.S72

**ALWAYS CONSULT MAIN SCHEDULES. USE NUMBER ASSIGNED ONLY WHEN
SUBJECT REPRESENTS MAJOR EMPHASIS OF WORK BEING CLASSIFIED**

Staphylococcal Phages see Staphylococcus Phages
Staphylococcal Pneumonia see Pneumonia,
   Staphylococcal
Staphylococcal Protein A   QW 52
Staphylococcal Toxoid   WC 250
Staphylococcal Vaccines   WC 250
Staphylococcus   QW 142.5.C6
Staphylococcus Phages   QW 161.5.S8
Starch   QU 83
Starvation   WD 100
Stasis Ulcer see Varicose Ulcer
State Dentistry   W 260
State Government
   Special topics, by subject
State Health Planning and Development Agencies
   WA 540
State Health Planning, United States see Health
   Planning
State Health Plans   WA 540
State Medicine   W 225
State-of-the-Art Review see Review Literature
Statewide Health Coordinating Councils see Health
   Planning Councils
Statistical Computing see Mathematical Computing
Statistical Models see Models, Statistical
Statistical Regression see Regression Analysis
Statistics   HA
   Biometry (General)   QH 323.5
   Mathematical methods (General)   QA 276-280
   Medical   WA 900
      As a form subdivision (Form number 16 in
         any NLM schedule where applicable)
      Theory and methods   WA 950
        By specialty (Form number 25 in any NLM
         schedule where applicable)
   Nursing   WY 31
   Periodical government documents   W2
   Vital see Vital statistics   HB, etc.
   Special topics, by subject
Status Asthmaticus   WF 553
Status Dysraphicus see Spinal Dysraphism
Status Lymphaticus see Lymphatic Diseases
Stealing see Theft
Steam   TJ 268-280.7
   See also Baths, Finnish   WB 525; Sterilization
      WX 165, etc.
Steatorrhea see Celiac Disease
Steatorrhea, Idiopathic see Celiac Disease
Steele-Richardson-Olszewski Syndrome see
   Supranuclear Palsy, Progressive
Stegomyia see Aedes
Stein-Leventhal Syndrome see Polycystic Ovary
   Syndrome
Stellate Ganglion   WL 600
Stem Cell Assay see Colony-Forming Units Assay
Stem Cell Assay, Tumor see Tumor Stem Cell Assay
Stem Cells   QH 581.2
Stem Cells, Hematopoietic see Hematopoietic Stem
   Cells
Stem Cells, Neoplastic see Tumor Stem Cells
Stenocardia see Angina Pectoris
Stenosis see Constriction, Pathologic; names of
   various types of stenosis, e.g., Pulmonary Valve

Stenosis
Step Test see Exercise Test
Stereognosis   WR 102
Stereophotogrammetry see Photogrammetry
Stereopsis see Depth Perception
Stereoscopic Vision see Depth Perception
Stereoscopy see Optics
Stereotaxic Techniques   WL 368
Stereotyped Behavior   WM 165
   In a particular situation, with the situation
Stereotypic Movement Disorder   WM 197
Stereotyping   BF 323.S63
Sterility see Infertility
Sterility, Female see Infertility, Female
Sterility, Male see Infertility, Male
Sterilization
   In dentistry   WU 300
   In hospitals   WX 165
   In mortuary practice   WA 840
   In organ transplantation   WO 665
   In preventive medicine   WA 240
   In surgery   WO 113
Sterilization, Involuntary
   Social aspects   HV 4989
Sterilization, Sexual
   Family planning   HQ 767.7
   Female   WP 660
      See also Castration   WP 660; Sterilization,
        Tubal   WP 660
   Insect   QX 600
   Male   WJ 868
      See also Castration   WJ 868; Vasectomy
        WJ 780
Sterilization, Tubal   WP 660
Sternum   WE 715
Steroid Receptors see Receptors, Steroid
Steroidal Anti-Inflammatory Agents see
   Anti-Inflammatory Agents, Steroidal
Steroids
   Biochemistry   QU 85
   Organic chemistry   QD 426-426.7
   Hormones   WK 150
   See also names of specific steroids, e.g., Anabolic
      Steroids   WK 150, etc.
Steroids, Anabolic see Anabolic Steroids
Sterols   QU 95
Stethoscopes   WB 26
   See also Auscultation   WB 278
Stethoscopy see Auscultation
Stevens-Johnson Syndrome   WR 150
Sticklebacks see Fishes
Stigmatization   BV 5091.S7
Stilbenes
   As contraceptives   QV 177
   Organic chemistry   QD 341.H9
Stilbestrol see Diethylstilbestrol
Stillbirth see Fetal Death
Still's Disease, Juvenile-Onset see Arthritis, Juvenile
   Rheumatoid
Stimulants see Analeptics; Convulsants;
   Parasympathomimetics; Sympathomimetics;
   Xanthines; names of specific stimulants
Stimulation, Chemical   QV 38

**ALWAYS CONSULT MAIN SCHEDULES. USE NUMBER ASSIGNED ONLY WHEN
SUBJECT REPRESENTS MAJOR EMPHASIS OF WORK BEING CLASSIFIED**

Stimulation, Electric see Electric Stimulation
Stings see Bites and Stings
Stippled Epiphyses see Chondrodysplasia Punctata
STLV–III see SIV
Stochastic Processes   QA 274–274.76
  Special topics, by subject
Stockings, Compression see Bandages
Stockings, Elastic see Bandages
Stoicism see Philosophy
Stokes–Adams Attacks see Adams–Stokes Syndrome
Stomach   WI 300–387
  Acidity see Gastric Acidity Determination   QY 130; Gastric Juice   WI 302, etc.; Antacids   QV 69
  Analysis   QY 130
  Desiccated see Tissue Extracts   QV 370, etc.
Stomach Dilatation   WI 300
  Veterinary   SF 851
Stomach Diseases   WI 300–387
  General works   WI 300
  Veterinary   SF 851
Stomach Neoplasms   WI 320
Stomach, Ruminant   QL 862
  Domestic animals   SF 851
Stomach Rupture   WI 300
Stomach Ulcer   WI 360
Stomach Volvulus   WI 300
Stomas
  General   WI 900
  Nursing   WY 161
  Created for a specific organ, with the organ, e.g., Colon   WI 520
Stomatitis
  General works for the dentist   WU 140
  General works for the gastroenterologist   WI 200
  Veterinary   SF 852
Stomatitis, Aphthous
  General works for the dentist   WU 140
  General works for the gastroenterologist   WI 200
Stomatitis, Herpetic   WC 578
Stomatitis, Ulcerative see Gingivitis, Necrotizing Ulcerative
Stomatognathic Diseases   WU 140
Stomatognathic System
  Anatomy   WU 101
  Abnormalities see Stomatognathic System Abnormalities   WU 101.5
  Pathology   WU 140
  Physiology   WU 102
  Surgery   WU 600
Stomatognathic System Abnormalities   WU 101.5
Stomatology see Oral Medicine
Storerooms see Materials Management, Hospital
Strabismus   WW 415
Strabismus, Convergent see Esotropia
Strains see Sprains and Strains
Stramonium   QV 134
Strapping, Wounds see Bandages
Stratigraphy, X-Ray see Tomography, X-Ray
Stream Pollution see Water Pollution
Street Drug Testing see Substance Abuse Detection

Street Drugs
  Abuse   WM 270
  General works   QV 55
  Pharmacology   QV 38
Street People see Homeless Persons
Streetcars, Public Health Aspects see Public Health Aspects   WA 810 under Transportation
Strepsirhini   QL 737.P95
  Diseases   SF 997.5.P7
Streptococcal Infections   WC 210
  Food poisoning   WC 268
Streptococcal OK–432 see Picibanil
Streptococcal Preparation OK–432 see Picibanil
Streptococcus   QW 142.5.C6
Streptococcus mutans   QW 142.5.C6
Streptococcus oralis   QW 142.5.C6
Streptococcus pneumoniae Infections see Pneumococcal Infections
Streptodornase see Deoxyribonucleases
Streptodornase and Streptokinase   QU 136
Streptomyces   QW 125.5.S8
Streptomycetaceae   QW 125.5.S8
Streptomycin   QV 356
Streptozocin Diabetes see Diabetes Mellitus, Experimental
Streptozotocin Diabetes see Diabetes Mellitus, Experimental
Stress   QZ 160
  Physiology   QT 162.S8
  Special topics, by subject
Stress Disorders, Post-Traumatic   WM 170
Stress Fractures see Fractures, Stress
Stress, Mechanical
  Biophysics   QT 34
  Bone   WE 140
  Other special topics, by subject
Stress Proteins see Heat–Shock Proteins
Stress, Psychological   WM 172
  Child   WS 350
  In aviation medicine   WD 730
  In space medicine   WD 754
  Infant   WS 350
Stress Test see Exercise Test
Stressful Events see Life Change Events
Striate Cortex see Visual Cortex
Striated Border see Microvilli
Stridor see Respiratory Sounds
Strikes, Employee   HD 5306–5450.7
  Hospital personnel   WX 159.8
  Occupational health services   WA 412
    Mental health services   WA 495
  Nurses   WY 30
    Dealings with hospitals   WX 159.8
  Special fields, by profession, industry, or specialty
  See also Labor Unions
Stroke see Cerebrovascular Disorders; Heat Exhaustion; Lightning; Sunstroke
Stroke Volume   WG 106
Strongyloidea   QX 243
Strongyloidiasis   WC 865
Strontium
  Inorganic chemistry   QD 181.S8
  Metabolism   QU 130

Pharmacology   QV 275
Strontium Isotopes
  Inorganic chemistry   QD 181.S8
  Pharmacology   QV 275
Strontium Radioisotopes   WN 420
  Nuclear physics   QC 796.S8
  See also special topics under Radioisotopes
Strophanthins   QV 153
Structure–Activity Relationship
  Biochemistry   QU 34
  Pharmaceutical chemistry   QV 744
Structure, Molecular see Molecular Structure
Struma see Goiter
Struma Ovarii   WP 322
Strychnine   QV 103
  Toxicology   QV 628
Student Dropouts   LC 142–145
  Adolescent psychology and psychiatry   WS
    462–463
Student Health Services   WA 350–353
  Universities and colleges   WA 351
    Mental health   WA 353
  See also Mental Health Services   WM 30, etc.;
    School Health Services   WA 350, etc.
Student Loans see Training Support
Student Selection see School Admission Criteria
Students
  Substance abuse   WM 270, etc.
  School mental health services   WA 352–353
  School public health services   WA 350–351
  Sexual behavior   HQ 27–29
  See also Adolescence   WS 460, etc.; Child
    WS, etc.
Students, Dental   WU 18
Students, Health Occupations   W 18
Students, Medical   W 18
  Supervision of student assistants in a mental
    hospital   WM 30
  Other special topics, by subject
Students, Nursing   WY 18
  Supervision in hospitals   WY 105
    In mental hospitals   WM 30
Students, Premedical   W 18
Stuttering   WM 475
Stye see Hordeolum
Styrenes
  Organic chemistry   QD 341.H9
  Toxicology   QV 633
Subacromial Impingement Syndrome see Shoulder
  Impingement Syndrome
Subacute Care   WX 162–162.5
  Nursing   WY 152
    Pediatric   WY 159
  Of a particular disease, with the disease
Subarachnoid Hemorrhage   WL 200
Subarachnoid Pressure see Intracranial Pressure
Subarachnoid Space   WL 200
Subcellular Fractions   QH 581–581.2
Subchondral Cysts see Bone Cysts
Subclavian Artery   WG 595.S8
Subclavian Steal Syndrome   WL 355
Subclavian Vein   WG 625.S8
Subconscious see Unconscious (Psychology)

Subcorneal Pustular Dermatosis see Skin Diseases,
  Vesiculobullous
Subcutaneous Tissue, Medication by see Injections,
  Subcutaneous
Subdiaphragmatic Abscess see Subphrenic Abscess
Subject Headings   Z 695–695.1
  Medicine   Z 695.1.M48
Sublimation   WM 193.5.S8
  Adolescence   WS 463
  Child   WS 350.8.D3
Sublimation, Drugs see Drug Compounding
Subliminal Perception see Subliminal Stimulation
Subliminal Projection see Subliminal Stimulation
Subliminal Stimulation   BF 323.S8
  In psychoanalysis   WM 460
  Perception   WL 705
  Suggestion   BF 1156.S8
Sublingual Gland   WI 230
Sublingual Region see Mouth Floor
Submandibular Gland   WI 230
Submarine Medicine   WD 650
Submaxillary Gland see Submandibular Gland
Submersion see Immersion
Subphrenic Abscess   WI 575
Subsidies, Educational see Training Support
Subsidies, Government see Financing, Government
Subsidies, Health Planning see Health Planning
  Support
Subsidies, Research see Research Support
Substance Abuse see Substance–Related Disorders
Substance Abuse Detection   HV 5823–5823.5
  Of specific substance, with the substance
  Through urine screening   QY 185
Substance Abuse, Intravenous   WM 270
  Special topics, by subject
Substance Abuse Testing see Substance Abuse
  Detection
Substance Abuse Treatment Centers   WM 29
Substance Dependence see Substance–Related
  Disorders
Substance–Related Disorders   WM 270–290
  Autopsy to determine   WM 270–290
  Cannabis   WM 276
  Narcotics   WM 284
  Nicotine   WM 290
  Opium alkaloids   WM 286
  Social aspects   HV 5800–5840
  See also Alcohol–Related Disorders   WM 274;
    Cocaine–Related Disorders   WM 280; Doping
    in Sports   QT 261; Heroin Dependence   WM
    288; Marijuana Abuse   WM 276; Morphine
    Dependence   WM 286; Opioid–Related
    Disorders   WM 284; Tobacco Use Disorder
    WM 290
Substance Use Disorders see Substance–Related
  Disorders
Substance Withdrawal, Neonatal see Neonatal
  Abstinence Syndrome
Substance Withdrawal Syndrome   WM 270–290
Substantia Nigra   WL 310
Substrate Specificity   QU 135
Subtrochanteric Fractures see Hip Fractures
Suburban Health   WA 300

Suburban Health Services   W 84–84.8
    See also Community Health Services   WA 546
Success see Achievement
Succinate Dehydrogenase   QU 140
Succinates   QU 98
    Organic chemistry
        Aliphatic compounds   QD 305.A2
Succinbromimide see Bromosuccinimide
Succinic Oxidase see Succinate Dehydrogenase
Succinimides   QV 85
Succinylcholine   QV 140
Succinyldicholine see Succinylcholine
Sucralfate   QV 66
Sucrase   QU 136
Sucrose   QU 83
Sucrose, Dietary see Dietary Sucrose
Suction
    Drainage in surgery   WO 188
    Puncture technique in diagnosis   WB 373
Suction Curettage see Vacuum Curettage
Suction Lipectomy see Lipectomy
Sudden Deafness see Deafness, Sudden
Sudden Infant Death   WS 430
Sudeck's Atrophy   WE 250
Sudorifics see Sweating
Suffocating Gases see Phosgene; names of other
    specific gases
Suffocation see Asphyxia
Sugar Acids   QU 84
Sugar Alcohol Dehydrogenases   QU 140
Sugar Alcohol Oxidoreductases see Sugar Alcohol
    Dehydrogenases
Sugar Alcohols
    Biochemistry   QU 75
    Organic chemistry   QD 305.A4
    Pharmacology   QV 82
Sugar Phosphates   QU 75
    See also Glycerophosphates   QU 93
Sugar Substitutes see Sweetening Agents
Sugars see Carbohydrates
Sugars, Dietary see Dietary Sucrose
Suggestion   WM 415
    See also Counseling   WM 55, etc.; Mental
        Healing   WB 880–885; related special topics
Suicide   HV 6543–6548
    Medicolegal aspects   W 864
    Specific mental disorders associated with suicide,
        with the disorder
    See also Crisis Intervention   WM 401
Suicide, Assisted   W 50
Suicide, Attempted   HV 6543–6548
    Psychiatric aspects   WM 165
    Specific disorders associated with attemped
        suicide, with the disorder
    See also Crisis Intervention   WM 401
Suipoxvirus   QW 165.5.P6
Sulbactam   QV 350
Sulfadiazine   QV 265
Sulfadoxine   QV 265
Sulfamethoxazole   QV 265
Sulfamethoxypyridazine   QV 265
Sulfamethylisoxazole see Sulfamethoxazole
Sulfamyl Diuretics see Diuretics, Sulfamyl

Sulfanilamides   QV 265
Sulfaninylbutylurea see Carbutamide
Sulfates   QV 280
Sulfates, Inorganic see Sulfates
Sulfates, Organic see Sulfuric Acids
Sulfathiazoles   QV 265
Sulfhydryl Compounds
    Biochemistry   QU 130
    Organic chemistry
        Aliphatic compounds   QD 305.S3
        Aromatic compounds   QD 341.S3
Sulfhydryl Compounds Antagonists see Sulfhydryl
    Reagents
Sulfhydryl Compounds Inhibitors see Sulfhydryl
    Reagents
Sulfhydryl Reagents   QU 143
Sulfides   QV 280
    Inorganic chemistry   QD 181.S1
Sulfobromophthalein   QV 240
Sulfonamides   QV 265
Sulfones
    Biochemistry   QU 130
    Organic chemistry
        Aliphatic compounds   QD 305.S6
        Aromatic compounds   QD 341.S6
    Pharmacology   QV 265
Sulfonethylmethane see Hypnotics and Sedatives
Sulfonic Acids   QU 98
    Inorganic chemistry   QD 181.S1
    Organic chemistry
        Aliphatic   QD 305.S3
        Aromatic   QD 341.S3
Sulfonmethane see Hypnotics and Sedatives
Sulfonyldianiline see Dapsone
Sulfonylurea Compounds
    As hypoglycemic agents   WK 825
    Organic chemistry
        Aliphatic compounds   QD 305.S6
Sulformethoxine see Sulfadoxine
Sulforthomidine see Sulfadoxine
Sulfoxides
    Organic chemistry
        Aliphatic compounds   QD 305.S3
        Aromatic compounds   QD 341.S6
    Pharmacology   QV 265
Sulfur
    Inorganic chemistry   QD 181.S1
    Pharmacology   QV 265
    Mineral waters   WB 442
Sulfur Amino Acids see Amino Acids, Sulfur
Sulfur Compounds   QV 265
Sulfur Dioxide
    Inorganic chemistry   QD 181.S1
    Toxicology   QV 618
Sulfur Isotopes
    Inorganic chemistry   QD 181.S1
    Pharmacology   QV 265
Sulfur Mustard see Mustard Gas
Sulfur Oxides
    As air pollutants   WA 754
    Inorganic chemistry   QD 181.S1
Sulfuric Acids   QD 181.S1
    Toxicology   QV 612

Sulindac
    As an anti–inflammatory analgesic QV 95
Sulph–
    For words beginning thus, see those beginning
      with Sulf–
Sulpiride QV 77.5
Sumac see Toxicodendron
Sun Baths see Sunlight; Heliotherapy
Sun Fever see Dengue
Sunbathing see Heliotherapy
Sunburn WR 160
Sunlight
    As an aid to health QT 230
    Therapeutic use see Heliotherapy WB 480, etc.
Sunscreening Agents QV 63
Sunspots see Solar Activity
Sunstroke WD 610
    See also Heat Exhaustion WD 610
Superantigens QW 573
Superego WM 460.5.R3
    Adolescence WS 463
    Child WS 350.5
    Infant WS 350.5
Superfecundation see Pregnancy, Multiple
Superfetation WQ 235
Superior Vena Cava Obstruction see Superior Vena
  Cava Syndrome
Superior Vena Cava Syndrome WG 625.V3
Superior Vena Cava Thrombosis see Superior Vena
  Cava Syndrome
Superiority Complex see Personality Disorders
Supernumerary Organs see Abnormalities
Superoxide Dismutase QU 140
Superoxides QV 312
Superpalite see Phosgene
Supersonic Waves see Ultrasonic Therapy;
  Ultrasonics
Superstitions
    Curiosities WZ 308
    Medical WZ 309
    Occult sciences BF 1405–1999
    Popular delusions AZ 999
    Religion BL 490
Supplementary Medical Insurance Program,
  Medicare see Medicare Part B
Supplies, Pharmaceutical see Equipment and
  Supplies; Pharmacy; Catalogs, Drug; specific
  types of pharmaceutical supplies, e.g., Drug
  packaging
Supply Catalogs see Catalogs, Commercial; names
  of other specific types of catalogs
Suppositories
    Administration of medicines WB 344
    Drug forms QV 785
Suppressor Cells see T–Lymphocytes,
  Suppressor–Effector
Suppressor–Effector T–Lymphocytes see
  T–Lymphocytes, Suppressor–Effector
Suppressor Factor, T–Cell, Glioblastoma–Derived
  see Transforming Growth Factor beta
Suppressor Transfer RNA see RNA, Transfer
Suppuration QZ 150
    Clinical examination QY 210

See also Infection WC 195, etc.
Supranuclear Palsy, Progressive WL 359
Suprarenal Glands see Adrenal Glands
Suprarenalin see Epinephrine
Suprasellar Cyst see Craniopharyngioma
Supratentorial Neoplasms WL 358
Suprofen QV 95
Surface–Active Agents QV 233
    See also Pulmonary Surfactant WF 600; Surface
      Tension QC 183
Surface Anesthesia see Anesthesia, Local
Surface Antigens see Antigens, Surface
Surface Glycoproteins see Membrane Glycoproteins
Surface Markers, Immunological see Antigens,
  Surface
Surface Properties QD 506.A1A–508
    Dental chemistry WU 170
    In other areas, by subject
Surface Proteins see Membrane Proteins
Surface Tension QC 183
    See also Pulmonary Surfactant WF 600; Surface
      Active Agents QV 233
Surfactants see Surface–Active Agents
Surfactants, Pulmonary see Pulmonary Surfactants
Surgeon–Patient Relations see Physician–Patient
  Relations
Surgeons see Biography WZ 112.5.S8, etc., and
  Directories WO 22 under Surgery
Surgeons, Oral, Directories see Directories WU
  22 under Surgery, Oral
Surgery WO
    Abdominal see Surgery WI 900–970 under
      Abdomen
    Adolescence WO 925
    Aged WO 950
    Animal see Surgery, Veterinary SF 911–914.4
    Atlases WO 517, etc.
    Biography
      Collective WZ 112.5.S8
        Military WZ 112.5.M4
      Individual WZ 100
    Care plans see Insurance, Health W 100–275
    Case studies WO 16
    Child WO 925
    Colorectal see Colorectal Surgery WI 650
    Cosmetic see Surgery, Plastic WO 600–640
    Cryogenic see Cryosurgery WO 510
    Dental see Dentistry, Operative WU 300–360,
      etc.
    Directories WO 22
    Emergency WO 700–820
    Experimental WO 50
    Exploratory WO 141
    Gynecological WP 660
    Humor about WZ 305.5
    Industrial WO 700–820
    Infant WO 925
    Insurance see Insurance, Health W 100–275
    Military WO 800
    Naval WO 800
    Neurological see Neurosurgery WL 368
    Obstetrical WQ 400–450
    Ophthalmological WW 168

Oral see Surgery, Oral   WU 600–640, etc.

Orthopedic see Orthopedics   WE 168–190, etc.

Otorhinolaryngologic   WV 168

Proctological see Colorectal Surgery   WI 650

Reconstructive see Surgery, Plastic   WO 600–640

Thoracic see Thoracic Surgery   WF 980

Traumatic   WO 700–820

Urologic   WJ 168, etc.

Veterinary see Surgery, Veterinary   SF 911–914.4

See also Surgical Procedures, Operative   WO 500–517, etc.; names of specific types of surgery and surgical procedures; and surgery under various organ, disease, and specialty terms

Surgery, Cosmetic see Surgery, Plastic

Surgery Department, Hospital   WO 27–28

Surgery, Esthetic see Surgery, Plastic

Surgery, Laser see Laser Surgery

Surgery, Office see Ambulatory Surgical Procedures

Surgery, Oral   WU 600–640

Child   WU 480

Directories of oral surgeons   WU 22

Infant   WU 480

See also Oral Surgical Procedures   WU 600–640, etc.

Surgery, Orthopedic see Orthopedics

Surgery, Outpatient see Ambulatory Surgical Procedures

Surgery, Plastic   WO 600–640

Specific locations, by site

See also Cosmetic Techniques; Reconstructive Surgical Procedures; names of specific procedures, e.g., Blepharoplasty   WW 205; Mammaplasty   WP 910; Rhinoplasty   WV 312

Surgery, Repeat see Reoperation

Surgery, Veterinary   SF 911–914.4

Surgical Anastomosis see Anastomosis, Surgical

Surgical Atlases see Surgery, Operative

Surgical Blood Loss see Blood Loss, Surgical

Surgical Care Plans see Insurance, Health

Surgical Diathermy see Electrocoagulation

Surgical Diseases see Surgery

Surgical Equipment   WO 162–170

Catalogs   W 26

Surgical Errors see Medical Errors

Surgical Flaps   WO 610

Used in surgery for a particular condition, with the condition

Surgical Infection see Surgical Wound Infection

Surgical Instruments   WO 162

Catalogs   W 26

Surgical Mesh   WO 162

Surgical Nursing see Perioperative Nursing

Surgical Pathology see Pathology, Surgical

Surgical Procedures, Endoscopic

General works   WO 505

For specific diseases or regions, with the disease or region

Surgical Procedures, Laparoscopic

General works   WO 505

For specific diseases, with the disease

Surgical Procedures, Minimally Invasive

General works   WO 505

For specific diseases or regions, with the disease or region

Surgical Procedures, Minor   WO 192

Surgical Procedures, Operative   WO 500–517

Atlases   WO 517, etc.

Adolescence   WO 925

Aged   WO 950

Biliary tract see Biliary Tract Surgical Procedures   WI 770

Cardiac see Cardiac Surgical Procedures   WG 169, etc.

Cardiac problems in general surgery and dentistry   WG 460

Cardiovascular see Cardiovascular Surgical Procedures   WG 168–169.5

Case studies   WO 16

Child   WO 925

Cryogenic see Cryosurgery   WO 510

Dental   WU 300–360, etc.

Digestive system see Digestive System Surgical Procedures   WI 900

Diseases   WO 140

Emergency   WO 700–820

Endocrine system see Endocrine Surgical Procedures   WK 148

Experimental   WO 50

Exploratory   WO 141

Gynecologic see Gynecologic Surgical Procedures   WP 660

Infant   WO 925

Infection   WO 184–185

See also Surgical Wound Infection   WO 185

Military   WO 800

Naval   WO 800

Nervous system see Neurosurgical Procedures   WL 368

Obstetrical see Obstetric Surgical Procedures   WQ 400–450

Ophthalmological see Ophthalmologic Surgical Procedures   WW 168

Oral see Oral Surgical Procedures   WU 600–640, etc.

Orthopedic see Orthopedic Procedures   WE 168–190, etc.

Otologic see Otologic Surgical Procedures   WV 200; Surgery   WV 200 under Ear

Otorhinolaryngologic see Otorhinolaryngologic Surgical Procedures   WV 168; Surgery   WV 168 under Otorhinolaryngologic Diseases; Surgery   WV 300 under Nose; Surgery   WV 540 under Larynx

Proctological see Surgery   WI 650 under Rectum

Pulmonary see Pulmonary Surgical Procedures   WF 668; Surgery   WF 668 under Lung

Reconstructive see Reconstructive Surgical Procedures   WO 600–640

Thoracic see Thoracic Surgical Procedures   WF 980

Urologic see Surgery   WJ 168 under Urinary Tract; Surgery   WJ 168 under Urogenital

System; Urogenital Surgical Procedures   WJ
168; Urologic Surgical Procedures   WJ 168;
Urologic Surgical Procedures, Male   WJ 700
Vascular see Vascular Surgical Procedures   WG
170, etc.
Veterinary see Surgery, Veterinary   SF
911–914.4
Localized, by site
See also Ambulatory Surgical Procedures   WO
192; Diagnostic Techniques, Surgical   WO
141; Electrosurgery   WO 198, etc.; Surgery
WO; Surgery under specific disease and organ
terms, and terms for specific surgical
procedures
Surgical Replantation see Replantation
Surgical Revision see Reoperation
Surgical Scrub see Handwashing
Surgical Staplers   WO 162
Surgical Wound Dehiscence   WO 185
Surgical Wound Infection   WO 185
Surrogate Markers see Biological Markers
Surrogate Mothers   HQ 759.5
Special topics, by subject
Surveillance, Immunologic see Immunologic
Surveillance
Survey Methods see Data Collection
Surveys see Dental Health Surveys; Health Surveys;
Library Surveys; Nutrition Surveys; subject of
other specific surveys, e.g., Nursing
Survival
Arctic and antarctic   QT 160
Atomic warfare   WN 650
Aviation accidents   WD 740
Civil defense   UA 926–929
First aid   WA 292
Shipwrecks
Navies and merchant marines   VK 1250–1299
Private ships   G 525–530
Space flight   WD 740
Wilderness   WA 250
From other accidents and disasters, by subject
Survival Analysis   WA 950
Special topics, by subject
Survival Rate   WA 900
Special topics, by subject
Survivorship see Survival Rate
Suspending Agents see Excipients
Suspensions   QV 785
Sustained–Release Preparations see Delayed–Action
Preparations
Suture Techniques   WO 166
Sutures   WO 166
Suxamethonium see Succinylcholine
SV40 Virus see Polyomavirus macacae
Swallowing see Deglutition
Swamp Fever see Equine Infectious Anemia
Sweat   WR 400
Sweat Gland Diseases   WR 400
Sweat Gland Neoplasms   WR 400
Sweat Glands   WR 400
Sweating   WR 102
Drugs inducing   QV 122
Swedish Gymnastics see Gymnastics; Exercise

Therapy
Sweetening Agents   WA 712
Swimbladder see Air Sacs
Swimming   QT 260.5.S9
Accidents   QT 260.5.S9
Swimming Pools   WA 820
Swine
Anatomy   SF 767.S95
Culture   SF 391–397.83
As laboratory animals   QY 60.S8
Physiology   SF 768.2.S95
Swine Diseases   SF 971–977
Swine Herpesvirus 1 see Herpesvirus 1, Suid
Swine Influenza Virus see Influenza A Virus, Porcine
Swinepox Virus see Suipoxvirus
Swing Beds see Bed Conversion
Swiss Mice see Mice
Sydnones
Organic chemistry   QD 401
Used for particular diseases, with the disease
Sylvian Vein see Cerebral Veins
Symbiosis
Ecology and general   QH 548
Microbial   QW 52
Plant   QK 918
Symbiotes see Rickettsiaceae
Symbiotic Relations (Psychology) see Object
Attachment
Symbolism   BF 458
Psychoanalysis   WM 460.5.D8
See also Emblems and Insignia   WZ 334, etc.
Sympathectomy   WL 610
Sympathetic–Blocking Agents see Sympatholytics
Sympathetic Ganglia see Ganglia, Sympathetic
Sympathetic Nerve Block see Autonomic Nerve
Block
Sympathetic Nervous System   WL 610
Child   WS 340
Infant   WS 340
Sympathetic Transmitter Releasers see
Sympathomimetics
Sympathins see Catecholamines
Sympatholytics   QV 132
Sympathomimetics   QV 129
Symphalangus see Hylobates
Symphysiotomy   WQ 430
Symptomatology see Signs and Symptoms
Synapses   WL 102.8
Synaptic Membranes   WL 102.8
Synaptic Potentials see Synaptic Transmission
Synaptic Receptors see Receptors, Neurotransmitter
Synaptic Transmission   WL 102.7–102.8
Synaptosomes   WL 102.8
Syncope   WB 182
Syndactyly   WE 835
Syndrome   QZ 140
Of specific disorders, with the disorder
Synergism see Drug Synergism
Synostosis   WE 250
Synovia see Synovial Fluid
Synovial Fluid   WE 300
Synovial Membrane   WE 300
Synovioma see Sarcoma, Synovial

Synovitis   WE 300
Synovitis, Pigmented Villonodular   WE 300
Synstigmin see Neostigmine
Synthetases see Ligases
Synthetic Vaccines see Vaccines, Synthetic
Syphacia see Oxyuroidea
Syphilids see Syphilis, Cutaneous
Syphilis   WC 160–170
   Antisyphilitics   QV 261–262
   Cerebrospinal see Neurosyphilis   WC 165
   Drug therapy   WC 170
   Pregnancy   WQ 256
Syphilis, Cardiovascular   WC 168
Syphilis, Congenital   WC 161
Syphilis, Cutaneous   WC 160
Syphilis, Latent   WC 160–164
Syphilis Serodiagnosis   QY 275
Syphilis, Spinal Cord see Tabes Dorsalis
Syringadenoma see Adenoma, Sweat Gland
Syringe Sharing see Needle Sharing
Syringes   W 26
Syringomyelia   WL 400
Syrup of Ipecac see Ipecac
Systematics see Classification
Systeme International d'Unites see International
  System of Units
Systemic Capillary Leak Syndrome see Capillary
  Leak Syndrome
Systemic Poisons see Poisons
Systems Analysis
   Analytical methods connected with physical
    problems   QA 402–402.37
   Industrial engineering   T 57.6–57.97
Systems Theory   QA 402–402.37
   Of other special topics, by subject
Systole   WG 280
Systolic Click-Murmur Syndrome see Mitral Valve
  Prolapse
Systolic Time Interval see Systole
Szondi Test   WM 145.5.S9
   Adolescence   WS 462
   Child   WS 105.5.E8
   In psychology   BF 698.8.S85

T

T Antigens see Antigens, Viral, Tumor
T-Cell Growth Factor see Interleukin-2
T-Cell Growth Factor Receptors see Receptors,
  Interleukin-2
T-Cell Leukemia Virus I, Human see HTLV-I
T-Cell Leukemia Viruses, Human see HTLV-BLV
  Viruses
T-Cell Receptors see Receptors, Antigen, T-Cell
T-Cells see T-Lymphocytes
T-Cells, Suppressor-Effector see T-Lymphocytes,
  Suppressor-Effector
T-Groups see Sensitivity Training Groups
T-Lymphocytes   WH 200
   Cellular immunity   QW 568
T-Lymphocytes, Cytotoxic   WH 200
   In cellular immunity   QW 568
T-Lymphocytes, Suppressor-Effector   WH 200

   In cellular immunity   QW 568
T-Lymphotropic Virus Type III Antibodies, Human
see HIV Antibodies
T-Lymphotropic Virus Type III Infections, Human
see HIV Infections
T-Lymphotropic Virus, Type III, Simian see SIV
T-Phages   QW 161.5.C6
Tabacosis see Pneumoconiosis
Tabes Dorsalis   WC 165
Tables
   (Form number 16 in any NLM schedule where
    applicable or appropriate LC number, e.g.,
    tables illustrating general science   Q 199)
   Nutrition   QU 145
   Nutrititive value   QU 145.5
   See also name of specific subject of the table
Tablets   QV 787
   As medication for particular diseases, with the
    disease
Tablets, Enteric-Coated   QV 787
Taboo   GN 471.4
Tac Peptide see Receptors, Interleukin-2
Tac P55 Peptide see Receptors, Interleukin-2
Tachyarrhythmia see Tachycardia
Tachycardia   WG 330
Tachycardia, Paroxysmal   WG 330
Tachypleus see Horseshoe Crabs
Taenia   QX 400
Taenia Infections see Taeniasis
Taeniacides see Anticestodal Agents
Taeniarhynchus see Taenia
Taeniasis   WC 838
   Veterinary   SF 810.C5
Tahyna Virus see California Group Viruses
Talampicillin   QV 354
Talc
   Adverse effects   WF 654
   Dosage form   QV 785
Talipes Cavus see Foot Deformities
Talipes Equinovarus see Clubfoot
Tamarin, Golden see Callitrichinae
Tamias see Sciuridae
Tamoxifen
   As an estrogen antagonist   WP 522
   Used in the treatment and prevention of breast
    neoplasms   WP 870
Tampons
   In surgery   WO 162
Tanning
   Occupational medicine   WA 400–495
Tannins   QV 65
Tantalum
   Inorganic chemistry   QD 181.T2
   Pharmacology   QV 290
Tape Recording
   Catalogs and works about (Form number 18.2
    in any NLM schedule where applicable)
   Recordings, by subject
Tape Recording, Video see Videotape Recording
Tapetoretinal Degeneration see Retinitis Pigmentosa
Tapeworm Infection see Cestode Infections
Tapeworms see Cestoda
Tapioca see Cassava

Tapping see Punctures
Tarantulas see Spiders
Targeted Toxins see Immunotoxins
Tars   QV 241
    As dermatologic agents   QV 60
    See also Coal Tar   QV 60, etc.
Tarsal Joint   WE 880
Tartar see Dental Calculus
Tartar Emetic see Antimony
Taste   WI 210
Taste Buds   WI 210
TAT see Thematic Apperception Test
Tattooing   GN 419.3
Taurine   QU 60
    Organic chemistry   QD 305.A8
Tax Exemption   HJ 2336–2337
    Hospitals   WX 157
    In other fields, in practice management or
      economics number by subject
Taxes
    General   HJ 2240–7390
    Dentistry   WU 77
    Hospitals   WX 157
    Medicine   W 74
    Nursing   WY 77
    Pharmacy   QV 736
    Tax aspects of legislation, in number for
      discussion of legislation, e.g., of black lung
      legislation   WF 33
Taxonomy see Classification
Tc–99m MDP see Technetium Tc 99m Medronate
TCGF see Interleukin–2
TDE see DDD
Tea
    As a beverage used as a dietary supplement in
      health or disease   WB 438
    As a medicinal plant   QV 766
    Chemical technology   TP 650
    Cultivation of plant   SB 271–272
    See also Theophylline   QV 107
Teachers' Manuals see Teaching Materials
Teaching
    (Form number 18 in any NLM schedule where
      applicable)
    As a medical profession   W 88
    Nursing   WY 105
    Of the blind   HV 1618–2349
    Of the deaf   HV 2417–2990.5
    Of the deaf-mute   HV 2417–2990.5
    Of other groups in education, number for the
      group
Teaching Materials   LB 1027
    (Form number 18.2 in any NLM schedule where
      applicable)
    Physiology   QT 200
    Special topics, by subject
Team Nursing see Nursing, Team
Tear Gases   QV 665
Tears   WW 208
    Secretion   WW 208
      See also Crying   WS 105.5.E5, etc.
Tears, Artificial see Ophthalmic Solutions
Teas, Herbal see Beverages

Teas, Medicinal see Beverages
Technetium   WN 420
    Nuclear physics   QC 796.T35
    See also special topics under radioisotopes
Technetium Methylene Diphosphonate see
    Technetium Tc 99m Medronate
Technetium Tc 99m Medronate   WN 420
    Diagnostic use   WN 445
Technical Services, Library see Library Technical
    Services
Technology   T–TX
    Chemical (General)   TP 144–145
    General works   T 44–51
    Special topics, by subject
Technology Assessment, Biomedical
    General   W 74
    Special topics, by subject
Technology, Dental   WU 150
Technology, Educational see Educational
    Technology
Technology, Food see Food Technology
Technology, High–Cost
    Medicine   W 74
    Other topics, class by subject if specific; if general,
      in economics number where available
Technology, Medical
    General works   W 82
    Diagnostic and therapeutic techniques   WB 365
    Economic aspects   W 74
    Instrumentation (General)   W 26
      In special fields (Form number 26 in any NLM
        schedule where applicable)
    Special topics, by subject
Technology, Medical Laboratory
    As a profession   QY 21
    Clinical pathology   QY
    Diagnostic and therapeutic techniques   QY 25
    See also Laboratory Techniques and Procedures
      QY, etc.
Technology, Pharmaceutical   QV 778
Technology, Radiologic   WN 160
    Instrumentation   WN 150
    Veterinary   SF 757.8
Tectum Mesencephali see Corpora Quadrigemina
Tedelparin   QV 193
Teenage Pregnancy see Pregnancy in Adolescence
Teeth see Tooth
Teeth–Straightening see Orthodontics
Teething see Tooth Eruption
Tegafur   QV 269
Telangiectasia, Hereditary Hemorrhagic   WG 700
Telangiectasis   WG 700
Telecommunication Networks see Computer
    Communication Networks
Telecommunications   TK 5101–5105.9
Teleconference see Telecommunications
Telemedicine
    General works   W 83
    In private practice   WB 50
    In particular subjects, by subject
Telemetry
    Biomedical (General)   QT 34
    General   TK 399

Space flight   WD 750
  Monitoring special systems, in the diagnosis
    number for the system
Telencephalon   WL 307
Teleological Ethics see Ethics
Telepathology   QY 25
Telepathy   BF 1161–1171
Telephone Hotlines see Hotlines
Teleradioisotope Therapy see Radioisotope
  Teletherapy
Teleradiology   WN 160
Teletherapy, Radioisotope see Radioisotope
  Teletherapy
Television
  Educational (General)   LB 1044.7–1044.8
  Effect on adolescents   WS 462
  Effect on children   WS 105.5.E9
  In special fields of education
    (Form number 18.2 in any NLM schedule
      where applicable)
  Special topics, by subject
Tellurium
  Inorganic chemistry   QD 181.T4
  Metabolism   QU 130
Temefos
  Agriculture   SB 952.P5
  Public health   WA 240
Temperament   BF 795–811
Temperance   HV 5701–5722
Temperature
  Medical climatology   WB 700
  Meteorology   QC 901–913.2
  Physiological effects on animals   QP 82.2.T4
  Physiological effects on humans   QT 145–160
  See also Body Temperature   WB 270, etc.; Cold
    Climate   QT 160, etc.; Desert Climate   QT
    150, etc.; Heat   QZ 57, etc.
Temperature Sense   WL 103
Templates
  Biochemistry   QU 58
  Dental see Dental Materials   WU 190
  Genetics   QH 450.2
Temporal Arteries   WG 595.T3
Temporal Arteritis   WG 595.T3
Temporal Bone   WE 705
  For the otolaryngologist   WV 201
Temporal Lobe   WL 307
Temporary Threshold Shift, Auditory see Auditory
  Fatigue
Temporomandibular Joint   WU 101–102
Temporomandibular Joint Disk   WU 101–102
Temporomandibular Joint Disorders   WU 140.5
Temporomandibular Joint Dysfunction Syndrome
  WU 140.5
Tendinitis   WE 600
Tendon Injuries   WE 600
  Veterinary   SF 901
Tendon Reflex see Reflex, Tendon
Tendon Sheaths see Tendons
Tendon Transfer   WE 600
Tendons   WE 600
  Achilles see Achilles Tendon   WE 880
Teniasis see Taeniasis

Tenicides see Anticestodal Agents
Tennis   QT 260.5.T3
Tenosynovitis   WE 600
  Veterinary   SF 901
TENS see Transcutaneous Electric Nerve
  Stimulation
Tensile Strength
  Biophysics   QT 34
  Bone   WE 103
Tension–Discharge Disorders see Personality
  Disorders
Tension, Intraocular see Intraocular Pressure
Tensor Tympani   WV 230
Teratogenesis see Etiology   QS 675 under
  Abnormalities; Abnormalities, Drug-Induced;
  Chromosome Abnormalities
Teratogens   QS 675–679
Teratoid Tumor see Teratoma
Teratology see Abnormalities
Teratoma   QZ 310
  Localized, by site
Teratoma, Cystic see Dermoid Cyst
Teratoma, Mature see Dermoid Cyst
Terminal Addition Enzyme see DNA
  Nucleotidylexotransferase
Terminal Care
  Child   WS 200
  Infant   WS 200
  Medical aspects   WB 310
  Nursing   WY 152
  Of patients with particular disease, with the
    disease
  See also Attitude to Death   BF 789.D4;
    Hospices   WX 28.6–28.62
Terminal Deoxyribonucleotidyltransferase see DNA
  Nucleotidylexotransferase
Terminally Ill
  Child   WS 200
  Infant   WS 200
  Medical aspects   WB 310
  Nursing   WY 152
  With a particular disease, with the disease
Terminals, Computer see Computer Terminals
Terminology
  (Form number 15 in any NLM schedule where
    applicable)
Terpene Phosphates see Polyisoprenyl Phosphates
Terpenes
  Biochemistry   QU 85
  Toxicology   QV 633
Territoriality
  Animal   QL 756.2
  Human   HM
Terrorism see Violence
Test–Tube Fertilization see Fertilization in Vitro
Testicular Diseases   WJ 800–875
  General Works   WJ 830
  Monorchidism   WJ 840
Testicular Feminization   WJ 712
Testicular Hormones   WJ 875
Testicular Neoplasms   WJ 858
Testicular Torsion see Spermatic Cord Torsion
Testing, Biocompatible Materials see Materials

Testing
Testis   WJ 830
  Abnormalities   WJ 840
  Diseases see Testicular Diseases   WJ 830, etc.
  Feminization see Testicular Feminization   WJ 712
  Hormones see Testicular Hormones   WJ 875
  Neoplasms see Testicular Neoplasms   WJ 858
  Surgery   WJ 868
  Tunica Vaginalis   WJ 800
  See also Castration   WJ 868, etc.; Epididymis   WJ 800
Testis, Undescended see Cryptorchidism
Testosterone   WJ 875
Testosterone Propionate see Testosterone
Tests see Laboratory Techniques and Procedures; Psychological Tests; Serodiagnosis; names of other specific tests
Tetanus   WC 370
  Veterinary   SF 804
Tetanus Antitoxin   WC 370
Tetanus Toxoid   WC 370
Tetanus Vaccine see Tetanus Toxoid
Tetany   WD 200.5.C2
  Veterinary   SF 910.T47
Tethered Cord Syndrome see Spina Bifida Occulta
Tetracaine   QV 115
Tetracemate see Edetic Acid
Tetrachlorodibenzodioxin
  As an herbicide   WA 240
Tetrachloroethylene   QV 253
Tetracycline   QV 360
Tetradecanoylphorbol Acetate
  As a carcinogen   QZ 202
Tetraethylammonium Compounds   QV 132
Tetraethylthiuram Disulfide see Disulfiram
Tetragastrin Receptors see Receptors, Cholecystokinin
Tetrahydrocannabinol   QV 77.7
Tetrahydrofolate Dehydrogenase   QU 140
Tetrahydronaphthalenes
  Organic chemistry   QD 391
  Pharmacology   QV 241
Tetrahymena   QX 151
Tetrakain see Tetracaine
Tetralins see Tetrahydronaphthalenes
Tetralogy of Fallot   WG 220
Tetramon see Tetraethylammonium Compounds
Tetraplegia see Quadriplegia
Tetrylammonium see Tetraethylammonium Compounds
Textbooks, Programmed see Programmed Instruction
Textile Industry
  Occupational accidents   WA 485
  Occupational medicine   WA 400-495
  Industrial waste   WA 788
Textiles
  Fire prevention   WA 250
TGF-beta see Transforming Growth Factor beta
Thalamencephalon see Diencephalon
Thalamic Nuclei   WL 312
Thalamostriate Vein see Cerebral Veins

Thalamus   WL 312
Thalassemia   WH 170
Thalassotherapy   WB 750
Thalidomide   QV 85
  Adverse effects   QS 679
Thalidomide Children see Abnormalities, Drug-Induced
Thallium
  Toxicology   QV 618
Thallium Radioisotopes   WN 415-450
Thanatology   HQ 1073-1073.5
THC see Tetrahydrocannabinol
Thea see Tea
Thebaine   QV 92
Theca Cell Tumor see Thecoma
Thecoma   WP 322
Theft
  Special topics, by subject
Theileriasis   SF 809.T5
Thematic Apperception Test   WM 145.5.T3
Theobroma see Cacao
Theobromine   QV 107
Theology see Religion
Theophylline   QV 107
Theophylline Receptors see Receptors, Purinergic
Therapeutic Abortion see Abortion, Therapeutic
Therapeutic Community   WM 440
Therapeutic Cults see Alternative Medicine
Therapeutic Equivalency   QV 38
Therapeutic Touch   WB 890
Therapeutics   WB 300-962
  Aged   WT 166
  Animals (General works)   SF 743-745
    See also Drug Therapy   SF 915-919.5
  Anesthetics   WO 375
  Biological see Biological Therapy   WB 365
  Cardiovascular diseases   WG 166
  Child   WS 366
  Eye diseases   WW 166
  Gynecologic diseases   WP 650
  Home remedies   WB 120
  Hormones   WK 190
    See also Hormone Replacement Therapy   WK 190; Estrogen Replacement Therapy   WP 522; and names of specific hormones
  Infant   WS 366
  Mental disorders   WM 400-460.7
    Child   WS 350.2
    Infant   WS 350.2
  Mouth diseases   WU 166
  Neoplasms   QZ 266-269
  Physical see Physical Therapy   WB 460-545, etc.
  Radioisotopes   WN 450
  Radium   WN 340
  Roentgen ray see X-Ray Therapy   WN 250.5.X7
  Skin diseases   WR 650-660
  Special systems see Alternative Medicine   WB 890-962, etc.; other specific types of therapy, by name
  Tooth diseases   WU 166
  Urologic diseases   WJ 166

ALWAYS CONSULT MAIN SCHEDULES. USE NUMBER ASSIGNED ONLY WHEN SUBJECT REPRESENTS MAJOR EMPHASIS OF WORK BEING CLASSIFIED

For therapy of other diseases see general works number for disease, organ, or system

Therapy, Combined Modality see Combined Modality Therapy

Therapy, Computer-Assisted   WB 365
   Special topics, by subject

Thermocoagulation see Electrocoagulation

Thermodynamics
   Biochemistry   QU 34
   Physical and theoretical chemistry   QD 504
   Physics   QC 310.15-319

Thermoelectric Power Plants see Power Plants

Thermography   WN 205
   Used for diagnosis of specific diseases, with the disease

Thermogravimetry   QD 79.T4
   In clinical pathology   QY 90

Thermoluminescent Dosimetry   WN 660

Thermometers
   As equipment   WB 26
   In physical examination   WB 270

Thermopenetration see Diathermy

Thermoreceptors   WL 102.9

Thermoregulation see Body Temperature Regulation QT 165, etc

Thermotherapy see Hyperthermia, Induced;
   Therapeutic use   WB 469 under Heat

Theropithecus   QL 737.P93
   Diseases   SF 997.5.P7
   As laboratory animals   QY 60.P7

Theropithecus gelada see Theropithecus

Thesaurus see Vocabulary, Controlled

Theses see Dissertations, Academic

Thiabendazole   QV 253

Thiamine   QU 189

Thiamine Deficiency   WD 122
   Veterinary   SF 855.V58

Thiamine Diphosphate see Thiamine Pyrophosphate

Thiamine Pyrophosphate   QU 135

Thiamphenicol   QV 350.5.C5

Thiazines
   Dyes   QV 240
      Chemical technology   TP 918
      Chemistry   QD 441
   Organic chemistry   QD 403

Thienamycins   QV 350

Thigh   WE 865

Thin Sectioning see Microtomy

Thinking   BF 441-449.5
   Adolescence   WS 462
   Child   WS 105.5.D2
   Infant   WS 105.5.D2

Thinness
   Anthropology   GN 66-67.5
   Nutrition disorders   WD 100
   Signs and symptoms   WB 146

Thio-Tepa see Thiotepa

Thiobacillus   QW 135

Thiobacteriaceae see Gram-Negative Chemolithotrophic Bacteria

Thioctic Acid   QU 135

Thiocyanates   WK 202

Thioethers see Sulfides

Thiols see Sulfhydryl Compounds

Thiomebumal see Thiopental

Thiopental   QV 88

Thiopentobarbital see Thiopental

Thiophenes
   Acting on the nervous system   QV 76.5
   As anthelmintics   QV 253
   Organic chemistry   QD 403

Thiophenicol see Thiamphenicol

Thiophosphamide see Thiotepa

Thioredoxin   QU 55

Thiosemicarbazones   QV 268

Thiosulfates
   Inorganic chemistry   QD 181.S1
   Pharmacology   QV 280

Thiotepa   QV 269

Thiothixene   QV 77.9

Thiourea   WK 202

Third-Party Payments see Insurance, Health, Reimbursement

Thirst
   Neurophysiology   WI 102

Thomsonian Medicine see Alternative Medicine

Thoracentesis see Punctures

Thoracic Arteries   WG 595.T4

Thoracic Cyst see Mediastinal Cyst

Thoracic Diseases   WF 970-985
   Child   WS 280
   Infant   WS 280
   See also Empyema   WF 745

Thoracic Duct   WH 700

Thoracic Injuries   WF 985

Thoracic Neoplasms   WF 970

Thoracic Nerves   WL 400

Thoracic Outlet Syndrome   WL 500

Thoracic Radiography see Radiography, Thoracic

Thoracic Surgery   WF 980
   See also Thoracic Surgical Procedures   WF 980

Thoracic Surgical Procedures   WF 980

Thoracic Vertebrae   WE 725

Thoracoplasty   WF 980

Thoracotomy   WF 980

Thorax
   Anatomy and physiology   WE 715
   Bone structure and abnormalities   WE 715
   Diseases of the organs within (General)   WF 970-975
   Funnel see Funnel Chest   WE 715
   Mass X-ray see Mass Chest X-Ray   WF 225
   Radiography see Radiography, Thoracic   WF 975
   Surgery see Thoracic Surgery   WF 980;
      Thoracic Surgical Procedures   WF 980
   Wounds see Thoracic Injuries   WF 985

Thorium   WN 420
   Nuclear physics   QC 796.T5
   See also special topics under Radioisotopes

Thornapple see Stramonium

Thorny-Headed Worms see Acanthocephala

Threadworms see Nematoda

Three-Day Fever see Phlebotomus Fever

Three-Day Sickness see Ephemeral Fever

Threshold Limit Values see Maximum Permissible

Exposure Level
Throat see Pharynx
Thrombase see Thrombin
Thrombelastography   QY 410
Thrombin   QV 195
   In the mechanism of blood coagulation   WH 310
Thromboangiitis Obliterans   WG 520
Thrombocytapheresis see Plateletpheresis
Thrombocytes see Blood Platelets
Thrombocytopathy see Blood Platelet Disorders
Thrombocytopenia   WH 300
Thromboelastography see Thrombelastography
Thromboembolism   QZ 170
   Venous   WG 610
Thromboendarterectomy see Endarterectomy
Thrombolysis, Therapeutic see Thrombolytic Therapy
Thrombolytic Agents see Fibrinolytic Agents
Thrombolytic Therapy   QZ 170
   See also Fibrinolytic Agents   QV 190
Thrombopenia see Thrombocytopenia
Thrombopenic Purpura see Purpura, Thrombopenic
Thrombophilia   QZ 170
Thrombophlebitis   WG 610
Thromboplastin   WH 310
   Clinical analysis   QY 410
Thrombosis   QZ 170
   Arterial   WG 540
   Cerebral see Cerebral Embolism and Thrombosis   WL 355
   Carotid artery see Carotid Artery Thrombosis   WL 355
   Coronary see Coronary Disease   WG 300
   Meningeal vessels   WL 200
   Pulmonary see Pulmonary Embolism   WG 420
   Sinus see Sinus Thrombosis   WL 355
   Venous see Venous Thrombosis   WG 610
Thrombosis, Coronary see Coronary Thrombosis
Thrombosis, Venous see Venous Thrombosis
Thrombospondins   QU 55
Thrombotest see Prothrombin Time
Thromboxane–A Synthase   QU 137
Thromboxane A2   QU 90
Thromboxane Synthetase see Thromboxane–A Synthase
Thromboxanes   QU 90
   Perinatology   WQ 210–211
Thrombus see Thrombosis
Thrush see Moniliasis, Oral
Thulium
   Inorganic Chemistry   QD 181.T8
   Pharmacology   QV 290
Thumb   WE 835
Thumbsucking see Fingersucking
Thyme see Lamiaceae
Thymectomy   WK 400
Thymic Cyst see Mediastinal Cyst
Thymic Factor, Circulating   WK 400
Thymic Group Viruses see Herpesviridae
Thymidine   QU 57
   Pharmacology   QV 185
Thymidine Kinase   QU 141

Thymine   QU 58
Thymins see Thymopoietins
Thymoanaleptics see Antidepressive Agents
Thymol   QV 250
Thymoleptics see Antidepressive Agents
Thymoma   WK 400
   Veterinary   SF 910.T8
Thymopoietins   WK 400
Thymosin   WK 400
Thymotaxin see beta 2–Microglobulin
Thymus–Dependent Lymphocytes see T–Lymphocytes
Thymus Extracts
   Pharmacology   QV 370
   Therapeutic use (General)   WB 391
   Used for treatment of particular disorders, with the disorder or system
Thymus Gland   WK 400
Thymus Hyperplasia   WK 400
Thymus Neoplasms   WK 400
Thyrocalcitonin see Calcitonin
Thyroglobulin   WK 202
Thyroglossal Cyst   WK 270
Thyroid Antagonists see Antithyroid Agents
Thyroid Diseases   WK 200–280
Thyroid Function Tests   WK 202
Thyroid Gland   WK 200–280
Thyroid Hormone Receptors see Receptors, Thyroid Hormone
Thyroid Hormones   WK 202
   Deficiency   WK 250
   As a cause of particular disorders, with the disorder
   See also Hypothyroidism   WK 250
Thyroid Neoplasms   WK 270
Thyroid Peroxidase see Iodide Peroxidase
Thyroid–Stimulating Hormone see Thyrotropin
Thyroidectomy   WK 280
Thyroiditis   WK 200
Thyroliberin see Protirelin
Thyrotoxicosis see Hyperthyroidism   WK 265
Thyrotropin   WK 515
Thyrotropin–Releasing Hormone see Protirelin
Thyroxine   WK 202
Thyroxine–Binding Globulin see Thyroxine–Binding Proteins
Thyroxine–Binding Prealbumin see Thyroxine–Binding Proteins
Thyroxine–Binding Proteins   WK 202
Thyroxine Receptors see Receptors, Thyroid Hormone
Thyroxine 5'–Deiodinase see Iodide Peroxidase
Thyroxine 5'–Monodeiodinase see Iodide Peroxidase
Tiabendazol see Thiabendazole
Tibia   WE 870
Tibial Fractures   WE 870
Tibial Menisci see Menisci, Tibial
Tic see Tic Disorders
Tic Disorders   WM 197
   Neurologic manifestation   WL 340
Tic Douloureux see Trigeminal Neuralgia
Ticarcillin   QV 354
Tick–Borne Diseases   WC 600

Tick–Borne Rickettsial Fevers see Rickettsia
    Infections
Tick Control   QX 600
    Animal culture   SF 810.T5
Tick Infestations   WC 900
    Disinfestation   WC 900
    Veterinary   SF 810.T5
Ticks   QX 479
Time   QB 209–224
    Factor in ability to infect   QW 700
    In relation to particular topics, by subject
Time and Motion Studies
    Special topics, by subject
Time Factors
    Factor in ability to infect   QW 700
    In relation to particular topics, by subject
Time Perception   BF 468
    Child   WS 105.5.D2
    Infant   WS 105.5.D2
Time–Resolved Immunofluorometric Assay see
    Fluoroimmunoassay
Timed–Release Preparations see Delayed–Action
    Preparations
Timidity see Shyness
Timolol   QV 132
Tin
    As a trace element   QU 130.5
    Dental use   WU 180
    Toxicology   QV 618
    Used in particular procedures, with the procedure
Tinctures, Pharmacy see Solutions
Tinea   WR 310
    Veterinary   SF 809.R55
Tinea Capitis   WR 330
Tinea Favosa   WR 330
Tinea Pedis   WR 310
Tinidazole   QV 254
Tinnitus   WV 272
Tiotixene see Thiothixene
TIPSS see Portasystemic Shunt, Transjugular
    Intrahepatic
Tissue Adhesives   WO 166
Tissue Banks   QS 523–524
    Organ banks   WO 23–24
    Tooth banks   WU 24.5
    See also Eye Banks   WW 23–24
Tissue Compatibility see Histocompatibility
Tissue Culture
    General works   QS 530
    Plant   QK 725
    Technique   QS 525
Tissue Distribution   QV 38
Tissue Donors   QS 523–524
Tissue Expansion
    General   WO 600
    Localized, by site
    For specific conditions, with the condition
Tissue Extracts
    Pharmacology   QV 370
    Therapeutic use (General)   WB 391
    Used for the treatment of particular disorders,
    with the disorder or system
Tissue Factor see Thromboplastin

Tissue Grafts see Transplants
Tissue Plasminogen Activator
    Enzymology   QU 142
    Blood coagulation   WH 310
Tissue Preservation
    Histology   QS 525
    Transplantation   WO 665
Tissue Therapy   WB 391
Tissue Thromboplastin see Thromboplastin
Tissue Transplantation   WO 660–690
Tissue Transplants see Transplants
Tissue–Type Plasminogen Activator see Tissue
    Plasminogen Activator
Tissue Typing see Histocompatibility Testing
Tissues
    Aging   WT 104
    Composition   QU 100
    Specific types   QS 532–532.5
    Susceptibility to infection   QW 700
    Transplantation   WO 660–690
    See also Histology   QS 504–539, etc.
Titanium
    Inorganic chemistry   QD 181.T6
    Dentistry   WU 180
Titration, Conductometric see Conductometry
TLV see Maximum Permissible Exposure Level
TMJ Disorders see Temporomandibular Joint
    Disorders
TMJ Syndrome see Temporomandibular Joint
    Dysfunction Syndrome
Tn Elements see DNA Transposable Elements
TNF–alpha see Tumor Necrosis Factor
Toad, Fire–Bellied see Anura
Toad Venoms see Amphibian Venoms
Toads and Frogs see Anura
Toads, True see Bufonidae
Tobacco
    Cultivation   SB 273–278
    Dependence   WM 290
        See also Smoking   WM 290
    Pharmacology   QV 137
        See also Nicotine   QV 137; Smoking   WM
        290, etc.
Tobacco Dependence see Tobacco Use Disorder
Tobacco Industry   HD 9130–9149
Tobacco Mosaic Virus   QW 163
Tobacco Smoke see Smoke; Tobacco
Tobacco Smoke Pollution   WA 754
Tobacco, Smokeless
    Dependence   WM 290
    Pharmacology   QV 137
Tobacco Use Cessation   WM 290
Tobacco Use Disorder   WM 290
Tobramycin   QV 350
Tocodynamometry see Uterine Monitoring
Tocography see Uterine Monitoring
Tocolysis   WQ 330
Tocolytic Agents
    Pharmacology   WK 102
Tocolytic Therapy see Tocolysis
Tocopherol see Vitamin E
Tocopherols see Vitamin E
Toenails see Nails

**ALWAYS CONSULT MAIN SCHEDULES. USE NUMBER ASSIGNED ONLY WHEN
SUBJECT REPRESENTS MAJOR EMPHASIS OF WORK BEING CLASSIFIED**

Toothbrushing   WU 113
Topectomy see Psychosurgery
Topical Infiltration see Topical Anesthesia   WO 340 under Anesthesia, Local
Topographic Brain Mapping see Brain Mapping
Topography, Medical   WB 700–710
　Of specific diseases, with the disease
　See also Epidemiology   WA 900, etc.
Topography, Moire see Moire Topography
Tornadoes see Natural Disasters
Torsion   QZ 150
　Ovarian   WP 320
　Testicular see Spermatic Cord Torsion   WJ 780
Torsion Dystonia see Dystonia Musculorum Deformans
Torticollis   WE 708
Torture
　As a form of punishment   HV 8593–8599
Torula see Cryptococcus
Torulopsis see Candida
Torulosis see Cryptococcosis
Total Body Clearance Rate see Metabolic Clearance Rate
Total Body Irradiation see Whole–Body Irradiation
Total Communication Methods see Communication Methods, Total
Total Parenteral Nutrition see Parenteral Nutrition, Total
Total Quality Management   HD 62.15
　In special fields by subject, in number for professions where available
Touch   WR 102
Tourette Syndrome   WM 197
Tourette's Disorder see Tourette Syndrome
Tourniquet Pain Test see Pain Measurement
Town Planning see City Planning
Toxaphene
　Agriculture   SB 952.C44
　Public health   WA 240
Toxemia   WC 240
　In pregnancy see Pregnancy Toxemias   WQ 215
　Intestinal   WI 405
Toxic Shock Syndrome see Shock, Septic
Toxic Substances, Environmental see Hazardous Substances
Toxicity Tests   QV 602
　For specific drugs, with the drug
Toxicodendron   WD 500
　See also Dermatitis, Toxicodendron
Toxicodendron Dermatitis see Dermatitis, Toxicodendron
Toxicology   QV 600–667
　Industrial   WA 465
　Laboratory manual   QV 602
　Medicolegal aspects   W 750
　Methods   QV 602
　Nursing texts   QV 600
　Public health aspects   WA 730
　Veterinary   SF 757.5
　See also Poisoning   QV 600–667, etc.; Toxicity Tests   QV 602; names of types of poisoning, e.g. Plant poisoning   WD 500–530; names of particular poisons

Toxin–Antibody Conjugates see Immunotoxins
Toxin–Antibody Hybrids see Immunotoxins
Toxin–Antitoxin Reaction see Antitoxins; Toxins
Toxin Carriers see Immunotoxins
Toxin Conjugates see Immunotoxins
Toxins   QW 630
　See also names of specific toxins
Toxins, Chimeric see Immunotoxins
Toxins, Deactivated see Toxoids
Toxins, Targeted see Immunotoxins
Toxoids   QW 805
　Used for particular diseases, with the disease
　See also names of specific toxoids
Toxoplasma   QX 140
Toxoplasma gondii see Toxoplasma
Toxoplasma gondii Infection see Toxoplasmosis
Toxoplasmosis   WC 725
Toxoplasmosis, Animal   SF 809.T6
Toxoplasmosis, Congenital   WC 725
Toxoplasmosis, Ocular   WW 140
Toys see Play and Playthings
Trabeculectomy
　For glaucoma   WW 290
Trabeculoplasty see Trabeculectomy
Trace Elements
　Biochemistry   QU 130.5
　Analytical chemistry   QD 139.T7
Tracers, Radioactive see Radioisotopes
Trachea   WF 490
Tracheal Cyst see Mediastinal Cyst
Tracheal Diseases   WF 490
Tracheal Neoplasms   WF 490
Tracheal Stenosis   WF 490
Tracheitis   WF 546
Tracheoesophageal Fistula   WI 250
Tracheotomy   WF 490
Trachoma   WW 215
Track and Field   QT 260.5.T7
Traction   WE 190
Trade Unions see Labor Unions
Trades, Diseases see Occupational Diseases
Traditional Birth Attendant see Midwifery
Traditional Medicine, Chinese see Medicine, Chinese Traditional
Traditional Medicine, Oriental see Medicine, Oriental Traditional
Traffic Accidents see Accidents, Traffic
Training, Athletic see Sports
Training of Children see Child Care; Child Rearing
Training Programs see Education
Training Support
　(Form number 18 in any NLM schedule where applicable)
　Directories (Form number 22 in any NLM schedule where applicable)
　Science   Q 181–183.4
Tranquilizing Agents   QV 77.9
　In anesthesia   WO 297
Tranquilizing Agents, Major see Antipsychotic Agents
Tranquilizing Agents, Minor see Anti–Anxiety Agents
Transactional Analysis   WM 460.6

ALWAYS CONSULT MAIN SCHEDULES.   USE NUMBER ASSIGNED ONLY WHEN SUBJECT REPRESENTS MAJOR EMPHASIS OF WORK BEING CLASSIFIED

Special topics, by subject
Transaminases   QU 141
Transcendental Meditation see Meditation
Transcriptases see DNA–Directed RNA Polymerase
Transcription, Genetic   QH 450.2
Transcriptional Regulatory Elements see Genes, Regulator
Transcultural Nursing   WY 107
Transcultural Studies see Cross–Cultural Comparison
Transcutaneous Administration see Administration, Cutaneous
Transcutaneous Blood Gas Monitoring see Blood Gas Monitoring, Transcutaneous
Transcutaneous Capnometry see Blood Gas Monitoring, Transcutaneous
Transcutaneous Electric Nerve Stimulation   WB 495
Transcutaneous Oximetry see Blood Gas Monitoring, Transcutaneous
Transdermal Administration see Administration, Cutaneous
Transdermal Electrostimulation see Transcutaneous Electric Nerve Stimulation
Transducers, Pressure   QT 26
Transduction, Genetic   QW 51
Transfection   QW 51
Transfer Factor
   In cellular immunity   QW 568
   Other special topics, by subject
Transfer (Psychology)   LB 1059
Transfer RNA see RNA, Transfer
Transfer RNA, Amino Acyl see RNA, Transfer, Amino Acyl
Transferases   QU 141
Transference (Psychology)   WM 62
Transferrin   WH 400
   Clinical analysis   QY 455
Transformation, Bacterial   QH 448.4
Transformation, Genetic   QW 51
Transforming Genes see Oncogenes
Transforming Growth Factor Alpha Receptors see Receptors, Epidermal Growth Factor–Urogastrone
Transforming Growth Factor beta   QU 107
Transforming Growth Factors   QU 107
Transforming Region see Base Sequence
Transfusion see Blood Transfusion
Transgenic Animals see Animals, Transgenic
Transgenic Mice see Mice, Transgenic
Transgenic Organisms see Organisms, Transgenic
Transglutaminase see Protein–Glutamine gamma–Glutamyltransferase
Transient Ischemic Attack see Cerebral Ischemia, Transient
Transient Situational Disturbance see Adjustment Disorders
Transient Tic Disorder see Tic Disorders
Transients and Migrants
   Demography   HB 1951–2577
   Labor   HD 5855–5856
   Health problems   WA 300, etc.
   See also Emigration and immigration   JV

6008–6348
Transillumination   WW 143
   Used for other special purposes, by subject
Transketolase   QU 141
Translating   PN 241–245
   Directories of translators   PN 241
   Machine translating   P 307–310
   Science   Q 124
   Technology   T 11.5
   See also Automatic Data Processing   W 26.55.A9, etc.
Translation, Genetic   QH 450.5
Translations
   Bibliography   Z 6514.T7
      Classical   Z 7018.T7
      Medical NLM subject number preceded by Z
      National
         Great Britain and Ireland   Z 2014.T7
         Latin and South America   Z 1609.T7
         United States   Z 1231.T7
   Individual works, with the original work, by subject
Translocation, Chromosomal see Translocation (Genetics)
Translocation (Genetics)   QH 462.T7
Transluminal Coronary Balloon Dilatation see Angioplasty, Transluminal, Percutaneous Coronary
Transmembrane Potentials see Membrane Potentials
Transmissible Gastroenteritis of Swine see Gastroenteritis, Transmissible, of Swine
Transmission Electron Microscopy see Microscopy, Electron
Transmission of Infectious Diseases see Carrier State; Disease Outbreaks; Epidemiology; Infection; specific types of vectors, e.g., Insect Vectors; names of particular diseases
Transmitter Uptake Inhibitors, Neuronal see Neurotransmitter Uptake Inhibitors
Transphosphorylases see Phosphotransferases
Transplacental Exposure see Maternal–Fetal Exchange
Transplantation   WO 660–690
   Legal, ethical, or religious aspects   WO 690
   (Laws   WO 32)
   Skin   WO 610
   Tube grafts   WO 610
   Specific organs, with the organ
   See also Tissue preservation   WO 665
Transplantation, Allogeneic see Transplantation, Homologous
Transplantation, Autologous   WO 660
Transplantation, Bone see Bone Transplantation
Transplantation, Bone Marrow see Bone Marrow Transplantation
Transplantation, Brain Tissue see Brain Tissue Transplantation
Transplantation, Cardiac see Heart Transplantation
Transplantation Conditioning   WO 680
   Used for special purposes, by subject, e.g., Bone Marrow Transplantation   WH 380
Transplantation, Heart see Heart Transplantation
Transplantation, Heart–Lung see Heart–Lung

Transplantation
Transplantation, Hepatic see Liver Transplantation
Transplantation, Heterologous   WO 660
Transplantation, Homologous   WO 660
    Veterinary   SF 911
Transplantation Immunology   WO 680
Transplantation, Islets of Langerhans see Islets of
    Langerhans Transplantation
Transplantation, Kidney see Kidney Transplantation
Transplantation, Liver see Liver Transplantation
Transplantation, Lung see Lung Transplantation
Transplantation, Organ see Organ Transplantation
Transplantation, Pancreas see Pancreas
    Transplantation
Transplantation, Pancreatic Islets see Islets of
    Langerhans Transplantation
Transplantation, Renal see Kidney Transplantation
Transplantation, Skin see Skin Transplantation
Transplantation, Tissue see Tissue Transplantation
Transplants   WO 660-690
    Specific organs, tissues, or cells; with the organ,
      tissue or cell
Transport, Biological see Biological Transport
Transport of Wounded and Sick see Transportation
    of Patients
Transport Proteins see Carrier Proteins
Transportation
    Hazardous materials   WA 810
    Mentally disabled   HV 3005.5
    Nursing services   WY 143
    Of elderly   WT 30
    Physically disabled   HV 3022
    Public health aspects   WA 810
    See also Automobiles   TL 1-390, etc.;
      Wheelchairs   WB 320, etc.; names of other
      modes of transportation
Transportation of Patients
    Ambulance service (general or hospital)   WX
      215
    War   UH 500-505
    See also Ambulances   WX 215 etc.
Transposable Elements see DNA Transposable
    Elements
Transposition of Great Vessels   WG 220
Transsexualism   WM 611
Transudates see Exudates and Transudates
Transvestism   WM 610
Tranylcypromine   QV 77.5
Trauma see Wounds and Injuries
Trauma Centers   WX 215
Trauma, Multiple see Multiple Trauma
Trauma Severity Indices
Traumatology   WO 700
Travel   QT 250
    First aid   WA 292
    Medical   W 10
    See also Expeditions   W 10, etc.
Trazodone
    As an antidepressant   QV 77.5
Treacher-Collins Syndrome see Mandibulofacial
    Dysostosis
Treadmill Test see Exercise Test
Treatment Costs see Health Care Costs

Treatment Protocols see Clinical Protocols
Trees
    Botany   QK 475-493.5
    Conservation   SD 411-428
    Damage from natural elements   SB 781-795
    Diseases   SB 761-767
    Forestry   SD
    Toxic   WD 500
Trematoda   QX 353
Trematode Infections   WC 805-810
    Veterinary   SF 810.F3
Tremor   WL 340
    Veterinary   SF 895
Trench Fever   WC 602
Trench Foot see Immersion Foot
Trench Mouth see Gingivitis, Necrotizing Ulcerative
Trephining   WE 705
Treponema   QW 155
Treponemal Infections   WC 422
Tretamine see Triethylenemelamine
Tretinoin   QU 167
    Used in treating a particular skin disease, with
      the disease
Triacylglycerol Lipase see Lipase
Triacylglycerols see Triglycerides
Trials, Medicolegal see Forensic Medicine
Triamcinolone   WK 757
Triamcinolone Acetonide   WK 757
Triamterene   QV 160
Triazines
    As analgesics   QV 95
    As herbicides   WA 240, etc.
    Organic chemistry   QD 401
Triazoles
    Organic chemistry   QD 401
Tribavirin see Ribavirin
Tributyrinase see Lipase
Tricarboxylic Acid Cycle see Citric Acid Cycle
Trichina see Trichinella
Trichinella   QX 207
Trichinelliasis see Trichinosis
Trichinelloidea see Trichuroidea
Trichinosis   WC 855
    Veterinary   SF 810.T7
Trichlorbutanol see Chlorobutanol
Trichlormethane see Chloroform
Trichloroacetic Acid   QU 98
    Organic chemistry   QD 305.A2
Trichloroethanes
    Toxicology   QV 633
Trichloroethylene   QV 81
Trichloromethylchloroformate see Phosgene
Trichobezoars see Bezoars
Trichocephaliasis see Trichuriasis
Trichocephalus see Trichuris
Trichomonas   QX 70
Trichomonas Infections   WC 700
    Veterinary   SF 810.T73
    Localized, by site
Trichomonas vaginalis   QX 70
Trichomonas Vaginitis   WP 258
Trichomoniasis see Trichomonas Infections
Trichophytosis see Tinea

Trichosanthin
  As an abortifacient agent   QV 175
Trichostrongyloidea   QX 248
Trichothecene Epoxides see Trichothecenes
Trichothecenes
  As mycotoxins   QW 630.5.M9
Trichuriasis   WC 860
Trichuris   QX 207
Trichuris trichiura see Trichuris
Trichuroidea   QX 207
Tricuspid Incompetence see Tricuspid Valve
  Insufficiency
Tricuspid Regurgitation see Tricuspid Valve
  Insufficiency
Tricuspid Valve   WG 268
Tricuspid Valve Incompetence see Tricuspid Valve
  Insufficiency
Tricuspid Valve Insufficiency   WG 268
Tricuspid Valve Stenosis   WG 268
Triethylenemelamine   QV 269
Triethylenethiophosphoramide see Thiotepa
Trifluoperazine   QV 77.9
Trifluoroperazine see Trifluoperazine
Trifluperidol   QV 77.9
Trifluralin
  Public health aspects   WA 240
  Toxicology   QV 633
Triftazin see Trifluoperazine
Trigeminal Nerve   WL 330
Trigeminal Neuralgia   WL 544
Trigeminal Nuclei   WL 310
Trigger Points, Myofascial see Myofascial Pain
  Syndromes
Triglyceride Lipase see Lipase
Triglycerides   QU 85
Triiodobenzoic Acids
  Biochemistry   QU 98
  As plant growth regulators   QK 745
Triiodothyronine   WK 202
Triiodothyronine Receptors see Receptors, Thyroid
  Hormone
Trimepranol   QV 132
Trimeprimine see Trimipramine
Trimethoprim   QV 256
Trimethoxyphenethylamine see Mescaline
Trimipramine   QV 77.5
Triolein   QU 85
Trional see Ethyl Methanesulfonate
Triparanol   QU 95
Triphosphopyridine Nucleotide see NADP
Triple-Symptom Complex see Behcet's Syndrome
Triplets   WQ 235
  Embryology   QS 642
  Psychology   WS 105.5.F2
Tris Buffer see Tromethamine
Trisaccharides   QU 83
Trisamine see Tromethamine
Trismus   WC 370
Trisomy   QH 461
  Associated with abnormalities, with the
    abnormality, e.g., Chromosome Abnormalities
    QS 677
Trisomy 21 see Down Syndrome

Triterpenes
  Organic chemistry   QD 416
  Pharmacognosy   QV 752
  Pharmacology   QV 66
Triticum see Wheat
Tritium   WN 420
  Inorganic chemistry   QD 181.H1
  See also special topics under Radioisotopes
Trituration see Drug Compounding
tRNA see RNA, Transfer
tRNA-Amino Acyl see RNA, Transfer, Amino Acyl
Trochanter see Femur
Trochanteric Fractures see Hip Fractures
Trombicula see Trombiculid Mites
Trombiculiasis   WC 900
Trombiculid Mites   QX 483
Trombidiidae see Mites
Trometamol see Tromethamine
Tromethamine
  In acid-base equilibrium   QU 105
Trophoblast   QS 645
Trophoblastic Neoplasms   WP 465
  Pathology   QZ 310
Trophoblastic Tumor see Trophoblastic Neoplasms
Tropical Climate
  Hygiene   QT 150
  Meteorology   QC 993.5
  Physiological effects   QT 150
Tropical Hygiene see Tropical Climate
Tropical Medicine   WC 680
  Child   WC 680
  Infant   WC 680
  Of the skin   WR 350
  See also names of particular diseases
Trunk see Musculoskeletal System
Trusses   WO 162
Trustees
  Hospitals   WX 150
  Of other organizations and institutions, in the
    administration number for the agency or lacking
    that, in the general number, e.g., Trustees of
    the American Medical Association   WB 1.
Truth Disclosure
  In drug research   QV 20.5
  In medical research   W 20.5
  In other fields, in research number if applicable
    and available; elsewhere, by subject
Trypanosoma   QX 70
Trypanosomiasis   WC 705
  Veterinary   SF 807
Trypanosomiasis, African   WC 705
  Veterinary   SF 807
Trypanosomiasis, Bovine   SF 967.T78
Trypanosomiasis, Cardiovascular see Chagas
  Cardiomyopathy
Trypanosomiasis, South American see Chagas
  Disease
Tryparsamide   QV 254
Trypsin   WI 802
Trypsin Inhibitor, alpha 1-Antitrypsin see alpha
  1-Antitrypsin
Trypsin Inhibitor, Kunitz, Pancreatic see Aprotinin
Trypsin Inhibitors   WI 802

Tryptamines
  Biochemistry QU 61
  Organic chemistry QD 401
  Serotonin antagonists QV 126
Tryptophan QU 60
Tryptophan Oxygenase QU 140
Tryptophan Pyrrolase see Tryptophan Oxygenase
Tsetse Flies QX 505
Tsetse Fly Disease see Trypanosomiasis, African
TSH see Thyrotropin
Tsutsugamushi Disease see Scrub Typhus
Tsutsugamushi Fever see Scrub Typhus
Tuba Uterina see Fallopian Tubes
Tubal Embryo Transfer see Embryo Transfer
Tubal Ligation see Sterilization, Tubal
Tubal Pregnancy see Pregnancy, Tubal
Tube Feeding see Enteral Nutrition
Tube Grafts see Transplantation
Tube Ileostomy see Ileostomy
Tubercle Bacillus see Mycobacterium tuberculosis
Tuberculin WF 250
Tuberculin Test WF 220
  Veterinary SF 808
Tuberculin-Type Hypersensitivity see
  Hypersensitivity, Delayed
Tuberculoid Infections see Mycobacterium
  Infections, Atypical
Tuberculoma WF 200
  Localized (other than the lungs), by site or
  associated disease
Tuberculosis WF 200–415
  Drugs for see Antitubercular Agents QV 268,
  etc.
  Genital see Tuberculosis, Female Genital WP
  160, etc.; Tuberculosis, Male Genital WJ 700,
  etc.
  ndustrial WF 405
  Laws WF 200
  Nursing WY 163
  Oral see Tuberculosis, Oral WI 200, etc.
  Pregnancy WQ 256
  Skin see Tuberculosis, Cutaneous WR 245
  Veterinary SF 808
    See also Paratuberculosis SF 809.J6
  Other localities, by site
  See also Silicotuberculosis WF 654
Tuberculosis, Avian SF 995.6.T8
Tuberculosis, Bovine SF 967.T8
Tuberculosis, Cardiovascular WG 100
  Localized, by site
Tuberculosis, Cutaneous WR 245
Tuberculosis, Endocrine WK 140
  Localized, by site
Tuberculosis, Female Genital WP 160
  Localized, by site
Tuberculosis, Gastrointestinal WI 140
  Localized, by site
Tuberculosis, Hepatic WI 700
Tuberculosis in Childhood WF 415
Tuberculosis, Laryngeal WV 500
Tuberculosis, Lymph Node WF 290
Tuberculosis, Male Genital WJ 700
  Localized, by site

Tuberculosis, Meningeal WL 200
Tuberculosis, Miliary WF 380
Tuberculosis, Ocular WW 160
  Localized, by site
Tuberculosis, Oral WI 200
  For the dentist WU 140
Tuberculosis, Osteoarticular WE 253
  Localized, by site
Tuberculosis, Peritoneal WI 575
Tuberculosis, Pleural WF 390
Tuberculosis, Pulmonary WF 300–360
  Rehabilitation
    At home WF 315
    At hospital WF 330
Tuberculosis, Renal WJ 351
Tuberculosis Societies WF 1
Tuberculosis, Spinal WE 253
Tuberculosis, Splenic WH 600
Tuberculosis, Urogenital WJ 140
  Localized, by site
Tuberculostatic Agents see Antitubercular Agents
Tuberous Sclerosis QS 675
Tubocurarine QV 140
Tubulin QU 55
Tuftsin QW 806
  As Immunologic Factors WH 400
Tularemia WC 380
Tullidora see Rhamnus
Tumescence, Penile see Penile Erection
Tumor Antibodies see Antibodies, Neoplasm
Tumor Antigens see Antigens, Neoplasm
Tumor Antigens, Viral see Antigens, Viral, Tumor
Tumor-Associated Carbohydrate Antigens see
  Antigens, Tumor-Associated, Carbohydrate
Tumor Cells, Cultured
  Special topics, by subject
Tumor Cells, Embolic see Neoplasm Circulating
  Cells
Tumor Initiators see Carcinogens
Tumor Markers, Biochemical see Tumor Markers,
  Biological
Tumor Markers, Biological
  In the diagnosis of neoplasms QZ 241
Tumor Metabolite Markers see Tumor Markers,
  Biological
Tumor Necrosis Factor QW 630
  See also Antibiotics, Antineoplastic QV 269;
  names of toxins specific to particular cells, e.g.,
  Enterotoxins QW 630.5.E6
Tumor Necrosis Factor-alpha see Tumor Necrosis
  Factor
Tumor Promoters see Carcinogens
Tumor Staging see Neoplasm Staging
Tumor Stem Cell Assay
  Used in testing antineoplastic agents QV 269
Tumor Stem Cells QZ 202
Tumor Suppressor Genes see Genes, Suppressor,
  Tumor
Tumor Vaccines see Cancer Vaccines
Tumor Virus Infections QZ 200
Tumor Viruses see Oncogenic Viruses
Tumor Viruses, Murine QW 166
Tumoricidal Activity, Immunologic see

Cytotoxicity, Immunologic
Tumorigenicity Tests see Carcinogenicity Tests
Tumors see Neoplasms
Tungsten
    Inorganic chemistry   QD 181.W1
    Metabolism   QU 130
    Pharmacology   QV 290
Tunica Vaginalis see Testis
Tunnel Anemia see Ancylostomiasis
Turbellaria   QX 352
Turbidimetry see Nephelometry and Turbidimetry
Turbinates   WV 301
Turkeys
    Culture   SF 507
    Diseases   SF 995.4
Turkish Baths see Baths
Turner's Syndrome   QS 677
Turpentine   QV 65
Turtles   QL 666.C5–666.C587
    Diseases   SF 997.5.T87
Twenty-Four Hour Rhythm see Circadian Rhythm
Twilight Sleep see Anesthesia, Obstetrical
Twinning see Embryology
Twins   WQ 235
    Embryology   QS 642
    Psychology   WS 105.5.F2
Twins, Conjoined   QS 675
Twins, Dizygotic   WQ 235
    Special topics, by subject
    See also Twins
Twins, Fraternal see Twins, Dizygotic
Twins, Identical see Twins, Monozygotic
Twins, Monozygotic   WQ 235
    Special topics, by subject
    See also Twins
Two-Parameter Models see Models, Statistical
Tympanic Cavity see Ear, Middle
Tympanic Membrane   WV 225
Tympanometry see Acoustic Impedance Tests
Tympanoplasty   WV 225
Tympanostomy Tube Insertion see Middle Ear
    Ventilation
Tympanum see Ear, Middle
Type A Personality   BF 698.3
    Medical aspects, with the disease
Type I Hypersensitivity see Hypersensitivity,
    Immediate
Type III Hypersensitivity see Immune Complex
    Diseases
Type IV Hypersensitivity see Hypersensitivity,
    Delayed
Typhoid   WC 270
Typhoid Bacillus see Salmonella typhi
Typhoid-Paratyphoid Vaccines
    For paratyphoid   WC 266
    General and for typhoid   WC 270
Typhus see Typhus, Epidemic Louse-Borne
Typhus, Abdominal see Typhoid
Typhus, Endemic Flea-Borne   WC 615
Typhus, Epidemic Louse-Borne   WC 605
    Epidemics   WC 610
Typhus, Murine see Typhus, Endemic Flea-Borne
Typhus, Sao Paulo see Rocky Mountain Spotted

Fever
Typhus, Scrub see Scrub Typhus
Typing, Bacteriophage see Bacteriophage Typing
Typology see Somatotypes
Tyramine   QV 174
Tyrocidine   QV 220
Tyrosine   QU 60
Tyrosine Aminotransferase see Tyrosine
    Transaminase
Tyrosine Transaminase   QU 141
Tyrothricin   QV 350
T3 Receptors see Receptors, Thyroid Hormone
T4 Antigens, T-Cell see Antigens, CD4
T4 Receptors see Receptors, Thyroid Hormone

U

Ubiquinone   QU 135
Ubiquitin   QU 56
Udder see Mammae
UDP Glucose see Uridine Diphosphate Glucose
UDP Sugars see Uridine Diphosphate Sugars
UDPG see Uridine Diphosphate Glucose
Ulcer
    Corneal see Corneal Ulcer   WW 220
    Decubitus see Decubitus Ulcer   WR 598
    Duodenal see Duodenal Ulcer   WI 370
    Gastric see Stomach Ulcer   WI 360
    Leg see Leg Ulcer   WE 850
    Oral see Oral Ulcer   WU 140
    Pathology   QZ 150
    Peptic see Peptic Ulcer   WI 350–370
    Skin see Skin Ulcer   WR 598
    Varicose see Varicose Ulcer   WG 620
Ulcer, Aphthous see Stomatitis, Aphthous
Ulna   WE 820
Ulnar Nerve   WL 400
    See also names of organs innervated, e.g.,
    Forearm   WE 820
Ultracentrifugation
    Biological research   QH 324.9.C4
    Chemical engineering   TP 159.C4
    Chemical techniques   QD 54.C4
    Clinical chemistry   QY 90
    See also Centrifugation   QD 54.C4, etc.
Ultradian Cycles see Activity Cycles
Ultramicrotomy see Microtomy
Ultrasonic Diagnosis see Ultrasonography
Ultrasonic Endoscopy see Endosonography
Ultrasonic Imaging see Ultrasonography
Ultrasonic Lithotripsy see Lithotripsy
Ultrasonic Therapy   WB 515
Ultrasonics
    Biophysics   QT 34
    Diagnostic use (General) see Ultrasonography
    WN 208
    Physics   QC 244
    Used for other special purposes, by subject
Ultrasonography   WN 208
    Used for special purposes, by subject
Ultrasonography, Endoscopic see Endosonography
Ultrasonography, Fetal see Ultrasonography,
    Prenatal

**ALWAYS CONSULT MAIN SCHEDULES. USE NUMBER ASSIGNED ONLY WHEN
SUBJECT REPRESENTS MAJOR EMPHASIS OF WORK BEING CLASSIFIED**

I-268

Ultrasonography, Mammary   WP 815
Ultrasonography, Prenatal   WQ 209
Ultraviolet Microscopy see Microscopy, Ultraviolet
Ultraviolet Rays
    Adverse effects (General)   WD 605
    Diagnostic use   WB 288
    General physiological effects   QT 162.U4
    Medical use (General)   WB 117
    Meteorology   QC 976.U4
    Therapeutic use see Ultraviolet Therapy   WB
    480
Ultraviolet Therapy   WB 480
Umbilical Arteries   WG 595.U6
Umbilical Cord   WQ 210
Umbilical Hernia see Hernia, Umbilical
Umbilical Veins   WI 720
    Embryology   QS 604
    Obstetrics   WQ 210
Umbilicus   WI 940
    See also Umbilical Cord   WQ 210
Umbra see Salmonidae
Uncinaria see Hookworms
Uncinaria stenocephala see Ancylostomatoidea
Uncinariasis, Human see Necatoriasis
Unconscious (Psychology)   BF 315
    Adolescence   WS 462
    Child   WS 105
    Infant   WS 105
    Psychoanalysis   WM 460.5.U6
Unconsciousness
    General diagnosis   WB 182
    Neurological manifestation   WL 341
Underachievement   BF 637.U53
    Academic   LC 4661
        Relation to personality   BF 698.9.A3
Underpopulation see Population Density
Undertaking see Mortuary Practice
Undulant Fever see Brucellosis
Unemployment   HD 5707.5–5710.2
Union Lists
    Books or general   Z 695.83
    Nonbook material   Z 6851
    Serials   Z 6945
    On particular subjects, in bibliography number
    for the subject
Unipolar Depression see Depressive Disorder
United States National Health Insurance see National
    Health Insurance, United States
Universal Coverage   W 100–275
    See also names of specific types of insurance, e.g.,
    Medicare   WT 31
Universal Precautions
    Precaution against a specific communicable
    disease, by disease
Universities   LB 2301–2430
University Health Services see Student Health
    Services
Unknown Primary Tumors see Neoplasms,
    Unknown Primary
Unsaturated Dietary Fats see Dietary Fats,
    Unsaturated
Unsaturated Fats see Fats, Unsaturated
Unsaturated Oils see Fats, Unsaturated

Unventilated Spaces see Confined Spaces
Unwed Fathers see Illegitimacy
Unwed Mothers see Illegitimacy
Uphill Transport see Biological Transport, Active
Upper Extremities see Extremities; names of
    particular parts
Upper Extremity see Arm
Upper Respiratory Infections see Respiratory Tract
    Infections
Urachus   WQ 210.5
Uracil
    In nucleic acids   QU 58
Uralenic Acid see Glycyrrhetinic Acid
Uranium   WN 420
    Nuclear physics   QC 796.U7
    See also special topics under Radioisotopes
Urban Development see Urban Renewal
Urban Health   WA 380
Urban Health Services   WA 380
Urban Planning see City Planning
Urban Population
    Demography   HB 2161–2367
    Health problems   WA 380
    Other aspects, by subject
    See also Housing   HD 257, etc.; Public Housing
        HD 7288.77–7288.78
Urban Renewal   HT 170–178
    Architecture and engineering   NA 9000–9428
    Public health aspects in   WA
Urea
    In animal nutrition   SF 98.U7
    In blood   QY 455
    In protein metabolism   QU 55
    In urine   QY 185
    Organic chemistry   QD 315
Urease   QU 136
Uremia   WJ 348
Ureter   WJ 400
Ureteral Calculi   WJ 400
Ureteral Diseases   WJ 400
Ureteral Neoplasms   WJ 400
Ureteral Obstruction   WJ 400
Ureteritis see Ureteral Diseases
Ureterolithiasis see Ureteral Calculi
Urethane   QV 269
Urethra   WJ 600
    Surgery   WJ 600
Urethral Diseases   WJ 600
Urethral Stenosis see Urethral Stricture
Urethral Stricture   WJ 600
    Child   WS 320
    Infant   WS 320
Urethritis   WJ 600
Urethrotomy see Surgery   WJ 600 under Urethra
Uric Acid   WJ 303
    In urine   QY 185
    Organic chemistry   QD 401
Uricosuric Agents   QV 98
Uridine   QU 57
Uridine Diphosphate Glucose
    Biochemistry   QU 57
    Pharmacology   QV 185

Uridine Diphosphate Sugars
   Biochemistry   QU 57
   Pharmacology   QV 185
Uridine Diphosphoglucose see Uridine Diphosphate
   Glucose
Urinalysis   QY 185
Urinary Calculi   WJ 140
   See also Bladder Calculi   WJ 500; Kidney
      Calculi   WJ 356; Ureteral Calculi   WJ 400
Urinary Catheterization   WJ 141
Urinary Diversion
   Surgery of the kidney   WJ 368
   Surgery of the penis   WJ 790
   Surgery of the ureter   WJ 400
   Surgery of the urethra   WJ 600
   By organ used as conduit if more appropriate
      for the work
Urinary Fistula   WJ 140
   See also Bladder Fistula   WJ 500; Vesicovaginal
      Fistula   WP 180
Urinary Incontinence   WJ 146
Urinary Incontinence, Stress   WJ 146
Urinary Tract   WJ
   Animals, Domestic   SF 871
   Antiseptics see Anti-Infective Agents, Urinary
      QV 243
   Child   WS 320–322
   Drugs affecting see Diuretics   QV 160;
      Vasopressin   QV 160, etc.
   Infant   WS 320–322
   Physiology see Urinary Tract Physiology   WJ
      102
   Surgery   WJ 168
Urinary Tract Diseases see Urologic Diseases
Urinary Tract Infections   WJ 151
   Child   WS 320
   Infant   Ws 320
   Veterinary   SF 871
Urinary Tract Physiology   WJ 102
Urination   WJ 146
Urination Disorders   WJ 146
   Veterinary   SF 871
Urine
   Analysis   See Urinalysis   QY 185
   Secretion   WJ 303
   Sugars see Diabetes Mellitus   WK 810–850;
      Glycosuria   WK 870
   Urine therapy see Alternative Medicine   WB
      890, etc.
Urine Concentrating Ability see Kidney
   Concentrating Ability
Urodela   QL 668.C2–668.C285
   As laboratory animals   QY 60.A6
Urodynamics   WJ 102
Urogastrone see Epidermal Growth
   Factor-Urogastrone
Urogastrone Receptors see Receptors, Epidermal
   Growth Factor-Urogastrone
Urogenital Abnormalities   WJ 101
Urogenital Diseases
   General   WJ 140
Urogenital Neoplasms   WJ 160
   Localized, by site

See also names of specific urogenital neoplasms
Urogenital Surgical Procedures   WJ 168
Urogenital System   WJ
   Animals, Domestic   SF 871
   Child   WS 320–322
   Infant   WS 320–322
   Surgery   WJ 168
      See also Urogenital Surgical Procedures   WJ
         168; Urologic Surgical Procedures   WJ 168;
         Urologic Surgical Procedures, Male   WJ
         700
Urography   WJ 141
   Child   WS 320
   Infant   WS 320
   Pyelography   WJ 302
Urokinase   QU 142
Urokinase-Type Plasminogen Activator see
   Urokinase
Urolithiasis see Urinary Calculi
Urologic Diseases   WJ
   General   WJ 140
   Child   WS 320–322
   Diagnosis   Wj 141
   Gynecology   WJ 190
   Infant   WS 320–322
   Nursing   WY 164
   Pregnancy   WQ 260
   Therapy   WJ 166
   Veterinary   SF 871
Urologic Neoplasms   WJ 160
   Localized, by site
Urologic Surgical Procedures   WJ 168
Urologic Surgical Procedures, Male
   General works   WJ 700
   See also Urogenital Surgical Procedures   WJ
      168
Urology   WJ
   Pediatric   WS 320–322
   See also Urogenital Surgical Procedures   WJ
      168; Urologic Surgical Procedures   WJ 168;
      Urologic Surgical Procedures, Male   WJ 700
Urology Department, Hospital   WJ 27–28
Uropepsin   QU 136
Urotropin see Methenamine
Ursodeoxycholic Acid
   Bile acid   WI 703
   As a Cholagogue and choleretic   QV 66
Urticaria   WR 170
Urticaria, Giant see Angioneurotic Edema
Urticaria Pigmentosa   WR 267
User-Computer Interface   QA 76.9.U83
Uterine Contraction   WQ 305
Uterine Diseases   WP 440–480
   General works   WP 440
Uterine Endoscopy see Hysteroscopy
Uterine Hemorrhage   WP 440
Uterine Inertia   WQ 330
Uterine Inversion   WP 454
Uterine Monitoring   WQ 209
Uterine Muscle see Myometrium
Uterine Neoplasms   WP 458–465
   Leiomyoma   WP 459
Uterine Prolapse   WP 454

Uterus WP 400–480
 Anatomy & histology WP 400
 During puerperium WQ 500
 Drugs affecting QV 170–174
 See also Oxytocics QV 173–174
Utilitarianism see Ethics
Utilization and Quality Control Peer Review
 Organizations see Professional Review
 Organizations
Utilization Review WX 153
 Of special hospitals, by type
Utopias HX 806–811
Uvea WW 240–245
Uveal Diseases WW 240
Uveal Neoplasms WW 240
Uvcitis WW 240
Uveitis, Sympathetic see Ophthalmia, Sympathetic
Uvula WV 410
U1 Small Nuclear RNA see RNA, Small Nuclear
U2 Small Nuclear RNA see RNA, Small Nuclear
U3 Small Nuclear RNA see RNA, Small Nuclear
U4 Small Nuclear RNA see RNA, Small Nuclear
U5 Small Nuclear RNA see RNA, Small Nuclear
U6 Small Nuclear RNA see RNA, Small Nuclear
U7 Small Nuclear RNA see RNA, Small Nuclear

V

v–Ha–ras Genes see Genes, ras
v–Ki–ras Genes see Genes, ras
Vaccination QW 806
 BCG see BCG Vaccine WF 250
 Child WS 135
 Infant WS 135
 Poliomyelitis see Prevention & control WC 556
  under Poliomyelitis
 Smallpox see Prevention & control WC 588
  under Smallpox
 Veterinary medicine SF 757.2
 Other diseases, with the disease
 See also Vaccines and particular types of vaccines
Vaccination Encephalitis see Encephalomyelitis,
 Acute Disseminated
Vaccine Therapy see Immunotherapy, Active
Vaccines QW 805
 Bacterial see Bacterial Vaccines WC 200
 BCG see BCG Vaccine WF 250
 Brucella see Brucella Vaccine WC 310
 Cancer see Cancer Vaccines QZ 266
 Chickenpox see Chickenpox Vaccine WC 572
 Cholera see Cholera Vaccine WC 262
 Fungal see Fungal Vaccines WC 450
 Influenza see Influenza Vaccine WC 515
 Measles see Measles Vaccine WC 580
 Mumps see Mumps Vaccine WC 520
 Pertussis see Pertussis Vaccine WC 340
 Plague see Plague Vaccine WC 350
 Poliovirus see Poliovirus Vaccine WC 556
 Rabies see Rabies Vaccine WC 550
 Rickettsial see Rickettsial Vaccines WC 600
 Rubella see Rubella Vaccine WC 582
 Smallpox see Smallpox Vaccine WC 588
 Staphylococcal see Staphylococcal Vaccines

 WC 250
 Tuberculosis see BCG Vaccine WF 250
 Typhoid–Paratyphoid see Typhoid–Paratyphoid
  Vaccines WC 270, etc.
 Viral scc Viral Vaccines WC 500
Vaccines, Cancer see Cancer Vaccines
Vaccines, DNA QW 805
Vaccines, Neoplasm see Cancer Vaccines
Vaccines, Recombinant see Vaccines, Synthetic
Vaccines, Recombinant DNA see Vaccines, DNA
Vaccines, Synthetic
 As a vaccine QW 805
 As an antigen QW 573
Vaccines, Tumor see Cancer Vaccines
Vaccinia WC 584
Vaccinia Virus QW 165.5.P6
Vacuolating Agent see Polyomavirus macacae
Vacuoles QH 591
 In plant cells QK 725
Vacuum Curettage WP 470
 Used for special purposes, by subject
Vagina WP 250–258
Vaginal Birth after Cesarean WQ 415
Vaginal Discharge WP 255
Vaginal Diseases WP 250–258
 General works WP 250
Vaginal Fistula WP 250
 See also Rectovaginal Fistula WP 180;
  Vesicovaginal Fistula WP 180
Vaginal Neoplasms WP 250
Vaginal Prolapse see Uterine Prolapse
Vaginal Smears WP 141
Vaginismus see Dyspareunia; Hyperesthesia; Vaginal
 Diseases
Vaginismus see Sexual Dysfunctions, Psychological
Vaginitis WP 255
 See also Trichomonas Vaginitis WP 258;
  Vulvovaginitis WP 200
Vagotomy WL 330
Vagotomy, Parietal Cell see Vagotomy, Proximal
 Gastric
Vagotomy, Proximal Gastric WL 330
Vagotomy, Selective Proximal see Vagotomy,
 Proximal Gastric
Vagus Nerve WL 330
 Vagotonia WL 330
Valerates QU 90
Valerian QV 767
 As sedative QV 85
Validity of Results see Reproducibility of Results
Valine QU 60
Valproic Acid QV 85
Vanadium
 Inorganic chemistry QD 181.V2
 Metabolism QU 130.5
 Pharmacology QV 290
Vanillin QV 810
Vanylglycol see Methoxyhydroxyphenylglycol
Vapor Baths see Baths
Vaporization, Laser see Laser Surgery
Vaporizers see Nebulizers and Vaporizers
Vaquez's Disease see Polycythemia Vera
Variation (Genetics) QH 401–411

Animal   QH 408
Microbial genetics
   Bacteria   QW 51
   Fungi   QW 180
   Viruses   QW 160
  Plants   QK 983
Varicella see Chickenpox
Varicella Vaccine see Chickenpox Vaccine
Varicella–Zoster Virus see Herpesvirus 3, Human
Varices see Varicose Veins
Varicocele   WJ 780
Varicose Ulcer   WG 620
Varicose Veins   WG 620
  Pregnancy   WQ 244
Variola see Smallpox
Variola Virus   QW 165.5.P6
Varnish see Paint
Vas Deferens   WJ 780
Vascular Access Ports see Catheters, Indwelling
Vascular–Assist Devices see Heart–Assist Devices
Vascular Capacitance   WG 106
Vascular Dementia see Dementia, Vascular
Vascular Diseases   WG 500–700
  General works   WG 500
  Child   WS 290
  Infant   WS 290
  Varices   WG 620
  Veterinary   SF 811
  See also Cardiovascular Diseases   WG, etc.;
   names of specific organs or systems (for their
   blood supply) or specific vascular diseases
Vascular Diseases, Peripheral see Peripheral
  Vascular Diseases
Vascular Endothelium see Endothelium, Vascular
Vascular Fistula
  General   WG 500
Vascular Headache   WL 344
  See also specifics, e.g., Migraine   WL 344y
Vascular Neoplasms
  General works   WG 500
  In arteries   WG 510
  In veins   WG 600
  In coronary vessels   WG 300
Vascular Permeability see Capillary Permeability
Vascular Prosthesis see Blood Vessel Prosthesis
Vascular Resistance   WG 106
Vascular Surgical Procedures   WG 170
  Child   WS 290
  Infant   WS 290
Vasculitis   WG 515
  Of the veins only   WG 610
Vasculitis, Allergic Cutaneous   WG 515
  Emphasis on skin hypersensitivity   WR 160
Vasculitis, Churg–Strauss see Churg–Strauss
  Syndrome
Vasectomy   WJ 780
Vasoactive Agonists see Vasoconstrictor Agents
Vasoactive Antagonists see Vasodilator Agents
Vasoactive Intestinal Peptide   WK 170
  As a Peptide   QU 68
  As a Vasopressin   WK 520
Vasoconstriction   WG 106
  See also Constriction, Pathologic   WG 560, etc.

Vasoconstrictor Agents   QV 150
Vasoconstrictor Agents, Nasal see Nasal
  Decongestants
Vasodilation   WG 106
  See also Dilatation, Pathologic   WG 578, etc.
Vasodilator Agents   QV 150–156
Vasodilator Disorders see Dilatation, Pathologic
Vasomotor Disorders see Vasomotor System; names
  of specific disorders
Vasomotor Regulation see Vasomotor System
Vasomotor Rhinitis see Rhinitis, Vasomotor
Vasomotor System   WL 610
  Disorders   WG 560
   Spastic see Raynaud's Disease   WG 570
   Vasodilator   WG 578
   See also Constriction, Pathologic   WG 560,
   etc.
  Regulation   WG 560
Vasopressin, Arginine see Argipressin
Vasopressin, Deamino Arginine see Desmopressin
Vasopressin, Isoleucyl–Leucyl see Oxytocin
Vasopressin, Lysine see Lypressin
Vasopressins   WK 520
  Diuretic   QV 160
Vasopressor Agents see Vasoconstrictor Agents
Vasospastic Disorders see Raynaud's Disease
Vasotocin, Leucyl see Oxytocin
Vater's Ampulla   WI 750
Vectorcardiography   WG 140
Vectors see Disease Vectors
Vectors, Genetic see Genetic Vectors
Vecuronium see Vecuronium Bromide
Vecuronium Bromide   QV 140
Vegetable Oils see Plant Oils
Vegetable Proteins   QU 55
  As a supplement in health or disease   WB 430
  Cookery   WB 430
Vegetables
  As a dietary supplement in health and disease
   WB 430
  Cultivation   SB 320–353.5
  Drugs see Plants, Medicinal   QV 766, etc.
  Poisonous see Plants, Toxic   WD 500–530
  Processing   TX 801–807
  Purgatives see Cathartics   QV 75
  Sanitation and other public health aspects   WA
   703
  See also names of specific vegetables
Vegetarianism   WB 430
Vegetative Nervous System see Autonomic Nervous
  System
Vegetative State, Persistent see Persistent Vegetative
  State
Vehicle Emissions   WA 754
Vehicles   QV 800
Vehicles, Motor see Motor Vehicles
Veiled Cells see Dendritic Cells
Vein Anesthesia see Anesthesia, Local
Vein of Galen see Cerebral Veins
Veins   WG 600–625
  Coronary see Coronary Vessels   WG 300
  Medication by see Injections, Intravenous   WB
   354

Portal see Portal Vein   WI 720
Velocimetry see Rheology
Velopharyngeal Insufficiency   WV 410
Vena Cava, Inferior   WG 625.V3
Vena Cava, Superior   WG 625.V3
Venae Cavae   WG 625.V3
Venereal Diseases see Sexually Transmitted Diseases
Venereology   WC 140–185
Venesection see Phlebotomy
Venesection see Phlebotomy
Venipuncture see Phlebotomy
Venipuncture see Phlebotomy
Venoclysis, Medication see Injections, Intravenous
Venography see Phlebography
Venoms
   Poisoning   WD 400–430
  Therapeutic use see name of disease being treated;
    Alternative Medicine   WB 890, etc.
   See also specific venoms, e.g., Bee Venoms   WD 430
Venous Catheterization, Peripheral see Catheterization, Peripheral
Venous Insufficiency   WG 600
Venous Pressure   WG 106
Venous Pressure, Central see Central Venous Pressure
Venous Thrombosis   WG 610
Venous Ulcer see Varicose Ulcer
Venovenous Hemofiltration see Hemofiltration
Ventilation   WA 770
   Hospitals   WX 165
   Industrial   WA 450
Ventilation, High Frequency Jet see High–Frequency Jet Ventilation
Ventilation, Intermittent Positive–Pressure see Intermittent Positive–Pressure Ventilation
Ventilation, Mechanical see Respiration, Artificial
Ventilation, Middle Ear see Middle Ear Ventilation
Ventilation–Perfusion Ratio   WF 141
Ventilation Tests see Pulmonary Ventilation
Ventilation Tests see Respiratory Function Tests
Ventilators, Mechanical   WF 26
Ventilators, Pulmonary see Ventilators, Mechanical
Ventilatory Muscles see Respiratory Muscles
Ventral Hernia see Hernia, Ventral
Ventricle–Assist Device see Heart–Assist Devices
Ventricular Dysplasia, Right, Arrhythmogenic see Arrhythmogenic Right Ventricular Dysplasia
Ventricular Ejection Fraction see Stroke Volume
Ventricular End–Diastolic Volume see Stroke Volume
Ventricular End–Systolic Volume see Stroke Volume
Ventricular Fibrillation   WG 330
Ventricular Puncture see Punctures
Ventricular Remodeling
   General   WG 202
   Following a particular disease, with the disease
Ventricular System see Cerebral Ventricles
Ventriculography, Cerebral see Cerebral Ventriculography
Verapamil   QV 150
Veratrum   QV 150

Veratrum Alkaloids   QV 150
Verbal Behavior
   Adolescence   WS 462
   Child   WS 105.5.C8
   General psychology   BF 455
   Infant   WS 105.5.C8
   Physiological aspects   WV 501
   Social psychology   HM
   Verbal ability   BF 463.V45
   Verbal self–defense   BF 637.V47
   Speech disorders   WM 475, etc.
Verbal Learning   LB 1139.L3
Vermifuges see Anthelmintics
Vermin, Public Health Aspects see Parasites
Veronal see Barbiturates
Verruga Peruana see Bartonella Infections
Verse's Disease see Calcinosis; Intervertebral Disk
Version, Fetal   WQ 415
Vertebrae see Spine
Vertebral Artery   WG 595.V3
Vertebral Artery Insufficiency see Vertebrobasilar Insufficiency
Vertebrate Viruses
   General works   QW 164
   DNA see DNA Viruses   QW 165
   RNA see RNA Viruses   QW 168
   See also names of other specific vertebrate viruses
Vertebrate Viruses, Unclassified   QW 169
Vertebrates
   Anatomy
     Domestic animals   SF 761–767
     Fishes   QL 639
     Wild animals   QL 801–950.9
       Specific animals or groups of animals, with animal or group
   Diseases   SF 600–997.5, etc.
   Human see specific topics
   Physiology   QP
     Domestic animals   SF 768–768.2
     Fishes   QL 639.1
     Wild animals   QP
   See also other specific topics relating to vertebrates, e.g., Embryology   QL 959, etc.
Vertebrobasilar Insufficiency   WL 355
Vertigo   WV 255
   Aural see Ménire's Disease   WV 258
   Manifestation of disease   QZ 140
Vertigo, Aural see Meniere's Disease
Vervet Monkey see Cercopithecus aethiops
Vesical Calculi see Bladder Calculi
Vesical Fistula see Bladder Fistula
Vesicants see Irritants
Vesication see Blister
Vesico–Ureteral Reflux   WJ 500
   Child   WJ 500
   Infant   WJ 500
Vesicovaginal Fistula   WP 180
Vesicular Exanthema of Swine   SF 977.V3
Vesicular Palmoplantar Eczema see Eczema, Dyshidrotic
Vesicular Skin Diseases see Skin Diseases, Vesiculobullous
Vesiculitis, Seminal see Seminal Vesicles

Vesiculobullous Skin Diseases see Skin Diseases, Vesiculobullous
Vespid Venoms see Wasp Venoms
Vestibular Apparatus see Vestibule
Vestibular Aqueduct   WV 255
Vestibular Diseases   WV 255
Vestibular Function Tests   WV 255
Vestibular Nerve   WL 330
  Physiology of hearing   WV 272
Vestibular Nuclei   WV 255
Vestibule   WV 255
Vestibulo–Ocular Reflex see Reflex, Vestibulo–Ocular
Veterans   UB 356–405
  Hospitalization   UH 460–485
  Lists of veterans   UA 37–39
  Provision for veterans   UB 356–405, etc.
Veterans Disability Claims   UB 368–369.5
Veterans Hospitals see Hospitals, Veterans
Veterans Nursing see Hospitals, Veterans; Military Nursing
Veterinary Anatomy see Anatomy, Veterinary
Veterinary Bacteriology see Veterinary Science QW 70 under Bacteriology
Veterinary Clinics see Hospitals, Animal
Veterinary Drugs   SF 917
  See also Veterinary   SF 915 under Pharmacology
Veterinary Education see Education, Veterinary
Veterinary Histology see Histology
Veterinary Hospitals see Hospitals, Animal
Veterinary Medicine   SF 600–1100
  Education   SF 756.3–756.37
  Immunology   SF 757.2
  Military see Veterinary Service, Military   UH 650–655
  Surgery see Surgery, Veterinary   SF 911–914.4
  See also Veterinary under particular topics and specific animals being treated
Veterinary Microbiology see Microbiology
Veterinary Pathology see Pathology, Veterinary
Veterinary Schools see Schools, Veterinary
Veterinary Service, Military   UH 650–655
Veterinary Toxicology see Toxicology
Vibration
  Adverse effects (General)   WD 640
  As a cause of disease   QZ 57
  In aviation   WD 735
  In industry
    Diseases   WA 400
    Prevention & control   WA 470
  Therapeutic use   WB 535
Vibrio   QW 141
Vibrio fetus see Campylobacter fetus
Vibrio Infections   WC 200
  Veterinary   SF 809.V52
  See also Cholera   WC 262–264
Vibrio parahaemolyticus   QW 141
Vibrionaceae   QW 141
Vibrocardiography see Kinetocardiography
Vicarious Menstruation see Menstruation Disorders
Vichy Water see Mineral Waters
Victimization see Crime Victims

Vidarabine   QU 57
  As an antiviral agent   QV 268.5
Video Display Terminals see Computer Terminals
Video Games
  Child psychology   WS 105.5.P5
  Effects on children   WS 105.5.E9
Video Recording   TK 6655.V5
  Recording by subject
Videodisc Recording   TK 6685
  Catalogs and works about (Form number 18.2 in any NLM schedules where applicable)
  Actual recordings, by subject
Videotape Recording
  Catalogs and works about (Form number 18.2 in any NLM schedule where applicable)
  Actual recordings, by subject
Videotherapy
  In psychiatry   WM 450.5.V5
Vidine see Choline
Vigilance see Attention
Vigilance, Cortical see Arousal
Village Health Worker see Community Health Aides
Vinblastine   QV 269
Vinca Alkaloids   QV 269
Vincaleukoblastine see Vinblastine
Vincent's Angina see Gingivitis, Necrotizing Ulcerative
Vincent's Infection see Gingivitis, Necrotizing Ulcerative
Vincristine   QV 269
Vinyl Chloride
  As carcinogen   QZ 202
Vinyl Chloride Polymer see Polyvinyl Chloride
Vinyl Compounds
  Organic chemistry   QD 305.H7
  Toxicology   QV 633
Vinyl Ether   QV 81
Vinylidene Chlorides see Dichloroethylenes
Violence
  Adolescence   WS 463
  Child   WS 350.8.A4
    Influence of television   WS 105.5.E9
  Criminal (Medicolegal aspects)   W 860
  Infant   WS 350.8.A4
  Political theory   JC 328.6
  Psychology (General)   BF 575.A3
  Sociology   HM
Viper Venoms   WD 410
Viral Antibodies see Antibodies, Viral
Viral Antigens see Antigens, Viral
Viral DNA see DNA, Viral
Viral Gene Expression Regulation see Gene Expression Regulation, Viral
Viral Gene Products see Viral Proteins
Viral Gene Proteins see Viral Proteins
Viral Genes see Genes, Viral
Viral Hepatitis Vaccines   WC 536
Viral Interference   QW 160
Viral Markers see Biological Markers
Viral Physiology   QW 160
Viral Proteins   QW 160
Viral RNA see RNA, Viral
Viral Tumor Antigens see Antigens, Viral, Tumor

Vitamin B 12   QU 194
Vitamin B 12 Deficiency   WD 120
Vitamin B 2 see Riboflavin
Vitamin B 6 see Pyridoxine
Vitamin C see Ascorbic Acid
Vitamin Content of Food see Analysis   QU 160
  under Vitamins; Nutrition
Vitamin D   QU 173
Vitamin D Deficiency   WD 145
Vitamin D 2 see Ergocalciferols
Vitamin D 3 see Cholecalciferol
Vitamin Deficiency see Avitaminosis
Vitamin E   QU 179
Vitamin E Deficiency   WD 150
Vitamin G see Riboflavin
Vitamin H see Biotin
Vitamin K   QU 181
Vitamin K Deficiency   WD 155
Vitamin K 1 see Phytonadione
Vitamin M see Folic Acid
Vitamin P Complex see Bioflavonoids
Vitamin PP see Niacinamide
Vitamins   QU 160–220
  Analysis   QU 160
    Clinical assay   QY 350
  Animal nutrition   SF 98.V5
  Animal physiology
    Domestic   SF 768–768.2
    Wild   QP 771–772
  Fat soluble   QU 165–181
  Plant constituents   QK 898.V5
  Water soluble   QU 185–210
  See also names of specific vitamins
Vitiligo   WR 265
Vitrectomy   WW 250
Vitreous Body   WW 250
  Opacity   WW 250
Vitreous Detachment   WW 250
Vitreous Fluorophotometry see Fluorophotometry
Vivisection
  Experimental surgery   WO 50
  Sociological aspects   HV 4915
Vocabulary   P 305
  Special topics, by subject
Vocabulary, Controlled   Z 695–695.1
  Medicine   Z 695.1.M48
Vocabulary Tests see Language Tests
Vocal Cord Paralysis   WV 535
Vocal Cords   WV 530–535
Vocal Fold see Vocal Cords
Vocalization, Animal   QL 765
Vocational Education   LC 1041–1048
  Exceptional children   LC 3976
Vocational Guidance   HF 5381–5382.5
  Dentistry   WU 21
  Dietetics   WB 400
  For the blind   HV 1652–1658
  For the deaf   HV 2452–2458
  For the mentally disabled   HV 3005
  For the physically disabled   HD 7255–7256; HV
    3018–3019
  Hospital administration   WX 155
  Hospital work (General)   WX 159

  Nurses' aides   WY 193
  Nursing   WY 16
    See also special types of nursing
  Ophthalmology   WW 21
  Opticianry   WW 721
  Optometry   WW 721
  Physicians   W 21
  Psychiatry   WM 21
  Surgery   WO 21
  In other areas, with the number for the profession
    or lacking that, in a general works number
Vocational Rehabilitation see Rehabilitation,
  Vocational
Vocations see Occupations
Voice
  Care   WV 500
  Physiology   WV 501
Voice Disorders   WV 500
  Psychogenic   WM 475
Voice Production, Alaryngeal see Speech,
  Alaryngeal
Voice Prosthesis see Larynx, Artificial
Voice Quality   WV 501
Voice Training   WV 500
Volatile Oils see Oils, Volatile
Volatile Poisons see Poisons
Volcanic Ash see Volcanic Eruption
Volcanic Eruption
  First aid   WA 292
  Hospital emergency service   WX 215
  Medical emergencies   WB 105
Volcanic Gases see Volcanic Eruption
Voles see Microtinae
Volhynia Fever see Trench Fever
Volition   BF 608–635
Volkmann Contracture see Compartment Syndromes
Volkmann's Contracture see Compartment
  Syndromes
Volume Index see Blood Volume
Voluntary Health Agencies   WA 1
  (Form number 1 in any NLM schedule where
    applicable)
  See also Red Cross   HV 560–583, etc.; names
    of specialties
Voluntary Health Insurance see Insurance, Health
Voluntary Sterilization see Sterilization, Sexual
Voluntary Workers
  In hospitals see Hospital Volunteers   WX 159.5,
    etc.
  In psychiatry   WM 30.5
  In social service   HV 41
  In other areas, by subject
Volunteers see Voluntary Workers
Volvulus see Intestinal Obstruction
Volvulus, Stomach see Stomach Volvulus
Vomer see Nasal Septum
Vomiting   WI 146
  Drugs promoting see Emetics   QV 73
  Pregnancy   WQ 215
  See also Adverse effects   WO 245 under
    Anesthesia
Von Gierke's Disease see Glycogen Storage Disease
  Type I

**ALWAYS CONSULT MAIN SCHEDULES. USE NUMBER ASSIGNED ONLY WHEN
SUBJECT REPRESENTS MAJOR EMPHASIS OF WORK BEING CLASSIFIED**

von Willebrand Disease   WH 312
von Willebrand Factor   WH 310
Voyages see Expeditions; Travel
VP 16-213 see Etoposide
Vulva   WP 200
Vulvar Neoplasms   WP 200
Vulvitis   WP 200
Vulvovaginal Glands see Bartholin's Glands
Vulvovaginitis   WP 200
VZ Virus see Heepesvirus 3, Human

W

Wages see Salaries and Fringe Benefits
Waiting Lists
    In hospitals   WX 159
    Practice management
        Dental   WU 77
        Medical   W 80
Wakefulness   WL 108
    In personal hygiene   QT 265
Waldenstrom Macroglobulinemia   WH 400
    Clinical pathology   QY 455
Walking
    As locomotion   WE 103
    As a sport   QT 260.5.W2
Wallabies see Kangaroos
War   U; V
    Adolescent psychology   WS 462
    Atomic warfare   U 263
    Bacterial warfare   UG 447.8
        For the bacteriologists   QW 300
    Biological warfare   UG 447.8
        For the bacteriologists   QW 300
    Chemical warfare   UG 447-447.65
    Child psychology   WS 105.5.E9
    Civil defense   UA 926-929
    Combat psychiatry   UH 629-629.5
    Military dentistry   UH 430-435
        Naval   VG 280-285
    Military medical services   UH 201-630
    Morale   U 22
    Naval medical services   VG 100-475
    Psychiatry see Military Psychiatry   UH 629-629.5
    Psychological warfare   UB 275-277
    Psychology see Psychology, Military   U 22.3
    Rehabilitation   UB 360-366
    Surgery   WO 800
    Veterinary services   UH 650-655
    War crimes   JX 5419.5
    Wounded, Transportation   UH 500-505
    See also Military Hygiene   UH 600-627;
        Military Medicine   UH 201-515, etc.
War Gases see Chemical Warfare Agents
War Neuroses see Combat Disorders
Ward Administration see Hospital Administration
Ward Attendants see Nurses' Aides; Personnel,
    Hospital; Psychiatric Aides
Ward Secretaries see Personnel, Hospital
Wards, Hospital see Hospital Units; also special
    topics under Manuals and Nursing, Supervisory
Warfare, Biological see Biological Warfare

Warfarin   QV 193
Wart-Hog Disease Virus see African Swine Fever
    Virus
Warthin Tumor see Adenolymphoma
Wasp Venoms   WD 430
Wasps   QX 565
Waste Disposal, Fluid   WA 785
Waste Disposal, Industrial see Industrial Waste
Waste Disposal, Solid see Refuse Disposal
Waste Products   WA 670
    Utilization   TP 995-996
    Special topics, by subject
    See also names of particular products, e.g.,
        Radioactive Pollutants   WN 615, etc.
Wasting Disease see Wasting Syndrome
Wasting Disease, HIV see HIV Wasting Syndrome
Wasting Syndrome   WB 146
    Associated with nutrition disorders   WD 100
        Child   WS 115
        Infant   WS 115
    In connection with specific diseases, with the
        disease
    See also HIV Wasting Syndrome   WC 503.5
Wasting Syndrome, HIV see HIV Wasting
    Syndrome
Water
    Analysis   WA 686-689
        Bacteriological see Water Microbiology   QW
            80
        Pharmacology   QV 270-273
    As a beverage   WB 442
        See also Drinking   WI 102; Water Supply
            WA 675-690
    Bacteriology see Water Microbiology   QW 80
    Balance see Water-Electrolyte Balance   QU 105
    Imbalance see Water-Electrolyte Imbalance
        WD 220
    Metabolism   QU 120
    Mineral see Mineral Waters   WB 442
    Officinal   QV 785
    Pharmacology   QV 270-273
    Therapeutic use see Hydrotherapy   WB 520;
        Balneology   WB 525
    See also Seawater   WB 525, etc.
Water Buffaloes see Buffaloes
Water Consumption see Drinking
Water Deprivation
    Experimental biochemistry   QU 34
    Experimental pharmacology   QV 34
    Experimental physiology   QT 25
    See also Dehydration   WD 220, etc.; Thirst
        WI 102
Water-Electrolyte Balance   QU 105
Water-Electrolyte Imbalance   WD 220
Water Intake see Drinking
Water Microbiology   QW 80
Water Pollutants   WA 689
    See also names of specific pollutants
Water Pollutants, Chemical   WA 689
Water Pollutants, Radioactive   WN 615
Water Pollution   WA 689
    See also Sewage   WA 785, etc.
Water Pollution, Chemical   WA 689

Water Pollution, Radioactive   WN 615
Water Softening   TP 263
   Public health aspects   WA 675–689
Water Supply   WA 675–690
   Analysis
      Bacteriological see Water Microbiology   QW 80
      General works   WA 686
   Purification   WA 690
   Sanitation   WA 675
Waterborne Diseases see Communicable Diseases; Water Pollution
Waterhouse-Friderichsen Syndrome   WC 245
Waxes   QU 85
Weaning   WS 125
Weather
   Meteorology (Physics)   QC 980–999
   Relation to disease   WB 700–710
      Of animals   SF 760.C55
   See also Acclimatization   QT 145–160
Weaver Mice see Mice, Neurologic Mutants
Webbed Fingers and Toes see Abnormalities   WE 835 under Fingers and under Toes
Weber-Christian Disease see Panniculitis, Nodular Nonsuppurative
Wechsler Scales
   For adults   BF 432.5.W4
   For children   BF 432.5.W42
Wegener's Granulomatosis   WF 600
Weight Gain
   Child   WS 103
   Infant   WS 103
Weight Lifting   QT 260.5.W4
Weight Loss
   Child   WS 103
   Infant   WS 103
Weight-Loss Agents see Anti-Obesity Agents
Weight Perception   WE 104
Weight Reduction see Weight Loss
Weight Tables for Children see Tables   WS 16 under Body Weight
Weightlessness   WD 752
Weights and Measures   QC 81–114
   Pharmaceutical   QV 16
   See also Metric System   QC 90.8–94
Weil's Disease   WC 420
   Veterinary   SF 809.L4
Welding
   Occupational accidents   WA 485
   Occupational medicine   WA 400–495
Welfare Work see Social Work; Social Welfare
Wellness Centers see Fitness Centers
Wellness Programs see Health Promotion
Wens, Sebaceous see Epidermal Cyst
Werner Syndrome   QZ 45
Wernicke Area see Temporal Lobe
Wernicke's Encephalopathy   WD 122
West Syndrome see Spasms, Infantile
Western Blotting see Blotting, Western
Western Immunoblotting see Blotting, Western
Wet Lung see Pulmonary Edema
Whales   QL 737.C4
   Diseases   SF 997.5.M35

Wheat
   As a dietary supplement in health or disease   WB 431
   Cultivation   SB 191.W5
   See also Bread   WB 431, etc.
Wheelchairs   WB 320
   Catalogs   W 26
   For particular disability, by the disability
Wheezing see Respiratory Sounds
Whiplash Injuries   WE 725
Whirlpool Baths see Hydrotherapy
White Blood Cell Count see Leukocyte Count
White Blood Cell Transfusion see Leukocyte Transfusion
White Blood Cells see Leukocytes
White Spots see Dental Caries
Whitefish see Salmonidae
Whites
   Anthropology   GN 537
   Other special topics, by subject, e.g., Alcohol problem   WM 274
Whitmore's Disease see Melioidosis
Whole-Body Counting   WN 660
Whole-Body Irradiation
   Adverse effects   WN 620
   Therapeutic use   WN 450
   Other aspects, by subject
Whooping Cough   WC 340
Widowers see Widowhood
Widowhood   HQ 1058–1058.5
   Special topics, by subject
Widows see Widowhood
Widows and Widowers see Widowhood
Wife Abuse see Spouse Abuse
Wild Animals see Animals, Wild
Will see Volition
Wilms' Tumor see Nephroblastoma
Wilson's Disease see Hepatolenticular Degeneration
Wind   QC 930.5–959
Wine
   As a dietary supplement in health or disease   WB 444
   Chemical technology   TP 544–561
Wing   QL 950.7
   Birds   QL 697–698.9
   Insects   QX 500
Wirsung's Duct see Pancreatic Ducts
Wit and Humor   PN 6147–6231
   Medicine and related subjects   WZ 305–305.5
   Satire on medicine   WZ 305–305.5
Withdrawal Symptoms see Substance Withdrawal Syndrome
Wittenborn Scales see Psychiatric Status Rating Scales
Wolff-Parkinson-White Syndrome   WG 330
Wolfram see Tungsten
Wolves   QL 737.C22
Women
   As physicians see Physicians, Women   W 21; WZ 80.5.W5
   As dentists see Dentists, Women   WU 21
   In industry   HD 6050–6220.7
   In history of medicine   WZ 80.5.W5

ALWAYS CONSULT MAIN SCHEDULES. USE NUMBER ASSIGNED ONLY WHEN SUBJECT REPRESENTS MAJOR EMPHASIS OF WORK BEING CLASSIFIED

Protection WA 491
In marriage HQ
In medicine see Physicians, Women W 21, etc.
Psychoanalysis WM 460.5.W6
See also Gynecology WP, etc.; Obstetrics
    WQ, etc.; other specific subjects
Women Physicians see Physicians, Women
Women, Working
    Special topics, by subject
Women's Health WA 309
Women's Health Services
    General WA 309
Women's Liberation see Women's Rights
Women's Rights HQ 1236–1236.5
    As executives HD 6054.3–6054.4
    As educators LB 2837
    In industry HD 6050–6220.7
    U.S. HQ 1236.5.U6
    See also Physicians, Women W 21, etc.
Wood
    Industrial accidents among wood workers WA 485
    Occupational disease of wood workers WA 400–495
Wool SF 377
    Animal anatomy QL 942
        Domestic animals SF 761–767
    Textile fibers TS 1547
Woolly Monkey see Cebidae
Woolsorters' Disease see Anthrax
Word Association Tests
    Psychiatry WM 145.5.W9
    Psychology BF 698.8.A8
Word Processing
    In particular fields (Form number 26.5 in any NLM schedule where applicable)
    Used for special purposes, by subject
Work
    Health see Occupational Health WA 400–495, etc.
    Physical effects WE 103
    Psychology BF 481
Work Capacity Evaluation
    Medicolegal aspects W 925
    Special topics, by subject
Work of Breathing WF 102
Work Satisfaction see Job Satisfaction
Work Schedule Tolerance
    Occupational health aspects WA 400–495
    Physiological effects WE 103
    Psychological aspects BF 481
Workers' Compensation HD 7103.6–7103.65
    Medicolegal aspects W 925
Working Women see Women, Working
Workmen's Compensation see Workers' Compensation
World Health WA 530
World Wide Web see Internet
Worms see Helminths
Wound Healing WO 185
    Pathology QZ 150
    Surgical wounds WO 185
Wound Infection WC 255

See also Surgical Wound Infection WO 185
Wounded, Transportation see Transportation of Patients
Wounds and Injuries WO 700–820
    As a cause of disease QZ 55
    Closure WO 188
    General systemic reaction QZ 160
    Local reaction QZ 150
    Medicolegal aspects in death W 843
    Minor injuries WA 292
    Minor surgery WO 192
    Veterinary SF 914.3–914.4
    See also Surgical Wound Dehiscence WO 185; Surgical Wound Infections WO 185; Wound Infection WC 255; names of various types of injury, by cause or site, e.g., Blast Injuries WO 820; Facial Injuries WE 706
Wounds, Gunshot WO 807
Wounds, Multiple see Multiple Trauma
Wounds, Penetrating WO 700–820
WPW Syndrome see Wolff–Parkinson–White Syndrome
WR–2721 see Amifostine
Wrestling QT 260.5.W9
Wrist WE 830
Wrist Injuries WE 830
Wrist Joint WE 830
Writing
    English (General) PE 1402–1497
    In psychotherapy WM 450.5.W9
    Medical WZ 345
    Rules (English) PE 1411
    See also Handwriting Z 105–115.5, etc.
Wryneck see Torticollis
Wuchereria QX 301

X

X Chromosome QH 600.5
X–Linked Lymphoproliferative Syndrome see Lymphoproliferative Disorders
X–Ray Departments see Radiology Department, Hospital
X–Ray Diagnosis see Radiography
X–Ray, Diagnostic see Radiography
X–Ray Emission Spectrometry see Spectrometry, X–Ray Emission
X–Ray Emission Spectrometry, Electron Microscopic see Electron Probe Microanalysis
X–Ray Emission Spectrometry, Electron Probe see Electron Probe Microanalysis
X–Ray Film WN 150
    Used for specific purpose, by subject
X–Ray Film–Screen Systems see X–Ray Intensifying Screens
X–Ray Fluorescence Spectrometry see Spectrometry, X–Ray Emission
X–ray Information Systems see Radiology Information Systems
X–Ray Intensifying Screens WN 150
    Used for specific purpose, by subject
X–Ray Measurement in Obstetrics see Pelvimetry
X–Ray Microanalysis, Electron Microscopic see

Electron Probe Microanalysis
X–Ray Microanalysis, Electron Probe see Electron
Probe Microanalysis
X–Ray Service, Hospital see Radiology Department,
Hospital
X–Ray Therapy   WN 250.5.X7
X–Ray Tomography see Tomography, X–Ray
X–Ray Tomography, Computed see Tomography,
X–Ray Computed
X–Rays
General works   WN 105
Diagnostic use (General)   WN 200
Therapeutic use   WN 250.5.X7
Physics   QC 480.8–482.3
Xanthines   QV 107
Xanthinol Niacinate   QV 150
Xanthinol Nicotinate see Xanthinol Niacinate
Xanthomatosis   WD 205.5.X2
Xanthotoxin see Methoxsalen
Xantinol Nicotinate see Xanthinol Niacinate
Xenarthra   QL 737.E2
Xenoantibodies see Antibodies, Heterophile
Xenobiotics
As carcinogens   QZ 202
Metabolism   QU 120
Xenograft see Transplantation, Heterologous
Xenograft Bioprosthesis see Bioprosthesis
Xenograft Dressings see Biological Dressings
Xenon
Inorganic chemistry   QD 181.X4
Pharmacology   QV 310
Xenopus   QL 668.E265
As laboratory animals   QY 60.A6
Xeroderma see Ichthyosis
Xeroderma Pigmentosum   WR 265
Xeromammography   WP 815
Xerophthalmia   WW 208
Xeroradiography, Breast see Xeromammography
Xerostomia   WI 230
Xiphosura see Horseshoe Crabs
Xylenes
As antiseptics   QV 223
Organic chemistry   QD 341.H9
Xylitol
Organic chemistry   QD 305.A4
Pharmacology   QV 82
Xylose   QU 75
XYY Karyotype   QS 677

Y

Y Chromosome   QH 600.5
Yaws   WC 425
Yeast, Budding see Saccharomycetales
Yeast, Dried   WB 447
Yeast, Fission see Schizosaccharomyces
Yeasts
As a dietary supplement in health or disease
WB 447
Microbiology   QW 180.5.Y3
Processing   TP 433
Yellow Fever   WC 530–532
Yellow Jackets see Wasps

Yellow Marrow see Bone Marrow
Yersinia   QW 138.5.Y3
Yersinia enterocolitica   QW 138.5.Y3
Yersinia Infections   WC 350–355
Yersinia pseudotuberculosis   QW 138.5.Y3
Yersinia pseudotuberculosis Infections   WC
350–355
Yoga   QT 255
Philosophy   B 132.Y6
Therapeutics see Alternative Medicine   WB 890,
etc.
Yogurt   SF 275.Y6
As a dietary supplement in health or disease
WB 428
Bacteriology   QW 85
Sanitation   WA 715
Yohimbans
As cardiovascular agents   QV 150
Organic chemistry   QD 421
Yohimbine   QV 132
Yolk Proteins see Egg Proteins
Yolk Sac Tumor see Endodermal Sinus Tumor
Youth see Adolescence
Yttrium Isotopes
Inorganic chemistry   QD 181.Y1
Pharmacology   QV 290

Z

Z–DNA see DNA
Zea see Corn
Zearalenone
As a mycotoxin   QW 630.5.M9
As an estrogen   WP 522
Special topics, by subject
Zebrafish   QL 638.C94
Zidovudine   QV 185
Special topics, by subject
Zimeldine
As an antidepressant   QV 77.5
Zimelidine see Zimeldine
Zimmermann's Corpuscles see Blood Platelets
Zinc
Inorganic chemistry   QD 181.Z6
Pharmacology   QV 298
Zinc Isotopes
Inorganic chemistry   QD 181.Z6
Pharmacology   QV 298
Zingiberaceae see Zingiberales
Zingiberales
As dietary supplements in health and disease
WB 430
As medicinal plants   QV 766
Botany   QK 495.A14
Zingiberaceae (Ginger)   QK 495.Z65
Ziram
As an industrial fungicide   WA 240
Toxicology   QV 298
Zirconium
Inorganic chemistry   QD 181.Z7
Pharmacology   QV 290
Zollinger-Ellison Syndrome   WK 885
Of the duodenum   WI 505

ALWAYS CONSULT MAIN SCHEDULES. USE NUMBER ASSIGNED ONLY WHEN
SUBJECT REPRESENTS MAJOR EMPHASIS OF WORK BEING CLASSIFIED

Zona see Herpes Zoster
Zona Pellucida   WQ 205
    Animal   QL 965
Zone Therapy see Massage
Zonography see Tomography, X–Ray
Zoology   QL
    Biography
        Collective   QL 26
        Individual   WZ 100
    Societies   QL 1
Zoonoses   WC 950
    Prevention & control   WA 110
    See also names of specific diseases
Zoophaginae see Viruses
Zoster see Herpes Zoster
Zuclomifene see Clomiphene
Zygote   WQ 205
Zymogens see Enzyme Precursors
Zymosan   QU 83

1

1–Oxacephalosporin see Moxalactam
1–Propanol
    Organic chemistry   QD 305.A4
    Pharmacology   QV 82
1–Sar–8–Ala Angiotensin II see Saralasin
1–Sarcosine–8–Alanine Angiotensin II see Saralasin
1,2–Benzopyrones see Coumarins
1,2–Dibromoethane see Ethylene Dibromide
1,8–Dihydroxy–9–anthrone see Anthralin
13–cis–Retinoic Acid see Isotretinoin
17 beta–Estradiol see Estradiol
17–Ketosteroids   WK 755
    Synthetic   WK 757
17–Oxosteroids see 17–Ketosteroids

2

2–Acetamidofluorene see 2–Acetylaminofluorene
2–Acetylaminofluorene   QZ 202
2–Aminoethylisothiuronium Bromide see AET
2–Bromoergocryptine see Bromocriptine
2–Chlorethanol see Ethylene Chlorohydrin
2–Chloroacetophenone see
    omega–Chloroacetophenone
2–Chloroethyl Alcohol see Ethylene Chlorohydrin
2–Hydroxyphenethylamine   QU 61
2–Mercaptoethanesulfonate see Mesna
2–Phenylethanolamine see
    2–Hydroxyphenethylamine
2–Propanol
    Pharmacology   QV 82
2',3'–Cyclic–Nucleotide Phosphodiesterases   QU 136
2,4–D see 2,4–Dichlorophenoxyacetic Acid
2,4–Dichlorophenoxyacetic Acid
    As a herbicide
        Agriculture   SB 951.4
        Public health   WA 240
    Organic chemistry   QD 341.A2
2',5'–Oligoadenylate Polymerase see
    2',5'–Oligoadenylate Synthetase
2',5'–Oligoadenylate Synthetase   QU 141

2–5A Synthetase see 2',5'–Oligoadenylate Synthetase
21–Hydroxyprogesterone see Desoxycorticosterone

3

3–Isoleucine,8–Leucine Vasopressin see Oxytocin
3,4–Benzopyrene see Benzo(a)pyrene
3,4–Methylenedioxyamphetamine   QV 102

4

4–Aminobutyrate Transaminase   QU 141
4–Aminobutyric Acid see GABA
4–Aminohippuric Acid see p–Aminohippuric Acid

5

5–HT see Serotonin
5–HT Antagonists see Serotonin Antagonists
5–Hydroxytryptamine see Serotonin
5–Hydroxytryptamine Antagonists see Serotonin
    Antagonists
5,12–diHETE see Leukotriene B4
5,12–HETE see Leukotriene B4

6

6–Mercaptopurine   QV 269

7

7S RNA see RNA, Small Nuclear

8

8–Hydroxyquinoline see Oxyquinoline
8–Methoxypsoralen see Methoxsalen
8–Quinolinol see Oxyquinoline

ALWAYS CONSULT MAIN SCHEDULES. USE NUMBER ASSIGNED ONLY WHEN
SUBJECT REPRESENTS MAJOR EMPHASIS OF WORK BEING CLASSIFIED

Appendix 1

Numbers Added or Deleted

The following is a list of new classification numbers added to the *NLM Classification* since the publication of the fourth edition, revised in 1981. It also includes numbers added since the publication of the 5th edition, which appear in italics, and were previously announced in *NLM Technical Bulletins* beginning with 1996. It does not include those numbers added for general coverage following a Table G number or for "Special topics, etc."

The column on the right reflects where materials on the subject were most often classified. "Various places" indicates that no "most often used" number was found. "None" identifies new numbers for concepts new to the *Classification*.

Although a notation may indicate that a subject was formerly classed in a particular number, that number may still be acceptable for material that represents another aspect of the subject.

Added Numbers

New	Subjects	Old
QS Human Anatomy		
QS 18.2	Educational materials	QS 18
QS 39	Handbooks	None
QS 518.2	Educational materials [Histology]	QS 518
QS 529	Handbooks [Histology]	QS 539
QS 618.2	Educational materials [Embryology]	QS 618
QS 629	Handbooks [Embryology]	QS 639
QT Physiology		
QT 18.2	Educational materials	QT 18
QT 29	Handbooks	QT 39
QT 36	Biomedical engineering	QT 34
QT 37	Biomedical and biocompatible materials	QT 34
QT 37.5	Specific materials, A-Z	QT 34
QT 260.5	Specific activities, A-Z [Athletics. Sports]	QT 260
QT 261	Sports medicine	QT 260
QU Biochemistry		
QU 18.2	Educational materials	QU 18
QU 39	Handbooks	None
QU 54	Nitrogen and related compounds	QU 55
QU 56	Nucleoproteins	QU 58
QU 57	Nucleosides. Nucleotides	QU 58
QU 58.5	DNA	QU 58
QU 58.7	RNA	QU 58
QU 61	Amines. Amidines	QU 60
QU 62	Amides	QU 60
QU 86	Fats. Oils	QU 85
QU 107	Growth substances. Growth inhibitors	QU 100
QU 130.5	Trace elements	QU 130

New	Subjects	Old
	QU Biochemistry – Continued	
QU 145.5	Nutritive values of food	QU 145
	QV Pharmacology	
QV 18.2	Educational materials	QV 18
QV 39	Handbooks	None
QV 77.2	Psychotropic drugs	QV 77
QV 350.5	Specific drugs, A-Z	QV 350
	QV 600 Toxicology	
QV 607	Handbooks	None
	QV 700 Pharmacy and Pharmaceutics	
QV 715	Classification. Nomenclature. Terminology	Various places
QV 717	Atlases. Pictorial works	QV 17
QV 722	Directories	QV 22
QV 732	Laws	QV 32
QV 733	Discussions of law. Jurisprudence	QV 33
QV 735	Handbooks	None
QV 760	Materia medica	None
	QW Microbiology and Immunology	
QW 18.2	Educational materials	QW 18
QW 25.5	Specific techniques, A-Z [Laboratory manuals. Technique]	Various places
QW 39	Handbooks	None
QW 50	Bacteria. Bacteriology	QW 4
QW 55	Environmental microbiology	None
QW 518.2	Educational materials [Immunology]	QV 518
QW 525.5	Specific techniques, A- Z [Laboratory manuals. Technique]	Various places
QW 539	Handbooks [Immunology]	None
QW 540	Immunity (General)	QV 504
QW 545	Autoimmunity	QV 504
QW 573.5	Specific antigens, A-Z	QV 573
QW 575.5	Specific antibodies, A-Z	QV 575
QW 630.5	Specific toxins and antitoxins, A-Z	QV 530
	QX Parasitology	
QX 18.2	Educational materials	QX 18
QX 39	Handbooks	None
QX 45	Host-parasite relations	Various places
	QY Clinical Pathology	
QY 18.2	Educational materials	QY 18
QY 39	Handbooks	None
	QZ Pathology	
QZ 18.2	Educational materials	QZ 18
QZ 39	Handbooks	None
QZ 275	Pediatric oncology. Adolescent oncology	QZ 200-269

Added Numbers

New	Subjects	Old
	W Health Professions	
W 18.2	Educational materials	W 18
W 20.55	Special topics, A-Z [Medical research]	Various places
W 26.55	Special topics, A-Z [Medical informatics …]	Various places
W 49	Handbooks	W 39
W82	*Medical technology (General)*	*Various places*
W 83	*Telemedicine (General) (Table G)*	*Various places*
W 83.1	*General Coverage (Not Table G)*	*Various places*
W 85.5	Right to die. Advance directives. Living wills	Various places
W 130	Managed care plans	Various places
W 132	Health maintenance organizations	W 125
W 160	Hospitalization insurance …	W 100-125
W 255	Nursing insurance	None
	W 600 Forensic Medicine and Dentistry	
W 618.2	Educational materials	W 618
W 639	Handbooks	None
	WA Public Health	
WA 18.2	Educational materials	WA 18
WA 30.5	*Environmental medicine. Environmental illness*	*Various places*
WA 39	Handbooks	None
WA 309	Women's health	Various places
WA 330	*Adolescent health services*	*Various places*
WA 530	International health administration	WA 540
WA 790	Medical waste. Dental waste	Various places
	WB Practice of Medicine	
WB 18.2	Educational materials	WB 18
WB 39	Handbooks	None
WB 101	Ambulatory care (General)	Various places
WB 102	Clinical medicine	None
WB 103	Behavioral medicine	None
WB 104	Medical Psychology	None
WB 327	Self care	None
WB 422	Macrobiotic diet	None
	WC Communicable Diseases	
WC 18.2	Educational materials	WC 18
WC 39	Handbooks	None
WC 501	RNA virus infections	WC 500
WC 502	Retroviridae infections	WC 500
WC 503	Acquired immunodeficiency syndrome. HIV infections	WD 308
	WD 100 Nutrition Disorders	
WD 101	Handbooks	None
	WD 200 Metabolic Diseases	
WD 200.1	Handbooks	None

Added Numbers

New	Subjects	Old
	WD 300 Immunology and Collagen Diseases. Hypersensitivity	
WD 301	Handbooks	None
	WD Animal Poisons	
WD 401	Handbooks	None
	WD 500 Plant Poisons	
WD 501	Handbooks	None
	WD 600 Diseases and Injuries Caused by Physical Agents	
WD 601	Handbooks	None
	WD 700 Aviation	
WD 701	Handbooks	WD 704
WD 704	Research	None
	WD 750 Space Medicine	
WD 751	Research	WD 704
WD 751.6	Medical informatics. Automatic data processing. Computers	None
	WE Musculoskeletal System	
WE 18.2	Educational materials	WE 18
WE 39	Handbooks	None
WE 304	Joint diseases	WE 300
	WF Respiratory System	
WF 18.2	Educational materials	WF 18
WF 39	Handbooks	None
WF 141.5	Specific techniques, A-Z [Examination. Diagnosis ...]	Various places
	WG Cardiovascular System	
WG 18.2	Educational materials	WG 18
WG 39	Handbooks	None
WG 120	Cardiovascular diseases	WG 100
WG 166.5	Specific therapeutic methods, A-Z	Various places
WG 210	Heart diseases	WG 200
	WH Hemic and Lymphatic Systems	
WH 18.2	Educational materials	WH 18
WH 39	Handbooks	None
WH 120	Hematologic diseases	WH 100
	WI Digestive System	
WI 18.2	Educational materials	WI 18
WI 39	Handbooks	None
WI 140	Diseases	WI 100
WI 529	Neoplasms. Polyps [Colon]	WI 520
WI 715	*Hepatitis (General or not elsewhere classified)*	*Various places*
WI 830	Surgery (General) [Pancreas]	WI 800

Added Numbers

New	Subjects	Old
	WJ Urogenital System	
WJ 18.2	Educational materials	WJ 18
WJ 39	Handbooks	None
WJ 140	Urologic diseases	WJ 100
WJ 706	Neoplasms (General) [Male genitalia]	WJ 700
	WK Endocrine System	
WK 18.2	Educational materials	WK 18
WK 39	Handbooks	None
WK 140	Endocrine diseases	WK 100
WK 148	*Endocrine surgical procedures (General)*	*WK 140*
	WL Nervous System	
WL 18.2	Educational materials	WL 18
WL 39	Handbooks	None
WL 103.5	Neuropsychology	WL 103
WL 103.7	Psychoneuroimmunology	None
WL 105	Neuroendocrinology	None
WL 140	Nervous system diseases	WL 100
WL 160	Nervous system Neoplasms	Various places
WL 340.2	Communicative disorders. Speech-language pathology	WL 340
	WM Psychiatry	
WM 18.2	Educational materials	WM 18
WM 34	Handbooks	None
WM 102	Biological psychiatry	WM 100
WM 140	Mental disorders	WM 100
WM 145.5	Specific tests, A-Z [Psychologic]	WM 145
WM 165	Behavioral symptoms	Various places
WM 284	Narcotics	WM 270
WM 290	Nicotine	Various places
WM 420.5	Special types, A-Z [Psychotherapy]	WM 420
WM 425.5	Special types, A-Z [Behavior therapy]	WM 425
WM 475.5	Aphasia [Psychogenic]	WM 475
WM 475.6	Dyslexia [Psychogenic]	WM 475
	WN Radiology. Medical Imaging	
WN 18.2	Educational materials	WN 18
WN 39	Handbooks	None
WN 105	Ionizing radiation	WN 100
WN 180	Diagnostic imaging	Various places
WN 185	Magnetic resonance imaging	Various places
WN 203	Radionuclide imaging	WN 445
WN 205	Thermography	WB 270
WN 206	Tomography	WN 160
WN 208	Ultrasonography	WB 289
WN 250.5	Special types, A-Z [Radiotherapy]	WN 250
WN 600	Radiobiology	WN 610
WN 660	Radiometry	WN 650
WN 665	Radiation dosage	WN 650

Added Numbers

New	Subjects	Old
	WO Surgery	
WO 18.2	Educational materials	WO 18
WO 39	Handbooks	None
	WO 200 Anesthesia	
WO 218.2	Educational materials	WO 218
WO 231	Handbooks	None
	WO 500 Operative Surgery and Surgical Techniques	
WO 505	*Endoscopic surgery*	*WO 500*
WO 511	Laser surgery	WO 500
	WP Gynecology	
WP 18.2	Educational materials	WP 18
WP 34	Malpractice	WP 32-33
WP 39	Handbooks	None
WP 440	Uterine diseases	WP 400
	WQ Obstetrics	
WQ 18.2	Educational materials	WQ 18
WQ 34	Malpractice	WQ 32-33
WQ 39	Handbooks	None
WQ 152	Natural childbirth	WQ 150
WQ 155	Home childbirth	WQ 145
	WR Dermatology	
WR 18.2	Educational materials	WR 18
WR 39	Handbooks	None
WR 141	Diagnosis. Monitoring	WR 140
	WS Pediatrics	
WS 18.2	Educational materials	WS 18
WS 39	Handbooks	None
WS 104	Growth disorders. Failure to thrive	Various places
WS 201	Pediatric emergencies	WS 200
WS 421	Diseases of newborn infants	WS 420
	WT Geriatrics. Chronic Disease	
WT 18.2	Educational materials	WT 18
WT 31	Medical care plans. Long term care	WT 30
WT 39	Handbooks	None
WT 115	Nutritional requirements. Nutrition disorders	QU 145
WT 116	Longevity. Life expectancy. Death	WT 104
WT 141	Physical examination and diagnosis	Various places
WT 145	Geriatric psychology. Mental health	WT 150
WT 155	Senile dementia. Alzheimer's disease	WT 150, WM 220
WT 166	Therapeutics	WT 100

Added Numbers

New	Subjects	Old
	WU Dentistry. Oral Surgery	
WU 18.2	Educational materials	WU 18
WU 49	Handbooks	WU 39
WU 105	Dental emergencies	WU 100
WU 140.5	Jaw diseases	WU 140
WU 141.5	Specific diagnostic methods, A-Z [Examination. Diagnosis …]	WU 141
WU 317	Atlases [Operative Dentistry]	WU 17
WU 417	Atlases [Orthodontics]	WU 17
WU 426	Orthodontic appliances	WU 400-440
WU 460	*Dental care for the chronically ill*	*Various places*
WU 470	Dental care for the disabled	Various places
WU 507	Atlases [Prosthodontics]	WU 17
WU 600.7	Atlases [Oral Surgery]	WU 17
	WV Otolaryngology	
WV 18.2	Educational materials	WV 18
WV 39	Handbooks	None
WV 140	Otorhinolaryngologic diseases	WV 100
WV 190	Otorhinolaryngologic neoplasms	WV 100
	WW Ophthalmology	
WW 18.2	Educational materials	WW 18
WW 21.5	Ophthlamic assistants	Various places
WW 39	Handbooks	None
	WX Hospitals and Other Health Facilities	
WX 18.2	Educational materials	WX 18
WX 39	Handbooks	None
WX 157.8	Diagnosis-related groups	Various places
	WY Nursing	
WY 15	Classification. Nomenclature. Terminology	None
WY 18.2	Educational materials	WY 18
WY 26.5	Medical informatics. Automatic data processing. Computers	None
WY 49	Handbooks	WY 39
WY 86.5	Holistic nursing	Various places
WY 100.4	Nursing assessment. Nursing diagnosis	WY 100
WY 107	Transcultural nursing	None
WY 150.5	*Rehabilitation nursing*	*WY 150*
WY 153	AIDS/HIV nursing	Various places
WY 158.5	Otolaryngological nursing	WY 158
WY 160.5	Neurological nursing	WY 160
	WZ History of Medicine	
WZ 18.2	Educational materials	WZ 18
WZ 39	Handbooks	WZ 29

Deleted Numbers

Deleted	Subject	Moved to
QS 539	Handbooks [Histology]	QS 529
QS 639	Handbooks [Embryology]	QS 629
QT 39	Handbooks [Physiology]	QT 29
QW 167	Oncolytic viruses	QW 160
QW 168.5.R6	RNA rodent viruses	QW 168
W 39	Handbooks [Health Professions]	W 49
WB 289	Diagnostic use of ultrasonics	WN 208
WG 595.I6	Innominate artery	WG 595.B72
WG 625.I6	Innominate vein	WG 625.B7
WM 612	Masturbation	HQ 447; WM 611
WM 615	Homosexuality	HQ 75-76.8; WM 611
WU 39	Handbooks [Dentistry]	WU 49
WY 39	Handbooks [Nursing]	WY 49
WZ 29	Handbooks [History of Medicine]	WZ 39

Appendix 2

Bibliography of Principal Sources
for
Classification Decisions

Bergey's manual of determinative bacteriology. 9th ed. Baltimore: Williams & Wilkins; c1994. 787 p.

Bergey's manual of systematic bacteriology. 1st ed. Baltimore: Williams & Wilkins; c1984- v.

Diagnostic and statistical manual of mental disorders: DSM-IV. 4th ed. Washington, D.C.: American Psychiatric Association; 1994. 886 p.

Diagnostic and statistical manual of mental disorders: DSM-III-R. 3rd ed., rev. Washington, D.C.: American Psychiatric Association; 1987. 567 p.

Dorland's illustrated medical dictionary. 27th ed. Philadelphia: Saunders; 1988. 1888 p.

The International classification of diseases: 9th revision, clinical modification: ICD-9-CM. 4th ed. Washington, D.C.: U.S. Dept. of Health and Human Services, Public Health Service, Health Care Financing Administration: For sale by the Supt. of Docs., U.S. G.P.O.; 1991- v.

Medical subject headings: annotated alphabetical list, 1999. Bethesda, Md.: National Library of Medicine; 1998. I-230, 1066 p.

Medical subject headings: tree structures, 1999. Bethesda, Md.: National Library of Medicine; 1998. I-124, 865 p.

The Merck index; an encyclopedia of chemicals and drugs. 11th ed. Rahway, N.J.: Merck and Co.; 1989. 1 v. (various pagings)

National Library of Medicine classification. 5th ed. 1964. Bethesda, Md.: U.S. Dept. of Health and Human Services, Public Health Service, National Institutes of Health, National Library of Medicine; Washington, D.C.: For sale by the Supt. of Docs., U.S. G.P.O.; 1995. [551] p.

Shortliffe, Edward H.; Perreault, Leslie E., editors. *Medical informatics: computer applications in health care.* Reading, Mass.: Addison-Wesley Pub. Co.; c1990. 715 p.

The Systematized nomenclature of human and veterinary medicine: SNOMED international. Northfield, Ill.: College of American Pathologists; Schaumburg, Ill.: American Veterinary Medical Association; c1993. 4 v.

Walker, John M.; Cox, Michael. *The language of biotechnology, a dictionary of terms.* Washington, D.C.: American Chemical Society; 1988. 255 p.

Appendix 3

NLM Staff Contributors
to the
NLM Classification

Arenales, Duane W., Chief, Technical Services Division
Armstead, Karen, Former Librarian, Technical Services Division
Bain, Evelyn S., Librarian, Technical Services Division
Boehr, Diane, Librarian, Technical Services Division
Charen, Thelma G., Retired Technical Information Specialist, Medical Subject Headings Section
Charuhas, Joe C., Public Affairs Specialist, Office of Public Information
Chung, Chong C., Librarian, Technical Services Division
Clausen, Carol, Librarian, History of Medicine Division
Colaianni, Lois Ann, Retired Associate Director, Library Operations
Coleman, Ann D., Technical Information Specialist, Technical Services Division
Coligan, Nelda C., Librarian, Technical Services Division
Conkle, Yhorda, Secretary, Technical Services Division
Cox, John W., Retired Computer Specialist, Office of Computer and Communications Systems
DeAnna, Paul, Librarian, Technical Services Division
Demsey, Andrea M., Librarian, Technical Services Division
Detweiler, Victoria L., Library Technician, Technical Services Division
Eannarino, Judith C., Librarian, Technical Services Division
Feng, Margaret S.C., Librarian, Technical Services Division
Fitzgerald, Joe P., Visual Information Officer, Lister Hill Center
Freidin, Mark, Librarian, Technical Services Division
Gilkeson, Roger L., Retired Assistant Chief, Office of Public Information
Goodson, Luanne M., Former Librarian, Technical Services Division
Gordner, Ronald L., Librarian, Public Services Division
Harbart, Charles (Andy) Former Librarian, Technical Services Division
Hay, Miranda, Librarian, Technical Services Division
Hoffmann, Christa F.B., Head, Cataloging Section, Technical Services Division
Horan, Meredith L., Librarian, Technical Services Division
Humphreys, Betsy L., Associate Director, Library Operations
Jacobs, Alice E., Assistant Head, Cataloging Section, Technical Services Division
Jurgrau, Lora A., Library Technician, Technical Services Division
Kao, Wen-Min C., Retired Principal Cataloger, Technical Services Division
Kingsland, Lawrence C., Chief, Computer Sciences Branch, Lister Hill Center
Kraly, Karen A., Computer Specialist, Office of Computer and Communications Systems
Kurth, Sabra M., Former Librarian, Technical Services Division
Licht, Pamela C., Former Librarian, Technical Services Division
Lindsay, Schendell A., Clerk, Former, Technical Services Division
Mandic, Christine, Librarian, Technical Services Division
Murtagh, Eileen, Librarian, Technical Services Division
Nguyen, Hien P., Librarian, Technical Services Division
Nguyen, Janet C., Librarian, Technical Services Division
Pothier, Patricia, Senior Research Analyst, Bibliographic Services Division
Powell, Tammy, Technical Information Specialist, Medical Subject Headings Section
Rawsthorne, Grace C., Former Librarian, Technical Services Division
Savage, Allan G., Technical Information Specialist, Medical Subject Headings Section
Schuyler, Peri L., Retired Head, Medical Subject Headings Section, Technical Services Division
Sinn, Sally K., Former Deputy Chief, Technical Services Division
Van Lenten, Elizabeth J., Technical Information Specialist, Bibliographic Services Division

White, Dorothy C., Librarian, Technical Services Division
Willis, Sharon R., Former Librarian, Technical Services Division
Wright, Nancy D., Former Head, Index Section, Bibliographic Services Division
Zellner, Varonica, Library Technician, Technical Services Division

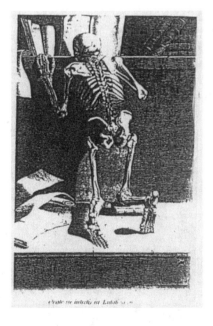

ISBN 0-16-050261-6

9 780160 502613

90000